Pediatric
Decision-Making
Strategies

Pediatric Decision-Making Strategies

Second Edition

Albert J. Pomeranz, MD

Professor
Medical College of Wisconsin
Children's Hospital of Wisconsin
Milwaukee, Wisconsin

Svapna Sabnis, MD

Associate Professor
Medical College of Wisconsin
Children's Hospital of Wisconsin
Milwaukee, Wisconsin

Sharon L. Busey, MD

Associate Professor
Medical College of Wisconsin
Children's Hospital of Wisconsin
Milwaukee, Wisconsin

Robert M. Kliegman, MD

Professor
Medical College of Wisconsin
Children's Hospital of Wisconsin
Milwaukee, Wisconsin

ELSEVIER
SAUNDERS

1600 John F. Kennedy Blvd.
Ste 1800
Philadelphia, PA 19103-2899

PEDIATRIC DECISION-MAKING STRATEGIES, SECOND EDITION ISBN: 978-0-323-29854-4

Library of Congress Cataloging-in-Publication Data

Pomeranz, Albert J., author.
  Pediatric decision-making strategies / Albert J. Pomeranz, Svapna Sabnis, Sharon L. Busey, Robert M. Kliegman. -- 2nd edition.
      p. ; cm.
  Preceded by Pediatric decision-making strategies to accompany Nelson Textbook of Pediatrics, 16th ed. / Albert J. Pomeranz ... [et al.]. c2002.
  Includes bibliographical references and index.
  ISBN 978-0-323-29854-4 (pbk. : alk. paper)
  I. Sabnis, Svapna, author. II. Busey, Sharon L., author. III. Kliegman, Robert, author. IV. Title.
  [DNLM: 1. Pediatrics. 2. Diagnosis. WS 200]
  RJ50.5
  618.92'0075--dc23
                    2014038049

Senior Content Strategist: James Merritt
Content Development Specialist: Lisa Barnes
Publishing Services Manager: Anne Altepeter
Senior Project Manager: Cindy Thoms
Book Designer: Steve Stave

Printed in United States of America

Last digit is the print number: 9   8   7

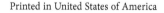

Preface

We are very pleased to be given the opportunity to produce a second edition of *Pediatric Decision-Making Strategies* 12 years after the original publication. The purpose and basic algorithmic format of the text has not changed, but each chapter has been updated to reflect the latest medical information available. As with the original text, the purpose is to assist the student, house officer, and clinician in the evaluation of common pediatric signs and symptoms and abnormal laboratory findings. The algorithmic format provides a rapid and concise stepwise approach to a diagnosis. The text accompanying each algorithm helps to clarify certain approaches to diagnoses and supplies additional useful information regarding various medical conditions.

The information in the book is the most up to date available. The literature has been extensively reviewed, and many of the algorithms have been discussed with the appropriate specialists. We believe that we have created algorithms that are accurate and easy to follow. There is rarely a single acceptable approach to any given problem, and not all diagnoses can fit neatly into an algorithm. Even though the algorithms cannot be considered all-inclusive, the goal is to facilitate a logical and efficient stepwise approach to reasonable differential diagnoses for the common clinical problems discussed. This task could not have been completed without the generous help of many of the faculty members of the Medical College of Wisconsin and Children's Hospital of Wisconsin.

Acknowledgments

We wish to thank the many physicians and staff at the Medical College of Wisconsin and Children's Hospital of Wisconsin who were asked a multitude of questions to ensure the accuracy and completeness of this text. They have all been extremely helpful and patient. We would like to extend special thanks to the following faculty members for their help: Jay Nocton and James Verbsky for Musculoskeletal System; Amanda Brandow for Hematology; Anoop Singh and Shanelle Clark for Cardiology; Scott Van Why and Cynthia Pan for Fluids and Electrolytes; Omar Ali and Patricia Donohoue for Endocrine System; Alisha Mavis for Gastrointestinal System; Lynn D'Andrea for Respiratory System; and Larry Greenbaum of Emory School of Medicine for Fluids and Electrolytes.

We also wish to thank Lisa Barnes and James Merritt at Elsevier for their support and encouragement.

Special thanks to Kelsie Birschbach for her invaluable assistance in the manuscript preparation.

Abbreviations

ABG — arterial blood gases
ALT — alanine aminotransferase
ALTE — apparent life-threatening event
ANA — antinuclear antibody
AP — anteroposterior
ARF — acute rheumatic fever
AST — aspartate aminotransferase
AVN — avascular necrosis
BP — blood pressure
BUN — blood urea nitrogen
CBC — complete blood count
CMV — cytomegalovirus
CNS — central nervous system
Cr — creatinine
CRP — C-reactive protein
CSF — cerebrospinal fluid
CT — computed tomography
CXR — chest x-ray
DTP — diphtheria-tetanus-pertussis
EBV — Epstein-Barr virus
ECF — extracellular fluid
ECMO — extracorporeal membrane oxygenation
EEG — electroencephalogram
EKG — electrocardiogram
EMG — electromyogram
ENT — ear, nose, and throat
ESR — erythrocyte sedimentation rate
FSH — follicle-stimulating hormone
GER — gastroesophageal reflux
GGT — γ-glutamyl transferase
GI — gastrointestinal
GU — genitourinary
H and P — history and physical
HEENT — head, eyes, ears, nose, and throat
Hgb — hemoglobin

HIV — human immunodeficiency virus
I and D — incision and drainage
ICP — intracranial pressure
IV — intravenous
JRA — juvenile rheumatoid arthritis
KUB — kidney, ureter, bladder (x-ray study)
LFT — liver function test
LH — luteinizing hormone
LP — lumbar puncture
MRI — magnetic resonance imaging
O&P — ova and parasites
OM — otitis media
PCR — polymerase chain reaction
PPD — purified protein derivative (of tuberculin)
PT — prothrombin time
PTT — partial thromboplastin time
RBC — red blood cell
RF — rheumatoid factor
RSV — respiratory syncytial virus
RTA — renal tubular acidosis
SCIWORA — spinal cord injury in the absence of radiographic abnormalities
SI — sacroiliac
Sp gr — specific gravity
s/p — status post
T_4 — thyroxine
Td — tetanus-diphtheria toxoid
TSH — thyroid-stimulating hormone
UA — urinalysis
UGI — upper gastrointestinal series
URI — upper respiratory infection
US — ultrasound
UTI — urinary tract infection
WBC — white blood cell

Contents

Head, Neck, and Eyes

Chapter 1
EAR PAIN

Ear pain is common, particularly in the first few years of life. Acute otitis media (AOM) accounts for most cases. Over 80% of children have at least one episode of AOM by the age of 3 years.

1. Signs of AOM may be nonspecific in the child younger than age 2 (e.g., fever, irritability, vomiting). Ear tugging is not a specific sign. AOM usually occurs with preceding or concomitant upper respiratory symptoms. The presence of a middle ear effusion is most accurately predicted by determining altered mobility of the tympanic membrane (TM) with an insufflator.

2. A swollen red auricle may be due to a contusion from blunt trauma (e.g., wrestling or boxing). It is important to recognize development of a hematoma with subperichondrial collection of blood in order to correctly treat and prevent the formation of a "cauliflower ear." Perichondritis of the ear cartilage may also lead to deformity if untreated. Swelling of the ear may be due to sunburn, frostbite, or an allergic reaction to insect bites or contact irritants.

3. The diagnosis of AOM is usually made based on the presence of middle ear inflammation (i.e., redness, opacity, and bulging of TM), middle ear effusion, and recent acute illness. About two thirds of AOM episodes are a result of bacterial infection. The major pathogens are nontypable *Haemophilus influenzae*, *Streptococcus pneumoniae*, and *Moraxella catarrhalis*. Inappropriate diagnosis of AOM contributes to the overuse of antibiotics and the serious problem of antimicrobial resistance.

4. Otitis media with effusion (OME) is the presence of fluid in the middle ear space without signs of inflammation or infection. It is commonly associated with URI or a successfully treated AOM. In general, OME should not be treated with antibiotics. Mild discomfort or a feeling of "fullness" is not unusual. Diagnosis can be aided by the use of tympanometry and acoustic reflectometry. These diagnostic tools determine the presence or absence of effusion but not infection.

5. With periostitis, infection within the mastoid air cells has spread to the periosteum that covers the mastoid process. Further spread of infection results in osteitis, which involves destruction of mastoid air cells and abscess formation. Resultant swelling is often severe enough to cause outward displacement of the pinna.

6. A cholesteatoma is a collection of squamous cells in the middle ear and should be suspected if retraction or perforation of the TM with white caseous debris is noted. The increasing size of the tumor results in destruction of the middle ear and temporal bone, in addition to intracranial spread.

7. The main clue to the diagnosis of a furuncle in the canal, although uncommon, is the severe pain elicited when the otoscope tip is placed in the canal. The canal appears generally normal, except for the erythematous papule or pustule.

8. The ear canal is protected by cerumen, a waxy, water-repellent coating. Excessive wetness or trauma or various skin dermatoses (e.g., eczema) can disrupt this cerumen. Frequent water exposure (e.g., swimming), hearing aids, eczematous skin lesions, and aggressive use of cotton-tipped swabs or other devices in the canal are risks for development of otitis externa. Edema, erythema, and discharge are common. Occasionally the disease is due to drainage from a perforated tympanic membrane or to infection in the presence of tympanostomy tubes. The moist, irritant nature of the purulent drainage results in superinfection from bacterial colonization. Pathogens include *Pseudomonas aeruginosa*, *Staphylococcus aureus*, other gram-negative organisms, and occasionally fungi.

Bibliography

American Academy of Pediatrics: Diagnosis and management of acute otitis media, *Pediatrics* 113:1451–1465, 2004.

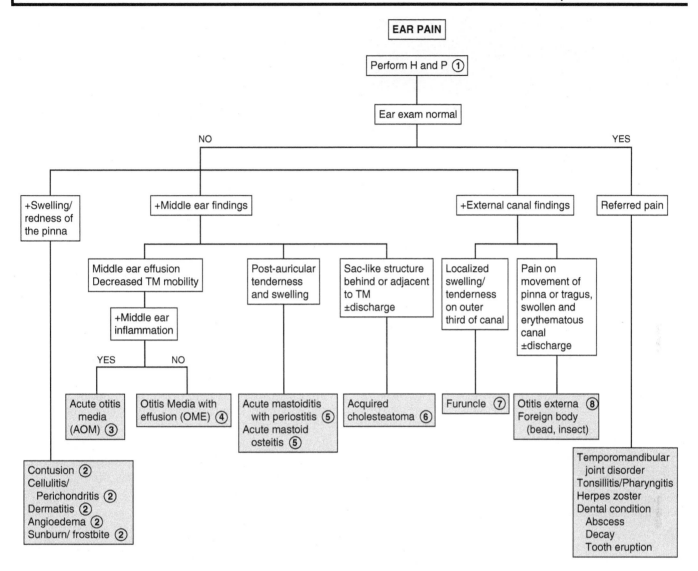

Nelson Textbook of Pediatrics, 19e. Chapters 631, 632, 634
Nelsons Essentials, 6e. Chapter 105

Chapter 2
RHINORRHEA

Rhinorrhea is a common complaint in childhood. It is most frequently due to a viral URI but must be distinguished from allergies and other less common etiologies.

1. A careful HEENT examination is essential. Stigmata suggestive of genetic syndromes should be noted because congenital nasal anomalies (e.g., atresia, stenosis, hypoplasia) are frequently associated with other anomalies. Examination of the nose should include the appearance of the mucosa (e.g., swelling, pallor, erythema, degree of patency), character of secretions, and presence of any obvious obstructing lesions (e.g., polyps, foreign bodies).

2. Acute rhinosinusitis or the "common cold" is the most common cause of rhinorrhea. It is a relatively common illness in children and adolescents. A viral etiology is far by the most common; bacterial etiology is less common. (See footnote 9.)

3. Allergic rhinitis is an immunoglobulin (Ig)E-mediated condition that may be seasonal (e.g., hay fever) or perennial. The nasal mucosa is typically boggy and pale or bluish. The rhinorrhea is clear and watery. Other allergic signs and symptoms, such as upward rubbing of the nose (i.e., allergic salute), allergic shiners, sneezing, and eye symptoms are common. Atopic disorders may be present (e.g., asthma, eczema). Fever suggests an alternative (infectious) diagnosis. Nonallergic inflammatory rhinitis with eosinophils (NARES) has a similar presentation to allergic rhinitis but without elevated IgE antibodies.

4. The vasomotor responses of increased secretion and mucosal swelling are the normal responses of the nasal mucosa to a variety of stimuli. These responses are exaggerated in those with vasomotor rhinitis. External stimuli (e.g., cold temperature, change in humidity, cigarette smoke, spicy food) are the most common. The autonomic system response, hormones, and stress are other triggers.

5. Bronchiolitis, roseola infantum, measles, mononucleosis, hepatitis, pertussis, and erythema infectiosum may appear with a prodromal acute watery rhinorrhea.

6. Rhinorrhea due to leakage of CSF is clear and usually unilateral, and it may vary noticeably with a change in head position, Valsalva maneuver, or jugular compression. Detection of glucose (50 mg/100 mL or higher) in the fluid is highly suggestive. The condition may occur acutely with head trauma or chronically with congenital conditions (e.g., fistulas, encephaloceles) or tumors.

7. When the clinical course and examination are not specific for a diagnosis, especially when considering sinusitis versus allergic rhinitis, a microscopic examination of the nasal secretions may be helpful. An eosin–methylene blue stain of these secretions can help to identify eosinophils, WBCs, and bacteria. A predominance of WBCs and bacteria suggests sinusitis, and at least 5% eosinophils suggests allergic rhinitis. The two diseases may occur together.

8. Foreign bodies usually have a unilateral foul-smelling, purulent, or bloody discharge.

9. Clinical diagnosis of bacterial rhinosinusitis is made by findings of prolonged symptoms of rhinorrhea without improvement for more than 10 to 14 days. Other suggestive symptoms include halitosis, fever, nocturnal cough, and post-nasal drip. Older children may have headache, facial pain, tooth pain, and periorbital swelling. Radiologic studies such as CT do not help differentiate bacterial from viral causes.

10. Rhinitis medicamentosa results from overuse of vasoconstrictor nose drops or sprays. A rapid toxic reaction of the nasal mucosa causes rebound swelling and obstruction.

11. Cocaine, marijuana, and inhaled solvents may result in mucoid or purulent rhinorrhea. Medications causing rhinorrhea include oral contraceptives, aspirin, nonsteroidal antiinflammatory and antihypertensive drugs. In the uncommon ASA triad (Samter's triad), nasal polyps are associated with aspirin sensitivity and asthma.

12. Symptoms of nasal obstruction with increasing frequency of episodes of epistaxis, particularly unilateral, in boys are suggestive of juvenile nasopharyngeal angiofibroma.

13. Bilateral choanal atresia presents early in the newborn period with respiratory distress. Unilateral choanal atresia presents later with chronic unilateral rhinorrhea that can be clear or purulent. Feeding difficulties are also common, since most newborns are nose breathers. Inability to pass a nasal catheter suggests this diagnosis. An ENT consultation should be obtained whenever choanal atresia is suspected.

14. Infants with congenital syphilis may present between the second week and third month of life with a watery nasal discharge that progresses to a mucopurulent or bloody discharge. Significant obstruction results in noisy breathing ("snuffles"). Chronic mucopurulent rhinorrhea, septal perforation, and saddle nose deformity are late complications. Serologic tests for treponemal antibodies and specimens for dark field microscopy examination should be obtained whenever this diagnosis is suspected.

Bibliography

DeMuri G, Wald ER: Acute bacterial sinusitis in children, *N Engl J Med* 367:1128–1134, 2012.

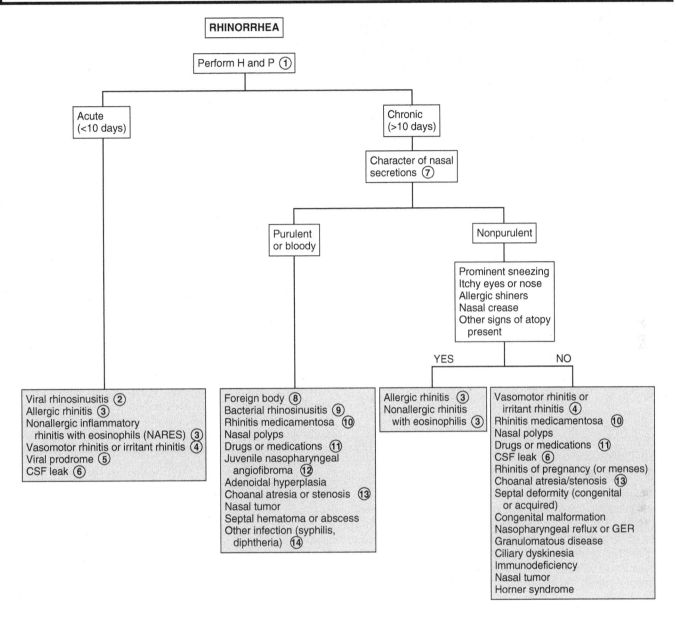

Nelson Textbook of Pediatrics, 19e. Chapters 137, 210, 368, 371, 372
Nelsons Essentials, 6e. Chapters 102, 184

Chapter 3
SORE THROAT

Most sore throats are benign, self-limiting viral illnesses. The practitioner should always consider the likelihood of group A β-hemolytic streptococcus (*Streptococcus pyogenes*), which is important to identify and treat because of its potentially serious complications. Other less common causes should be considered when symptoms are worrisome or prolonged.

1. A history of exposure to a family member or classmate with a cold or documented group A streptococcal infection is helpful. A history of sexual activity or abuse should raise the suspicion for pharyngeal gonococcal infection. The degree of pharyngeal inflammation is not always consistent with the severity of the complaint. Tonsillar exudates are suggestive of streptococcus but also of mononucleosis and adenovirus. Many patients with streptococcal pharyngitis have only mild erythema without tonsillar enlargement or exudates. Small ulcers or vesicles on the soft palate suggest a viral etiology.

2. Acute onset of illness with associated symptoms of stridor, drooling, and air hunger or an unwillingness to recline suggests impending airway obstruction. The patient warrants emergent management for airway stabilization and treatment for potentially life-threatening conditions such as epiglottitis and retropharyngeal abscess. (See Chapter 12.) A lateral neck film may be helpful but should be done only if the airway is stable.

3. *Corynebacterium diphtheriae* is a rare but serious cause of pharyngitis. The disease is suggested by a systemic illness and grayish membrane over the tonsils and pharyngeal walls. It should be suspected in unimmunized persons or in persons from underdeveloped countries. Culture of the organism and confirmation of its toxin are necessary to confirm the diagnosis. Soft tissue swelling and enlarged lymph nodes can cause a bull-neck appearance.

4. Even when the clinical picture is highly suggestive of streptococcal pharyngitis, laboratory confirmation is strongly recommended. Rapid antigen detection tests (RST) are highly specific, with sensitivities that are more variable. Throat cultures are the standard for diagnosis whenever the RST results are negative. The RST and the most commonly used culture methods do not identify organisms other than group A streptococcus. In cases in which another family member has a positive culture finding, or in which a typical scarlatina rash is present, group A streptococcus should still be considered despite negative test results.

5. Group A streptococcal pharyngitis is most common between 5 and 11 years of age and unlikely under 3 years of age. The occurrence of conjunctivitis, rhinitis, cough, and hoarseness is more indicative of a virus than group A streptococcus. Significant diarrhea also makes streptococcal disease unlikely. Some patients demonstrate the features of scarlet fever, including circumoral pallor, strawberry tongue, and a red, sandpaper-like scarlatina rash.

6. Viral pharyngitis is most commonly accompanied by "common cold" symptoms such as rhinitis and cough.

The most common etiologies are rhinovirus, coronavirus, adenovirus, enterovirus, RSV, and metapneumovirus. Viral pharyngitis is usually gradual in onset with early signs of fever, malaise, and anorexia generally preceding the sore throat.

7. Adenovirus may cause an exudative pharyngitis. Diarrhea and conjunctivitis are also common.

8. Exudative pharyngitis is often a manifestation of infectious mononucleosis. Patients can experience an abrupt onset of fatigue, malaise, fever, and headache preceding the pharyngitis. Hepatosplenomegaly and generalized lymphadenopathy are common. Preadolescents tend to have milder symptoms than adolescents and young adults. Atypical lymphocytosis is suggestive of the disorder, and a positive "Monospot" (heterophile antibody) test finding confirms EBV mononucleosis. The test is not considered reliable in children younger than age 5 because of a low titer of heterophile antibody. EBV serology should be used in young patients or in patients with heterophile-negative cases. CMV serology should also be considered because CMV causes approximately 5% to 10% of cases.

9. Primary infection with HIV can also manifest with pharyngitis and a mononucleosis-like syndrome.

10. *Arcanobacterium haemolyticum* may cause a scarlet fever–like illness but requires special culture methods. It is not routinely sought in the evaluation of pharyngitis. Although non–group A streptococci have been implicated in pharyngitis, they cause a self-limiting illness, are not associated with complications, and require no treatment. Gonococcal pharyngeal infections are usually asymptomatic but can cause acute pharyngitis with fever and cervical lymphadenitis.

11. Coxsackie A16 is responsible for hand-foot-mouth disease, a characteristic outbreak of vesicles on the palms and soles, with accompanying ulcerating vesicles throughout the oropharynx. Herpangina is a disorder characterized by fever and discrete painful, vesicular lesions of the posterior pharynx. A variety of enteroviruses cause herpangina, including enterovirus 71, although coxsackie A viruses are implicated most often.

12. Primary herpes simplex virus infection can cause gingivostomatitis characterized by painful ulcerating vesicles in the anterior portion of the oral cavity, including the lips. An exudative tonsillitis may occur. Fevers and impaired fluid intake are common. Herpetic gingivostomatitis may last up to 2 weeks.

13. Pharyngitis characterized by intense erythema but absent tonsillar enlargement or exudate is an early finding in measles. Fever, cough, coryza, conjunctivitis, and Koplik spots (i.e., blue-white enanthema on buccal mucosa) suggest the diagnosis. These are followed by development of a maculopapular rash that begins on the forehead then spreads downward. Laboratory criteria for diagnosis include positive serologic test for measles immunoglobulin (Ig)M, seroconversion (a significant rise in measles IgG), isolation of measles virus, or identification by PCR of measles virus RNA from a clinical specimen (blood, urine, or respiratory secretions).

14. Immunocompromised patients are at risk for fungal oropharyngeal infections. *Candida* is the most common pathogen. Diagnosis is made by examination of a specimen treated with potassium hydroxide or by culture.

15. Agranulocytosis may manifest as pharyngitis with a white or yellow exudate with underlying necrosis and ulceration.

Bibliography

Gereige R, Cunill-De Sautu B: Throat infections, *Pediatr Rev* 32:459–468, 2011.

Kenna MA: Sore throat in children. In Bluestone CD, Stool SE, Kenna MA, editors: *Pediatric otolaryngology*, ed 4, Philadelphia, 2003, WB Saunders, pp 1120.

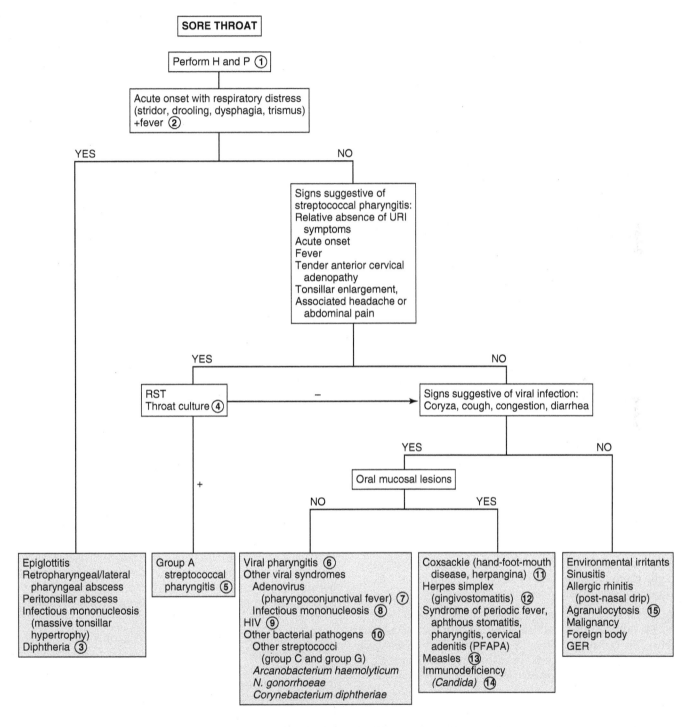

Nelson Textbook of Pediatrics, 19e. Chapters 176, 180, 238, 242, 244, 246, 254, 373
Nelsons Essentials, 6e. Chapter 103

Chapter 4
NECK MASSES

Most neck masses are benign, but it is important not to miss rare malignant masses. A directed H and P examination allows for successful diagnosis and, if necessary, referral for further evaluation and treatment.

1. Neck masses may be distinguished broadly into two categories: congenital and acquired. Masses present since birth, or with chronic drainage or recurrent episodes of swelling, are usually congenital. History of fever may indicate inflammation or infection. Constitutional symptoms such as fever, night sweats, and weight loss may indicate a malignancy or a granulomatous process. Rapidly enlarging, painless masses may be malignant. Those due to infection are often painful. Symptoms indicating compression of the trachea, esophagus, or recurrent laryngeal nerve should be elicited because rapid progression of the mass may be life threatening. A history of recurrent infections such as thrush, sinopulmonary infections, or cellulitis may indicate an immunodeficiency syndrome.

   The location of the mass is helpful in making the diagnosis. The neck is divided into two triangles: the anterior triangle, which is bounded by the mandible, the sternocleidomastoid, and the anterior midline; and the the posterior triangle, which is bounded by the sternocleidomastoid, the distal two thirds of the clavicle, and the posterior midline. It is also important to determine the consistency of the lesion. Cystic lesions may show fluctuance and transilluminate. A bruit may be heard with vascular lesions.

2. Thyroglossal duct cysts are the most common congenital neck masses. However, they rarely manifest in the newborn period and occur more commonly in children aged 2 to 10 years. Approximately one third are not diagnosed until after the age of 20. Thyroglossal duct cysts are usually painless and often move with tongue protrusion. They may occur with recurrent inflammation associated with a URI. Their location can be anywhere from the base of the tongue to behind the sternum but are usually near or below the hyoid bone. US may be done to confirm the diagnosis. A thyroid scan is important to identify ectopic gland tissue in the cyst (found in one third of cases), because excision may lead to hypothyroidism.

3. Dermoid cysts are benign congenital neoplasms located in the midline. They are nontender, smooth, and doughy or rubbery in consistency. They may be difficult to distinguish from thyroglossal duct cysts. In cases where the diagnosis is difficult to make, imaging studies and aspiration of the cyst may be considered.

4. Thymic cysts result from implantation of thymic tissue during its embryologic descent and are usually in a midline position.

5. In newborn infants, a goiter may be associated with hypothyroidism. This may occur with defects in thyroid hormone synthesis, administration of goitrogenic substances to the mother (e.g., antithyroid drug, iodides, amiodarone, radioiodine), or iodine deficiency, causing endemic goiter, which is rare in the United States. Congenital hyperthyroidism in infants born to mothers with Graves disease may cause a goiter that usually resolves in 6 to 12 weeks.

6. Teratomas are usually midline but may be paramedian. They are firm and irregular and do not transilluminate. Teratomas have classic radiologic findings of calcifications.

7. Laryngoceles are cystic dilations of the laryngeal ventricle located between the true and false vocal cords. They appear as soft, compressible masses just lateral to the midline. Laryngoceles may enlarge with Valsalva maneuver. They may cause hoarseness or stridor. Air-fluid levels may be seen radiographically.

8. Branchial cleft anomalies include cysts, sinuses, and fistulas. They are located in the lateral aspect of the anterior triangle. Most anomalies arise from the second branchial arch along the anterior border of the sternocleidomastoid. Some may arise from the first branchial arch at the angle of the mandible or in the postauricular region. These may not be present at birth but may manifest when older as drainage or a mass, if infected. Ultrasound, CT, or MRI may confirm the diagnosis.

9. Congenital torticollis is usually noted within the first few weeks of life. There is a firm, nontender, fibrous mass within the body of the sternocleidomastoid. It results in tilting of the head toward the mass, with the chin in the opposite direction. It is believed to be caused by trauma or abnormal positioning in utero. Prolonged, severe, untreated torticollis may result in a deformed face and skull.

10. Cystic hygromas (lymphangiomas) are cystic masses formed by dilated anomalous lymphatic channels. These are most common in the posterior triangle but may occur in the submandibular or submental region. They are soft, nontender, diffuse, and compressible masses that may increase in size with straining or crying. Most transilluminate. Diagnosis may be confirmed by US. A CXR may be considered to look for mediastinal extension in patients with stridor or respiratory compromise. Chromosomal aberrations are found in a significant percentage of infants who have cystic hygromas, and these lesions are associated frequently with Turner, Noonan, and Down syndromes. Cystic hygromas may be diagnosed as early as the second trimester of pregnancy by US.

11. Hemangiomas are vascular anomalies that appear at birth, often enlarging in the first year of life, followed by involution. They are soft, compressible, red or purple-colored masses. They may increase in size with crying or Valsalva maneuver. They do not transilluminate. Bruits may be heard, particularly over large hemangiomas. The diagnosis can usually be made on physical findings, but US is a good initial test to confirm the diagnosis.

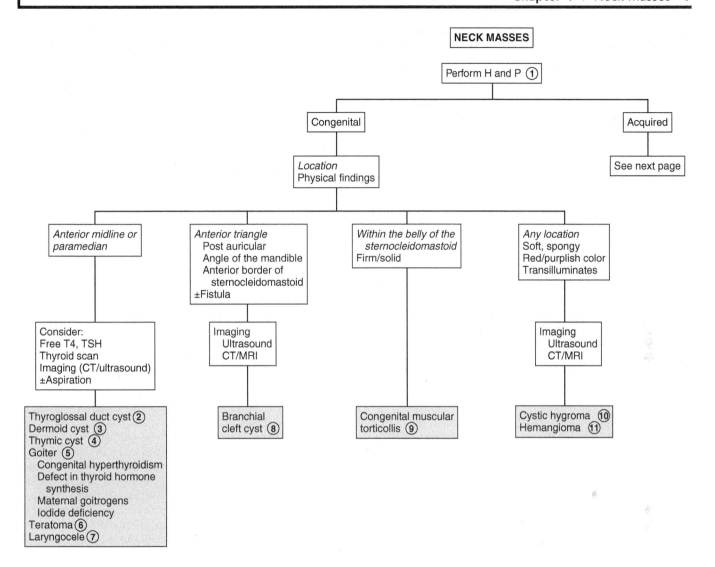

NECK MASSES

Perform H and P ①

Congenital

Acquired

See next page

Location
Physical findings

Anterior midline or paramedian

Anterior triangle
Post auricular
Angle of the mandible
Anterior border of
    sternocleidomastoid
±Fistula

Within the belly of the sternocleidomastoid
Firm/solid

Any location
Soft, spongy
Red/purplish color
Transilluminates

Consider:
Free T4, TSH
Thyroid scan
Imaging (CT/ultrasound)
±Aspiration

Imaging
Ultrasound
CT/MRI

Imaging
Ultrasound
CT/MRI

Thyroglossal duct cyst ②
Dermoid cyst ③
Thymic cyst ④
Goiter ⑤
    Congenital hyperthyroidism
    Defect in thyroid hormone
        synthesis
    Maternal goitrogens
    Iodide deficiency
Teratoma ⑥
Laryngocele ⑦

Branchial
cleft cyst ⑧

Congenital muscular
torticollis ⑨

Cystic hygroma ⑩
Hemangioma ⑪

Nelson Textbook of Pediatrics, 19e. Chapters 240, 308, 494, 497, 559, 560, 561, 562, 614, 640, 642, 672
Nelsons Essentials, 6e. Chapter 175

12 Salivary gland enlargement most commonly involves the parotid that obscures the angle of the mandible but may involve the submandibular or minor glands. Parotitis occurs with tender, swollen parotid glands classically caused by mumps but also associated with coxsackie A and HIV. In suppurative parotitis caused by *Staphylococcus aureus*, pus can be expressed from the gland's duct.

13 Bilateral enlargement of submaxillary glands may occur in AIDS, cystic fibrosis, and malnutrition. Parotid enlargement occurs with chronic emesis as in bulimia. Salivary calculus formation may be associated with anticholinergic antihistamine drugs. Recurrent idiopathic parotitis occurs at times lasting 2 to 3 weeks. It is usually unilateral with little pain. The condition is believed to be allergic in etiology. Tumors of the salivary gland are rare, and they are usually benign (e.g., hemangiomas, hamartomas, pleomorphic adenoma).

14 A goiter is an enlargement of the thyroid. It is a midline mass that moves with swallowing. A hard, rapidly growing nodule in the thyroid area should be assessed using a thyroid scan. "Cold" nodules may indicate malignancy. US or CT may also be done. Histologic examination of specimens obtained by fine needle aspiration or open biopsy are diagnostic indicators of carcinoma of the thyroid, including papillary, follicular, mixed differentiated, and medullary. Benign adenomas may also appear as solitary nodules.

15 Thyroid function tests should be obtained in all cases of thyroid enlargement. These enable classification into euthyroid, hyperthyroid, or hypothyroid goiters. Antithyroid antibodies (i.e., antiperoxidase antibodies and antithyroglobulin antibodies) may indicate an autoimmune etiology. Radiographic studies may be useful in defining the nature of the mass. US helps to differentiate cystic from solid lesions. Thyroid scan demonstrates "hot" or "cold" areas, which indicate increased or decreased activity. If the etiology cannot be determined, fine-needle aspiration or biopsy should be done to exclude malignancy.

16 Autoimmune thyroiditis (also known as lymphocytic or Hashimoto thyroiditis) is the most common cause of thyroid disease in children. It occurs most commonly during adolescence. Most children are asymptomatic and euthyroid. Although a significant proportion of patients eventually become hypothyroid, an occasional patient has hyperthyroidism. Antithyroid antibodies are usually present. Endemic goiter due to iodine deficiency is rare in the United States, with iodized salt availability. Goitrogenic drugs include lithium, amiodarone, and iodides in cough medicines. Defects in thyroid hormone synthesis may also cause hypothyroid goiters.

17 Children with Pendred syndrome (i.e., goiter and congenital deafness) are often euthyroid but may be hypothyroid. It is believed to be caused by a defect in hormone synthesis. Simple colloid goiters are of unknown etiology. The thyroid scans are normal, and thyroid antibodies are absent.

18 Hyperthyroidism is most commonly due to Graves disease. In addition to the thyroid, there is increase in size of the thymus, spleen, and retroorbital tissue (exophthalmos). Patients exhibit classic signs and symptoms of hyperthyroidism, such as heat intolerance, weight loss, palpitations, and tremor. TSH level is decreased, T_3, T_4, free T_3 and free T_4 are increased, and antiperoxidase antibodies are present. Thyroid scan is not usually needed but shows rapid and diffuse concentration of radioiodine in the thyroid. Hyperthyroidism may rarely be seen with McCune-Albright syndrome and hyperfunctioning thyroid carcinoma.

19 Rhabdomyosarcoma may occur with cervical node enlargement with or without pain. The diagnosis should be considered in patients with enlarging and persistent neck masses and chronic ear or nose drainage that is refractory to therapy. Neuroblastoma should be suspected in patients with a cervical mass and Horner syndrome, which consists of homolateral miosis, mild ptosis, and apparent enophthalmos with slight elevation of the lower lid. Horner syndrome is due to oculosympathetic paresis. If it occurs before age 2, there may be hypopigmentation of the iris on the affected side (i.e., heterochromia of the iris). Orbital metastases can result in periorbital ecchymoses, resulting in a "raccoon eyes" appearance.

Bibliography

Beck AE, Scott P: Index of suspicion, *Pediatr Rev* 21:139–143, 2000.
Brown RL, Azizkhan RG: Pediatric head and neck lesions, *Pediatr Clin North Am* 45:889, 1998.

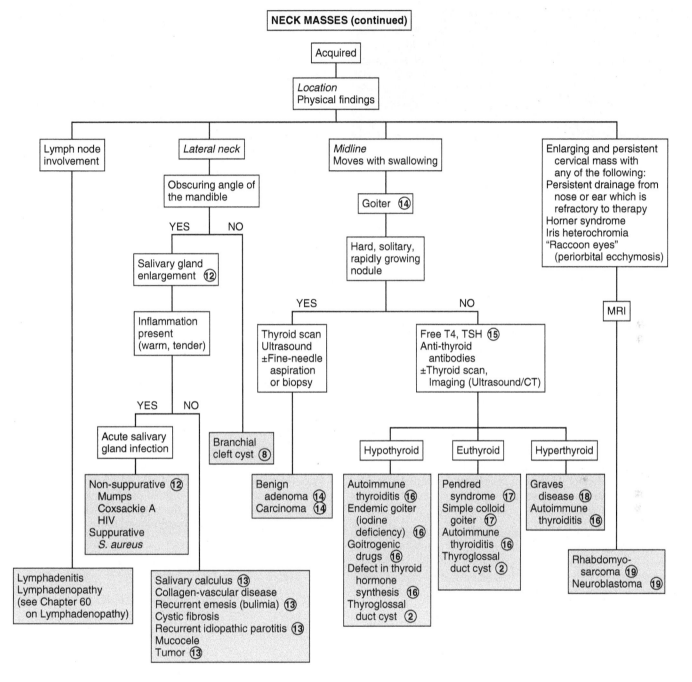

NECK MASSES (continued)

Acquired

Location
Physical findings

Lymph node involvement

Lateral neck

Obscuring angle of the mandible

YES — NO

Salivary gland enlargement ⑫

Inflammation present (warm, tender)

YES — NO

Acute salivary gland infection

Non-suppurative ⑫
Mumps
Coxsackie A
HIV
Suppurative
S. aureus

Branchial cleft cyst ⑧

Lymphadenitis
Lymphadenopathy
(see Chapter 60
on Lymphadenopathy)

Salivary calculus ⑬
Collagen-vascular disease
Recurrent emesis (bulimia) ⑬
Cystic fibrosis
Recurrent idiopathic parotitis ⑬
Mucocele
Tumor ⑬

Midline
Moves with swallowing

Goiter ⑭

Hard, solitary, rapidly growing nodule

YES — NO

Thyroid scan
Ultrasound
±Fine-needle aspiration or biopsy

Benign adenoma ⑭
Carcinoma ⑭

Free T4, TSH ⑮
Anti-thyroid antibodies
±Thyroid scan, Imaging (Ultrasound/CT)

Hypothyroid   Euthyroid   Hyperthyroid

Autoimmune thyroiditis ⑯
Endemic goiter (iodine deficiency) ⑯
Goitrogenic drugs ⑯
Defect in thyroid hormone synthesis ⑯
Thyroglossal duct cyst ②

Pendred syndrome ⑰
Simple colloid goiter ⑰
Autoimmune thyroiditis ⑯
Thyroglossal duct cyst ②

Graves disease ⑱
Autoimmune thyroiditis ⑯

Enlarging and persistent cervical mass with any of the following:
Persistent drainage from nose or ear which is refractory to therapy
Horner syndrome
Iris heterochromia
"Raccoon eyes" (periorbital ecchymosis)

MRI

Rhabdomyo-sarcoma ⑲
Neuroblastoma ⑲

Nelsons Essentials, 6e. Chapter 175

Chapter 5
ABNORMAL HEAD SIZE, SHAPE, AND FONTANELS

Macrocephaly is defined as an occipitofrontal circumference (OFC) greater than 2 standard deviations above the mean. Megalencephaly is a disorder of brain growth, usually accompanied by macrocephaly. An increase in growth rate with crossing of percentiles is of more concern than the case of a child with a large head growing at a normal rate. In microcephaly the OFC is 2 standard deviations below the mean.

(1) A birth history, developmental history and history of irritability, headaches, and visual problems are important components of the initial evaluation. For macrocephaly, inquire about familial head sizes (e.g., ask about hat sizes). It is important to note any features suggestive of specific syndromes.

(2) US can be done if the anterior fontanel (AF) is open. Otherwise, an MRI should be considered. A CT is preferred if there is suspicion of trauma (nonaccidental or accidental). Radiologic evaluation may not be necessary if development is normal, a parent is macrocephalic, and the child's head is growing at a normal rate. Further evaluation is directed by the history and physical examination. Plain long bone radiographs may be indicated for evaluation of skeletal dysplasia or trauma. Consider chromosome testing (fragile X) or metabolic tests (urine organic acids).

(3) Benign familial megalencephaly is the most common cause of anatomic megalencephaly. It is inherited as an autosomal dominant trait. These children may have mild neurodevelopmental dysfunction. It is diagnosed by careful family history and measurement of the parents' head circumferences.

(4) Hydrocephalus is caused by multiple conditions associated with impaired circulation and absorption of CSF or increased production of CSF. Causes of obstructive (noncommunicating) hydrocephalus include aqueductal stenosis, neonatal meningitis, subarachnoid hemorrhage in a premature infant, intrauterine viral infections, vein of Galen malformation, and posterior fossa lesions or malformations (tumors, Chiari malformation, Dandy-Walker syndrome). Subarachnoid hemorrhage in a premature infant can also cause nonobstructive (communicating) hydrocephalus. A rare cause is overproduction of CSF with choroid plexus papilloma.

(5) In hydranencephaly the cerebral hemispheres are absent or represented by membranous sacs. The cause of this condition is unknown.

(6) Occasionally, benign fluid collections (e.g., subarachnoid, subdural) cause macrocephaly without other clinical significance. A pediatric neurosurgeon should be consulted for recommendations.

(7) Various metabolic and degenerative disorders may cause megalencephaly. These include lysosomal diseases (Tay-Sachs disease, gangliosidosis, mucopolysaccharidoses), maple syrup urine disease, and leukodystrophies.

(8) Many syndromes are associated with microcephaly. If a chromosomal syndrome is suspected (child has abnormal facies, short stature, congenital anomalies) karyotype and/or array-comparative genomic hybridization (microarray) study and MRI may be considered.

(9) MRI can evaluate structural abnormalities of the brain (lissencephaly, pachygyria, and polymicrogyria) and both MRI and CT scanning may detect intracerebral calcification, which suggests congenital infection. Also consider TORCH titers (*to*xoplasmosis, *r*ubella, *C*MV, and *h*erpes simplex) and HIV testing of the mother and child, as well as a urine culture for CMV. Consider testing for maternal serum phenylalanine level (PKU), because high maternal levels can affect a nonphenylketonuric infant.

(10) Familial microcephaly is often associated with some degree of mental retardation.

(11) Secondary microcephaly results from exposure to noxious agents during periods of rapid brain growth in utero or during the first 2 years of life.

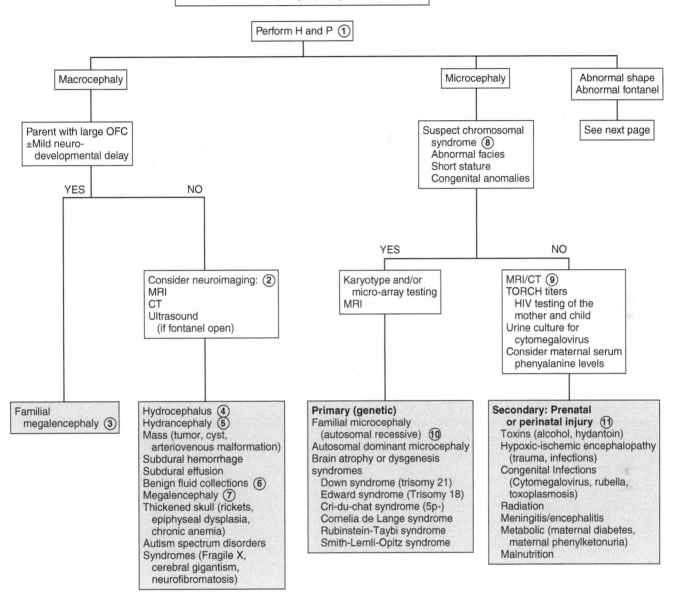

ABNORMAL HEAD SIZE, SHAPE, OR FONTANELS

Perform H and P ①

Macrocephaly

Parent with large OFC
±Mild neuro-
developmental delay

YES

Familial
megalencephaly ③

NO

Consider neuroimaging: ②
MRI
CT
Ultrasound
(if fontanel open)

Hydrocephalus ④
Hydrancephaly ⑤
Mass (tumor, cyst,
arteriovenous malformation)
Subdural hemorrhage
Subdural effusion
Benign fluid collections ⑥
Megalencephaly ⑦
Thickened skull (rickets,
epiphyseal dysplasia,
chronic anemia)
Autism spectrum disorders
Syndromes (Fragile X,
cerebral gigantism,
neurofibromatosis)

Microcephaly

Suspect chromosomal
syndrome ⑧
Abnormal facies
Short stature
Congenital anomalies

YES

Karyotype and/or
micro-array testing
MRI

Primary (genetic)
Familial microcephaly
(autosomal recessive) ⑩
Autosomal dominant microcephaly
Brain atrophy or dysgenesis
syndromes
Down syndrome (trisomy 21)
Edward syndrome (Trisomy 18)
Cri-du-chat syndrome (5p-)
Cornelia de Lange syndrome
Rubinstein-Taybi syndrome
Smith-Lemli-Opitz syndrome

NO

MRI/CT ⑨
TORCH titers
HIV testing of the
mother and child
Urine culture for
cytomegalovirus
Consider maternal serum
phenyalanine levels

**Secondary: Prenatal
or perinatal injury** ⑪
Toxins (alcohol, hydantoin)
Hypoxic-ischemic encephalopathy
(trauma, infections)
Congenital Infections
(Cytomegalovirus, rubella,
toxoplasmosis)
Radiation
Meningitis/encephalitis
Metabolic (maternal diabetes,
maternal phenylketonuria)
Malnutrition

**Abnormal shape
Abnormal fontanel**

See next page

Nelson Textbook of Pediatrics, 19e. Chapters 88, 584, 585
Nelsons Essentials, 6e. Chapter 187

12 Skull deformational malformations occur as the result of an alteration of the normal forces (in utero, perinatal, or postnatal) acting upon the growing cranium. Positional skull deformity, or plagiocephaly (skull asymmetry), is the most common type of deformational malformation. Its incidence has increased because of the recommendations to place infants on their backs while sleeping. Plagiocephaly is a benign condition that must be distinguished from true cranial suture synostosis. In plagiocephaly, sutures are open, and a frontal and temporal prominence occurs on the same side as the flat occiput. Frontal flattening occurs on the side opposite the flat occiput. Molding can occur with breech presentation or as the neonate passes though the birth canal; it resolves within a few weeks. Congenital muscular torticollis may restrict the infant's range of motion at the neck, leading to facial asymmetry and plagiocephaly. It is often not noticed in the newborn and is diagnosed when the infant develops better head control. The diagnosis of positional skull deformity is made based on H and P. Imaging studies are rarely necessary and should only be considered in refractory cases or children born with congenital deformities.

13 Cleidocranial dysostosis is a hereditary condition characterized by incomplete ossification of membranous bones, including the cranium, clavicle, and pelvis. Cranial sutures are often wide and contain wormian bones.

14 The anterior fontanel averages 2.5 cm in diameter. Average age of closure is between 7 and 19 months. As long as head growth is normal and sutural ridging is absent, early closure is not a concern.

15 In true synostosis of a lambdoidal suture, frontal and parietal bossing would occur on the opposite side because of compensatory growth. Symmetric occipital flattening that is believed to be positional does not require imaging. In craniosynostosis, there is often palpable ridging over the fused sutures. The condition may occur as a primary isolated disorder, which is most common, or as part of a syndrome. Common associated disorders include Crouzon, Apert, and Pfeiffer syndromes, congenital hyperthyroidism, and adrenal hyperplasia.

16 Imaging is recommended except in the case of a crying infant in whom the bulging resolves spontaneously or in an infant with a clinical picture of meningitis. An LP should be performed if meningitis is suspected.

17 Normal fullness occurs with crying in an infant with a normal fontanel. It should be distinguished from true bulging, such as occurs in hydrocephalic infants. Normally the fontanel is pulsatile even when full due to crying. In hydrocephalus, the anterior fontanel is usually not visibly pulsatile. Examination of the fontanel should be performed while the infant is in a sitting position.

18 Transient unexplained benign bulging of the fontanel may occur in normal infants. This, however, should be a diagnosis of exclusion.

Bibliography

Kiesler K, Ricer R: The abnormal fontanel, *Am Fam Physician* 67:2547–2552, 2003.

Purugganan OH: Abnormalities in head size, *Pediatr Rev* 27:473–476, 2006.

Ridgway EB, Weiner HL: Skull deformities, *Pediatr Clin North Am* 51: 359–387, 2004.

Robin NH: Congenital muscular torticollis, *Pediatr Rev* 17:374–375, 1996.

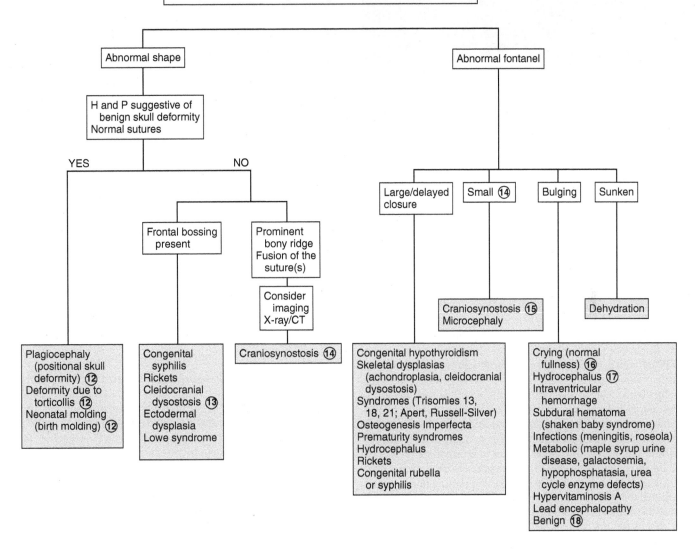

ABNORMAL HEAD SIZE, SHAPE, OR FONTANELS (continued)

Abnormal shape

H and P suggestive of benign skull deformity
Normal sutures

YES

NO

Frontal bossing present

Prominent bony ridge
Fusion of the suture(s)

Consider imaging X-ray/CT

Plagiocephaly (positional skull deformity) ⑫
Deformity due to torticollis ⑫
Neonatal molding (birth molding) ⑫

Congenital syphilis
Rickets
Cleidocranial dysostosis ⑬
Ectodermal dysplasia
Lowe syndrome

Craniosynostosis ⑭

Abnormal fontanel

Large/delayed closure

Small ⑭

Bulging

Sunken

Craniosynostosis ⑮
Microcephaly

Dehydration

Congenital hypothyroidism
Skeletal dysplasias (achondroplasia, cleidocranial dysostosis)
Syndromes (Trisomies 13, 18, 21; Apert, Russell-Silver)
Osteogenesis Imperfecta
Prematurity syndromes
Hydrocephalus
Rickets
Congenital rubella or syphilis

Crying (normal fullness) ⑯
Hydrocephalus ⑰
Intraventricular hemorrhage
Subdural hematoma (shaken baby syndrome)
Infections (meningitis, roseola)
Metabolic (maple syrup urine disease, galactosemia, hypophosphatasia, urea cycle enzyme defects)
Hypervitaminosis A
Lead encephalopathy
Benign ⑱

Chapter 6
RED EYE

Red eye is a common pediatric complaint. It can occur secondary to a wide range of etiologies.

(1) The age of onset of the red eye, the nature of any discharge, and the associated signs and symptoms are the most important components of the history. History of exposure to irritants (e.g., allergens, particulate matter, chemicals) and of trauma or infectious contacts (e.g., "pink-eye" in school or daycare settings) may also be helpful. For infants, inquire about the possibility of any maternal infections.

(2) Conjunctivitis within the neonatal period (4 weeks of birth) is also known as ophthalmia neonatorum. The most common causes in the United States are *Staphylococcus aureus*, *Staphylococcus epidermidis*, *Streptococcus pneumoniae*, and *Moraxella catarrhalis*.

(3) Ophthalmia neonatorum also can be caused by *Chlamydia trachomatis*, *Neisseria gonorrhoeae*, and herpes simplex virus (HSV). Gonococcal conjunctivitis typically appears as a fulminant purulent conjunctivitis in the first 2 to 6 days of life. Chlamydial conjunctivitis is more likely beyond the first 6 days of life and is often associated with a pneumonitis. It can develop in 30% to 40% of infants whose mothers had untreated chlamydia. Conjunctivitis caused by HSV characteristically occurs as a unilateral bright red eye with thin watery discharge. Vesicles or erosions are present on the lid or surrounding skin. These clinical findings are not specific, however, and prompt evaluation and treatment are always indicated to avoid serious sequelae. A Gram stain and culture will aid in the diagnosis of gonorrhea. Rapid antigen tests are available for chlamydial infections. HSV is usually cultured, but PCR may be helpful. Ophthalmologic consultation is indicated when herpes is suspected.

(4) Viral conjunctivitis may vary in presentation from mild redness and irritation with minimal watery drainage to severe conjunctival injection with purulent discharge. Adenovirus is the most common cause and may present with preauricular lymphadenopathy. Coxsackie and echoviruses may cause a hemorrhagic conjunctivitis.

(5) Dacryostenosis (i.e., congenital lacrimal duct stenosis) is a common disorder that occurs within 2 to 4 months of age but sometimes is not noticed until tear production with crying becomes evident. An excessive tear lake and overflow with crusting are seen on examination. Children so affected are at

(6) Tearing, photophobia, and blepharospasm make up the classic triad of presenting symptoms of infantile glaucoma. Conjunctival injection, corneal enlargement (>12 mm), and corneal clouding (edema) are the other findings.

(7) Conjunctivitis in the first 24 hours of life is probably a chemical conjunctivitis unless membranes were ruptured prematurely. Silver nitrate is more likely to produce this condition than other agents used for prophylaxis (e.g., erythromycin, tetracycline) and is no longer used in the United States. In older children, chemical irritants may include cosmetics or eye medications.

(8) Corneal abrasion presents with pain, tearing, photophobia, and eye redness. It is an important consideration in the diagnosis of an irritable infant. Diagnosis is by fluorescein staining and observation under blue light.

(9) Subconjunctival hemorrhage may occur with vomiting, coughing, or weight lifting. It may also occur in newborns after vaginal delivery.

(10) Allergic conjunctivitis is characterized by itching, chemosis, papillae of the tarsal conjunctivae, and white stringy discharge. In limbal vernal conjunctivitis, a ring of swollen conjunctiva surrounds the limbus of the cornea.

(11) Bacterial conjunctivitis may be unilateral or bilateral, but viral conjunctivitis is more commonly bilateral. Bacterial conjunctivitis is more likely to have purulent discharge than viral conjunctivitis, although significant overlap in the clinical presentation of the two etiologies does occur. Nontypable *Haemophilus influenzae*, pneumococci, staphylococci, and streptococci are common agents.

(12) Redness may be due to irritation from eye rubbing. Excessive television or computer use may cause decreased rate of blinking, with drying and irritation.

(13) Iritis and iridocyclitis may occur secondary to localized infection or trauma, or they may be manifestations of a rheumatic disorder (e.g., JRA, Reiter syndrome, Behçet's disease). Inflammatory bowel disease and Kawasaki disease are other associated conditions. Photophobia is typically a significant finding with iritis and iridocyclitis.

(14) Scleritis may accompany certain autoimmune disorders including systemic lupus erythematosus and Henoch-Schönlein purpura. Pain is present, eye discharge is absent, and dilated blood vessels are larger than in conjunctivitis.

(15) Parinaud's oculoglandular syndrome is a form of cat scratch disease caused by *Bartonella henselae*. Symptoms include a granulomatous conjunctivitis and preauricular lymphadenopathy.

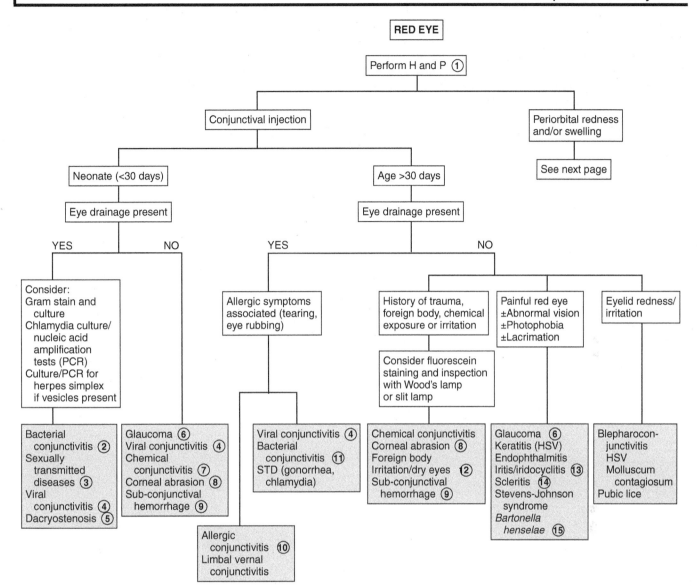

Nelson Textbook of Pediatrics, 19e. Chapters 611, 614, 618, 619, 624, 625
Nelsons Essentials, 6e. Chapter 119

16 Pain with extraocular eye movements may accompany orbital cellulitis. Proptosis and impaired extraocular movement and vision are other signs. Orbital cellulitis must be distinguished from preseptal (periorbital) cellulitis. Minimal conjunctival redness usually occurs in orbital cellulitis, and extraocular muscle movements are intact in preseptal cellulitis.

17 Orbital tumors, including rhabdomyosarcomas, neuroblastomas, and lymphangiomas, may have a similar presentation to orbital cellulitis.

18 Some systemic disorders, such as sarcoid, tuberculosis, and syphilis, may cause chronic dacryocystitis.

The lacrimal gland (i.e., the site of tear production) is located in the lateral aspect of the upper eyelid. Rarely, inflammation of the lacrimal gland (i.e., dacryoadenitis) can occur as a result of infections (e.g., *S. aureus*, infectious mononucleosis, mumps).

Bibliography

Greenberg MF, Pollard ZF: The red eye in childhood, *Pediatr Clin North Am* 50:105–124, 2003.

Richards A, Guzman-Cottrill JA: Conjunctivitis, *Pediatr Rev* 31:196–208, 2010.

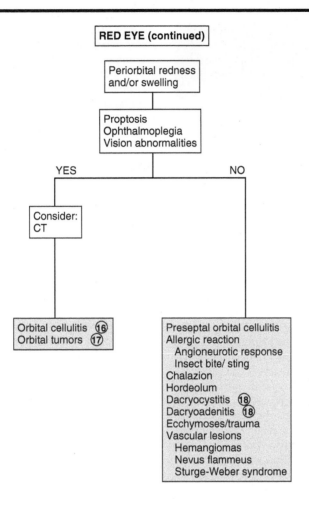

RED EYE (continued)

Periorbital redness and/or swelling

Proptosis
Ophthalmoplegia
Vision abnormalities

YES

NO

Consider:
CT

Orbital cellulitis ⑯
Orbital tumors ⑰

Preseptal orbital cellulitis
Allergic reaction
　Angioneurotic response
　Insect bite/ sting
Chalazion
Hordeolum
Dacryocystitis ⑱
Dacryoadenitis ⑱
Ecchymoses/trauma
Vascular lesions
　Hemangiomas
　Nevus flammeus
　Sturge-Weber syndrome

Chapter 7
STRABISMUS

Strabismus ("squint," "crossed eyes," "straying eyes") is a term used to describe any misalignment of the eyes. It affects 4% of children younger than age 6. It is usually an isolated problem in children but can occasionally indicate an underlying pathology. Early diagnosis, appropriate referral, and treatment are essential to prevent the development of amblyopia (i.e., visual loss), which occurs in 30% to 50% of children with strabismus.

1. The history should include age of onset, circumstances eliciting the deviation, and associated visual complaints. Prematurity, prenatal drug exposure (fetal alcohol syndrome), cerebral palsy, developmental delay, and chromosomal and genetic anomalies are risk factors for early-onset strabismus. A family history and evaluation of family photographs (for corneal light reflex and red reflex) may also be helpful.

Binocular alignment and ocular motility can be assessed using the corneal light reflex test, cover/uncover, and alternate cover tests. Corneal light reflex tests are useful in younger children; the examiner projects a light source onto the cornea of both eyes simultaneously. In straight eyes, the light reflection appears symmetric and slightly nasal to the center of each pupil. If strabismus is present, the reflected light is asymmetric. Cover tests for strabismus require a child's attention and cooperation. The alternate cover test differentiates tropias, or manifest deviations, from latent deviations, or phorias. Careful examination should result in being able to classify the problem as a heterophoria (latent, deviating under certain circumstances) or heterotropia (constant), paralytic or nonparalytic, and inward turning (eso-) or outward turning (exo-). Based on the nature of the defect and the child's age at the time the problem develops, many cases can be identified as a specific clinical entity.

2. Intermittent transient eye crossing is normal in infants in the first 3 months of life. It is also known as ocular instability of infancy and frequently occurs when infants are tired.

3. A wide, flat nasal bridge or prominent epicanthal folds may create an optical illusion of in- turning eyes (i.e., pseudostrabismus). Careful assessment of the corneal light reflexes confirms that the alignment is normal.

4. Heterophoria is a latent tendency to deviate; it often occurs with fatigue, illness, stress, or covering one eye and is often asymptomatic. If the heterophoria is significant, it may cause transient diplopia (double vision), headaches, or eyestrain and might require treatment.

5. Sensory strabismus occurs when there is severe vision loss (unilateral or bilateral) and there is subsequent loss of ocular alignment. It may be accompanied by sensory nystagmus in children with severe and early vision loss.

6. Strabismus may be a presenting symptom in children with retinoblastoma along with leukocoria.

7. The term *comitant strabismus* is used when the extraocular muscles and the nerves innervating them are normal. The degree of deviation is constant or relatively constant in all directions of gaze. There is usually no underlying neurologic, mechanical, sensory, or other deficit. Noncomitant strabismus is suggested by an eye misalignment that varies according to the direction of the gaze. The condition is produced by an underlying nerve palsy, muscle weakness, or mechanical restriction of eye movement. Compensatory head tilting often occurs.

8. Infantile (congenital) esotropia appears before 6 months of age. There is often a family history of strabismus.

9. Acquired esotropia is often accommodative; the eyes turn inward with attempt to focus. Onset is typically between 2 and 3 years of age. Acquired esotropia may follow a period of occlusion of one eye.

10. Infantile exotropia is less common than infantile esotropia and is more frequent in children with neurologic abnormalities.

11. Careful assessment of ocular motility and associated lid and pupillary functions should help identify cranial nerve palsies. Acquired cranial nerve palsies warrant careful evaluation to rule out CNS lesions. Compensatory head tilting often occurs.

In children, third nerve palsies are usually congenital and may be associated with a developmental anomaly or birth trauma. Acquired third nerve palsies in children are concerning and may indicate a neurologic abnormality (intracranial neoplasm or aneurysm). A third nerve palsy causes exotropia, downward deviation (hypotropia) of the affected eye, and ptosis of the upper lid due to the normal but unopposed action of the lateral rectus muscle and the superior oblique muscle. There may be dilation of the pupil if the internal branch of the third nerve is involved.

Fourth nerve palsies can be congenital or acquired; they result in weakness of the superior oblique muscle, resulting in upward deviation of the eye (hypertropia). The inferior oblique is relatively unopposed, and the affected eye demonstrates an upshoot when attempting to look toward the nose.

Sixth nerve palsies cause severely crossed eyes with limited ability to move the afflicted eye laterally.

12. In Duane syndrome there is a congenital absence of the sixth nerve nucleus and anomalous innervation of the lateral rectus muscle. Lateral movement of the affected eye is limited. Medial movement produces sharp upshoots or downshoots of the affected eye. These motions are also accompanied by globe retraction. They can have exotropia or esotropia. A defect of the sixth and seventh cranial nerve nuclei results in congenital facial diplegia and defective abduction in Möbius syndrome. Parinaud's syndrome is a palsy of vertical gaze, isolated or associated with pupillary or nuclear oculomotor (third cranial nerve) paresis. In Gradenigo syndrome, inflammation results in a sixth nerve palsy due to nerve entrapment along the petrosphenoidal ligament. Etiologies include otitis media, mastoiditis, and tumor. Monocular elevation deficiency is an inability to elevate the eye in both adduction and abduction. It may be due to paresis of the superior rectus and inferior oblique muscles, which are elevator muscles, or a restriction to elevation from a fibrotic inferior rectus muscle.

13. Myasthenia gravis is uncommon in children but should be considered when there is intermittent strabismus and ptosis.

14. Palsies of the third cranial nerves with resultant pupillary dilation and ptosis are characteristic of most ophthalmoplegic

migraines. The eye muscle paralysis may last for a few weeks following a headache.

15 Restrictive strabismus is due to mechanical forces such as inflammation, edema, trauma, or congenital disorders resulting in fibrosis.

16 Blunt trauma to the eye leading to a blowout fracture of the orbit may cause strabismus due to muscle entrapment as well as edema and hematoma of the muscle(s).

17 In Brown syndrome, an abnormality of the superior oblique tendon results in an inability to elevate the eye in the medial position.

18 Excessive fibrosis and anomalous insertion of extraocular muscles results in ptosis and external ophthalmoplegia. Convergence on attempted upward gaze, divergence on attempted downward gaze, and compensatory chin-up posturing are also characteristic of congenital fibrosis syndrome.

Bibliography

Magramm I: Amblyopia: Etiology, detection, and treatment, *Pediatr Rev* 13: 7–14, 1992.
Ticho BH: Strabismus, *Pediatr Clin North Am* 50:173–188, 2003.
Tingley DH: Vision screening essentials: Screening today for eye disorders in the pediatric patient, *Pediatr Rev* 28:54–61, 2007.

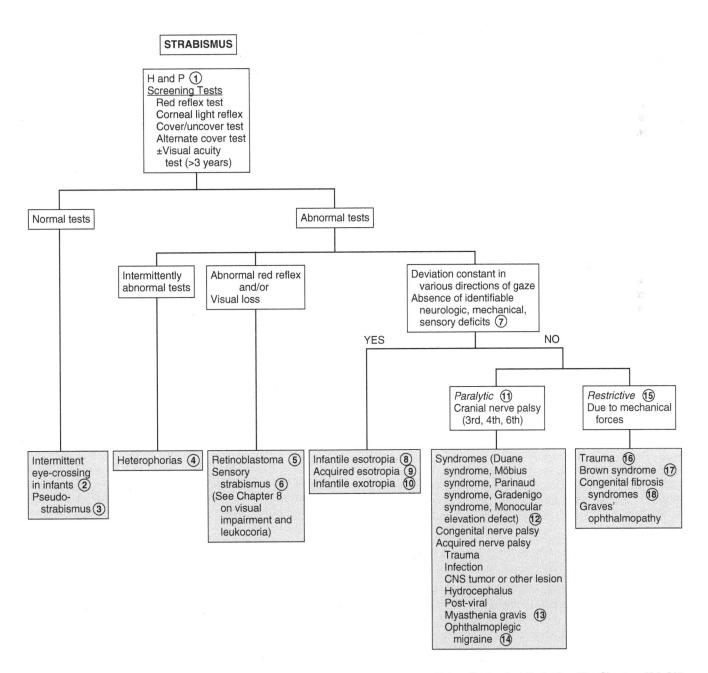

Chapter 8
VISUAL IMPAIRMENT AND LEUKOCORIA

When treating a child in whom there are visual concerns, consultation with a pediatric ophthalmologist or optometrist is frequently required, especially for a very young infant.

1 A detailed description of the visual complaint is helpful, but in infants and young children the history tends to be based primarily on the observations of family and caretakers. For older children, inquire about focal versus general blurring, double images, night vision, and abnormal sensations (e.g., spots, lines). The birth history is an important component of the medical history because asphyxia or trauma (i.e., forceps injury) may be contributory. Recent illness may aid in the diagnosis of sudden visual loss caused by acute optic neuritis. A family history of neurocutaneous disorders, metabolic disorders, cataracts, or other visual problems may also be helpful. The examination should include an assessment for visual acuity using a Snellen chart or one designed for preliterate children (e.g., tumbling E and picture tests). For infants and toddlers, referral for visual assessment using behavioral responses may be necessary. Visual fields should also be assessed. Examination of the pupils, ocular motility, and eye alignment is necessary. A thorough ophthalmologic examination should be done. Common findings that may be helpful in diagnosis include strabismus, corneal opacity, leukocoria, and nystagmus.

2 Leukocoria (i.e., white pupillary reflex) may be due to abnormalities in the retina, lens, or vitreous. Leukocoria is most common in the young infant, although it may occur with problems that develop at a later age. It is the most common presentation of retinoblastoma. Referral to an ophthalmologist for a thorough diagnostic evaluation is always indicated.

3 Cataracts are opacity of the lens and are a common cause of leukocoria. Common etiologies of cataracts include infections (e.g., rubella, toxoplasmosis, CMV), hereditary or metabolic disorders, chromosomal disorders (e.g., trisomy 18, trisomy 13, Turner syndrome), toxins, and trauma. They may also develop as a result of an intraocular processes such as retinopathy of prematurity. Metabolic and endocrine diseases associated with cataracts include galactosemia, galactokinase deficiency, hypoparathyroidism, Wilson disease, and juvenile-onset diabetes mellitus. Cataracts may also be seen in children of diabetic and prediabetic mothers.

4 Retinoblastoma is a malignancy of the retina and is the most common intraocular tumor in children.

5 Retinopathy of prematurity is a disease of developing retinal vasculature and occurs in premature infants. According to the American Academy of Pediatrics screening guidelines, infants with a birth weight of less than 1500 g or gestational age of 30 weeks or less, and selected high-risk infants with birth weight between 1500 and 2000 g or gestational age of over 30 weeks, should have retinal screening examinations.

6 Glaucoma is a progressive optic neuropathy associated with elevated pressure within the eye. Congenital glaucoma is present at birth, infantile glaucoma develops during the first 3 years of life, and juvenile glaucoma begins between 3 and 30 years of age. Glaucoma may be primary and due to an isolated anomaly of the drainage apparatus of the eye (trabecular meshwork) or secondary with other associated ocular or systemic abnormalities. In infantile glaucoma, signs and symptoms are different from adult glaucoma, because the infant eye is pliable, leading to enlargement of the cornea and globe. This is known as buphthalmos or "ox-eye." Only 30% of children with infantile glaucoma demonstrate the classic triad of glaucoma: tearing, photophobia, and blepharospasm (i.e., eyelid squeezing). Other signs include corneal haziness, conjunctival injection, and visual impairment.

7 Anterior uveitis involves inflammation of the iris and/or ciliary body. It may be associated with JRA, sarcoidosis, Kawasaki disease, Stevens-Johnson syndrome, viral infections (e.g., herpes simplex, herpes zoster), syphilis, tuberculosis, and many other conditions. Posterior uveitis involves the choroid and often the retina. Causes include parasites (e.g., toxoplasmosis, toxocariasis), viruses (e.g., rubella, herpes simplex, HIV, CMV), tuberculosis, and others.

8 Optic neuritis is an inflammation or demyelination of the optic nerve, leading to acute vision loss. It may be due to inflammatory diseases (e.g., systemic lupus erythematosus), infections (e.g., HIV, syphilis, Lyme disease, meningitis), toxin exposure (e.g., methanol, lead), or nutrient deficiency (e.g., B_{12}). Multiple sclerosis is also a possible etiology but is more common in adults.

9 Psychogenic vision loss (malingering, conversion reactions) is more likely to occur in older school-aged children. Complaints of visual loss or blurring may be accompanied by numerous other complaints (e.g., abnormal visual sensations, diplopia, polyopia, painful eyes, headaches). Diagnosis is suggested by normal examination findings and behavioral "red flags" such as inconsistent complaints in different situations, positive responses to examiner's suggestions of maneuvers to improve vision, and inappropriate affect (e.g., indifferent, belligerent, overdramatic) during the examination.

10 Amblyopia is a decrease in visual acuity despite correction of any refractive errors. It occurs in visually immature children and is due to the lack of a clear image projecting onto the retina. When this occurs during the critical period of development in the first decade of life, amblyopia may occur. The unformed image can occur secondary to a strabismus, a difference in refractive error between the eyes (anisometropic amblyopia), a high refractive error in both eyes (ametropic amblyopia), and image deprivation due to cataracts, corneal opacities, or occlusion (e.g., eye patch).

11 Optic gliomas are most commonly located in the optic chiasm but may occur anywhere along the optic pathway. They can occur with a variety of symptoms, including unilateral vision loss, proptosis, bitemporal hemianopia, and eye deviation. Craniopharyngiomas may occur with visual loss, pituitary dysfunction (e.g., diabetes insipidus, short stature, hypothyroidism), and increased ICP. Neuroimaging is indicated whenever a tumor is suspected.

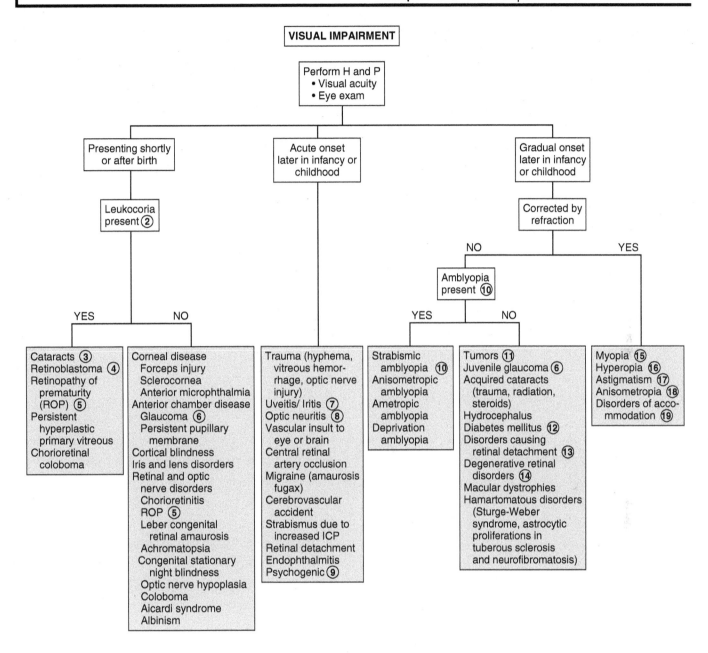

ROP = Retinopathy of prematurity

Nelson Textbook of Pediatrics, 19e. Chapters 496, 611-614, 620-624

12 Children with diabetes may develop retinopathy, optic neuropathy, or even cataracts, leading to vision loss.

13 Retinal detachment may be caused by trauma (child abuse), retinopathy of prematurity, congenital cataract surgery, diabetes, sickle cell disease, Coats disease, retinoblastoma, and ocular inflammation. The presenting signs may be loss of vision, strabismus, nystagmus, or leukocoria.

14 Degenerative disorders originating in the retina are Coats disease, retinoschisis, familial exudative vitreoretinopathy, and retinitis pigmentosa.

15 Myopia or near-sightedness is the most common refractive error in children for which glasses are prescribed; only near objects are seen in sharp focus.

16 Hyperopia (far-sightedness) is common at birth and improves with time. Accommodation is used to bring objects into focus; excessive accommodation may cause eyestrain.

17 Astigmatism is a refractive error usually due to irregularity of the surface of the cornea; a clear image requires accommodation or squinting, which may lead to eyestrain.

18 Anisometropia is when the refractive state of one eye is significantly different from the other eye.

19 Disorders of accommodation in children are rare; premature presbyopia is occasionally seen in children. Other causes of paralysis of accommodation in children may be iatrogenic (cycloplegics), neurogenic (oculomotor nerve lesions), and systemic disorders (botulism).

Bibliography

Curnyn KM, Kaufman LM: The eye examination in the pediatrician's office, *Pediatr Clin North Am* 50:25–40, 2003.

Fierson WM: AAP policy statement. Screening examination of premature infants for retinopathy of prematurity, *Pediatrics* 131:189–195, 2013.

Greenwald MJ: Refractive abnormalities in childhood, *Pediatr Clin North Am* 50:197–212, 2003.

Kipp MA: Childhood glaucoma, *Pediatr Clin North Am* 50:89–104, 2003.

Levin AV: Congenital eye anomalies, *Pediatr Clin North Am* 50:55–76, 2003.

Mittleman D: Amblyopia, *Pediatr Clin North Am* 50:189–196, 2003.

Stout AU, Stout JT: Retinopathy of prematurity, *Pediatr Clin North Am* 50: 77–88, 2003.

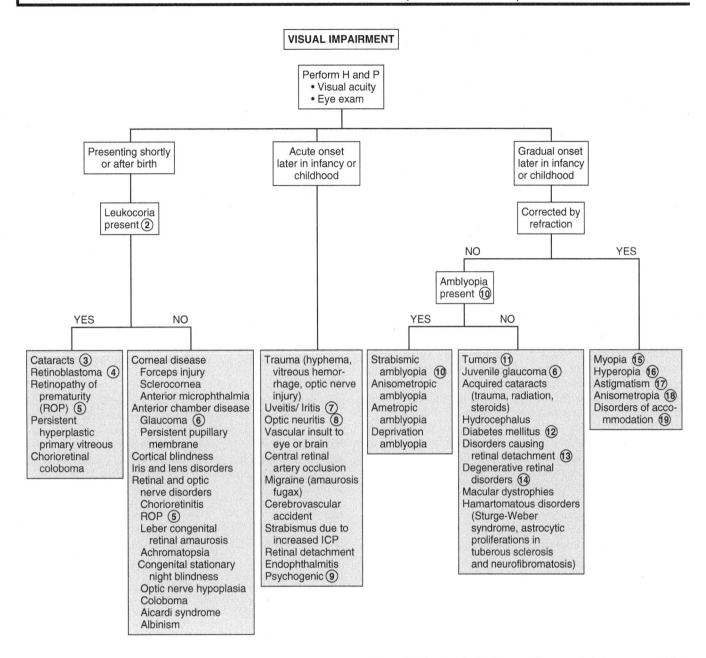

VISUAL IMPAIRMENT

Perform H and P
• Visual acuity
• Eye exam

Presenting shortly
or after birth

Acute onset
later in infancy or
childhood

Gradual onset
later in infancy
or childhood

Leukocoria
present ②

Corrected by
refraction

NO   YES

Amblyopia
present ⑩

YES   NO

YES   NO

Cataracts ③
Retinoblastoma ④
Retinopathy of
  prematurity
  (ROP) ⑤
Persistent
  hyperplastic
  primary vitreous
Chorioretinal
  coloboma

Corneal disease
  Forceps injury
  Sclerocornea
  Anterior microphthalmia
Anterior chamber disease
  Glaucoma ⑥
  Persistent pupillary
    membrane
Cortical blindness
Iris and lens disorders
Retinal and optic
  nerve disorders
  Chorioretinitis
  ROP ⑤
  Leber congenital
    retinal amaurosis
  Achromatopsia
  Congenital stationary
    night blindness
  Optic nerve hypoplasia
  Coloboma
  Aicardi syndrome
  Albinism

Trauma (hyphema,
  vitreous hemor-
  rhage, optic nerve
  injury)
Uveitis/ Iritis ⑦
Optic neuritis ⑧
Vascular insult to
  eye or brain
Central retinal
  artery occlusion
Migraine (amaurosis
  fugax)
Cerebrovascular
  accident
Strabismus due to
  increased ICP
Retinal detachment
Endophthalmitis
Psychogenic ⑨

Strabismic
  amblyopia ⑩
Anisometropic
  amblyopia
Ametropic
  amblyopia
Deprivation
  amblyopia

Tumors ⑪
Juvenile glaucoma ⑥
Acquired cataracts
  (trauma, radiation,
  steroids)
Hydrocephalus
Diabetes mellitus ⑫
Disorders causing
  retinal detachment ⑬
Degenerative retinal
  disorders ⑭
Macular dystrophies
Hamartomatous disorders
  (Sturge-Weber
  syndrome, astrocytic
  proliferations in
  tuberous sclerosis
  and neurofibromatosis)

Myopia ⑮
Hyperopia ⑯
Astigmatism ⑰
Anisometropia ⑱
Disorders of acco-
  mmodation ⑲

ROP = Retinopathy of prematurity

Nelson Textbook of Pediatrics, 19e. Chapters 496, 611-614, 620-624

Chapter 9
ABNORMAL EYE MOVEMENTS

Abnormal eye movements may occur as a benign finding or in association with other visual or ocular problems. They may, however, indicate an acquired, more severe underlying neurologic problem.

1. The history should include an accurate description of the eye movements, age of onset, and associated signs and symptoms. Specifically inquire about visual acuity, color vision, night vision, photophobia, abnormal head movements, tinnitus, and oscillopsia. Oscillopsia is a sensation of movement or swinging of the visual field.

Careful examination should yield an accurate description of the eye movements and other associated signs and symptoms. Eye movements should be initially classified as rhythmic (swinging, pendulum-like) or nonrhythmic. The association of any nonocular muscle movements should be discerned. Nystagmus is defined as repetitive rhythmic oscillations of one or both eyes. The waveform, direction, amplitude, frequency, and velocity of oscillations further help to classify the pattern of nystagmus. It should be noted whether the movements are symmetric or asymmetric between the two eyes. Some patterns have diagnostic implications. For example, vertical nystagmus is associated with posterior fossa lesions. Some drug-induced nystagmus may occasionally be vertical.

Frequently, neuroimaging and sometimes more specialized studies (e.g., electroretinogram, visual evoked potential test) are necessary to rule out underlying etiologies.

2. Ocular myoclonus describes rhythmic oscillating eye movements accompanied by nonocular movements of the soft palate, tongue, face, pharynx, larynx, and diaphragm.

3. Congenital sensory nystagmus is commonly associated with ocular abnormalities that lead to visual impairment. It is the most common type of nystagmus in infants. It generally occurs in children in the first 6 months of life and in children with congenital or perinatal vision defects. It may also be observed in children who develop blindness in the first few years of life. The cause is frequently evident on general or ophthalmoscopic examination. Electrophysiologic imaging may be necessary to rule out certain causes (e.g., achromatopsia, congenital stationary night blindness, Leber's congenital retinal amaurosis) that are not evident on funduscopic examination. (See Chapter 8.) Neuroimaging to rule out tumors is always recommended when the cause is not evident.

4. Congenital idiopathic nystagmus typically appears in the first 3 months of life and is associated with compensatory head tilting. A thorough examination, neuroimaging, and electrophysiologic studies are usually necessary to rule out underlying ocular or neurologic disorders.

5. Neurologic disorders must always be excluded as a cause of acquired nystagmus. Imaging should be considered to exclude intracranial neoplasms. Other etiologies include CNS infections, trauma, encephalopathy, and demyelination disorders.

6. Labyrinthitis is often caused by viral illness and may be an infrequent complication of otitis media. Manifestations can include vertigo, ear pain, nausea, vomiting, hearing loss, and nystagmus.

7. Spasmus nutans is usually a benign condition that occurs as a combination of bilateral asymmetric nystagmus, head nodding, and torticollis in the first years of life. The etiology is unknown. It generally resolves by age 3 years without sequelae. Despite the benign nature of the condition, neuroimaging is recommended to rule out the possibility of a CNS neoplasm.

8. Both children and adults can exhibit an occasional one to two beats of lateral nystagmus on side gaze that is not considered significant.

Bibliography
Curnyn KM, Kaufman LM: The eye examination in the pediatrician's office, *Pediatr Clin North Am* 50:25–40, 2003.
Ruttum MS: Eye disorders. In Kliegman RM, Lye PS, Greenbaum LA, editors: *Practical strategies in pediatric diagnosis and therapy*, ed 2, Philadelphia, 2004, Elsevier Saunders. Chapter 43.
Thompson L, Kaufman LM: The visually impaired child, *Pediatr Clin North Am* 50:225–239, 2003.

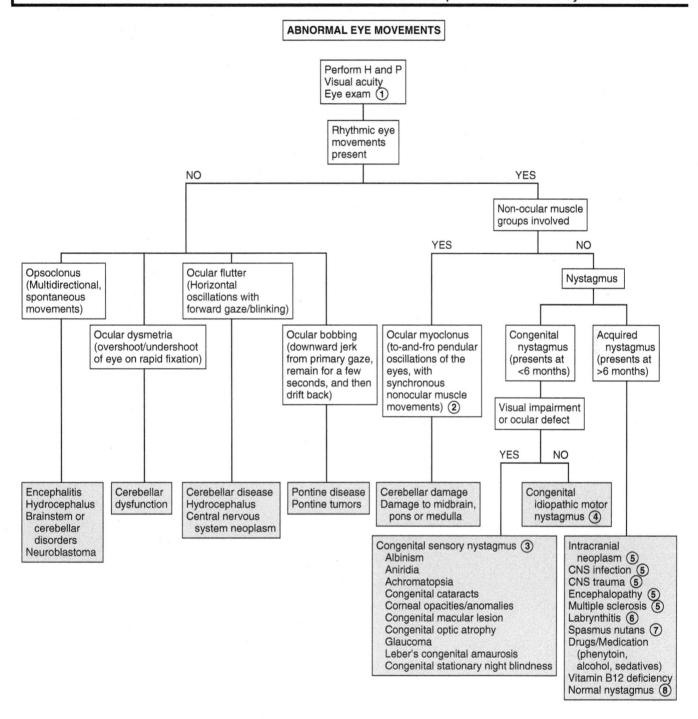

ABNORMAL EYE MOVEMENTS

Perform H and P
Visual acuity
Eye exam ①

Rhythmic eye movements present

NO / YES

Non-ocular muscle groups involved

YES / NO

Opsoclonus (Multidirectional, spontaneous movements)

Ocular flutter (Horizontal oscillations with forward gaze/blinking)

Ocular dysmetria (overshoot/undershoot of eye on rapid fixation)

Ocular bobbing (downward jerk from primary gaze, remain for a few seconds, and then drift back)

Ocular myoclonus (to-and-fro pendular oscillations of the eyes, with synchronous nonocular muscle movements) ②

Nystagmus

Congenital nystagmus (presents at <6 months)

Acquired nystagmus (presents at >6 months)

Visual impairment or ocular defect

YES / NO

Encephalitis
Hydrocephalus
Brainstem or cerebellar disorders
Neuroblastoma

Cerebellar dysfunction

Cerebellar disease
Hydrocephalus
Central nervous system neoplasm

Pontine disease
Pontine tumors

Cerebellar damage
Damage to midbrain, pons or medulla

Congenital idiopathic motor nystagmus ④

Congenital sensory nystagmus ③
  Albinism
  Aniridia
  Achromatopsia
  Congenital cataracts
  Corneal opacities/anomalies
  Congenital macular lesion
  Congenital optic atrophy
  Glaucoma
  Leber's congenital amaurosis
  Congenital stationary night blindness

Intracranial neoplasm ⑤
CNS infection ⑤
CNS trauma ⑤
Encephalopathy ⑤
Multiple sclerosis ⑤
Labrynthitis ⑥
Spasmus nutans ⑦
Drugs/Medication (phenytoin, alcohol, sedatives)
Vitamin B12 deficiency
Normal nystagmus ⑧

Nelson Textbook of Pediatrics, 19e. Chapter 615

Respiratory System

Chapter 10

COUGH

① The medical history should include a neonatal history and an assessment for immunodeficiency. An environmental history should include inquiries about potential irritants (e.g., wood burning stove, smoke, perfume, scented candles, incense). The review of systems should include respiratory and nonrespiratory symptoms (e.g, poor growth and malodorous stools could be associated with cystic fibrosis; halitosis and headache may be associated with sinusitis). Inquire specifically about any recent choking episodes as well as any seasonal variation of symptoms, and relationship of symptoms to feeding. A family history for asthma (and other atopic conditions) and cystic fibrosis may be helpful.

② Bronchitis is a frequently used but nonspecific term in pediatrics. Inflammation of the large airways (tracheobronchitis) commonly occurs and is due to multiple infectious agents. A viral URI complicated by a prolonged, possibly productive cough and malaise are common. These cases are typically self-limited (2 to 3 weeks) and unresponsive to antibiotics. Bacterial pneumonia may occur primarily or complicate a preceding URI. Fever and physical examination findings suggest this diagnosis. There is an emerging recognition of a persistent or protracted bacterial bronchitis, which will respond to antibiotics and may be associated with more significant pulmonary disease (i.e., chronic suppurative lung disease). However, this diagnosis should be made with caution, particularly in children with a relatively acute history of cough. Careful consideration of other underlying pulmonary or systemic disorders should be made in children with chronic or recurring cough.

③ Clinical diagnosis of acute bacterial rhinosinusitis is made by prolonged symptoms of rhinorrhea for 10 to 14 days. Halitosis, fever, nocturnal cough, and postnasal drip are other suggestive symptoms. Older children may experience headache, facial pain, tooth pain, and periorbital swelling.

④ Croup (i.e., laryngotracheobronchitis or laryngotracheitis) most commonly affects children age 3 months to 3 years. It classically presents with the abrupt onset of an acute barky cough following 1 to 2 days of nonspecific viral URI symptoms. The cough is described as seal-like or brassy; inspiratory stridor, hoarseness, and respiratory distress may be associated. Worsening of symptoms at night is typical. High fever may occur. Diagnosis should be clinical; imaging (anteroposterior and lateral neck films) should only be obtained when another diagnosis is suspected (e.g., epiglottitis), symptoms are severe, or there is lack of improvement with therapy.

Spasmodic croup refers to a clinically similar condition, but without evidence of airway inflammation. The clinical course is typically more abrupt and short-lived than cases that are obviously associated with URIs, plus the symptoms occur exclusively at night. Episodes can resolve and recur multiple times in one night and for a few nights in a row, with the child appearing completely well in between coughing episodes. A lack of consensus exists regarding whether a spasmodic croup presentation is a distinct entity (with an allergic component) or on the same spectrum as infectious croup because both have been associated with viral infections.

⑤ According to the Centers for Disease Control and Prevention (CDC) and the World Health Organization (WHO), a clinical diagnosis of pertussis can be made based on a cough history of 2 weeks' duration if one of the following is present: paroxysms of coughing (especially at night), inspiratory whoop, or posttussive vomiting. Children with pertussis generally appear well between paroxysmal coughing spells. The "whoop" may not occur in infants younger than 3 months of age or in partially immunized children. Conjunctival hemorrhages, upper body petechiae, and exhaustion are additional supportive symptoms; the *absence* of fever, myalgia, pharyngitis, and abnormal lung findings are also supportive. During epidemics or, in the case of close contact with a known case, a cough history ≥ 2 weeks is sufficient for diagnosis. Contact history is important; most cases of pertussis in infants and children can be traced to contact with a mildly symptomatic adolescent or adult whose only symptom may be a nonspecific prolonged cough. The timing of exposure to sick contacts can be helpful; the incubation period for pertussis is 7 to 10 days, as opposed to 1 to 3 days for most viral URIs. Nasopharyngeal cultures are still considered the gold standard for diagnosis; however, the sensitivity can be diminished by the fastidious nature of the organism and inappropriate handling of the specimen. PCR testing is more sensitive and is most useful during the first 3 weeks of illness; the risk of false-negative results increases after 4 weeks of illness. Testing after antibiotic treatment and early in the course of an illness when symptoms are still fairly nonspecific is not recommended. An elevated white blood cell count (15,000 to 100,000/μl) due to lymphocytosis supports the diagnosis, although it may not occur in very young infants or immunized children.

⑥ Aspiration of food or secretions in neurologically abnormal children may cause cough of varying frequency or severity. Cough due to aspiration may be produced by airway inflammation, bronchospasm, or pneumonia. Aspiration pneumonia may or may not be superinfected. If infection does occur, it is usually due to anaerobes or gram-negative organisms when chronic or nosocomial. Radionuclide scans or barium contrast studies may help to diagnose swallowing abnormalities. The intermittent nature of aspiration, however, frequently makes diagnosis difficult.

⑦ Rigid bronchoscopy is increasingly becoming the diagnostic and therapeutic procedure of choice when a choking episode was witnessed, or when the history and physical are strongly suggestive of an aspirated foreign body. In the absence of a witnessed choking episode, chest films will generally be obtained to rule out other etiologies; however, only 10% to 25% of foreign bodies are radiopaque. Expiratory or lateral decubitus views may be helpful in identifying air trapping acutely but can be difficult to obtain.

⑧ Foreign body aspiration is usually obvious immediately, but occasionally a delay of weeks to months may occur before symptoms develop. Aspiration of foreign bodies occurs most commonly in children under 4 years of age, with food (especially nuts) and small toys being the most commonly aspirated items. In cases where a delayed diagnosis is suspected based on clinical findings (e.g., chronic cough, wheezing, localized lung findings) the risk/benefit ratio of CT versus fluoroscopy versus performing a diagnostic flexible bronchoscopy must be considered.

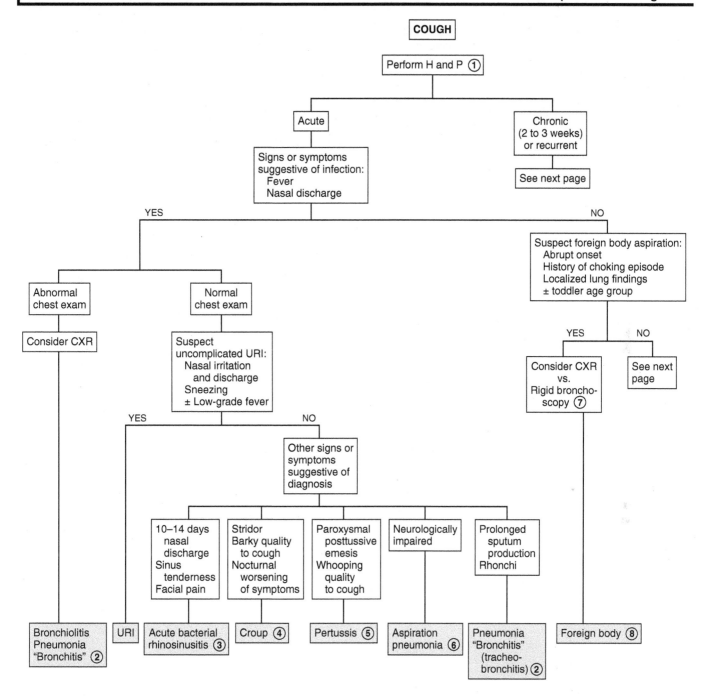

COUGH

Perform H and P ①

Acute

Chronic (2 to 3 weeks) or recurrent

See next page

Signs or symptoms suggestive of infection:
Fever
Nasal discharge

YES

NO

Suspect foreign body aspiration:
Abrupt onset
History of choking episode
Localized lung findings
± toddler age group

Abnormal chest exam

Normal chest exam

Consider CXR

Suspect uncomplicated URI:
Nasal irritation and discharge
Sneezing
± Low-grade fever

YES

NO

YES

NO

Consider CXR vs. Rigid broncho-scopy ⑦

See next page

Other signs or symptoms suggestive of diagnosis

10–14 days nasal discharge
Sinus tenderness
Facial pain

Stridor
Barky quality to cough
Nocturnal worsening of symptoms

Paroxysmal posttussive emesis
Whooping quality to cough

Neurologically impaired

Prolonged sputum production
Rhonchi

Bronchiolitis Pneumonia "Bronchitis" ②

URI

Acute bacterial rhinosinusitis ③

Croup ④

Pertussis ⑤

Aspiration pneumonia ⑥

Pneumonia "Bronchitis" (tracheo-bronchitis) ②

Foreign body ⑧

Nelson Texbook of Pediatrics, 19e. Chapters 138, 189, 315, 376, 377, 379, 383
Nelsons Essentials, 6e. Chapters 107, 133, 136

9. Pulmonary contusions can occur as a result of chest trauma. The onset of symptoms may be acute or delayed. Contusions may be visible on a chest x-ray; however, initial film findings are often negative.

10. Historically, gastroesophageal reflux disease (both symptomatic and asymptomatic) has been implicated as an etiology of chronic cough. Actual data supporting the role of reflux in chronic cough remains conflicting, except in children with neurologic impairment and a risk of aspiration.

11. Asthma is the most common cause of chronic and recurrent cough in children. Wheezing may not be evident. A suggestive history, such as significant cough with colds, exercise, hard laughter, crying, or exposure to cold air, smoke, or other environmental irritants or a frequent nocturnal cough, and an improvement of symptoms to therapy (e.g., bronchodilators, short courses of oral corticosteroids) are highly suggestive of the asthma diagnosis. Ideally, spirometry would be used to confirm the diagnosis, although young children are typically unable to perform the testing, and normal results do not always rule out the diagnosis. Chest x-rays are not necessary in the absence of respiratory distress; however, if obtained, hyperinflation and atelectasis are common findings.

12. The term postinfectious cough syndrome describes a prolonged cough (up to 8 weeks), which may follow certain otherwise uncomplicated respiratory infections, presumably due to extensive inflammation of airway epithelium or hypersensitivity of cough receptors. The term upper airway cough syndrome (previously "postnasal drip") describes cough symptoms made worse by lying down; sinusitis and allergic rhinitis may be contributors.

13. Habit cough (also called psychogenic cough or cough tic) is an infrequent cause of a prolonged cough in school-aged children that is often refractory to treatment. The harsh, barky cough occurs only during waking hours. It will disappear during sleep and with distraction. The child appears well and is typically not bothered by the coughing, even though it can frequently be significant enough to disrupt a classroom.

14. Mediastinal disorders include tumor, lymphadenopathy due to sarcoidosis, tuberculosis, histoplasmosis and coccidioidomycosis, pericardial cyst, and diaphragmatic hernia.

15. A large number of rare conditions can occur with cough, including interstitial lung disease, graft-versus-host disease, $\alpha 1$-antitrypsin deficiency, pulmonary hemosiderosis, alveolar proteinosis, heart failure, pulmonary edema, sarcoidosis, obliterative bronchiolitis, and follicular bronchiolitis.

16. Angiotensin-converting enzyme (ACE) inhibitors are recognized as a cause of chronic cough. A history of radiation to the chest or cytotoxic medications should raise suspicions for lung disease. Use of aspirin and other nonsteroidal pain relievers can exacerbate asthma symptoms in certain people who are sensitive to these drugs. Be conscious of illicit drug use in teens (including inhalants) as a cause of chronic cough.

Bibliography

American Academy of Pediatrics. Pertussis. In *Red Book: 2012 Report of the Committee on Infectious Diseases.* Pickering LK, ed. 29th ed. Elk Grove Village, IL: American Academy of Pediatrics; 2012: 553-566.

Bjornson C, Johnson DW: Croup, *Lancet* 371:329–339, 2008.

COUGH (continued)

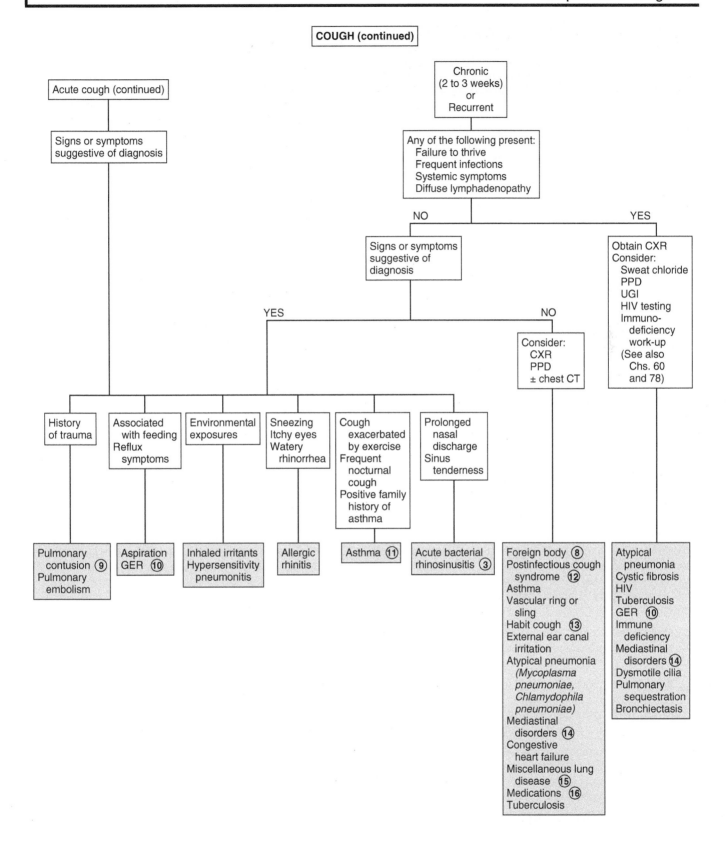

Chapter 11
HOARSENESS

Hoarseness is a change in the quality of the voice caused by alteration of the size, shape, or tension of the vocal cords. It is associated with vocalization, as opposed to stridor, which is associated with respiration; however, the two can occur together. Hoarseness is usually benign, but evaluation is indicated for hoarseness if the onset is congenital, associated with trauma, or if it persists longer than 1 to 2 weeks.

1. Congenital anomalies of the larynx causing hoarseness include subglottic stenosis, laryngoceles, and webs. Laryngeal fissures and clefts are rare conditions, but 20% of posterior fissures or clefts are associated with tracheoesophageal fistulas.

2. Dislocation of the cricothyroid or cricoarytenoid articulations may occur during a traumatic birth. Trauma related to neonatal intubation may also cause stenosis or dislocation of the laryngeal cartilages.

3. Congenital vocal cord paralysis is more commonly unilateral than bilateral; most cases are idiopathic. Unilateral vocal cord paralysis is more common than bilateral. When the disorder is unilateral, it is associated with a weak, breathy cry and may lead to feeding difficulties and aspiration. In bilateral cases, stridor is more predominant and the cry may not be obviously affected. Birth trauma may also produce vocal cord paralysis because of damage to the recurrent laryngeal nerve. Vocal cord paralysis may also be a manifestation of central neurologic disorders, including hydrocephalus, subdural hematomas, and other causes of brainstem compression (e.g., Dandy-Walker cysts, Arnold-Chiari malformations), as well as peripheral neurologic problems (due to recurrent laryngeal nerve trauma, cardiovascular abnormalities, mediastinal masses, myasthenia gravis, and other neuropathies). Neurologic problems are more likely to be associated with bilateral vocal cord paralysis.

4. Hoarseness commonly occurs as a result of overuse of the voice. Inquire about recent attendance at athletic events or rock concerts.

5. Benign vocal cord nodules ("screamer's nodules") may also be a complication of vocal overuse. Further evaluation is indicated if rest does not result in resolution. Reflux to the level of the larynx can exacerbate symptoms.

6. The most common cause of transient hoarseness is croup (laryngotracheobronchitis) in older infants and toddlers, and viral URIs causing laryngitis in older children. Sinus disease is another cause, though it is less common.

7. Allergic angioneurotic edema of the larynx may occur acutely with hoarseness and respiratory distress. Urgent evaluation and treatment are indicated.

8. One to two weeks is a reasonable interval to observe children prior to referring for an ENT evaluation if the etiology of hoarseness is unclear. There is no clear consensus regarding when children (beyond infancy) should undergo visualization of their vocal cords for symptoms of a hoarse voice; specialists will make the decision for laryngoscopy based on the severity of hoarseness or associated symptoms, suspected diagnosis, and procedural risk. Any element of respiratory distress, tachypnea, or decreased air entry warrants visualization.

9. Acquired vocal cord paralysis may occur as a result of polyneuropathy (e.g., Guillain-Barré syndrome), Arnold-Chiari malformation, compression from a mass or tumor, brainstem encephalitis, or neck or thoracic surgery.

10. Rare infectious causes of hoarseness include granulomatous lesions in the larynx due to syphilis, tuberculosis, and histoplasmosis. Immunologic disorders, including HIV infection, may predispose patients to fungal infections of the airways. Prolonged use of inhaled corticosteroids has been associated with *Candida* overgrowth. Diphtheria, rabies, and tetanus are other etiologies.

11. Respiratory papillomatosis develops as a progressive hoarseness anytime between the first several months and up to 5 years of age. The etiology is human papillomavirus (most commonly types 6 and 11) transmitted at birth from the mother's genital tract.

12. Cutaneous hemangiomas, especially of the head and neck, may be a marker for underlying airway hemangiomas that can present as progressive hoarseness or stridor over the first few months of life. Lymphangiomas, rhabdomyosarcomas, and leukemic infiltrations are other etiologies.

13. Congenital hypothyroidism is often not apparent until after the newborn period. If undetected by newborn screening, presenting signs include hoarseness, constipation, prolonged hyperbilirubinemia, hypotonia, and hypothermia. A lethargic, hoarse cry is not likely to be evident until after a few months of life. Hypothyroidism that develops later in childhood may also cause a hoarse voice.

14. Rarer causes of hoarseness include hypocalcemic tetany and thiamine deficiency, which can occur occasionally in breast-fed infants of thiamine-deficient mothers. Connective tissue disorders including JRA are rare causes of hoarseness in children. Metabolic disorders cause hoarseness because of the abnormal deposition of metabolites in the airways or vocal cords. Other causes include vincristine toxicity, laryngeal edema related to congestive heart failure, and dryness due to ectodermal dysplasia, cystic fibrosis, antihistamine therapy, and psychogenic causes.

Bibliography

Ahmad SM, Soliman AM: Congenital anomalies of the larynx, *Otolaryngol Clin North Am* 40:177–191, 2007.

Derkay CS, Wiatrak B: Recurrent respiratory papillomatosis: a review, *Laryngoscope* 118:1236–1247, 2008.

Friedberg J: Hoarseness. In Bluestone CD, Stool SE, Alper CM, et al, editors: *Pediatric otolaryngology*, ed 4, Philadelphia, 2003, WB Saunders, p 1413.

Hastriter EV, Olsson JM: In brief: hoarseness, *Pediatr Rev* 27:e47–48, 2006.

Schwartz SR, Dailey SH, Deutsch ES, et al: Clinical practice guideline: hoarseness (dysphonia), *Otolaryngol Head Neck Surg* 141:S1–S31, 2009.

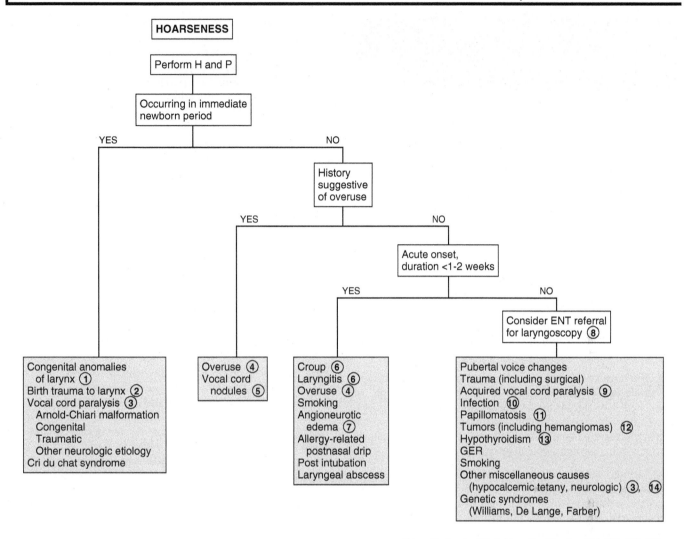

Nelson Textbook of Pediatrics, 19e. Chapters 311, 376, 377, 382
Nelson Essentials, 6e. Chapters 107, 135

Chapter 12
STRIDOR

Stridor is a predominantly inspiratory harsh, medium-pitched sound caused by obstruction in the upper (extrathoracic) airway. The most common cause is infectious croup.

1 Inquire about risk factors for respiratory problems, such as prematurity, intubation, chronic medical problems, and hospitalizations. The review of systems should include signs of infection and any obvious aggravating factors (e.g., position, agitation). Particularly important is a history of any recent choking episodes, which would raise the suspicion of a foreign body. Assess the child's level of illness, apparent anxiety, and respiratory distress (e.g., nasal flaring, grunting, accessory muscle use, retractions). A careful skin exam for cutaneous findings such as hemangiomas should be performed, particularly in infants in whom the stridor is gradually worsening over time.

2 The most common cause of congenital stridor is laryngomalacia. If present early in the newborn period or associated with significant dyspnea, ENT evaluation is necessary to rule out severe congenital laryngeal malformations that may require acute intervention. Milder cases of laryngomalacia do not require laryngoscopic diagnosis.

3 Laryngomalacia may be evident at birth but most commonly becomes notable at 2 to 4 weeks of age. Symptoms are characteristically worse when the infant is supine or agitated and typically resolve within the first year. Diagnosis is often clinical but may be confirmed by laryngoscopy. Laryngomalacia is often accompanied by tracheomalacia that may cause expiratory wheezing and cough as well as stridor.

4 Subglottic tracheal stenosis may be congenital or acquired. The latter may result from prolonged endotracheal intubation and manifest gradually in the first year of life. Symptoms are exaggerated in an acute respiratory illness. Recurrent croup may occur at young ages in these children.

5 The indication for x-rays will be determined by clinical judgment based on the degree of respiratory distress and the specific clinical presentation. A child with a clinical picture consistent with croup who is stable and responding well to therapy may be managed without imaging. For a child with severe respiratory distress and a clinical picture suggesting bacterial tracheitis or epiglottitis (e.g., high fever, anxiety, drooling, cyanosis, tripod position), imaging should be delayed and airway protection prioritized. If epiglottitis is suspected, arrangements should be made for immediate intubation in an operating room.

6 Infectious croup (laryngotracheobronchitis or laryngotracheitis) most commonly affects children age 3 months to 3 years. It classically presents with the abrupt onset of an acute barky cough following 1 to 2 days of nonspecific viral URI symptoms. The cough is described as seal-like or brassy; inspiratory stridor, hoarseness, and respiratory distress may be associated. Worsening of symptoms at night is typical. High fever may occur.

7 Epiglottitis is rare in developed countries because of widespread immunization against *Haemophilus influenzae*. Classic features include rapid progression from a sore throat and fever to severe respiratory distress, drooling, and dysphagia. Patients tend to assume a tripod position, with their neck hyperextended. Immediate intubation in an operating room is recommended because of the high risk of complete airway obstruction. Bacterial tracheitis should be suspected when an acute clinical worsening occurs (e.g., respiratory distress, toxicity, lack of improvement with therapy) following a few days of milder illness. (Drooling and the tripod position preference do not occur with bacterial tracheitis.)

8 Abscesses (e.g., peritonsillar, retropharyngeal) usually develop as a complication of a pharyngitis or URI. Retropharyngeal abscesses are more common in ages greater than 5 years and are more likely to present with neck pain, torticollis, hyperextension of the neck, and cervical adenopathy. Peritonsillar abscesses are more common in older children and adolescents and are more likely to present with trismus (pain and difficulty with opening the mouth), a muffled voice, and adenopathy; asymmetrical peritonsillar bulging may be evident on exam. Nonspecific signs and symptoms may include sore throat, fever, adenopathy, drooling, and refusal to move the neck.

9 Spasmodic croup is clinically similar to infectious croup but without evidence of airway inflammation. The clinical course is typically more abrupt and short-lived than cases that are obviously associated with URIs, plus the symptoms occur exclusively at night. Episodes can resolve and recur multiple times in 1 night and for up to 4 nights in a row, with the child appearing completely well in between coughing episodes. A lack of consensus exists regarding whether a spasmodic croup presentation is a distinct entity (with an allergic component) or on the same spectrum as infectious croup, because both have been associated with viral infections.

10 Stridor due to aspiration of a foreign body is generally an acute symptom of an object lodged in the larynx or trachea. Even if a choking or gagging episode was not observed, rigid bronchoscopy is increasingly becoming the diagnostic (and therapeutic) procedure of choice when the H and P are strongly suggestive (e.g., acute respiratory distress, cough, stridor, inability to speak). Posterior-anterior chest x-rays are frequently obtained, but only 10% to 25% of foreign bodies are radiopaque. Aspiration of objects small enough to reach the lower airways is more likely to present with cough and wheezing. (See Chapter 10.)

11 Airway lesions (e.g., hemangioma, cyst, tumor) may cause airway obstruction due to rapid enlargement (e.g., hemorrhage, infection). Congenital hemangiomas in a subglottic location are rare but potentially life-threatening. Symptoms usually develop between 1 and 2 months of age as gradual enlargement causes progressive airway obstruction. Cutaneous hemangiomas, particularly on the head and neck, should raise suspicion for this condition. Rarely, mediastinal lesions, thyroid enlargement, or esophageal foreign bodies may cause stridor by impinging on the larynx.

12 Vascular malformations, that compress the trachea or esophagus usually present in infancy with stridor, cough, or wheezing (or simply "noisy breathing" from a parent's perspective) from birth. Symptoms are usually worsened by crying and neck flexion; complete vascular rings may cause swallowing difficulties. Chest x-rays may suggest the diagnosis; barium esophagrams can be very useful. However, echocardiograms plus CT or MR angiography are increasingly preferred because of the enhanced anatomic detail provided.

13 Human papillomaviruses can cause recurrent respiratory tract papillomas. Papillomas develop primarily in the larynx; occasional spread to other sites in the aerodigestive tract occurs in severe cases. They can develop at any time from shortly after birth to several years of age, initially presenting as hoarseness (which may go unnoticed initially) and progressing to stridor.

14 Vocal cord paralysis in the newborn is most commonly due to birth trauma resulting in recurrent laryngeal nerve trauma. Other causes include neurologic syndromes (Arnold-Chiari malformation) and neck or chest surgery.

Bibliography

Bjornson C, Johnson DW: Croup, *Lancet* 337:329–339, 2008.
Sobol SE, Zapa1 S: Epiglottitis and croup, *Otolaryngol Clin North Am* 41: 551–566, 2008.

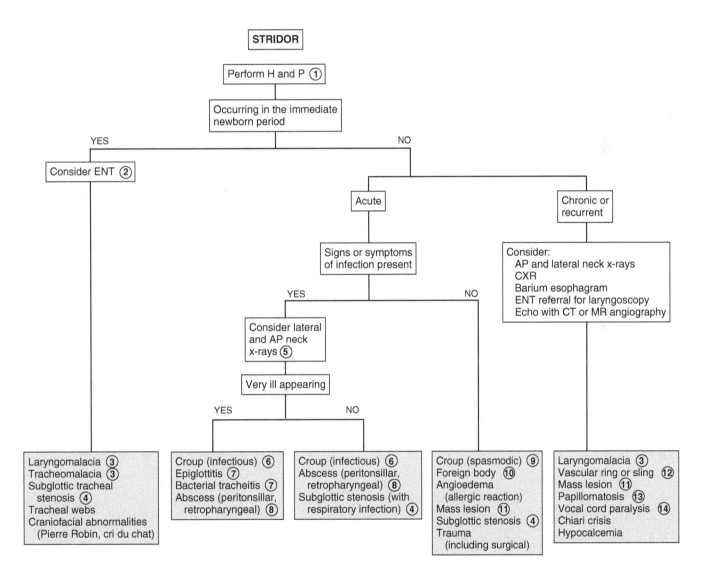

Nelson Textbook of Pediatrics, 19e. Chapters 258, 374, 376, 377, 378, 380
Nelsons Essentials, 6e. Chapters 107, 135, 136

Chapter 13
WHEEZING

Wheezing is a high-pitched musical sound caused by obstruction of the lower (intrathoracic) airways. The etiologies for wheezing are numerous. The clinical significance of the underlying problem can range from mild to severe.

1   Inquire about risk factors for respiratory problems, such as prematurity, intubation, chronic medical problems, and hospitalizations. The review of systems should include signs and symptoms such as fever, weight loss, night sweats, and dysphagia. Inquire specifically about any recent choking episodes and about medications (specifically inquire if the child was ever prescribed an inhaler in their past), as well as a family history of asthma and allergies. Signs of respiratory distress (e.g., nasal flaring, grunting, accessory muscle use, retractions) should be noted, as should chest wall asymmetry and chest excursion.

2   In patients with an uncomplicated illness consistent with bronchiolitis or a URI, a chest x-ray is not indicated. Depending on the level of illness, a chest x-ray could be considered to rule out a treatable pneumonia.

3   The most likely cause of recurrent wheezing in children is asthma. By definition, the diagnosis of asthma requires a history of recurrent or chronic symptoms of wheezing or airflow obstruction. An acute episode of wheezing can be the first manifestation of asthma, and a positive response to a trial of bronchodilator therapy confirms reversible airway obstruction. However, the diagnosis should not be made until the wheezing manifests itself as a recurrent disorder of airway obstruction supported by an appropriate history, physical examination, and diagnostic testing such as spirometry (if possible). A diagnosis of asthma is supported by: (1) a history of a prolonged cough with colds, (2) nocturnal cough (unassociated with illness), (3) symptoms of cough or shortness of breath, and (4) chest tightness induced by exercise, hard laughter, crying, or exposure to cold air, smoke, or other environmental irritants.

Chest x-rays will not aid in the diagnosis of asthma and should only be considered when the diagnosis is not clear or to rule out complications of an asthma attack (e.g., pneumothorax, atelectasis, pneumomediastinum).

4   Bronchiolitis is a common lower respiratory tract infection in infants. The classic presentation of acute bronchiolitis begins with nonspecific cold symptoms and progresses fairly rapidly to profuse rhinorrhea, harsh cough, wheezing, and tachypnea. Respiratory distress may occur, especially in younger infants. RSV is the most common cause. Parainfluenza, influenza, rhinovirus, human metapneumovirus, adenovirus, and human bocavirus are other etiologies.

5   *Mycoplasma pneumoniae* and *Chlamydophila pneumoniae* are exceptions to the "bacteria do not cause wheezing" generalization. These pathogens cause more clinically significant illness in school-aged children than in younger children. Cough that progresses over the first week of illness, fine crackles and wheezes, and nonspecific x-ray findings are characteristic.

6   Isolated episodes of wheezing or bronchospasm may occur with viral respiratory illnesses of milder clinical severity than bronchiolitis. Wheezing with certain viral infections early in life is predictive of the later development of asthma; less clear is whether these infections cause asthma or whether they are identifying children who have a predilection toward the later development of asthma. A positive response to a trial of bronchodilator therapy confirms reversible airway obstruction. Until the wheezing manifests itself as a recurrent disorder of airway obstruction, the term "asthma" should not be used. Most children who wheeze in infancy or early childhood will not wheeze later in childhood.

7   Diagnosis of foreign bodies can be difficult. Episodes of choking or gagging associated with aspiration are often unobserved. Posterior-anterior chest x-rays are frequently obtained, but only 10% to 25% of foreign bodies are radiopaque. Rigid bronchoscopy is increasingly becoming the diagnostic (and therapeutic) procedure of choice when the H and P examination are strongly suggestive. Localized lung findings or a history of recurrent or persistent pneumonia in a single lobe should arouse the clinician's suspicion for a retained foreign body. (See Chapter 10.) Foreign bodies in the esophagus can be mistaken as tracheal foreign bodies.

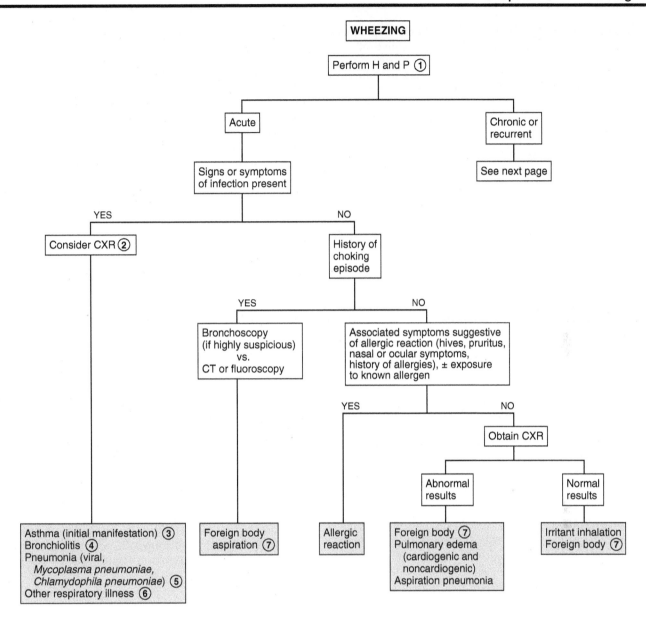

Nelson Textbook of Pediatrics, 19e. Chapters 138, 376, 378, 379, 381, 383, 396, 426
Nelson Essentials, 6e. Chapters 109, 136

8 Recurrent aspiration as a cause of chronic respiratory symptoms is most likely to occur in children with swallowing dysfunction, frequently associated with an underlying neurologic condition. Chronic aspiration may result in a diminished cough reflex, resulting in "silent aspiration." Although GER has been historically associated with chronic cough and wheezing, evidence supporting this association is inconclusive.

9 Primary tracheomalacia and bronchomalacia are characterized by wheezing that is located more centrally then peripherally, and is not responsive to bronchodilators. The wheezing is usually low pitched (not "musical"), expiratory, monophonic, and typically becomes evident after 2 to 3 months of life, although parents may describe the child as a "noisy breather" from birth. Cough may or may not be significant. The defect is insufficient cartilage to maintain airway patency throughout the breathing cycle. The problem can affect the trachea or bronchi in isolation, or it can affect the entire airway, including the larynx (laryngomalacia). (See Chapter 12.) Bronchomalacia can be bilateral or unilateral (usually on the left). Diagnosis is often clinically based, but it may be confirmed using bronchoscopy.

10 Primary ciliary dyskinesia (PCD) is a rare cause of wheezing. Abnormal structure of the cilia leads to impaired clearance of endobronchial secretions, resulting in chronic respiratory infections (upper and lower tract). PCD may present in the neonatal period with respiratory distress; the clinical manifestations in older children include chronic cough, recurrent wheezing and recurrent otitis, rhinosinusitis, and lower respiratory tract infections. Poor feeding and failure to thrive may also occur. Approximately 50% of patients with PCD have situs inversus totalis; when a patient with situs inverus totalis develops chronic sinusitis and bronchiectasis, they are described as having Kartagener triad (or syndrome).

11 Clinical diagnosis of cystic fibrosis occurs less frequently since newborn screening for cystic fibrosis has been implemented for all U.S. states. Although the screening is 95% sensitive, it is only a screen—additional evaluation is always appropriate when clinical suspicions are present.

12 Vocal cord dysfunction can mimic asthma by manifesting as periodic "wheezing" and dyspnea that is unresponsive to inhaled bronchodilators. During acute exacerbations, patients can experience dyspnea and stridor, but the pulmonary gas exchange rate is normal. The high-pitched respiratory sound created by vocal cord dysfunction is more correctly classified as stridor, although it is transmitted throughout the lung fields and is difficult to distinguish from peripheral wheezing (although it is primarily inspiratory). Pulmonary function tests during an episode demonstrate some degree of extrathoracic obstruction. Pulmonary function tests and supportive clinical history are adequate to make the diagnosis. Laryngoscopy (during an episode) may help to make the diagnosis in less clear cases. The disorder is most common in teenage girls, and underlying psychosocial stressors can often be identified.

13 Several environmental contaminants including inorganic dusts (e.g., talcum, asbestos, silica) and chemical fumes can cause interstitial lung disease and wheezing. Disease due to inhalation of organic dusts (particularly on farms or with exposure to birds) has been reported in children, although it is significantly more common in adults.

14 Chest x-ray findings may be suggestive in cases of vascular malformations that compress the airway. The barium esophagram (or UGI series) has been the traditional diagnostic test and is diagnostic in most cases, although it will not define the specific anatomy of a lesion. Barium studies are still frequently performed, although a CT or MR angiogram (where available) will provide more precise anatomic details. Echocardiograms may visualize some vascular rings but will miss atretic segments and do not reliably define anatomy; their value is to rule out any accompanying cardiac defects. Other congenital malformations that may present with recurrent wheezing or stridor in young infants include tracheoesophageal fistulas, laryngeal or tracheal webs, stenoses, clefts, cysts, or atresias; bronchoscopy would effectively diagnose all of these. Suspected diagnosis, availability, radiation risk, and need for sedation should all factor into the selection of a diagnostic test.

Bibliography

Weinberger M, Abu-Hasan M: Pseudo-asthma: when cough, wheezing, and dyspnea are not asthma, *Pediatrics* 120:855–864, 2007.

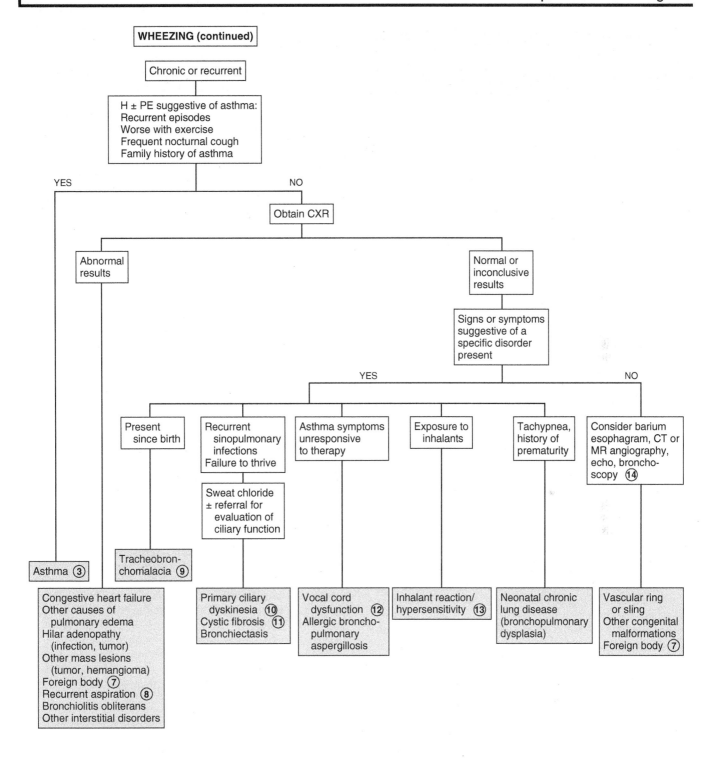

WHEEZING (continued)

Chronic or recurrent

H ± PE suggestive of asthma:
Recurrent episodes
Worse with exercise
Frequent nocturnal cough
Family history of asthma

YES

NO

Obtain CXR

Abnormal results

Normal or inconclusive results

Signs or symptoms suggestive of a specific disorder present

YES

NO

Present since birth

Recurrent sinopulmonary infections
Failure to thrive

Asthma symptoms unresponsive to therapy

Exposure to inhalants

Tachypnea, history of prematurity

Consider barium esophagram, CT or MR angiography, echo, broncho- scopy ⑭

Sweat chloride ± referral for evaluation of ciliary function

Asthma ③

Tracheobron- chomalacia ⑨

Congestive heart failure
Other causes of pulmonary edema
Hilar adenopathy (infection, tumor)
Other mass lesions (tumor, hemangioma)
Foreign body ⑦
Recurrent aspiration ⑧
Bronchiolitis obliterans
Other interstitial disorders

Primary ciliary dyskinesia ⑩
Cystic fibrosis ⑪
Bronchiectasis

Vocal cord dysfunction ⑫
Allergic broncho- pulmonary aspergillosis

Inhalant reaction/ hypersensitivity ⑬

Neonatal chronic lung disease (bronchopulmonary dysplasia)

Vascular ring or sling
Other congenital malformations
Foreign body ⑦

Chapter 14
CYANOSIS

Cyanosis refers to a bluish discoloration of the skin or mucous membranes. Central cyanosis affects the skin, mucous membranes, lips, and conjunctiva. It occurs secondary to significant arterial oxygen desaturation. A minimum of 5 g/dL of desaturated hemoglobin must be present in order for cyanosis to be clinically evident. Cyanosis can be due to pulmonary, cardiac, CNS (hypoventilation), neuromuscular (hypoventilation), or hematologic etiologies, or be a result of decreased oxygen in the environment (e.g., airtight space, suffocation). Peripheral cyanosis may be due to more benign etiologies; however, careful assessment is necessary to rule out central cyanosis. (The differential diagnosis of cyanosis in the neonate is not included in this algorithm.)

1 Pertinent elements of the history of the cyanotic patient vary according to age. For infants, the birth history and age of onset of cyanosis are important. For older children, a history of trauma, possible ingestion, or choking may be helpful. Any physical stigmata that may be suggestive of a genetic syndrome (e.g., trisomies, Turner syndrome, VATER) should be noted. Older children should be assessed for signs of chronic or progressive illness, including growth parameters, clubbing, vascular skin markings, and stigmata of neuromuscular disease (e.g., hypotonia, weakness, bell-shaped chest). Also inquire about potential exposure to any medications, drugs, or potential toxins (including food poisoning). Obtaining an oxygen saturation value early in the assessment of a cyanotic patient is recommended. ABGs may help to distinguish pulmonary from cardiac etiologies; pulmonary problems are likely to cause hypercapnea.

2 Acrocyanosis is a benign bluish discoloration of the hands and feet that occurs when peripheral O_2 extraction is increased because of sluggish blood flow in the peripheral vascular system. It is most common in young infants who have vasomotor instability. Systemic arterial saturation is normal; pulse oximetry is normal.

3 For young infants, maternal problems (e.g., diabetes mellitus, systemic lupus erythematosus, substance abuse, teratogenic medication use), and feeding difficulties (especially easy tiring with feeds) may suggest an increased risk of congenital heart disease (CHD). For older children, a history of poor growth, exercise intolerance, and findings of hypertension, hepatosplenomegaly, peripheral edema, or asynchronous upper and lower extremity pulses are suggestive of a cardiac problem.

4 Cyanotic CHD is almost always diagnosed early in the newborn period, although many lesions may not present until after hospital discharge. Preductal and postductal pulse oximetry performed after 24 hours of age has emerged as a very specific and acceptably sensitive (approximately 76%) method for detecting severe congenital heart disease in newborns. It is recommended to be performed routinely with other newborn screening tests, although implementation may vary by state.

5 Some cardiac diseases, most commonly tetralogy of Fallot, can present with cyanosis weeks to months after birth. If CHD is suspected, the hyperoxia test (obtaining preductal and postductal pulse oximetry or ABG values before and after the administration of 100% FIO_2) can help distinguish cardiac causes of cyanosis from pulmonary causes. Clinical status and oxygen saturation or arterial PO_2 (PaO_2) improve in respiratory disease; minimal changes occur with cyanotic heart lesions. A pediatric cardiologist should be consulted whenever the diagnosis of CHD is suspected. An echocardiogram will quickly help to establish most diagnoses.

6 Pulmonary hypertension may cause peripheral cyanosis if the patient has a patent foramen ovale allowing right-to-left shunting. Right-sided heart failure (cor pulmonale) occurring in advanced stages of the disease leads to cyanosis due to low cardiac output. Pulmonary hypertension has a number of causes (e.g., pulmonary, cardiac, idiopathic). Physical examination reveals a loud single or narrowly split S2.

7 Dyspnea, cough, chest pain, wheezing, snoring, hemoptysis, and abnormal physical findings on chest examination suggest a pulmonary etiology of cyanosis.

8 Methemoglobin is Hgb containing iron in an oxidized (or ferric [Fe^{+3}]) state compared to the normal reduced (or ferrous [Fe^{+2}]) state; it is normally present at a level of less than 1%. Its presence impairs oxygen delivery to tissue. Methemoglobinemia can be due to the presence of abnormal Hgb (the most common inherited variant is Hgb M) or a deficiency of enzymes involved in the normal reduction of heme; severe cases can be fatal. Certain drugs or toxins (oxidizing agents in drugs or anesthesia, nitrates in well water, and even nitrite-forming microorganisms causing diarrhea in infants) can also be responsible for the disorder, especially in young infants who have low levels of methemoglobin reductase activity and increased susceptibility to oxidation of Hgb F. Mild forms of congenital methemoglobinemia may appear later in infancy or childhood owing to exposure to precipitating agents. In methemoglobinemia, cyanosis will not improve with administration of 100% inhaled oxygen, and the (deoxygenated) blood has a brown or purple color (in contrast to the bright red color of oxygenated blood). ABG pO_2 values will be normal (because that is a measurement of O_2 dissolved in plasma). Pulse oximetry values will be low but rarely below 85%; O_2 saturation values tend to be overestimated, although newer devices may overcome this limitation. ABGs reporting *calculated* O_2 saturation values also yield misleadingly high values; *measured* O_2 saturations are more accurate. A methemoglobin level must be obtained to confirm the diagnosis.

9 Cyanosis commonly accompanies apnea in children of any age. Causes include infection (e.g., RSV, pertussis, sepsis, meningitis), seizures, ALTE, and neuromuscular disorders causing hypoventilation.

10 Breath-holding spells may cause cyanosis or pallor. Cyanotic or "blue" breath-holding spells are described as prolonged expiratory apnea or a sudden lack of inspiratory effort, often during crying. They are usually triggered by injury, anger, or frustration. Apnea, brief loss of consciousness, tonic posturing, and occasionally anoxic seizures can also occur. Breath-holding spells typically occur between ages 6 and 18 months, although they may be seen in children up to age 5 or 6 years. Children recover quickly from these events, and no diagnostic evaluation is indicated, although affected children should be assessed for iron deficiency and treated if it is present.

⑪ Cyanosis can occur with ingestion of agents that cause respiratory depression (e.g., narcotics, sedatives) or airway edema and obstruction (e.g., acid or alkali products).

Bibliography

Mahle WT, Martin GR, Beekman RH 3rd, et al: Endorsement of Health and Human Services recommendation for pulse oximetry screening for critical congenital heart disease, *Pediatrics* 129:190–192, 2012.

Sasidharan P: An approach to diagnosis and management of cyanosis and tachypnea in term infants, *Pediatr Clin North Am* 51:999, 2004.

Stack AM: Cyanosis. In Fleisher G, Ludwig S, editors: *Textbook of pediatric emergency medicine*, ed 6, Philadelphia, 2010, Lippincott Williams & Wilkins, pp 198–202.

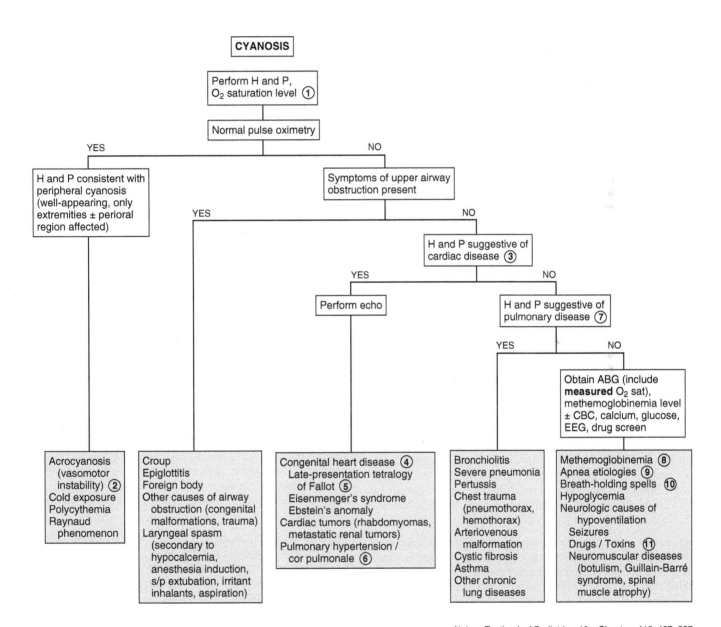

Nelson Textbook of Pediatrics, 19e. Chapters 416, 427, 587
Nelsons Essentials, 6e. Chapters 58, 139

Chapter 15
HEMOPTYSIS

Hemoptysis, the expectoration of blood from the lower respiratory tract, is typically foamy bright red, mixed with sputum, and has an alkaline pH. Respiratory infections, foreign body aspiration, and bronchiectasis are among the most common causes. It may be associated with coughing and in some cases chest pain or a sensation of gurgling or warmth. Pulmonary hemorrhage, particularly of a slow nature, may occur without hemoptysis. Hemoptysis must be distinguished from blood from the nasopharynx and the GI tract (hematemesis), which is often dark red or brown with an acidic pH. Hematemesis is also more likely to be associated with nausea or abdominal pain than with coughing. Bleeding from epistaxis may result in blood that is swallowed and coughed out.

1. The history should contain inquiries about associated respiratory symptoms, epistaxis, foreign body aspiration, recent procedures (e.g., tonsillectomy, laryngoscopy), and the possibility of a bleeding disorder. Children with certain underlying conditions are predisposed to pulmonary hemorrhage that, in some cases, can be severe. Children with cystic fibrosis have the greatest risk of hemoptysis. Other at-risk disorders include cardiac disease, hemoglobinopathies, connective tissue disorders, coagulation abnormalities, and immunodeficiency states. A chest x-ray (at minimum) and specialty consultation should be urgently obtained when children with these conditions present with hemoptysis.

2. Lung contusions may occur without evidence of external trauma. The chest x-ray may reveal a poorly defined density. Initial films, however, may appear normal.

3. If the child has spit up a minimal amount of blood, and if the clinical picture is consistent with a nonthreatening, self-limiting upper respiratory illness, it may not be necessary to obtain a chest x-ray or perform any further evaluation. Severe coughing may cause a small amount of hemoptysis in even mild cases of viral respiratory infections (tracheobronchitis) because the mucosa is inflamed and friable.

4. Infection is a common cause of hemoptysis. Children who have traveled internationally may be at risk for unusual parasitic infections. Uncomplicated pneumonias are unlikely to cause hemoptysis, but severe pneumonias, particularly in immunodeficient children, may result in hemoptysis due to erosion of bronchial wall vessels. Severe viral pneumonias (e.g., advenovirus, measles) and tuberculosis are other risk factors for hemoptysis.

5. Bleeding from a foreign body may appear weeks to months after aspiration. Often there is no recall of a choking episode. Organic foreign bodies are problematic because they cause an inflammatory reaction that can result in significant bleeding. They are radiolucent and typically yield only subtle x-ray findings, such as air trapping or atelectasis. In some cases, bronchoscopy may not be diagnostic if the object has worked its way into smaller airways. CT may reveal the diagnosis, or diagnosis may be delayed until the infected area is removed surgically. Sharp foreign bodies may cause acute hemoptysis because of airway laceration.

6. Cystic fibrosis is the most common chronic condition in children who experience hemoptysis. Bronchiectasis (dilation and weakening of the airway wall) occurs secondary to chronic inflammation and infection. Acute or chronic hemoptysis, which is usually mild, occurs due to leakage of these bronchial wall vessels. Anastomoses between pulmonary and bronchial arteries can occasionally result in significant bleeding. Coagulopathy due to vitamin K malabsorption may also be present.

7. The most common vascular anomalies leading to hemoptysis are arteriovenous malformations (AVM). Many children with pulmonary AVM have hereditary hemorrhagic telangiectasia (Osler-Weber-Rendu syndrome), an autosomal dominant condition; 80% of these will experience only epistaxis (not hemoptysis). Presentation is rare in childhood; a history of recurrent epistaxis, a positive family history, and development of mucocutaneous telangiectasias at puberty support this diagnosis. Large fistulas may be evident on chest x-ray; CT is the gold standard for diagnosis. Airway hemangiomas, unilateral pulmonary artery agenesis, and bronchial artery aneurysms are less common vascular anomalies.

8. Autoimmune disorders, which characteristically involve the lungs and the kidneys, are sometimes described as the "pulmonary-renal syndromes." Goodpasture syndrome (or anti–glomerular basement membrane antibody disease) occurs mostly in young adult males (rarely in children). Patients present abruptly with pulmonary hemorrhage and nephritis, both of which can be rapidly progressive and severe. Pathologically it is characterized by immunoglobulin deposition on alveolar and glomerular basement membranes, although diagnosis can be made by the finding of anti–glomerular basement membrane antibodies in the peripheral blood stream.

9. The term Wegener granulomatosis has been replaced by granulomatosis with polyangiitis. Bleeding from cavitation of pulmonary granulomas results in hemoptysis; specific diagnosis is based on the presence or absence of specific antinuclear cytoplasmic antibodies. Microscopic polyangiitis and Churg-Strauss syndrome are other ANCA (antineutrophil cytoplasmic antibodies) associated vasculitides that can result in pulmonary hemorrhage.

10. The term pulmonary hemosiderosis describes the accumulation of hemosiderin in the lungs that occurs when alveolar macrophages convert hemoglobin to hemosiderin when alveolar hemorrhage occurs. Previous classification systems for causes of pulmonary hemorrhage utilized primary and secondary causes of pulmonary hemosiderosis; newer systems divide the causes of diffuse alveolar hemorrhage based on the presence or absence of pulmonary capillaritis. There are a number of causes of diffuse alveolar hemorrhage (e.g., pulmonary-renal syndromes, cardiac disease). The clinical manifestations can be variable; patients may be asymptomatic, or they may exhibit cough, wheezing, or dyspnea. They may or may not develop hemoptysis, or they may present with shock and respiratory failure from massive hemoptysis. Iron deficiency anemia and poor growth are also common. Large numbers of hemosiderin-laden macrophages in gastric fluid, sputum, bronchial washings, or lung biopsy specimens are diagnostic indicators.

11 Other immune disorders include systemic lupus erythematous, Henoch-Schönlein purpura, and polyarteritis nodosa. Immunocompromised children (especially following a transplant of solid organs or bone marrow) are also at risk for pulmonary hemorrhage.

12 Secondary pulmonary hypertension due to congenital or acquired heart lesions can lead to hemoptysis due to dilation and angiomatoid changes of small pulmonary arteries. These changes develop slowly and present with hemoptysis in adolescence or young adulthood.

13 Heiner syndrome describes a condition of pulmonary hemosiderosis presumed to be due to cow's milk hypersensitivity. The condition has historically been reported to include pulmonary infiltrates, GI bleeding, anemia, and failure to thrive; it is characterized by high serum titers of precipitating antibodies to cow's milk proteins. There is, however, some controversy regarding the diagnosis because the role of the milk precipitins is unclear.

14 When no additional organ systems are involved and investigation excludes other causes of pulmonary hemorrhage,

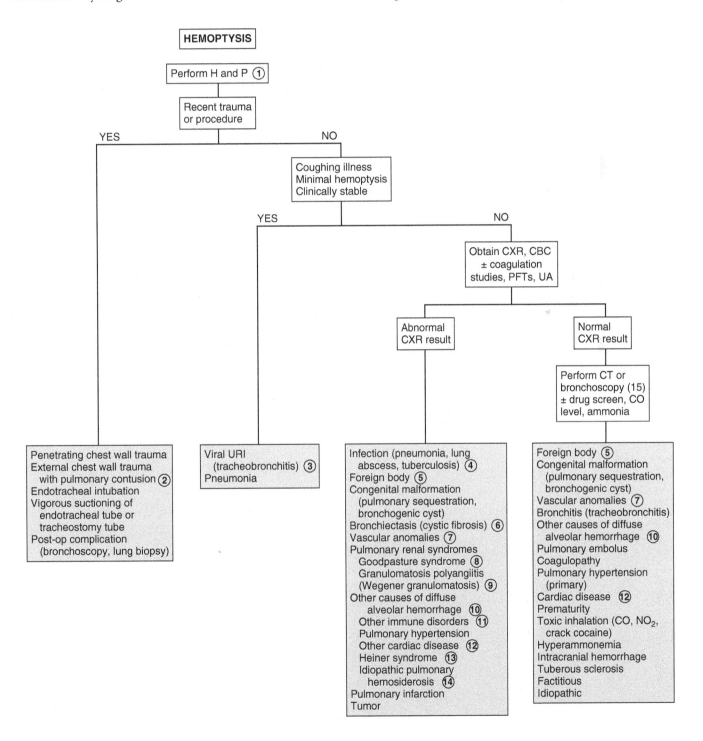

Nelson Textbook of Pediatrics, 19e. Chapters 161, 400, 401, 511, 642
Nelsons Essentials, 6e. Chapter 136

the condition is called idiopathic pulmonary hemosiderosis. There are rare reports of infants experiencing acute idiopathic pulmonary hemorrhage with no identifiable underlying disorder.

15 Rigid or flexible bronchoscopy may be indicated when bleeding is active to provide suction during the procedure. Bronchoscopy would also be the procedure of choice if aspiration of a foreign body is suspected because it provides the capability for extraction. Bronchoalveolar washings should be obtained if pulmonary hemosiderosis is a consideration. Chest CT with contrast or angiography is helpful in the diagnosis of AVM or other congenital lesions. Consider labs based on clinical suspicions.

Bibliography

Godfrey S: Pulmonary hemorrhage/hemoptysis in children, *Pediatr Pulmonol* 37:476–484, 2004.

Liechty KW, Flake AW: Pulmonary vascular malformations, *Seminars in Pediatric Surgery* 17: 9–16, 2008.

Susarla SC, Fan LL: Diffuse alveolar hemorrhage syndromes in children, *Curr Opin Pediatr*, 19(3):314–320, 2007.

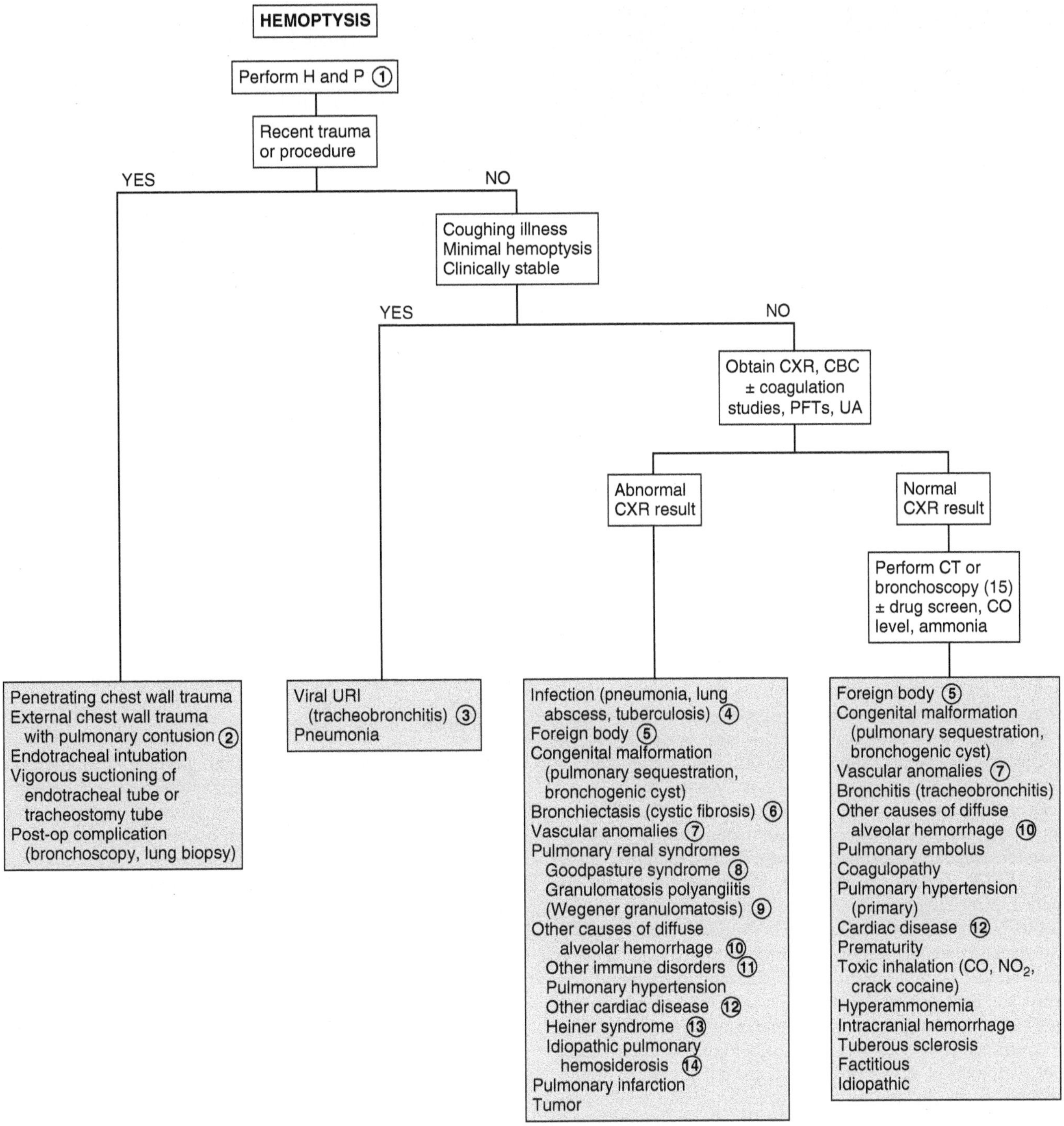

HEMOPTYSIS

Perform H and P ①

Recent trauma or procedure

YES

NO

Coughing illness
Minimal hemoptysis
Clinically stable

YES

NO

Obtain CXR, CBC
± coagulation
studies, PFTs, UA

Abnormal
CXR result

Normal
CXR result

Perform CT or
bronchoscopy (15)
± drug screen, CO
level, ammonia

Penetrating chest wall trauma
External chest wall trauma
  with pulmonary contusion ②
Endotracheal intubation
Vigorous suctioning of
  endotracheal tube or
  tracheostomy tube
Post-op complication
  (bronchoscopy, lung biopsy)

Viral URI
  (tracheobronchitis) ③
Pneumonia

Infection (pneumonia, lung
  abscess, tuberculosis) ④
Foreign body ⑤
Congenital malformation
  (pulmonary sequestration,
  bronchogenic cyst)
Bronchiectasis (cystic fibrosis) ⑥
Vascular anomalies ⑦
Pulmonary renal syndromes
  Goodpasture syndrome ⑧
  Granulomatosis polyangiitis
  (Wegener granulomatosis) ⑨
Other causes of diffuse
  alveolar hemorrhage ⑩
  Other immune disorders ⑪
  Pulmonary hypertension
  Other cardiac disease ⑫
  Heiner syndrome ⑬
  Idiopathic pulmonary
    hemosiderosis ⑭
Pulmonary infarction
Tumor

Foreign body ⑤
Congenital malformation
  (pulmonary sequestration,
  bronchogenic cyst)
Vascular anomalies ⑦
Bronchitis (tracheobronchitis)
Other causes of diffuse
  alveolar hemorrhage ⑩
Pulmonary embolus
Coagulopathy
Pulmonary hypertension
  (primary)
Cardiac disease ⑫
Prematurity
Toxic inhalation (CO, NO_2,
  crack cocaine)
Hyperammonemia
Intracranial hemorrhage
Tuberous sclerosis
Factitious
Idiopathic

Nelson Textbook of Pediatrics, 19e. Chapters 161, 400, 401, 511, 642
Nelsons Essentials, 6e. Chapter 136

Chapter 16
APNEA

Apnea is the cessation of breathing for a period of time (age dependent) or for any period if accompanied by pallor, cyanosis, bradycardia, and/or hypotonia. Apnea may be due to a central origin, an element of airway obstruction or a combination of both elements. (The differential diagnosis of apnea in neonates is extensive and includes many conditions unique to the neonate. Neither neonatal apnea nor apnea of prematurity is discussed here.)

When parents report that their child stopped breathing, benign conditions such as periodic breathing or breath-holding spells must be differentiated from more worrisome etiologies. Apnea can be a manifestation of a variety of serious conditions, and in children it is frequently part of a constellation of symptoms (including choking, gagging, or change in color or tone) described as an apparent life-threatening event (ALTE).

1 Because of the broad differential diagnosis of apneic events, there is no concensus regarding a standardized recommended evaluation. A careful history and physical remain the critical diagnostic elements; multiple experts agree that subsequent testing should be guided by the history and physical because at least 50% of ALTE cases will have an identifiable etiology. The history for an apneic event should include any associated illness, the relationship of the event to sleeping and eating, and the presence or absence of associated symptoms, such as cyanosis, bradycardia, altered level of consciousness, and posturing or abnormal tonic-clonic movements. A birth and developmental history, a history of previous similar events, and a family history inquiring about apnea, ALTE, genetic disorders or infant deaths should be obtained. A social history should ask about potentially toxic exposures, including drugs or medications in the home, tobacco smoke exposure, and potential carbon monoxide exposure. Careful questioning should be done regarding whether any intervention was needed and how quickly the child recovered from the event. For infants who were sleeping, inquire about sleep position, bedding, and coverings. The review of systems should include information about symptoms of airway obstruction, including chronic mouth breathing, noisy daytime respirations, snoring, and restlessness during sleep. The physical examination should be complete with careful attention to vital signs, head circumference (in infants), signs of airway obstruction, skin findings for bruising or signs of trauma, and facial dysmorphism. A careful ENT examination for fresh blood in the nose or mouth is important (it may suggest abuse). Dysmorphic features may be associated with craniofacial syndromes predisposing to airway obstruction (e.g., Pierre-Robin syndrome) or genetic or metabolic disorders. Airway hemangiomas are often associated with hemangiomas on the face, neck, or upper trunk.

2 Urine toxicology screens are simple to perform and may reveal a causative etiology for apnea. Barbiturates, salicylates, ipecac, boric acid, and cocaine are examples. Carbon monoxide poisoning can also be an etiology. Neuroimaging should be considered because child abuse is always part of the differential diagnosis of apnea in children. Hypoglycemia is likely to be the primary cause of apnea only in neonates, but it may accompany serious disorders leading to apnea in older children.

3 The possibility of child abuse should always be considered when evaluating an apneic event. Inflicted neurotrauma, deliberate suffocation, and poisoning attempts may be etiologies; a history of sudden infant death syndrome (SIDS) or recurrent ALTEs (especially at a late age) in a family or a history of recurrent events while in the care of a single caregiver could be suspicious for caregiver-fabricated illness (previously called Munchausen syndrome by proxy).

4 Congenital metabolic disorders (e.g., fatty acid oxidation disorders, urea cycle defects) are being increasingly recognized. A history of symptom onset occurring in association with fasting, altered mental status, recurrent episodes, a family history of infant deaths, and an occurrence beyond one year of age should raise suspicion for metabolic disorders. Serum glucose, ammonia, and pH should be obtained if suspicious of a metabolic disorder; if possible, samples of blood and urine should be obtained during the period of acute symptoms and frozen for future testing, if indicated.

5 Respiratory infections frequently associated with apnea include RSV (respiratory syncytial virus), bronchiolitis, and pertussis. Both central and obstructive apnea can occur with RSV bronchiolitis. In young infants, apnea can be the first sign of RSV infection; there may be minimal pulmonary findings. Localized upper airway infections (e.g., tonsillitis, peritonsillar or retropharyngeal abscesses, croup, epiglottitis) can result in obstructive apnea.

6 The term apparent life-threatening event (ALTE) describes an acute event that appears frightening to the caregiver and includes some combination of apnea, bradycardia, color change (usually cyanosis or pallor, occasionally plethora), and choking or gagging. The term replaces the previously used "near-miss SIDS"; scientific studies about the two conditions are difficult to compare because of the heterogeneity between them, but no clear association between SIDS and ALTEs has been demonstrated. ALTEs can be associated with a sleeping or awake state, may or may not be associated with feeding, and they are commonly reported to resolve quickly with intervention. Children frequently appear completely normal when they present for evaluation, which is why the evaluation decisions are so challenging.

7 Infants may appear to be choking or struggling to breathe during an event, suggesting an element of airway obstruction (obstructive apnea); they may exhibit absence of any respiratory effort (central apnea), or a mixture of both may occur.

8 Gastroesophageal reflux (GER) has been implicated in ALTEs, although its causal role is controversial since GER is so common in infancy, plus no clear temporal association between reflux events and apneic events has been demonstrated. Other etiologies should always be carefully considered, even when GER appears to be temporally associated with an event. Esophageal pH monitoring is a more sensitive diagnostic test for GER than an upper gastrointestinal series (UGI) but is still only useful in determining causality if an event is captured during the study.

9 Airway problems that may lead to apneic events include nasal obstruction (e.g., severe allergies, polyps, choanal stenosis [especially if exacerbated by upper respiratory infection or congestion]), laryngeal and subglottic abnormalities (e.g., cysts, webs, hemangiomas, laryngomalacia, vocal cord paralysis), and craniofacial syndromes (e.g., Pierre-Robin syndrome).

⑩ Obstructive sleep apnea (OSA) is a sleep-related airway obstruction. Children may demonstrate frequent, loud snoring that disrupts their sleep, long breathing pauses, and choking or gasping arousals. Both obese and normal weight children can be affected. Severe exacerbations of symptoms may rarely occur in the face of concurrent respiratory infections. Polysomnography is the best test to evaluate the severity of this problem.

⑪ No concensus exists for a standard evaluation of an ALTE; the importance of individualizing any testing based on a detailed history is emphasized. If a first-time episode was mild, brief, self-resolving, and a likely etiology is recognized (e.g., choking, GER, nasal congestion), no work up may be indicated. If the history suggests a particular diagnosis, initial evaluation should be focused on that. Blood counts, chemistries (e.g., electrolytes, BUN, calcium, phosphorus), CSF analysis and cultures, metabolic screening, screening for RSV and pertussis, screening for gastroesophageal reflux, chest x-ray, neuroimaging, skeletal survey, EEG, echocardiogram, and pneumogram have been useful studies in the face of a suggestive history or physical. When the history and physical are noncontributory,

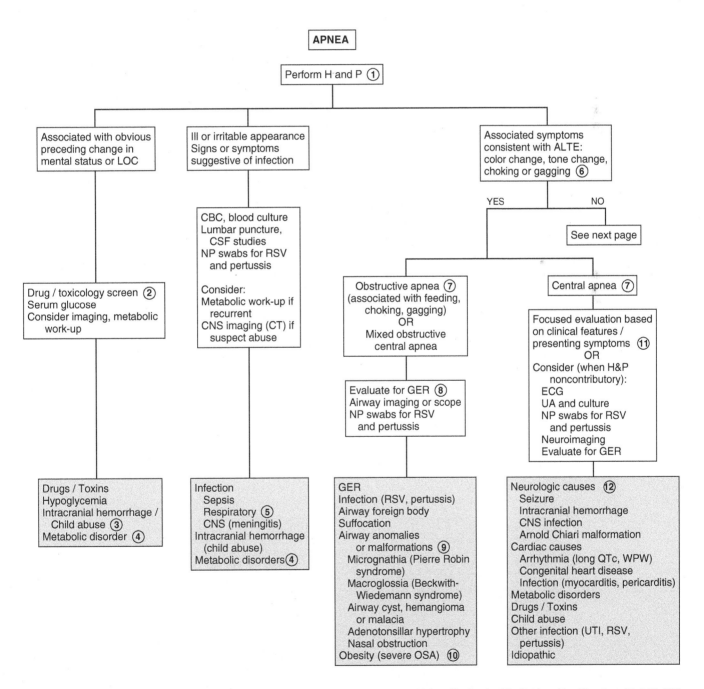

Nelson Textbook of Pediatrics, 19e. Chapters 17, 315, 587
Nelsons Essentials, 6e. Chapters 51, 109, 134

the studies listed on the algorithm could be considered. The severity of the event and subsequent clinical findings may indicate additional testing; careful judgment should be applied because up to half of ALTEs will be labeled as idiopathic with no identified etiology.

12 Neurologic causes are more likely in the absence of choking and in the presence of an alteration of tone. Children with neurologic problems (e.g., birth asphyxia, Arnold-Chiari malformation, neuromuscular disease) often experience pharyngeal hypotonia, which contributes to airway obstruction.

13 Laryngospasm can occur as a protective reflex during episodes of GER; these episodes are frequently limited, self-resolving, and associated with feeding. More significant episodes may be a component of an allergic reaction (e.g., insect bites, medication, other allergies).

14 The term "breath-holding spells" is somewhat of a misnomer because the episodes are not due to intentional breath holding. Cyanotic or "blue" breath-holding spells are described as prolonged expiratory apnea or a sudden lack of inspiratory effort, often during crying. In pallid breath-holding spells, a reflex vagal-bradycardia is responsible for the event. Both are usually triggered by injury, anger, or frustration. Apnea, brief loss of consciousness, tonic posturing, and occasionally anoxic seizures can follow. Breath-holding spells typically occur between ages 6 and 18 months, although they may be seen in children up to 6 years of age. Children recover quickly from these events and no diagnostic evaluation is indicated, although affected children should be assessed for iron deficiency and treated if it is present.

15 Periodic breathing is a nonpathologic breathing pattern that interrupts an infant's regular rhythmic breathing pattern. Brief, 5-10 second pause in breathing are followed by a period of rapid respirations for several seconds; no respiratory distress is associated. It is most common in premature infants but is also seen in full term infants until several months of age.

16 Congenital central hypoventilation syndrome (CCHS) is a rare but serious disorder of decreased central respiratory drive. It usually presents with apnea at birth, although late onset (LO-CCHS) milder cases may present with unexplained hypoventilation, particularly with anesthesia or sedation medication; these patients will likely manifest signs of chronic hypoventilation (e.g., pulmonary hypertension, polycythemia).

Bibliography

Brand DA, Altman RL, Purtill K, Edwards KS: Yield of diagnostic testing in infants who have had an apparent life-threatening event, *Pediatrics* 115:885–893, 2005.

Genizi J, Pillar G, Ravid S, Shahar E: Apparent life-threatening events: neurological correlates and the mandatory work-up, *J Child Neurol* 23:1305–1307, 2008.

Hoki R, Bonkowsky JL, Minich LL, et al: Cardiac testing and outcomes in infants after an apparent life-threatening event, *Arch Dis Child* 97:1034–1038, 2012.

Kahn A: Recommended clinical evaluation of infants with an apparent life-threatening event. Consensus document of the European Society for the Study and Prevention of Infant Death, *Eur J of Pediatr* 163:108–115, 2003.

Kahn A, Rebuffat E, Franco P, et al: Apparent life-threatening events and apnea of infancy. In Berckerman RC, Brouillette RT, Hunt CE, editors: *Respiratory control disorders in infants and children*, New York, 1992, Williams and Wilkins, pp 178.

McGovern MC, Smith MB: Causes of apparent life-threatening events in infants: a systematic review, *Arch Dis Child* 89:1043–1048, 2004.

Mousa H, Woodley FW, Metheney M, et al: Testing the association between gastroesophageal reflux and apnea in infants, *J Pediatr Gastroenterol Nutr* 41:169–177, 2005.

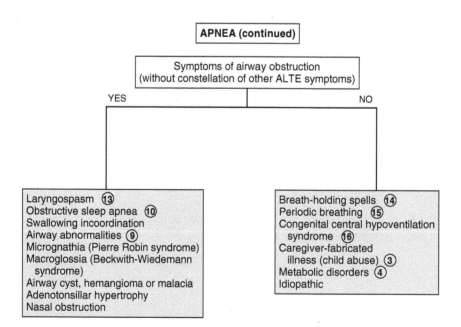

Cardiology

Chapter 17
CHEST PAIN

Chest pain is common in children and adolescents. Despite the degree of concern that it generates, the symptom is rarely associated with a serious cardiac problem. The epidemiology of chest pain in youth is not well understood, although available data suggest more cases are classified as idiopathic than are attributed to a more specific etiology (e.g., cardiac, respiratory). Studies approximate between 1% and 10% of pediatric chest pain cases are due to cardiac etiologies.

1. A properly done history and physical are often the only tools required in the evaluation of pediatric chest pain. Screening tests are not considered helpful unless specifically indicated. Eliciting the patient's or family's concerns about their complaint may be useful.

A medical history of asthma, sickle cell disease, collagen vascular disease, or a recent coughing illness may be helpful. Long-standing diabetes mellitus and chronic anemias are risk factors for ischemic chest pain. Inquire about a history of Kawasaki disease, including the possibility of an undiagnosed case. The review of systems should include inquiries about associated acute and chronic symptoms and any precipitating factors. Inquire about choking episodes, recent trauma, and exercise or activities that could cause pain from muscle strain or overuse. It is critical to distinguish a history of exercise (that could cause muscular chest wall pain) from exercise as a precipitating factor (which may be consistent with ischemic pain and mandates an urgent cardiac evaluation). Associated syncope is very worrisome and also mandates a cardiac evaluation. A medication history could provide clues to a potentially causative etiology (oral contraceptives) or the possibility of mucosal injury (e.g., tetracycline, NSAIDs); also investigate the possibility of substance abuse, especially cocaine and methamphetamine. Evaluation of psychosocial factors in the child's life is very important. Ask about school attendance and performance, relationships with friends and family, and any current stresses or conflicts.

The family history should inquire about hypercholesterolemia, Marfan syndrome, and cardiomyopathy. A family history of recurrent syncope or unexplained sudden death may suggest hypertrophic cardiomyopathy or long QT syndrome. Heart disease in an adult family member may provoke anxiety-related chest pain in a younger person.

A complete thorough physical exam is necessary; focusing on the chest exam may miss findings pertinent to a noncardiac underlying cause of chest pain.

2. Costochondritis is pain due to inflammation of the costochondral joints (where the bony rib meets the costal cartilage). It is a common cause of chest pain in children and is usually unilateral, sharp, transient in nature, and can be reproduced by palpation on examination. Tietze syndrome, a rare form of costochondritis, affects a single chostochondral, costosternal or sternoclavicular joint and causes notable swelling, tenderness, and warmth localized to the affected joint.

3. Other skeletal causes of chest pain include traumatic injury, spondyloarthritis, and stress fractures. The latter should be considered in athletes with repetitive upper extremity motions, especially in the absence of a recognized acute traumatic event; a bone scan should be considered if suspicion is high and x-rays are negative. Chest wall deformities (pectus carinatum, pectus excavatum) are rare causes of pediatric chest pain.

4. Muscular chest wall pain is common in weight-lifters, but carrying heavy back packs, severe coughing, and sports involving rotation or twisting can also be causative. Sharp pain in the intercostal muscles can occur with infection due to coxsackie and other enteroviruses. This pain (historically called pleurodynia or Bornholm disease) is sudden in onset, paroxysmal, and accompanied by fever and other systemic signs of enteroviral infection (e.g., vomiting, headache, sore throat). Sometimes the illness exhibits a biphasic pattern with a recurrence of the chest pain and fever several days after the initial presentation.

5. Early puberty may cause chest pain related to breast nodule development in males and females. Other breast disorders including infections, cystic disorders, pregnancy, and menstrual swelling may cause chest pain in females.

6. Pain related to shingles (herpes zoster) may precede the appearance of the rash. Children affected by hypersensitivity pain syndromes may complain of pain with light touch to their chest wall, or even with wearing certain clothing; other somatic complaints are typically present as well.

7. Chest pain is occasionally the initial presentation of asthma. A history of nocturnal cough, atopy or a remote history of bronchospasm may support the diagnosis. Bronchoconstriction is often reported by children as chest pain. Prolonged cough (due to acute exacerbations or poor control of asthma) can lead to soreness of chest wall muscles. Asthma also sometimes presents with a complaint of chest pain with running or exertion (with or without coughing). Chest x-ray findings are often normal, but may reveal hyperinflation, atelectasis, or peribronchial thickening.

8. It is difficult to clearly define the role of psychological disorders in cases of pediatric chest pain because of inconsistent use of valid psychological assessment tools and differences in research terminology in this area. Stress, anxiety, mood disorders, somatoform disorders, depression, and psychotic disorders have all been associated with chest pain; the validity of these diagnoses is impacted by the use (or misuse or nonuse) of appropriate psychological assessments. The psychological impact of organic causes of chest pain on patients is also poorly defined, even though it is likely very relevant to patients and families dealing with a serious medical diagnosis. Providers must be cognizant of the importance of using valid assessments to diagnose psychological disorders; psychogenic chest pain should never be a diagnosis of exclusion.

9. Hyperventilation typically presents with rapid breathing, dyspnea, anxiety, and sometimes with palpitations, chest pain, paresthesias, lightheadedness, and confusion. Careful evaluation often reveals anxiety or underlying psychological concerns.

10. Precordial catch syndrome (Texidor twinge) is classically described as a benign condition characterized by brief paroxysms of sharp, well-localized pains in the midsternal or precordial region. Episodes are brief (30 seconds to 3 minutes), self-resolving, and exacerbated by deep breathing. Expert opinions

vary regarding whether this phenomenon is a distinct entity, or if it should be considered an idiopathic etiology of chest pain.

11 Most children with mitral valve prolapse (MVP) do not complain of chest pain.

12 Infections are rare but serious causes of chest pain in children. Chest pain is frequently a prominent symptom in pericarditis; it is usually exacerbated by lying down or with inspiration. Physical examination findings include a friction rub,

muffled heart sounds, tachycardia, neck vein distention, and pulsus paradoxus. Myocarditis presents with a more subtle but progressive illness, including fever, chest pain, vomiting, and shortness of breath. Electrocardiograms are abnormal in each of these conditions, and cardiomegaly is evident on chest x-ray.

13 Asthma, cystic fibrosis, and connective tissue disorders (Marfan syndrome, Ehlers-Danlos syndrome, ankylosing spondylitis) are risk factors for pneumothoraces. Pneumonias

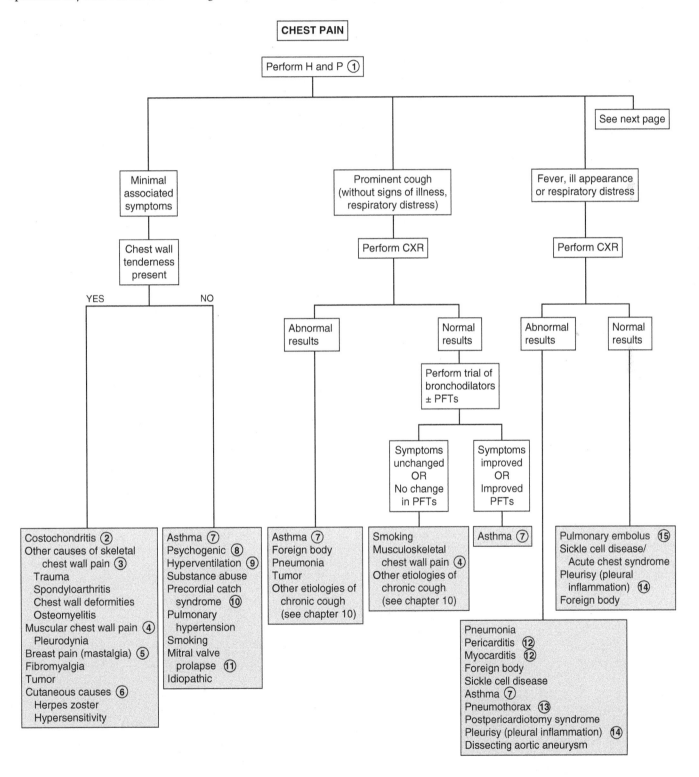

Nelson Textbook of Pediatrics, 19e. Chapters 405, 413, 416, 433
Nelsons Essentials, 6e. Chapters 128, 141, 147, 148

due to certain pathogens (e.g., *Pneumocystis jirovecii* in immunodeficient conditions or staphylococcal, anaerobic gram negative pathogens) also predispose to the development of pneumothoraces. Healthy children may also develop spontaneous pneumothorax; cocaine use is a risk factor. Forceful vomiting is a rare cause of esophageal rupture causing pneumomediastinum (Boerhaave syndrome). Traumatic or iatrogenic causes should also be considered.

14 Movement and deep breathing often aggravate the pain associated with pleurisy (pleuritis) or pleural effusions. Bacterial pneumonias are the most common cause of pleuritis in children; collagen vascular disorders can also be causative.

15 Risk factors for venous thrombosis (e.g., oral contraceptives, recent abortion or surgery [especially cardiac], the presence of a central venous line, immobilization, sepsis, hypercoagulable states, vascular malformations) should raise suspicion for pulmonary emboli. Associated symptoms include dyspnea, cough, hypoxia, and occasionally, hemoptysis. If emboli are suspected, appropriate labs and imaging (spiral CT or pulmonary angiography) should be performed.

16 Slipping rib syndrome is characterized by pain along the lower rib margin of the upper abdomen, sometimes associated with a slipping sensation and a popping or clicking sound. Although a clear consensus on the cause of the pain is lacking, a commonly presumed etiology is that trauma to the eighth, ninth, or tenth rib causes a sprain-like injury, which increases the mobility of the rib and allows impingement on an intercostal nerve. Reproduction of the pain by hooking the fingers under the anterior costal margins and pulling the ribs forward is characteristic.

17 Symptoms of GERD (gastroesophageal reflux disease) vary by age; common symptoms in older children and adolescents are abdominal or substernal pain, vomiting or regurgitation, increased pain after meals or when recumbent, and relief with antacids. A trial of empiric therapy is appropriate in children with typical symptoms, although a positive response is not confirmatory of GERD since spontaneous resolution of symptoms (due to any cause) can occur.

18 The value of an UGI contrast study is to rule out other GI disorders (e.g., esophageal abnormalities, intestinal obstruction); it will not diagnose GERD.

19 Peptic ulcer disease (PUD) frequently presents with a chronic intermittent history of dull or aching pain and often includes nighttime complaints. The pain may be epigastric or poorly localized abdominal pain; it may or may not be relieved by antacids.

20 Eosinophilic esophagitis (EoE) is diagnosed by endoscopic biopsies showing localized eosinophilic infiltrates of the esophagus. The condition is being increasingly recognized in all age groups; abdominal pain and vomiting are more common in younger children and dysphagia, chest pain, and food impaction are more likely in adolescents. Other atopic diseases and food allergies are commonly associated.

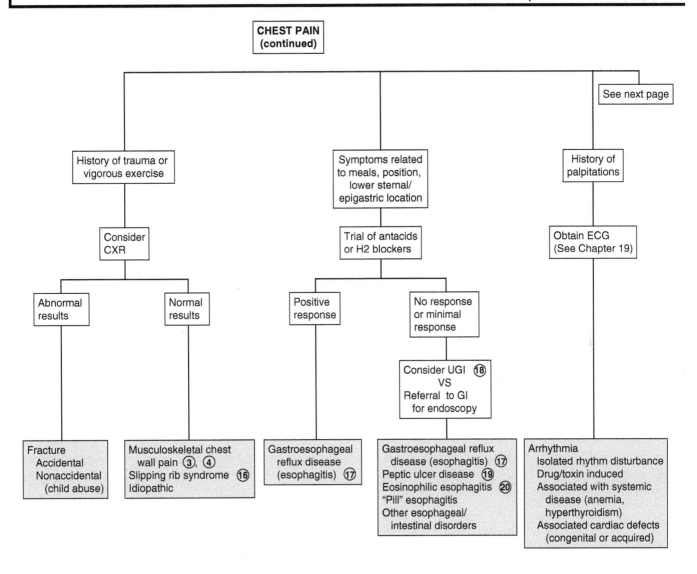

CHEST PAIN
(continued)

See next page

History of trauma or vigorous exercise

Symptoms related to meals, position, lower sternal/epigastric location

History of palpitations

Consider CXR

Trial of antacids or H2 blockers

Obtain ECG (See Chapter 19)

Abnormal results

Normal results

Positive response

No response or minimal response

Consider UGI ⑱
VS
Referral to GI for endoscopy

Fracture
Accidental
Nonaccidental
(child abuse)

Musculoskeletal chest
wall pain ③, ④
Slipping rib syndrome ⑯
Idiopathic

Gastroesophageal
reflux disease
(esophagitis) ⑰

Gastroesophageal reflux
disease (esophagitis) ⑰
Peptic ulcer disease ⑲
Eosinophilic esophagitis ⑳
"Pill" esophagitis
Other esophageal/
intestinal disorders

Arrhythmia
Isolated rhythm disturbance
Drug/toxin induced
Associated with systemic
disease (anemia,
hyperthyroidism)
Associated cardiac defects
(congenital or acquired)

21 Consultation with a cardiologist is recommended because of the potentially serious (ischemic) nature of chest pain caused by severe obstructive lesions; it is also considered a more cost-effective alternative to obtaining additional studies without consultation.

22 Hypertrophic cardiomyopathy is a genetic disorder transmitted in an autosomal dominant pattern, although a large proportion of cases are considered *de novo* mutations. Classic physical examination findings include a left ventricular lift and a harsh systolic ejection murmur that is increased with any maneuver that decreases venous return (Valsalva maneuver, rising from squatting to standing). As the development of hypertrophy is gradual over years, examination findings in children may be limited to nonspecific murmurs; cardiac evaluation is indicated whenever there is a known family history.

23 Unless suspected to be asthma, chest pain that is precipitated by exercise or running or is associated with syncope or palpitations warrants urgent cardiac consultation. Myocardial ischemia is rare in children overall, although an increasing number of children are at risk due to advances in care and treatment of congenital and acquired (Kawasaki) heart disease. Unlike adults with atherosclerotic heart disease, children do not experience classic angina-type pain (i.e., chest pressure or squeezing sensation with radiation to neck, jaws or arms); rather, the symptoms of myocardial ischemia in younger patients are nonspecific and include irritability, nausea, vomiting, abdominal pain, failure to thrive, shock, syncope, seizures, or sudden cardiac arrest. The presentation of congenital coronary artery abnormalities may be subtle or abrupt with few identifiable risk factors. However, children with a history of heart surgery (e.g., repair of tetralogy of Fallot or transposition of the great arteries), congenital heart conditions, or a history of Kawasaki disease warrant a higher threshold of awareness for risk of ischemic chest pain.

24 Coronary artery anomalies are rare but can be associated with severe ischemia. The physical examination may be normal or may include tachypnea, tachycardia, pallor, diaphoresis, distant heart tones, a murmur consistent with mitral regurgitation, or a gallop rhythm suggesting myocardial dysfunction. Echocardiogram and angiography are used in diagnosis.

Bibliography

Eslick GD, Selbst SM: Pediatric chest pain. Preface. *Pediatr Clin North Am* 57(6):xiii-xiv, 2010.

Reddy S, Singh H: Chest pain in children and adolescents, *Pediatr Rev* 31: e1-e9, 2010.

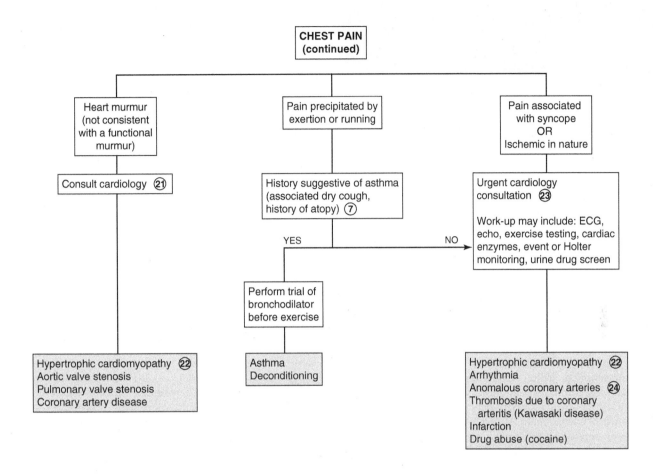

Chapter 18
SYNCOPE

Syncope is the temporary loss of consciousness and tone followed by a complete recovery after a brief period. It occurs due to inadequate cerebral perfusion. It is a common complaint in older children and adolescents (15% to 25% of children and adolescents report at least one episode before adulthood) but is unusual in children less than 6 years of age. Syncope is usually benign in children but must be carefully addressed because it may occasionally herald a life-threatening condition. When recurrent, it can generate a significant amount of stress for a patient and family. Presyncope is a constellation of symptoms associated with the sense that one is about to pass out but without a loss of consciousness. Presyncope should be approached in the same diagnostic manner as syncope.

1 When obtaining a history of the event, witnesses can be especially helpful. Inquire about events (e.g., eating, voiding, stretching) and position (including a change in position) prior to the episode, duration of loss of consciousness, associated symptoms (e.g., pallor, palpitations, headache, shortness of breath, nausea, diaphoresis, amnesia, vision changes), and time since the last meal. Environmental factors (e.g., warm temperature, crowded environment, noxious stimuli) may be helpful. Syncope associated with exertion or exercise is ominous because it may indicate a serious cardiac etiology; a thorough evaluation is always indicated. Syncope in the absence of presyncopal symptoms should be approached with a similar level of concern.

A family history of sudden death, sudden infant death syndrome (SIDS), heart disease (including congenital), arrhythmias, deafness, seizures, and metabolic disorders may be helpful in the diagnosis. Personal and family histories of prior episodes of fainting are often obtained in cases of benign (vasovagal) syncope. A menstrual history should be obtained in females to investigate the possibility of pregnancy. The social history should inquire about the possibility of ingestion or illicit drug use. Inquire about access to any potential toxins or medications, including medications of other family members that might be accessible. Diuretics, beta-blockers, other cardiac medications, and tricyclic anti-depressants are medications that may lead to syncopal events.

The physical examination findings are usually normal in children who experience syncope. The examination should include a thorough neurologic examination, and the cardiac examination should be performed with the patient supine and standing to rule out an obstructive lesion.

2 Assessment for orthostatic hypotension should be done by obtaining blood pressure (and heart rate) after resting supine for 5 minutes then after standing for 2 to 5 minutes. Most experts recommend that all children with syncope should have an electrocardiogram (ECG) done with careful attention to the PR, QRS, and QT/QTc intervals, abnormalities of which can suggest an underlying conduction or electrolyte abnormality. The ECG also indicates chamber enlargement or hypertrophy. Checking glucose and electrolyte levels is usually not helpful, especially in children who present for evaluation hours to days after the episode. Labs

may be indicated, however, whenever there is a history of an eating disorder, malnutrition, a known or suspected endocrine abnormality (e.g., thyromegaly on physical examination), or a possible pregnancy.

3 Depending on the symptomatology, further evaluation may include a Holter monitor (24-hour ambulatory ECG), an echocardiogram, or an exercise stress test. Cardiac catheterization and electrophysiologic studies with invasive monitoring may be necessary in some severe cases.

4 Supraventricular tachycardia (SVT), ventricular tachycardia, and heart block are the most common arrhythmias causing syncope. Heart block can be congenital, postsurgical, acquired (Lyme disease), or medication related. First- and second-degree heart block are unlikely to cause syncope.

5 Wolff-Parkinson-White (WPW) syndrome is a primary conduction abnormality that is characterized by an accessory conduction pathway that results in SVT. Atrial flutter may also occur.

6 Long QT syndrome and Brugada syndrome are inherited cardiac ion channel abnormalities with characteristic ECG findings; both can cause lethal ventricular arrhythmias. The heterozygous form of congenital long QT (Romano-Ward) syndrome is most common and milder than the homozygous form (Jervell-Lange-Nielsen). The latter is also associated with congenital deafness. Acquired long QT syndrome can occur secondary to myocarditis, mitral valve prolapse, electrolyte abnormalities, and medications (e.g., tricyclic antidepressants, antipsychotics, macrolide antibiotics, organophosphates, antihistamines, antifungals).

7 Worrisome elements of the history include syncope that either occurs in a recumbent position or is associated with exercise, chest pain, or palpitations. A history of heart disease (repaired or unrepaired) or a family history of unexplained death, drowning, hypertrophic cardiomyopathy (HCM), long QT syndrome (or other arrhythmias), or pacemaker placement are worrisome. Patients with abnormal cardiac examination findings should also be referred for an urgent cardiac evaluation.

8 Hypertrophic cardiomyopathy (HCM) is a rare but serious cause of syncope. Subaortic hypertrophied myocardium causes outflow tract obstruction; the subsequent murmur characteristically increases during a Valsalva maneuver and when a patient rises from a squatting up to a standing position (both maneuvers decrease preload). The condition can also cause arrhythmias leading to syncope. An evaluation is indicated whenever a murmur is present in a patient with syncope; a positive family history should raise the level of suspicion because the inheritance risk is high.

9 Seizures are the most likely neurologic cause of syncope in children; however, overall neurologic causes are rare in children and adolescents. A few tonic-clonic contractions are normal in cases of vasovagal syncope. They should not be considered true seizure activity. Characteristics that may help distinguish a seizure from a syncopal event include a postictal phase, a rigid (rather than limp) posture, a warm or flushed appearance (as opposed to pallor), and incontinence. Patients with seizures do not experience presyncopal symptoms, and they are usually unconscious for a longer period. Loss of consciousness with syncope is usually less than 1 minute. Seizures should also be suspected when the loss of consciousness occurs in the supine position.

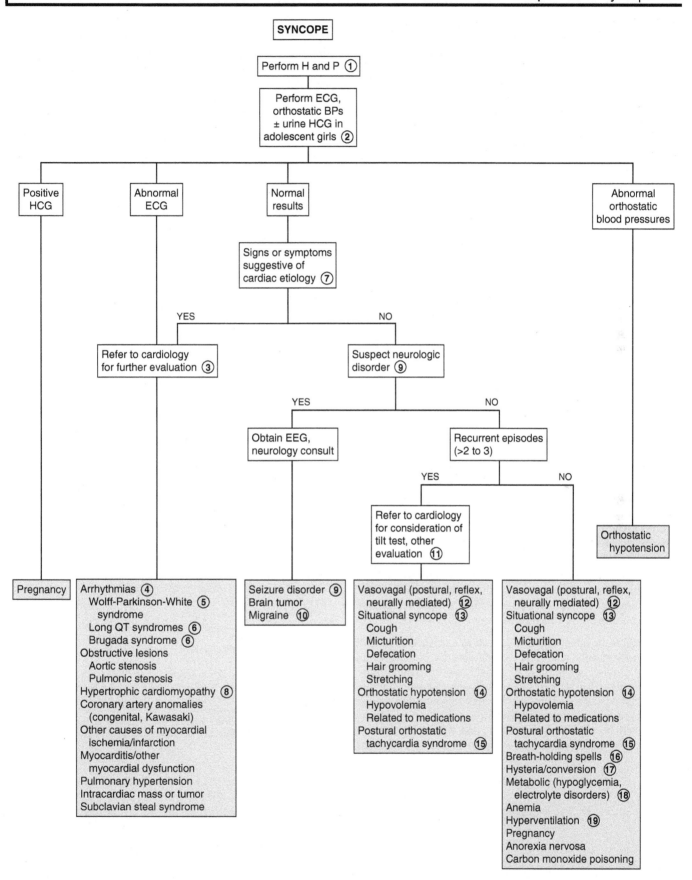

10 A rare migraine variant (basilar-type) can cause syncope. A severe occipital headache and unilateral visual changes are commonly associated; ataxia, vertigo, and vomiting may also occur.

11 Further evaluation may be indicated because frequent episodes of syncope are very distressing to a patient, even when the etiology is benign. A tilt table evaluation may aid in the diagnosis of syncope due to orthostatic intolerance (e.g., vasovagal, orthostatic hypotension, postural orthostatic tachycardia syndrome) and in the selection of therapy; there are, however, limitations to its sensitivity, specificity, diagnostic yield, and reproducibility.

12 Vasovagal syncope is also called postural, reflex, neurocardiogenic or neurally-mediated syncope, or simply "fainting"; some overlap in terminology is occurring with increasing understanding of the pathophysiology of orthostasis (the body's adjustment to upright posture). It is the most common type of syncope in normal children and adolescents; it occurs most frequently in the 15- to 19-year-old age group. A neurally-mediated decline in blood pressure (the exact mechanism of which is poorly understood) and heart rate are responsible for the transient decrease in cerebral blood flow leading to the syncopal episode. Recognizable precipitating factors (rising to stand, a prolonged period of standing, certain stressors like venipuncture, noxious stimuli, fasting, or a crowded location) and prodromal (presyncopal) autonomic symptoms (e.g., nausea, pallor, diaphoresis) are characteristic of this type of noncardiac syncope. The absence of a prodromal or presyncopal sensation is not consistent with a vasovagal etiology and should prompt consideration of more serious etiologies.

Also, vasovagal syncope can occur after vigorous, usually prolonged exertion (such as at the end of a long competitive run) due to a warm ambient temperature, venous pooling, and dehydration; it is distinct from "mid-stride" syncope, which should prompt an immediate cardiac evaluation. Most of these cases have a vasovagal (not cardiac) etiology, but sports participation should be curtailed until a worrisome cardiac etiology has been ruled out.

13 Autonomic responses triggered by certain bodily functions or movements (e.g., cough, micturition, defecation, hair grooming, stretching) can occasionally result in syncope; the mechanism is presumed to be vasovagal in nature.

14 Orthostatic hypotension is defined as a persistent fall of 20 mmHg systolic and/or 10 mmHg diastolic blood pressure within 3 minutes of assuming an upright position without moving the arms or legs. (Heart rates usually increase with standing but are not part of the diagnostic criteria.) In contrast to vasovagal syncope, true orthostatic hypotension is due to an inadequate vasoconstriction response to standing and will lead to syncope without the typical presyncopal symptoms seen with vasovagal syncope. Most cases in young people are nonneurogenic and caused by medications or hypovolemia (e.g., hemorrhage, dehydration). Neurogenic orthostatic hypotension is a significant disorder of the autonomic system and more likely to occur in older patients or in association with serious medical conditions (e.g., diabetes, amyloidosis, Parkinson's disease).

15 Postural orthostatic tachycardia syndrome (POTS) describes posturally-induced symptoms (e.g., lightheadedness, palpitations, nausea) accompanied by an increased heart rate of ≥ 30 bpm documented while obtaining blood pressures for orthostatic hypotension. (Some decrease in blood pressure may occur but is not part of the diagnostic criteria.) Recurrent near syncope is most common, but frank syncope can occur. Chronic fatigue and exercise intolerance are commonly present in this syndrome, which is most common in young women.

16 Breath-holding spells are the most common mechanism of syncope in children younger than 6 years of age. Children who are startled or upset hold their breath in expiration, collapse, and become cyanotic for a brief period.

17 Hysterical or conversion syncope is a diagnosis of exclusion. It is most common in adolescents; they typically have an audience for this event. Hemodynamic changes, sweating, pallor, and subsequent psychological distress regarding the episode are absent.

18 Hunger, weakness, sweating, agitation, and confusion may accompany hypoglycemia or electrolyte disorders. Supine position does not provide relief.

19 A history of preceding psychological distress, sensations of shortness of breath, chest pain, visual changes, and numbness or tingling of the extremities may be reported in children with syncope due to hyperventilation. The patient may be able to reproduce the episode when requested to hyperventilate.

Bibliography

Fischer JW, Cho CS: Pediatric syncope: Cases form the emergency department, *Emerg Med Clin N Am* 28:501–516, 2010.

Lewis DA, Chala A: Syncope in the pediatric patient: The cardiologist's perspective, *Pediatr Clin North Am* 46:205–219, 1999.

Park MK: Pediatric cardiology for practitioners [electronic resource]. Philadelphia, 2008, Mosby/Elsevier.

Stewart JM: Common syndromes of orthostatic intolerance, *Pediatrics* 131: 968–980, 2013.

Strickberger SA, Benson DW, Biaggioni I, et al: AHA/ACCF scientific statement on the evaluation of syncope: from the American Heart Association Councils on Clinical Cardiology, Cardiovascular Nursing, Cardiovascular Disease in the Young, and Stroke, and the Quality of Care and Outcomes Research Interdisciplinary Working Group; and the American College of Cardiology Foundation in collaboration with the Heart Rhythm Society, *J Am Coll Cardiol* 47(2):473–484, 2006.

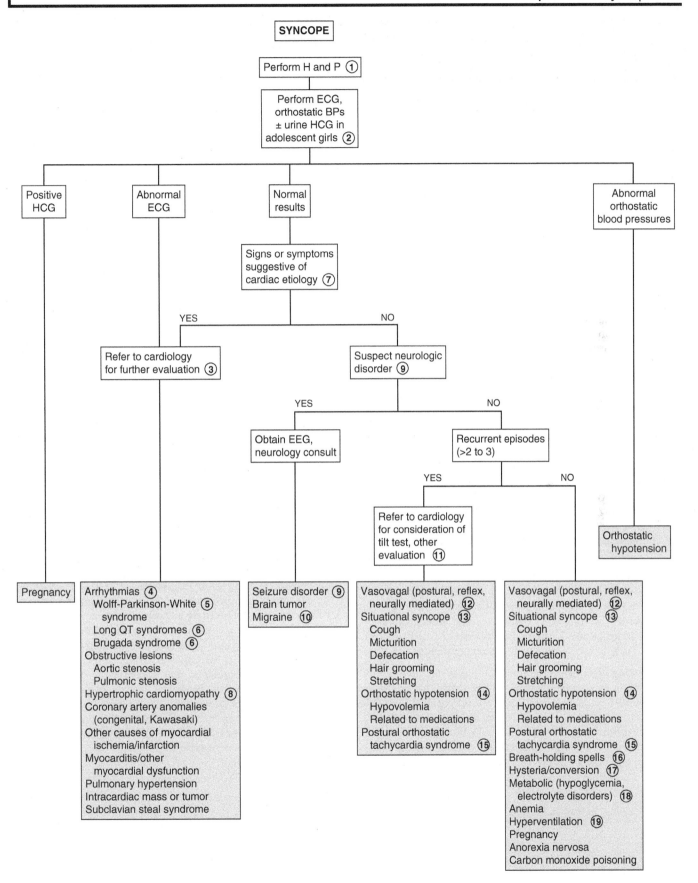

SYNCOPE

Perform H and P ①

Perform ECG, orthostatic BPs ± urine HCG in adolescent girls ②

Positive HCG

Abnormal ECG

Normal results

Abnormal orthostatic blood pressures

Signs or symptoms suggestive of cardiac etiology ⑦

YES — Refer to cardiology for further evaluation ③

NO — Suspect neurologic disorder ⑨

YES — Obtain EEG, neurology consult

NO — Recurrent episodes (>2 to 3)

YES — Refer to cardiology for consideration of tilt test, other evaluation ⑪

NO — Orthostatic hypotension

Pregnancy

Arrhythmias ④
  Wolff-Parkinson-White ⑤
    syndrome
  Long QT syndromes ⑥
  Brugada syndrome ⑥
Obstructive lesions
  Aortic stenosis
  Pulmonic stenosis
Hypertrophic cardiomyopathy ⑧
Coronary artery anomalies
  (congenital, Kawasaki)
Other causes of myocardial
  ischemia/infarction
Myocarditis/other
  myocardial dysfunction
Pulmonary hypertension
Intracardiac mass or tumor
Subclavian steal syndrome

Seizure disorder ⑨
Brain tumor
Migraine ⑩

Vasovagal (postural, reflex,
  neurally mediated) ⑫
Situational syncope ⑬
  Cough
  Micturition
  Defecation
  Hair grooming
  Stretching
Orthostatic hypotension ⑭
  Hypovolemia
  Related to medications
Postural orthostatic
  tachycardia syndrome ⑮

Vasovagal (postural, reflex,
  neurally mediated) ⑫
Situational syncope ⑬
  Cough
  Micturition
  Defecation
  Hair grooming
  Stretching
Orthostatic hypotension ⑭
  Hypovolemia
  Related to medications
Postural orthostatic
  tachycardia syndrome ⑮
Breath-holding spells ⑯
Hysteria/conversion ⑰
Metabolic (hypoglycemia,
  electrolyte disorders) ⑱
Anemia
Hyperventilation ⑲
Pregnancy
Anorexia nervosa
Carbon monoxide poisoning

Nelson Textbook of Pediatrics, 19e. Chapter 587
Nelsons Essentials, 6e. Chapter 140

Chapter 19
PALPITATIONS

Palpitations are sensations of the heart's actions. They may be described as rapid or slow, skipping or stopping, and regular or irregular. Most cases are not due to serious cardiac etiologies. The goal of the evaluation is to identify the small proportion of patients who are at risk for serious cardiac disease.

1. An accurate description of the sensation may aid in the diagnosis. For children old enough to articulate the sensation, racing, heart stopping or pausing, and skipping beats are common descriptors. Inquire about the duration of symptoms, whether the onset and termination of symptoms are subtle or abrupt, and the factors associated with onset (e.g., such as exercise) or termination (e.g., Valsalva maneuver). Infants may manifest nonspecific symptoms of irritability and poor feeding; some cases may progress to congestive heart failure prior to identification of an abnormal rhythm. When appropriate, consider instructing parents on how to take the child's pulse during future episodes.

Special attention should be paid to a history of structural cardiac abnormalities or cardiac surgery because those factors increase the risk of both arrhythmias and adverse outcomes associated with them. Certain medications can be responsible for arrhythmias. Symptoms suggestive of endocrine disorders may also indicate etiologies. A social history should investigate stress levels, caffeine intake, and tobacco use. Familial disorders that may be a cause of palpitations include Wolff-Parkinson-White syndrome, long QT syndrome (deafness is associated with one of these inherited syndromes), and Kearns-Sayre syndrome (e.g., retinal degeneration, ophthalmoplegia, muscle weakness).

2. An association of palpitations with syncope or exertion is ominous and warrants urgent cardiac consultation to direct an evaluation for an underlying cardiac etiology. Other worrisome history components include severe chest pain, a family history of long QT syndrome, and unexplained or aborted sudden death. If the history reveals any of these risk factors, an urgent cardiac evaluation is recommended.

3. A resting electrocardiogram (ECG) may identify an arrhythmia or suggest a cardiac abnormality that could be associated with an arrhythmia (e.g., cardiomyopathy, long QT syndrome). It can also reveal abnormalities that may cause symptoms other than palpitations (e.g., AV block, bradycardia). When the complaint of palpitations is a minor one and is associated with a likely causative condition (e.g., fever, anxiety),

an ECG may not be necessary acutely; clinical judgment should be applied.

4. Sinus tachycardia needs to be distinguished from supraventricular tachycardia (SVT). Both are narrow complex tachycardias. Sinus tachycardia is characterized by a normal P-wave axis, a gradual onset and termination, and a rate higher than the age-specific upper limit of normal (usually less than 230 to 240 beats per minute [bpm]); variability in the heart rate is a characteristic distinguishing it from SVT. Fever, pain, anemia, and dehydration are common causes of sinus tachycardia.

5. When drugs are responsible for palpitations, the most common mechanism is a transient increased heart rate, but they may occasionally cause more serious rhythm disturbances. Medications associated with palpitations include tricyclic antidepressants, aminophylline, stimulants (for ADHD treatment), and thyroid replacement medications. Drugs of abuse (e.g., cocaine, amphetamines) can also cause cardiac side effects ranging from benign palpitations to serious cardiac arrhythmias.

6. Clinical characteristics of hyperthyroidism include goiter, accelerated linear growth, failure to gain weight (or weight loss), abnormal eyelid retraction, exophthalmos, tremor, and weakness. Pallor on examination, a history of lethargy or easy fatigability, excessive blood loss, or a diet history suggestive of iron deficiency may be clues to anemia.

7. Holter monitoring is an extended rhythm recording (24 or 48 hours) recommended to attempt to capture an abnormal rhythm when a patient experiences frequent symptoms. If events are more intermittent, an incident or event recorder is preferable; these require activation by the patient when symptoms develop.

8. Sinus arrhythmia is a normal variation of the heart rate with a slowing during expiration and acceleration during inspiration. Occasionally it can be prominent; careful auscultation will identify the relationship to the respiratory phases and distinguish it from premature atrial contractions.

9. Premature ventricular complexes (PVCs) are common, occurring in approximately 25% of the general population. PVCs usually are followed by a compensatory pause preceding the next beat. They are often asymptomatic, although patients may describe a "skipped" beat followed by a strong beat or a sensation of the "heart turning over." Anxiety, fever, and certain drugs, especially stimulants, may increase the occurrence of PVCs. Although usually benign, a history of syncope, heart disease, chest pain or other symptoms, a family history of sudden death, aggravation by exercise, frequent or prolonged runs, or a nonuniform appearance of the QRS complex (suggesting a multifocal origin) are worrisome characteristics and warrant additional evaluation.

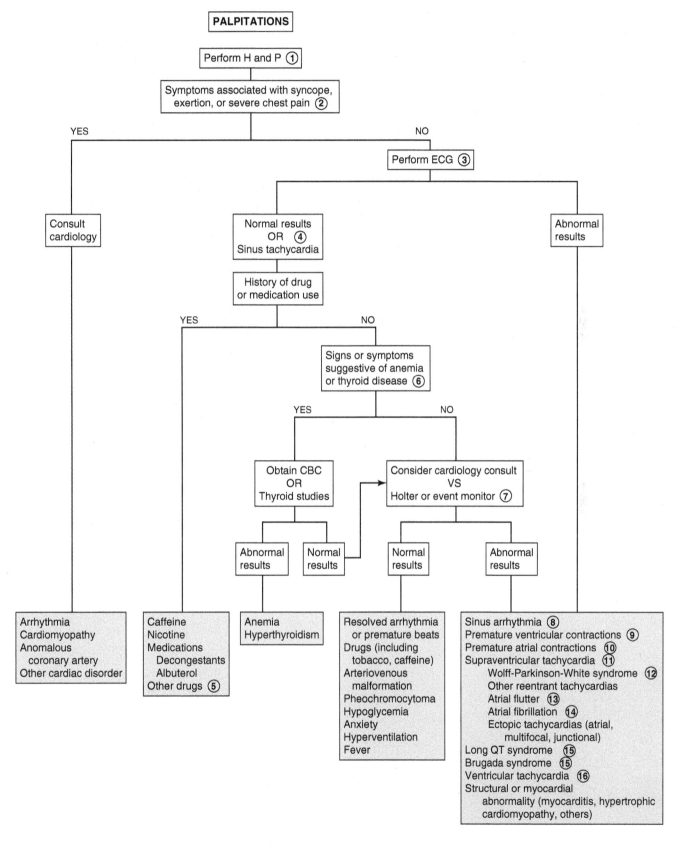

PALPITATIONS

Perform H and P ①

Symptoms associated with syncope, exertion, or severe chest pain ②

YES → Consult cardiology

NO → Perform ECG ③

Normal results OR ④ Sinus tachycardia

Abnormal results

History of drug or medication use

YES

NO → Signs or symptoms suggestive of anemia or thyroid disease ⑥

YES → Obtain CBC OR Thyroid studies

NO → Consider cardiology consult VS Holter or event monitor ⑦

Abnormal results

Normal results

Normal results

Abnormal results

Arrhythmia
Cardiomyopathy
Anomalous
  coronary artery
Other cardiac disorder

Caffeine
Nicotine
Medications
  Decongestants
  Albuterol
Other drugs ⑤

Anemia
Hyperthyroidism

Resolved arrhythmia
  or premature beats
Drugs (including
  tobacco, caffeine)
Arteriovenous
  malformation
Pheochromocytoma
Hypoglycemia
Anxiety
Hyperventilation
Fever

Sinus arrhythmia ⑧
Premature ventricular contractions ⑨
Premature atrial contractions ⑩
Supraventricular tachycardia ⑪
    Wolff-Parkinson-White syndrome ⑫
    Other reentrant tachycardias
    Atrial flutter ⑬
    Atrial fibrillation ⑭
    Ectopic tachycardias (atrial,
      multifocal, junctional)
Long QT syndrome ⑮
Brugada syndrome ⑮
Ventricular tachycardia ⑯
Structural or myocardial
  abnormality (myocarditis, hypertrophic
  cardiomyopathy, others)

Nelson Textbook of Pediatrics, 19e. Chapter 429
Nelsons Essentials, 6e. Chapter 142

(10) Premature atrial contractions (PACs) are also benign rhythm variations. They are usually asymptomatic; patients may occasionally complain of skipped beats or pauses in their heart rate.

(11) Supraventricular tachycardias (SVTs) originate in the atria, atrioventricular node, or one or more accessory pathways between the atria and ventricles or within the AV node (reentrant tachycardias). Reentrant tachycardias are characterized by an abrupt onset and cessation and tend to occur when the patient is at rest. They demonstrate a narrow QRS complex, an abnormal P-wave axis, and an unvarying rate that usually exceeds 180 bpm. It may be as high as 300 bpm. Congenital heart disease and use of over-the-counter decongestants are common causes of SVTs.

(12) Wolff-Parkinson-White syndrome is characterized by an SVT due to an accessory conduction pathway between the atria and the ventricles, which manifests (between episodes of SVT) with delta waves (a slow upstroke of the QRS) on the ECG.

(13) Atrial rates of 250 to 300 bpm occur in atrial flutter (higher rates can occur in infants); ventricular conduction can be 1:1 but some degree of heart block (2:1, 3:1) is more common, so QRS complexes may appear normal. It usually occurs in children with congenital heart disease, especially postoperatively, but may occur in neonates with normal hearts. Onset and termination are abrupt; the ECG shows atrial saw-toothed flutter waves.

(14) In atrial fibrillation, chaotic atrial excitation at a rapid rate (typically 350 to 400 bpm, sometimes higher) produces an irregular ventricular rhythm. It usually occurs in the presence of cardiac abnormalities. Otherwise healthy children experiencing atrial fibrillation should be evaluated for thyrotoxicosis, pulmonary emboli, and pericarditis.

(15) Long QT syndrome and Brugada syndrome are examples of inherited cardiac ion channel abnormalities with characteristic ECG findings. Genetic defects have been identified for several variations of long QT syndrome; these conditions can cause lethal ventricular arrhythmias. They may present with palpitations, syncope, drowning, or cardiac arrest. Calculation of the corrected QT interval (QTc) corrects the interval for the patient's heart rate. Jervell-Lange-Nielsen is a congenital long QT syndrome associated with congenital deafness. Acquired long QT syndrome can occur secondary to myocarditis, mitral valve prolapse, electrolyte abnormalities, and medications (e.g., tricyclic antidepressants, antipsychotics, macrolide antibiotics, antihistamines, antifungals, cisapride, multiple cardiac medications).

(16) Ventricular (wide QRS complex) tachycardia necessitates prompt treatment. It may be asymptomatic in children with normal hearts; children with structural heart disease are more likely to be symptomatic.

Bibliography

Anderson BR, Vetter VL: Arrhythmogenic causes of chest pain in children, *Pediatr Clin North Am* 57:1305–1330, 2010.
Biondi EA: Cardiac arrhythmias in children, *Pedatri Rev* 31:375–379, 2010.
Park MK: Cardiac arrhythmias. In Park MK, editor: *Pediatric cardiology for practitioners*, 5e, St. Louis, 2008, Mosby.

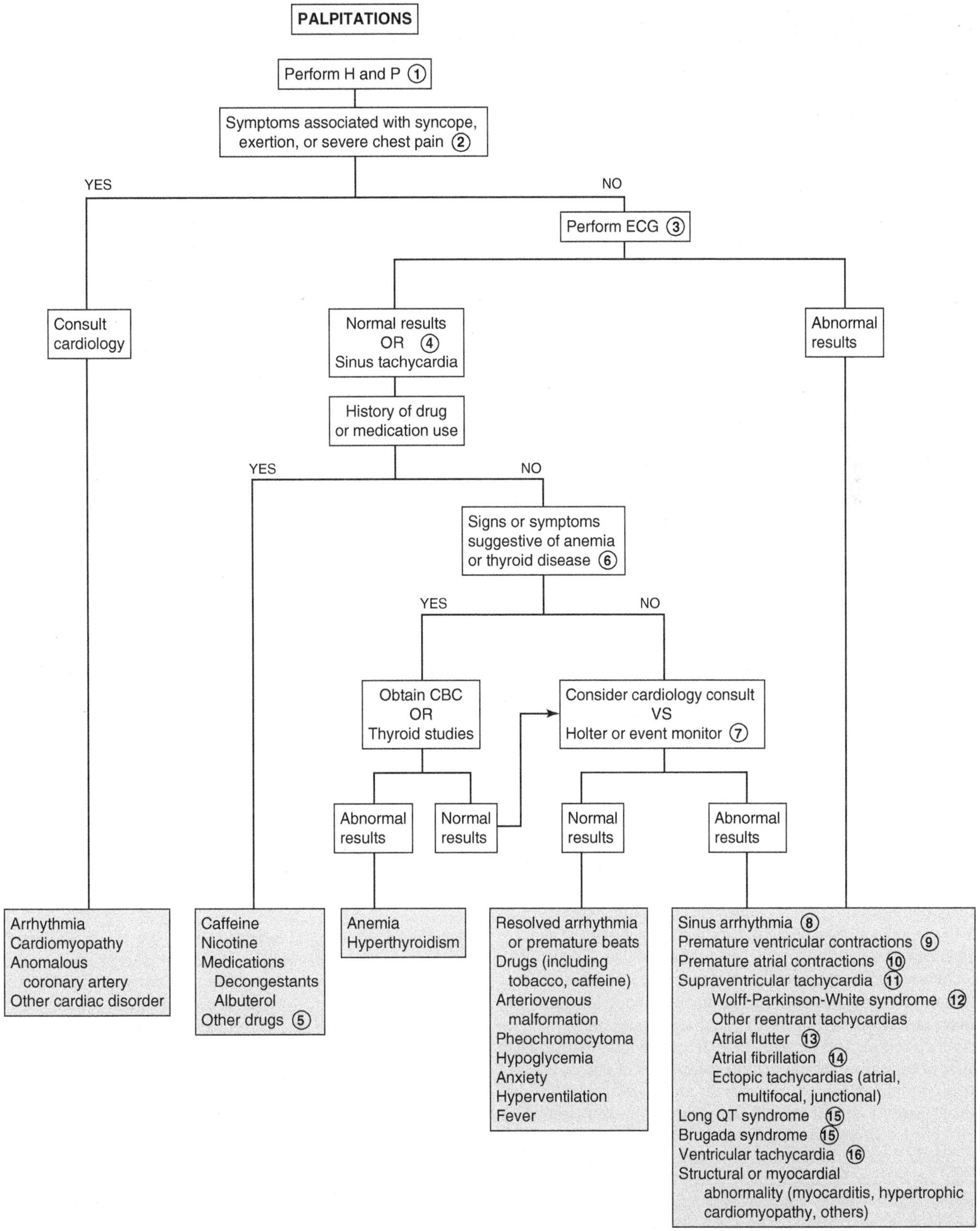

PALPITATIONS

Perform H and P ①

Symptoms associated with syncope, exertion, or severe chest pain ②

YES → Consult cardiology

Arrhythmia
Cardiomyopathy
Anomalous
  coronary artery
Other cardiac disorder

NO → Perform ECG ③

Normal results OR ④ Sinus tachycardia

Abnormal results

History of drug or medication use

YES →

Caffeine
Nicotine
Medications
  Decongestants
  Albuterol
Other drugs ⑤

NO →

Signs or symptoms suggestive of anemia or thyroid disease ⑥

YES → Obtain CBC OR Thyroid studies

Abnormal results → Anemia
Hyperthyroidism

Normal results →

NO → Consider cardiology consult VS Holter or event monitor ⑦

Normal results →

Resolved arrhythmia
  or premature beats
Drugs (including
  tobacco, caffeine)
Arteriovenous
  malformation
Pheochromocytoma
Hypoglycemia
Anxiety
Hyperventilation
Fever

Abnormal results →

Sinus arrhythmia ⑧
Premature ventricular contractions ⑨
Premature atrial contractions ⑩
Supraventricular tachycardia ⑪
  Wolff-Parkinson-White syndrome ⑫
  Other reentrant tachycardias
  Atrial flutter ⑬
  Atrial fibrillation ⑭
  Ectopic tachycardias (atrial,
    multifocal, junctional)
Long QT syndrome ⑮
Brugada syndrome ⑮
Ventricular tachycardia ⑯
Structural or myocardial
  abnormality (myocarditis, hypertrophic
  cardiomyopathy, others)

Nelson Textbook of Pediatrics, 19e. Chapter 429
Nelsons Essentials, 6e. Chapter 142

Chapter 20
HEART MURMURS

Most normal children (50% to 90%) have an audible heart murmur at some point prior to school age. The challenge to the practitioner is to ascertain which of these murmurs warrants additional evaluation. The clinical diagnosis of a normal or innocent murmur should be made only in the presence of a normal history and physical examination and characteristics consistent with a normal murmur. Despite the easy availability of echocardiography, the history and physical examination remain the accepted means of diagnosing normal murmurs. When the diagnosis of a murmur is unclear, it is generally more cost-effective to refer to a pediatric cardiologist than to order an echocardiogram.

1 The addition of preductal and postductal pulse oximetry performed in newborn nurseries is recognized as a fairly sensitive means of early identification of critical congenital heart disease. If not recognized in the newborn nursery, serious cardiac disorders may present with heart murmurs and congestive heart failure (CHF), the symptoms of which vary with age. In young infants with CHF, the feeding history may reveal limited intake, prolonged feeding times (but brief intervals between feeds because the infant is still hungry), diaphoresis, tachypnea or dyspnea, and possibly cyanosis with feeds. In older children, exercise or exertion can be assessed by inquiring about level of activity and tolerance to extended periods of play or activity (e.g., biking, gym class, walking, climbing stairs). Inquiring about how well older children keep up with their peers or siblings regarding exercise tolerance may also be helpful.

A history of fevers, lethargy, and recent dental work suggests possible endocarditis. Chronic mouth breathing, snoring, or obstructive sleep apnea may be clues to pulmonary hypertension.

A maternal history of gestational diabetes, infection, and use of certain drugs or medications may be risk factors for congenital heart disease. A family history of sudden death, rheumatic fever, sudden infant death syndrome, and structural cardiac defects in a first-degree relative may be significant. A family history of hypertrophic cardiomyopathy is sufficient to mandate an echocardiogram because of the autosomal dominant pattern of inheritance.

When assessing the child with a murmur, a complete physical examination is essential; growth parameters, peripheral edema, and hepatomegaly can be signs of CHF or chronic disease. The cardiac examination should include assessment of pulses, palpation of the precordium, auscultation, and blood pressures in both arms (involvement of a subclavian artery [most commonly the left] in a coarctation would cause a lower blood pressure in the ipsilateral arm) and a leg. Lower extremity blood pressure is usually 10-20 mmHg higher than upper extremity pressure. Diminished femoral pulses or a delay between the radial and femoral pulses suggest coarctation of the aorta (the simple presence of a femoral pulse does not rule out coarctation).

2 Noncardiac disorders that can cause a systolic outflow murmur include anemia, hyperthyroidism, and arteriovenous malformations (AVM). Hyperthyroidism is suggested by thyromegaly, tachycardia, a hyperdynamic precordium, slightly bounding pulses, and mild hypertension. Except for the thyromegaly, an AVM can cause similar findings; the examination may reveal localized continuous bruits over the head, neck, or liver. Pulmonary AVMs are generally not associated with bruits or murmurs. Anemia may manifest as pallor, tachycardia, exercise intolerance, or weakness.

3 A family history of sudden death or known hypertrophic cardiomyopathy is also significant and mandates further evaluation. Other physical examination findings that are worrisome include an abnormal rhythm, suprasternal thrill, prominent apical thrust, digital clubbing, wide or bounding pulses, and absent or weak femoral pulses. Signs of systemic disease (e.g., arthritis, fever, night sweats, embolic phenomena) should prompt consideration of acquired conditions, such as rheumatic heart disease or endocarditis.

4 When the diagnosis of a murmur is unclear, referral to a pediatric cardiologist is recommended; the severity of the clinical picture should determine the urgency of the referral. Discussion with a cardiologist may guide a clinician in obtaining studies (ECG, chest x-ray, echocardiogram) prior to a consultation visit, although postponing studies until a scheduled consultation will generally be more cost-effective, especially in an asymptomatic patient.

5 Rheumatic fever is an immunologically mediated inflammatory disorder following infection with group A streptococcus (GAS). 50% to 60% of rheumatic fever patients will experience carditis; in those cases, endocarditis (valvulitis) is universal and pericarditis or myocarditis may also develop. Patients typically present with murmurs of aortic or mitral regurgitation. The modified Jones criteria are used for diagnosis. Evidence of recent GAS disease (serologic or microbiologic) and either one major and two minor criteria or two major criteria are necessary to make the diagnosis. A history of fevers in the presence of a new or changing heart murmur should raise the suspicion for both rheumatic fever and endocarditis.

6 Ventricular septal defects (VSDs) are the most common congenital heart lesions. Symptoms depend on the size of the defect and pulmonary vascular resistance. Most VSDs are small and asymptomatic and close spontaneously in the first year or two of life. The murmur is classically described as a loud, usually holosystolic murmur with a harsh or blowing quality and is best heard at the left sternal border; a thrill or lift may be palpable with moderate lesions. In neonates the murmur may be heard best at the apex. Small defects may have soft murmurs that become softer over time as the lesion closes. In large defects, the left-to-right shunting increases over the first few weeks of life as pulmonary vascular resistance falls. Clinical symptoms of congestive heart failure develop gradually over this period. Referral for definitive diagnosis is recommended.

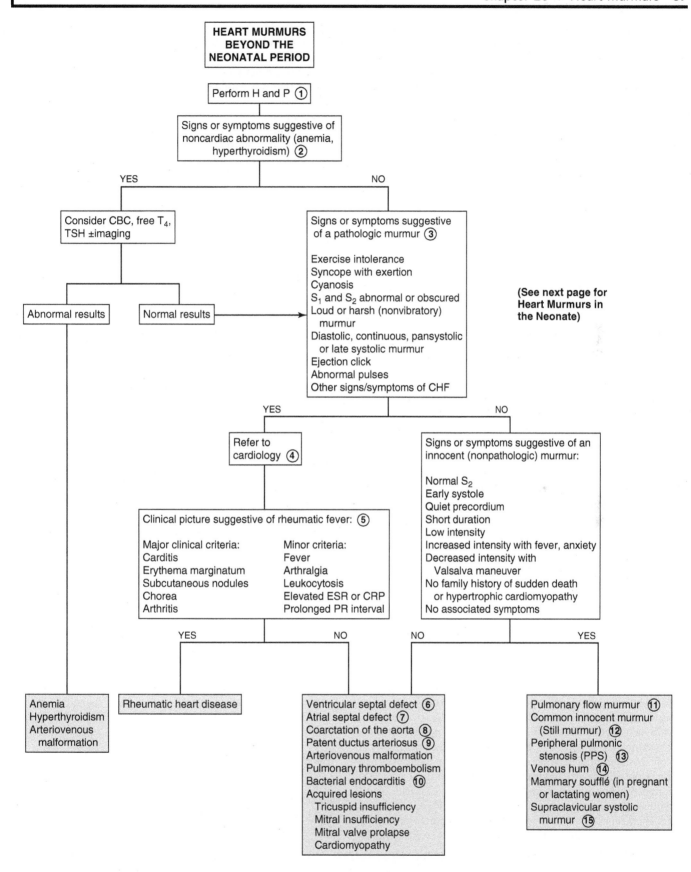

HEART MURMURS BEYOND THE NEONATAL PERIOD

Perform H and P ①

Signs or symptoms suggestive of noncardiac abnormality (anemia, hyperthyroidism) ②

YES → Consider CBC, free T₄, TSH ±imaging

- Abnormal results
- Normal results

NO → Signs or symptoms suggestive of a pathologic murmur ③

Exercise intolerance
Syncope with exertion
Cyanosis
S₁ and S₂ abnormal or obscured
Loud or harsh (nonvibratory) murmur
Diastolic, continuous, pansystolic or late systolic murmur
Ejection click
Abnormal pulses
Other signs/symptoms of CHF

(See next page for Heart Murmurs in the Neonate)

YES → Refer to cardiology ④

Clinical picture suggestive of rheumatic fever: ⑤

Major clinical criteria:	Minor criteria:
Carditis	Fever
Erythema marginatum	Arthralgia
Subcutaneous nodules	Leukocytosis
Chorea	Elevated ESR or CRP
Arthritis	Prolonged PR interval

NO → Signs or symptoms suggestive of an innocent (nonpathologic) murmur:

Normal S₂
Early systole
Quiet precordium
Short duration
Low intensity
Increased intensity with fever, anxiety
Decreased intensity with Valsalva maneuver
No family history of sudden death or hypertrophic cardiomyopathy
No associated symptoms

YES → Rheumatic heart disease

NO →
Ventricular septal defect ⑥
Atrial septal defect ⑦
Coarctation of the aorta ⑧
Patent ductus arteriosus ⑨
Arteriovenous malformation
Pulmonary thromboembolism
Bacterial endocarditis ⑩
Acquired lesions
  Tricuspid insufficiency
  Mitral insufficiency
  Mitral valve prolapse
  Cardiomyopathy

YES →
Pulmonary flow murmur ⑪
Common innocent murmur (Still murmur) ⑫
Peripheral pulmonic stenosis (PPS) ⑬
Venous hum ⑭
Mammary soufflé (in pregnant or lactating women)
Supraclavicular systolic murmur ⑮

Anemia
Hyperthyroidism
Arteriovenous malformation

Nelson Textbook of Pediatrics, 19e. Chapters 176, 416, 419, 420, 421, 431
Nelsons Essentials, 6e. Chapters 139, 143

7 Atrial septal defects (ASDs) are usually asymptomatic in infants and tend to be detected on routine physical examinations in the toddler or preschooler. They are characterized by a hyperdynamic right ventricular impulse and a characteristic fixed and widely split second heart sound. Murmurs are not always audible, but large defects may manifest a mid-systolic pulmonary flow murmur at the left upper sternal border or a mid-diastolic rumble at the left mid or lower sternal border due to increased flow over the tricuspid valve. When an ASD is suspected, a cardiology evaluation is warranted to identify the type of defect and the need for monitoring versus repair.

8 Coarctation of the aorta (COA) may present in infancy with congestive heart failure and lower extremity hypoperfusion. Children not diagnosed in infancy can remain asymptomatic (even with severe coarctation) and often present with hypertension later in childhood. The classic physical findings are diminished or delayed arterial pulses in the lower extremities compared to the upper extremities, with corresponding lower blood pressures in the lower extremities. A short systolic murmur at the third or fourth left intercostal spaces may be detected with transmission to the left infrascapular area or neck. A systolic ejection click or suprasternal thrill is consistent with a bicuspid aortic valve which occurs in 50% to 70% of patients with COA.

9 A small patent ductus arteriosus (PDA) in infants may be asymptomatic. Large ones tend to be symptomatic, causing congestive heart failure and failure to thrive. Classic findings of large PDA shunts are a wide peripheral pulse pressure (bounding pulses), a prominent apical impulse, a systolic thrill at the left upper sternal border, and a continuous harsh machinery-like murmur heard in the left infraclavicular region and at the left upper sternal border. The murmur characteristically becomes loudest during systole and softens during diastole. Large lesions may also produce a mid-diastolic apical rumble. Referral to cardiology is indicated for definitive diagnosis and treatment. The lesion is one of the cardiac anomalies frequently associated with prenatal maternal rubella infection; it is also common in congenital hypothyroidism.

10 Infective endocarditis can occur in children with healthy hearts but is most common in children with congenital heart disease or rheumatic heart disease; other risk factors include any valve malformation, patients who have had cardiac surgery, immunuosuppressed patients, patients with long-term intravascular catheters and IV drug users. Cases may present acutely or insidiously with intermittent fevers (classically occurring in the afternoons) and vague symptoms of fatigue, myalgias, joint pain, headache, and nausea or vomiting. New or changing murmurs, splenomegaly, and petechiae are common. Echocardiography is helpful in identifying vegetations, although results may be normal early in the disease. Adding transesophageal echocardiography to the transthoracic approach improves the diagnostic yield. Blood cultures are necessary to identify the pathogen. Three to five cultures from separate sites are recommended. Laboratories should be notified when endocarditis is suspected so that enriched media and prolonged incubation times are used.

11 The normal turbulence of ejection into the pulmonic root frequently generates an audible murmur of no hemodynamic significance. These murmurs are usually grade 1 to 3, short systolic murmurs with a slightly grating (rather than vibratory) quality. They are heard best over the left upper sternal border and may or may not transmit to the neck. Clicks and thrills associated with pulmonary valve stenosis are absent, and a normal S_2 distinguishes it from an ASD. The murmur can be accentuated by full exhalation and the supine position, and diminished by the upright posture and breath holding. It can occur in any age group (including neonates) but is most likely in older children and adolescents.

12 Some sources are replacing the classic "Still murmur" term with terms such as common innocent murmur, vibratory innocent murmur, or classic vibratory murmur. These normal murmurs are common in children (most commonly 3-7 years of age). The non-radiating murmur is usually a low-grade short systolic murmur heard best at the mid to lower left sternal border and also towards the apex. It has a characteristic vibratory or musical quality; commonly used descriptions include buzzing, a vibrating tuning fork, or a twanging cello string. Rarely, it can be surprisingly loud and ominous-sounding with transmission throughout the precordium. It may be heard best with the bell of a stethoscope, is usually loudest when the patient is supine and tends to diminish with an upright or a sitting position. This murmur is also exacerbated by fever, anxiety, excitement, or exercise.

13 Peripheral pulmonary artery stenosis (PPS) presents with a soft mid-systolic ejection murmur caused by flow through narrow pulmonary artery branches, which angle sharply off the main pulmonary artery. The murmur is loudest at the left upper sternal border with good transmission to the axillae and back. It generally disappears between 3 and 6 months of life as the pulmonary branches increase in size; persistence warrants cardiology evaluation to rule out true stenosis or constriction of the pulmonary arteries.

14 Venous hums are another common, normal murmur of childhood. These are medium frequency continuous murmurs heard in the infraclavicular region (right more common than left) and neck; their intensity increases slightly during diastole. The murmur typically is heard when the patient is sitting or standing, and it diminishes or disappears in the supine position, when the patient turns his or her head far to one side, and when gentle pressure is applied to the jugular veins in the neck. They are presumed to be due to the turbulence created as the internal jugular and subclavian veins enter the superior vena cava. The main differential diagnoses are PDA and arteriovenous malformations.

15 A supraclavicular systolic murmur (supraclavicular bruit) is a short systolic murmur heard best above the clavicles with minimal radiation to the neck. It is distinguished from aortic or pulmonary valve stenosis by the absence of an associated click and significant radiation to the neck. It is due to turbulence in the carotid arteries and may rarely be associated with a palpable thrill.

16 Congenital heart disease usually manifests in the first few days or weeks of life, depending on the lesion. Preductal and postductal pulse oximetry performed in newborn nurseries is identifying many cases of critical cardiac disease prior to symptom development. The development of a significant murmur in the neonatal period accompanied by cyanosis or congestive heart failure warrants an urgent evaluation. Congestive heart failure may manifest as poor feeding, disinterest in feeding, excessive fatigue, diaphoresis, and tachypnea or dyspnea. In cyanotic heart defects, a sudden deterioration in the first few days of life occurs coincident with the closing of the ductus. (See Chapter 14.) Many syndromes (e.g., Down, Turner, Williams) have characteristic cardiac anomalies.

Bibliography

Menashe V: Heart murmurs. *Pediatr Rev* 28(4):e19–22, 2007.
Park MK: Physical examination. In *Pediatric cardiology for practitioners*, St. Louis, 2008, Mosby.

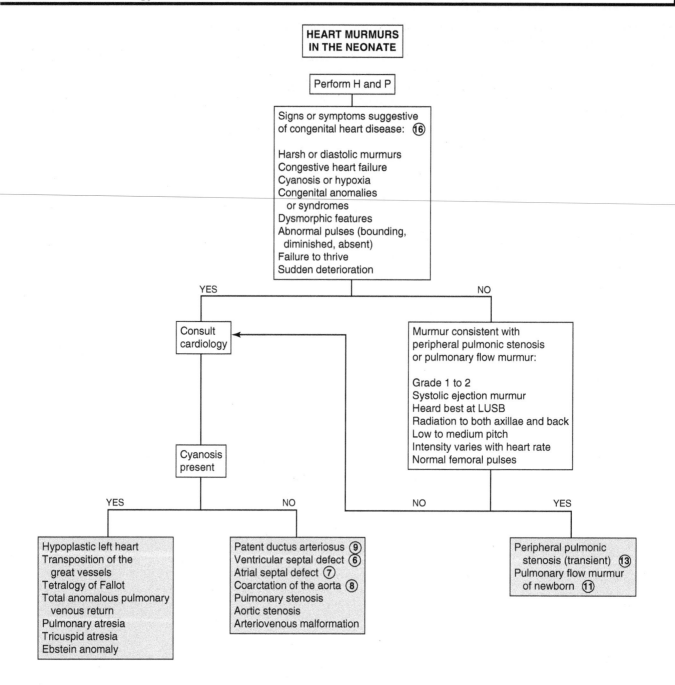

HEART MURMURS
IN THE NEONATE

Perform H and P

Signs or symptoms suggestive
of congenital heart disease: ⑯

Harsh or diastolic murmurs
Congestive heart failure
Cyanosis or hypoxia
Congenital anomalies
   or syndromes
Dysmorphic features
Abnormal pulses (bounding,
   diminished, absent)
Failure to thrive
Sudden deterioration

YES   NO

Consult
cardiology

Murmur consistent with
peripheral pulmonic stenosis
or pulmonary flow murmur:

Grade 1 to 2
Systolic ejection murmur
Heard best at LUSB
Radiation to both axillae and back
Low to medium pitch
Intensity varies with heart rate
Normal femoral pulses

Cyanosis
present

YES   NO   NO   YES

Hypoplastic left heart
Transposition of the
   great vessels
Tetralogy of Fallot
Total anomalous pulmonary
   venous return
Pulmonary atresia
Tricuspid atresia
Ebstein anomaly

Patent ductus arteriosus ⑨
Ventricular septal defect ⑥
Atrial septal defect ⑦
Coarctation of the aorta ⑧
Pulmonary stenosis
Aortic stenosis
Arteriovenous malformation

Peripheral pulmonic
   stenosis (transient) ⑬
Pulmonary flow murmur
   of newborn ⑪

Gastrointestinal System

Chapter 21
ABDOMINAL PAIN

Abdominal pain is a symptom of multiple disorders; this chapter includes disorders in which it is a predominant symptom. In children younger than 2 years, an organic cause of recurrent pain is more likely than a nonorganic cause.

1 A history of the nature and progression of abdominal pain is very helpful in arriving at a diagnosis but often difficult to obtain, especially in young children. Young patients may assume a protective posture and protect themselves from movement or cough, which may exacerbate the pain. The history should include a thorough review of symptoms, including a complete medication and diet history.

A thorough unhurried physical examination is essential in the evaluation of the child with abdominal pain. Inspection may reveal pallor, distention, jaundice, or pain with movement. A pelvic examination should be considered in any sexually active female (and may be helpful regardless of the patient's sexual history). A rectal examination should be performed unless the diagnosis is obvious.

Certain underlying medical conditions predispose a child to problems that may present primarily as abdominal pain. A child with sickle cell anemia is at risk for vasoocclusive crises, splenic sequestration, and cholelithiasis. Bacterial peritonitis should be carefully considered with nephrotic syndrome or cirrhosis. Children with previous surgeries may have strictures or adhesions that may cause obstructive symptoms.

2 The first challenge to the practitioner is to identify those cases that may be surgical or life threatening. Certain historical and physical criteria suggest an acute or surgical problem and mandate immediate surgical consultation. Worrisome signs and symptoms include sudden excruciating pain, point or diffuse severe tenderness on examination, bilious vomiting, involuntary guarding, a rigid voluntary wall, and rebound tenderness. After ruling out potential emergencies, the chronicity and location of the complaint should be considered to narrow the diagnosis.

3 US is a useful diagnostic aid for suspected disorders related to the gallbladder, pancreas, and urinary tract and for any abdominal mass. It provides a good assessment of the female reproductive organs and can also be used to visualize the appendix.

4 Acute pancreatitis presents as an intense, steady, epigastric and periumbilical pain that may radiate to the back. Bilious vomiting and fever may occur. Affected children look ill and often assume a knee-to-chest posture while sitting or lying on their side. The etiology may include trauma (including abuse), infection, congenital anomalies, medications, or systemic disorders (e.g., cystic fibrosis, diabetes mellitus, hemoglobinopathies); children dependent on total parenteral nutrition are also at risk due to gallstones. Diagnosis may be confirmed by an elevated amylase or lipase level; amylase may be normal initially (in 10% to 15% of cases); it normalizes sooner than lipase. US and CT are helpful imaging studies for confirming the diagnosis and in followup.

5 Cholelithiasis is characterized by episodic severe right upper quadrant pain that may radiate to the angle of the scapula or back. Risk factors include total parenteral nutrition, hemolytic disease, and cholestatic liver disease. Patients appear agitated and uncomfortable and may exhibit pallor, jaundice, tachycardia, nausea, weakness, and diaphoresis. On examination the tenderness is localized deep in the right upper quadrant. If superficial tenderness is present, an accompanying cholecystitis is suggested. Laboratory findings include elevated direct bilirubin and serum alkaline phosphatase levels. US is the preferred diagnostic imaging study.

6 Lower lobe pneumonia may present as abdominal pain and occasional vomiting. Cough may or may not be significant. In these cases the abdominal examination is nonspecific, but the lung examination should suggest the diagnosis.

7 X-ray studies are of limited usefulness in the routine evaluation of abdominal pain. KUB views (upright and lateral) are most likely to be helpful when suspected diagnoses include intestinal obstruction, renal or biliary tract calculi, calcified fecaliths, or intestinal perforation (e.g., pneumoperitoneum, free air). Ileus (i.e., diminished peristalsis in the absence of obstruction) occurs with infection, abdominal surgery, and metabolic abnormalities; it is demonstrated as multiple air-fluid levels on plain films. Plain films may also reveal large amounts of stool in the colon (often an incidental finding; should not always be presumed to be the cause of the pain).

8 Always consider obtaining a pregnancy test in an adolescent female with lower or diffuse abdominal pain. This should be done prior to imaging (x-ray or CT).

9 Appendicitis is a difficult diagnosis. It often presents as a nonspecific intermittent periumbilical pain. Nausea, anorexia, low-grade fever, and vomiting may occur. Diarrhea (small volume) and urinary frequency or dysuria may also occur. The pain gradually intensifies and shifts to the right lower quadrant (McBurney's point), usually within several hours of onset (but may take up to 3 days). Be aware that an atypical location of the appendix may cause pain in sites other than the right lower quadrant. The occurrence of emesis before pain makes the diagnosis of appendicitis unlikely. The total WBC count may be normal or elevated; a left shift is supportive of the diagnosis. UA may be normal or reveal some RBCs and WBCs. US or CT may aid in the diagnosis, although in many cases, observation and serial examinations will be the most useful diagnostic entities.

10 Mesenteric adenitis mimics appendicitis. Inflamed abdominal lymph nodes occur as a result of viral (adenovirus, measles) or bacterial (*Yersinia*) infections; diagnosis may be aided by accompanying upper respiratory symptoms, conjunctivitis, or pharyngitis. US or CT may make the diagnosis.

11 Acute unilateral back or flank pain, fever, dysuria, pyuria, and urinary frequency suggest pyelonephritis. Usually UA and culture is all that is needed to make a diagnosis. In certain circumstances, US obtained acutely may suggest pyelonephritis or identify obstructions or abscesses. A dimercaptosuccinic acid (DMSA) scan is a more sensitive test for pyelonephritis but is usually not needed if other diagnoses are being considered. CT can also be helpful.

12 The minimal diagnostic criteria for pelvic inflammatory disease include lower abdominal pain, adnexal tenderness,

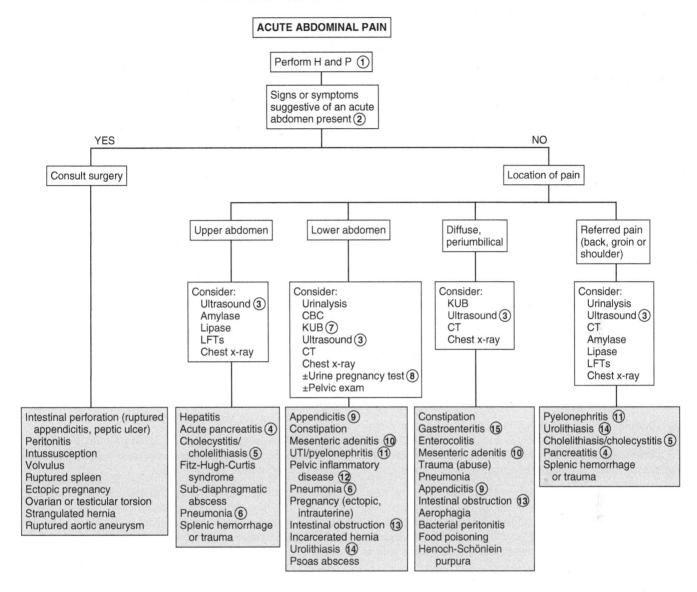

ACUTE ABDOMINAL PAIN

Perform H and P ①

Signs or symptoms suggestive of an acute abdomen present ②

YES — Consult surgery

NO — Location of pain

Upper abdomen

Consider:
Ultrasound ③
Amylase
Lipase
LFTs
Chest x-ray

Lower abdomen

Consider:
Urinalysis
CBC
KUB ⑦
Ultrasound ③
CT
Chest x-ray
±Urine pregnancy test ⑧
±Pelvic exam

Diffuse, periumbilical

Consider:
KUB
Ultrasound ③
CT
Chest x-ray

Referred pain (back, groin or shoulder)

Consider:
Urinalysis
Ultrasound ③
CT
Amylase
Lipase
LFTs
Chest x-ray

Intestinal perforation (ruptured appendicitis, peptic ulcer)
Peritonitis
Intussusception
Volvulus
Ruptured spleen
Ectopic pregnancy
Ovarian or testicular torsion
Strangulated hernia
Ruptured aortic aneurysm

Hepatitis
Acute pancreatitis ④
Cholecystitis/cholelithiasis ⑤
Fitz-Hugh-Curtis syndrome
Sub-diaphragmatic abscess
Pneumonia ⑥
Splenic hemorrhage or trauma

Appendicitis ⑨
Constipation
Mesenteric adenitis ⑩
UTI/pyelonephritis ⑪
Pelvic inflammatory disease ⑫
Pneumonia ⑥
Pregnancy (ectopic, intrauterine)
Intestinal obstruction ⑬
Incarcerated hernia
Urolithiasis ⑭
Psoas abscess

Constipation
Gastroenteritis ⑮
Enterocolitis
Mesenteric adenitis ⑩
Trauma (abuse)
Pneumonia
Appendicitis ⑨
Intestinal obstruction ⑬
Aerophagia
Bacterial peritonitis
Food poisoning
Henoch-Schönlein purpura

Pyelonephritis ⑪
Urolithiasis ⑭
Cholelithiasis/cholecystitis ⑤
Pancreatitis ④
Splenic hemorrhage or trauma

Nelson Textbook of Pediatrics, 19e. Chapters 298, 334
Nelsons Essentials, 6e. Chapter 126

or cervical motion tenderness. Additional diagnostic criteria include fever (>38.3°C [101°F]), abnormal cervical or vaginal discharge, elevated CRP or ESR, and positive cervical cultures for *Neisseria gonorrhoeae* or *Chlamydia trachomatis*. The role of US is not so much for definitive diagnosis as to identify tubo-ovarian abscesses, a common complication of pelvic inflammatory disease.

13 In intestinal obstruction, vomiting is usually a predominant symptom. Pain is a later finding and is crampy or colicky, and rushes of high-pitched "tinkling" bowel sounds may be noted. Plain x-ray films (KUB view) may reveal air-fluid levels or distended bowel loops above the obstruction; free air indicates an intestinal perforation. Contrast medium studies may aid in definitive diagnosis if malrotation or volvulus, distal small bowel obstruction, or intussusception is suspected.

14 Urolithiasis (i.e., kidney stones) presents as hematuria and acute colicky abdominal, flank, or back pain. The pain may radiate to the upper leg and groin. US and helical CT will detect both radiopaque and radiolucent stones.

15 When acute gastroenteritis is suggested based on a clinical presentation of vomiting and diarrhea preceding the complaint of diffuse abdominal pain and in the absence of any signs or symptoms of an acute abdomen, no additional workup is indicated. Parents should be counseled about worrisome signs and symptoms and supportive measures.

16 Chronic or recurrent abdominal pain is defined by recurrent or persistent bouts of pain that occur over a minimum of 3 months and may or may not interfere with daily activities. Chronic pain may be organic, nonorganic, or psychogenic.

17 If the diagnosis is in doubt, an abdominal film may help. Constipation is the most common cause of chronic and recurrent abdominal pain in children. It causes colonic distension and painful defecation. It may be functional or organic. However, presence of stool does not always mean the pain is from constipation.

18 Elements of the H and P examination that suggest an organic cause of abdominal pain include fever, weight loss or growth deceleration, joint symptoms, emesis (especially if blood or bile-stained), abnormal findings on physical examination (e.g., abdominal mass, perianal disease), and blood in the stool or other abnormal results of laboratory studies. An organic cause should be considered for pain or diarrhea that awakens a child from sleep, pain that is well localized away from the umbilicus, and pain that is referred to the back, flank, or shoulders.

19 Functional abdominal pain is the most common diagnosis after organic causes have been ruled out. It describes a pain that does not have a clear structural or biochemical basis but is recognized as genuine pain. Characteristics include onset at age older than 5 years, intermittent or episodic nature, periumbilical location, and a lack of association with activity, meals, or bowel pattern. The physical examination is always normal (although patients may appear tired or pale during episodes), and results of laboratory studies are normal. The entity remains a common yet poorly explained affliction of childhood.

20 Functional dyspepsia describes pain and discomfort in the upper abdomen. It is characterized by epigastric pain accompanied by early satiety, bloating, belching, and nausea or occasionally vomiting. One needs to rule out other diseases such as gastritis, ulcer, and eosinophilic gastroenteritis. Diagnosis is based on the presence of these symptoms of peptic ulcer disease in the presence of normal findings on upper endoscopy.

21 Inflammatory bowel disease is an important diagnosis to exclude when faced with the child with chronic abdominal pain. A thorough evaluation, including H and P and screening laboratory studies, will often suggest the disorder. Additional signs and symptoms that suggest inflammatory bowel disease are anorexia, growth failure, perianal disease, hematochezia, and diarrhea. The pain and diarrhea may awaken the child at night. Supportive laboratory results include anemia, increased ESR or CRP, thrombocytosis, hypoalbuminemia, heme-positive stools, and elevated stool calprotectin levels. Contrast medium studies (UGI series with small bowel follow-through) and barium enema may be helpful, although MRI enterography is often used because of concerns about radiation. CT with oral contrast can be helpful if an abscess is suspected. Endoscopy should be done for definitive diagnosis.

22 Celiac disease, or gluten-sensitive enteropathy, is becoming increasingly recognized as a cause of chronic abdominal pain. There is inflammation of the small intestine due to exposure to dietary gluten. It classically presents with diarrhea, steatorrhea, anemia, abdominal distention, failure to thrive, and often with nonspecific abdominal complaints. The tissue transglutaminase (tTG) antibody enzyme-linked immunoassay is a good screening test for celiac disease.

23 GER esophagitis in older children presents as substernal pain, increased pain after meals or when recumbent, and relief from pain with use of antacids.

24 Peptic ulcer disease includes gastric and duodenal ulcers, gastritis, and duodenitis. Unlike the classic adult presentation of epigastric pain, exacerbation with meals, and early morning occurrence, in children the pain may be more diffuse (epigastric or periumbilical) and unrelated to meals or time of day. If clinical presentation is consistent with the diagnosis, improvement with a trial of therapy is often diagnostic. If symptoms do not respond to treatment, a search for *Helicobacter pylori* with a urea breath test, serum antibodies, or stool antigens may be indicated. However, endoscopy with biopsy is the most reliable method.

25 Chronic pancreatitis is a rare cause of recurrent abdominal pain in children. Children experience intermittent epigastric abdominal pain, often with associated nausea and vomiting; symptoms are frequently precipitated by a large meal or stress. Serum lipase and amylase levels are not as likely to be elevated as with acute cases. US and CT may aid in diagnosis; x-ray studies may reveal calcifications consistent with chronic pancreatitis.

26 Irritable bowel syndrome is characterized by abdominal pain or discomfort and a variable defecation pattern. Bloating, flatulence, and mucus may be present. Either diarrhea or constipation may predominate in the disorder; the abdominal pain is usually relieved by defecation.

27 Lactose malabsorption causes symptoms of abdominal pain and cramping, bloating, diarrhea, and excess flatulence. In primary adult-type hypolactasia, symptoms may not develop until 3 to 5 years of age when lactase levels begin to decline. Breath hydrogen testing after an oral lactose load will make the diagnosis,

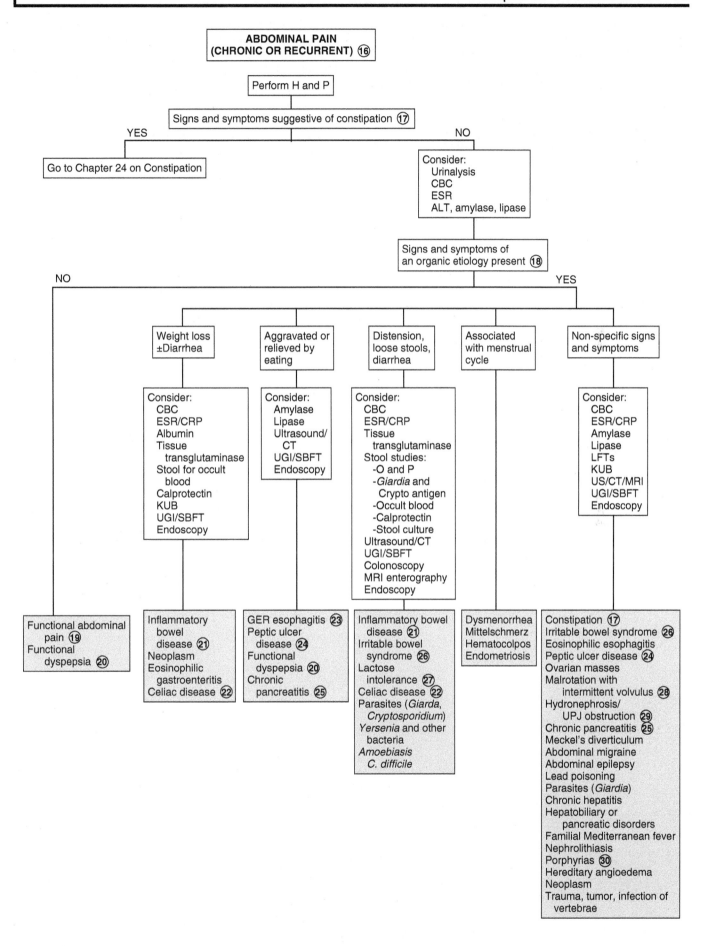

although resolution of symptoms after dietary restriction of lactose is strongly suggestive. Malabsorption of fructose and sorbitol may also cause symptoms of GI distress; a history of high fruit juice ingestion suggests the former, and frequent use of "sugar-free" products (sorbitol-containing) should raise suspicion of the latter.

28 A UGI series with small bowel follow-through is required to diagnose most cases of malrotation.

29 Ureteropelvic junction obstruction is an uncommon disorder, often presenting as abdominal pain in children and adolescents. Diagnosis in infants is often assisted by the presence of an abdominal mass or occurrence of a UTI. In older children, the physical examination and UA may be normal or may reveal a unilateral abdominal mass or hematuria. The chief complaint in over 70% of children older than 6 years with ureteropelvic junction obstruction is abdominal pain that is frequently referred to the groin or flank. In older children the disorder most commonly occurs in males and is on the left side. Symptoms tend to predominate during periods of fluid loading and diuresis. US is recommended if obstruction is suspected.

30 Acute intermittent porphyria is the most common of the porphyrias. It generally presents as abdominal pain; peripheral neuropathies are also common. In severe cases the urine may turn a port wine color. The diagnosis is made by demonstrating decreased porphobilinogen deaminase in erythrocytes and increased urinary levels of aminolevulinic acid and porphobilinogen.

Bibliography

Mahajan LA, Kaplan B: Chronic abdominal pain of childhood and adolescence. In Wyllie R, Hyams J, editors: *Pediatric gastrointestinal and liver disease,* ed 4, Philadelphia, 2010, WB Saunders, pp 64.

Ross A, LeLeiko NS: Acute abdominal pain, *Pediatr Rev* 31:135–144, 2010.

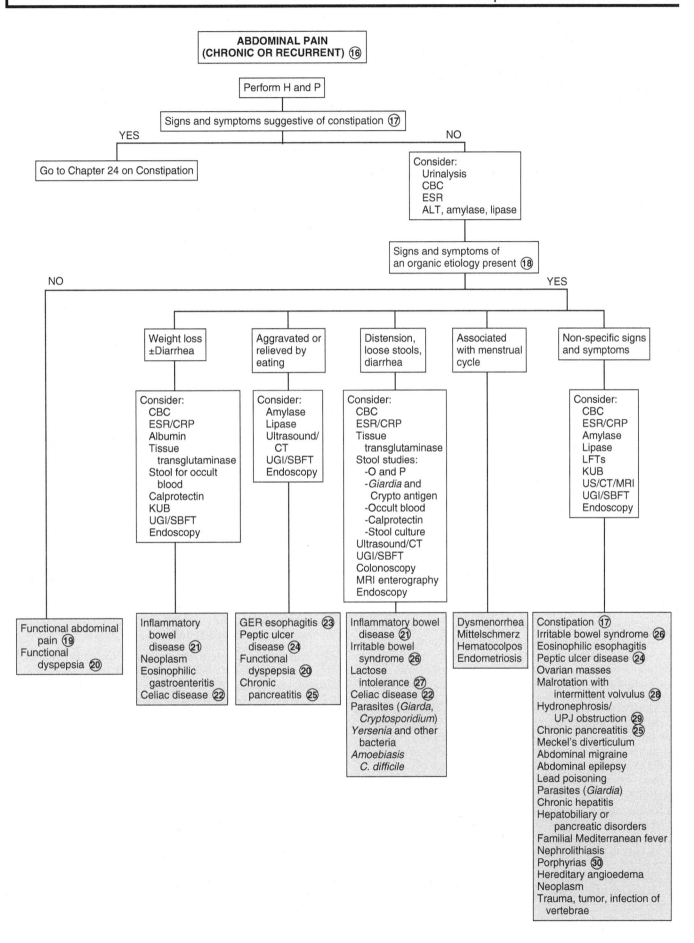

ABDOMINAL PAIN (CHRONIC OR RECURRENT) ⑯

Perform H and P

Signs and symptoms suggestive of constipation ⑰

YES

Go to Chapter 24 on Constipation

NO

Consider:
Urinalysis
CBC
ESR
ALT, amylase, lipase

Signs and symptoms of an organic etiology present ⑱

NO

YES

Weight loss ±Diarrhea

Aggravated or relieved by eating

Distension, loose stools, diarrhea

Associated with menstrual cycle

Non-specific signs and symptoms

Consider:
CBC
ESR/CRP
Albumin
Tissue
   transglutaminase
Stool for occult
   blood
Calprotectin
KUB
UGI/SBFT
Endoscopy

Consider:
Amylase
Lipase
Ultrasound/
   CT
UGI/SBFT
Endoscopy

Consider:
CBC
ESR/CRP
Tissue
   transglutaminase
Stool studies:
-O and P
-*Giardia* and
   Crypto antigen
-Occult blood
-Calprotectin
-Stool culture
Ultrasound/CT
UGI/SBFT
Colonoscopy
MRI enterography
Endoscopy

Consider:
CBC
ESR/CRP
Amylase
Lipase
LFTs
KUB
US/CT/MRI
UGI/SBFT
Endoscopy

Functional abdominal
   pain ⑲
Functional
   dyspepsia ⑳

Inflammatory
   bowel
   disease ㉑
Neoplasm
Eosinophilic
   gastroenteritis
Celiac disease ㉒

GER esophagitis ㉓
Peptic ulcer
   disease ㉔
Functional
   dyspepsia ⑳
Chronic
   pancreatitis ㉕

Inflammatory bowel
   disease ㉑
Irritable bowel
   syndrome ㉖
Lactose
   intolerance ㉗
Celiac disease ㉒
Parasites (*Giarda*,
   Cryptosporidium)
Yersenia and other
   bacteria
Amoebiasis
   C. difficile

Dysmenorrhea
Mittelschmerz
Hematocolpos
Endometriosis

Constipation ⑰
Irritable bowel syndrome ㉖
Eosinophilic esophagitis
Peptic ulcer disease ㉔
Ovarian masses
Malrotation with
   intermittent volvulus ㉘
Hydronephrosis/
   UPJ obstruction ㉙
Chronic pancreatitis ㉕
Meckel's diverticulum
Abdominal migraine
Abdominal epilepsy
Lead poisoning
Parasites (*Giardia*)
Chronic hepatitis
Hepatobiliary or
   pancreatic disorders
Familial Mediterranean fever
Nephrolithiasis
Porphyrias ㉚
Hereditary angioedema
Neoplasm
Trauma, tumor, infection of
   vertebrae

Chapter 22
VOMITING

True vomiting is a forceful ejection of stomach or esophageal contents from the mouth. It is often accompanied by nausea and retching. Regurgitation is an effortless or near effortless ejection and is not true emesis. Rumination is regurgitation with rechewing of food.

1. Vomiting should be approached by first identifying the pattern of vomiting. The review of systems should include other abdominal, respiratory, and neurologic complaints. Inquire about diet and medication use. In cases of chronic recurrent vomiting, the frequency is generally greater than two episodes; children are generally not acutely ill and vomit with a low intensity. In cyclic recurrent vomiting, episodes are infrequent ($\leq$2/week) but are characterized by acute severity and illness and forceful vomiting occurring at a high frequency (i.e., >4 to 6 times/h). Autonomic signs and symptoms such as pallor, lethargy, nausea, and abdominal pain are frequently associated. Initially, chronic and cyclic vomiting may appear to be acute problems until the pattern becomes evident. It is important to exclude pregnancy in a sexually active adolescent female.

2. When acute vomiting occurs in the context of an acute abdomen, immediate surgical consultation should be obtained. Signs and symptoms of an acute abdomen include sudden severe pain, bilious vomiting, point or diffuse tenderness on examination, diarrhea with abdominal distention, absent bowel sounds, involuntary guarding, rebound tenderness, a rigid abdomen, and pain with movement or cough.

3. Signs or symptoms suggestive of increased ICP include early morning occurrence, progressive headaches, absence of nausea, abnormal funduscopic examination, or a bulging fontanel in infants. A few causes are listed in the algorithm.

4. Volvulus, the twisting of bowel on the mesentery, generally occurs in the context of congenital intestinal malrotation. Many cases of malrotation present as volvulus (e.g., bilious vomiting, severe clinical toxicity) in the newborn period. Other cases present many years later as intermittent vomiting.

5. Obstruction can occur at any level of the GI tract and can appear as a surgical emergency or a chronic complaint of abdominal pain or vomiting. Congenital lesions (e.g., esophageal stenosis, volvulus, duodenal webs, annular pancreas) usually occur acutely in the newborn period but may occur later if the obstruction is partial. Many disorders (e.g., inflammatory bowel disease, mucosal disease, postoperative adhesions) may result in acquired obstructive lesions. Plain abdominal x-rays are recommended initially. US, CT, or fluoroscopy may provide a more definitive diagnosis but may not be necessary or recommended if a need for surgery has already been established.

6. Abdominal trauma occasionally results in an obstructive duodenal hematoma. Child abuse and seat belt injuries are recognized causes.

7. Superior mesenteric artery syndrome describes a condition of transient duodenal obstruction due to a trapping or compression in the duodenum by the superior mesenteric artery anteriorly and the aorta posteriorly. Clinically, bilious vomiting and epigastric pain occur and are relieved by a prone or knee-chest position. The condition is most commonly seen in cases of recent weight loss, lordosis, prolonged bed rest, or body casting.

8. In a child with acute-onset, large-volume emesis, fever, and/or diarrhea—a picture consistent with acute gastroenteritis—additional workup may not be necessary. With rotavirus in particular, vomiting often precedes diarrhea by 1 to 2 days. In other cases of acute severe vomiting, laboratory tests and a UA may aid in the assessment of dehydration and possible diagnosis. Further studies should be ordered based on suspected diagnoses.

9. Pyloric stenosis presents as nonbilious vomiting in the first few weeks of life and progresses in frequency and intensity. Clinical characteristics include projectile vomiting, later onset of "coffee ground" emesis (hematemesis), and poor weight gain. Patients are often dehydrated, with a metabolic alkalosis and hypochloremia by the time they present. Diagnosis is by physical examination and by US or a UGI study that shows the "string sign" of contrast medium through the narrowed pylorus.

10. Sinusitis may cause an acute, chronic, or cyclic pattern of vomiting. Associated nausea, congestion, postnasal drip, and early morning occurrence often preceded by coughing suggest the diagnosis.

11. Mental status changes and abnormal respirations may indicate ingestion of a toxic drug or poison.

12. Ureteropelvic junction obstruction results in hydronephrosis during fluid loading and diuresis. Congenital cases appear as an abdominal mass or UTI. Older children tend to present with intermittent abdominal or flank pain and often with vomiting. The physical examination and urinalysis may be normal or may reveal a unilateral abdominal mass or hematuria. A history of spontaneous resolution after several hours because of relief of the renal pelvic distention as dehydration develops is suggestive. US during an acute episode or after furosemide or an IV pyelogram should help provide the diagnosis.

13. Most inborn errors of metabolism appear early in the newborn period with vomiting and failure to thrive. Some disorders occur as chronic or cyclic vomiting at later ages after the addition of certain foods to the diet or in the context of acute stresses or illnesses. These children may experience acute intermittent episodes of vomiting accompanied by acidosis, mental deterioration, and coma. There may be a family history of the disorder or of unexplained mental retardation, failure to thrive, or neonatal deaths.

Consider a metabolic workup whenever neurologic symptoms (e.g., altered mental status, hypotonia, seizures, unexplained mental retardation), hepatosplenomegaly, or unusual odors (e.g., from breath, urine, ear wax) are present. For a metabolic workup, blood and urine should be obtained during episodes of suggestive symptoms. Blood tests should include a CBC, electrolytes, pH, glucose, ammonia, lactate, carnitine, acyl carnitine, and serum amino acids. Urine should be analyzed for ketones, reducing substances, organic acids, and amino acids.

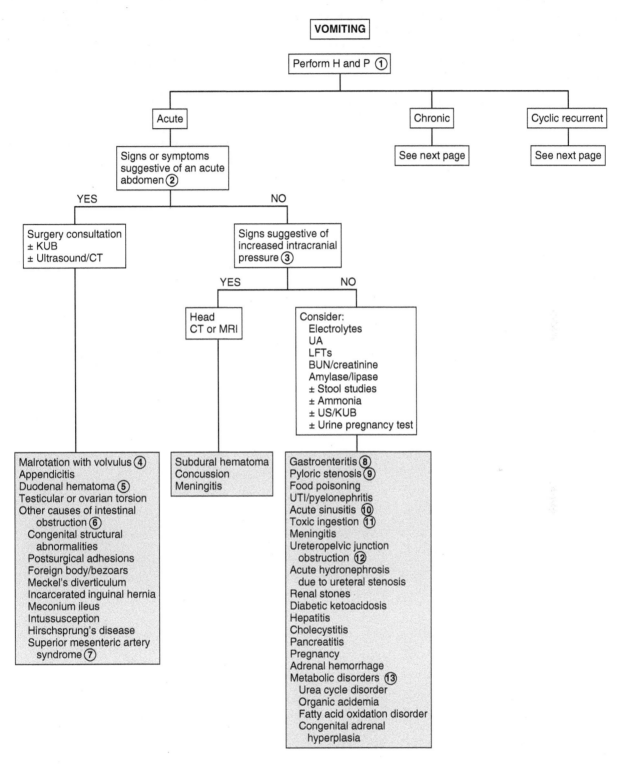

VOMITING

Perform H and P ①

Acute

Chronic
See next page

Cyclic recurrent
See next page

Signs or symptoms suggestive of an acute abdomen ②

YES

Surgery consultation
± KUB
± Ultrasound/CT

NO

Signs suggestive of increased intracranial pressure ③

YES

Head CT or MRI

NO

Consider:
  Electrolytes
  UA
  LFTs
  BUN/creatinine
  Amylase/lipase
  ± Stool studies
  ± Ammonia
  ± US/KUB
  ± Urine pregnancy test

Malrotation with volvulus ④
Appendicitis
Duodenal hematoma ⑤
Testicular or ovarian torsion
Other causes of intestinal
    obstruction ⑥
  Congenital structural
      abnormalities
  Postsurgical adhesions
  Foreign body/bezoars
  Meckel's diverticulum
  Incarcerated inguinal hernia
  Meconium ileus
  Intussusception
  Hirschsprung's disease
  Superior mesenteric artery
      syndrome ⑦

Subdural hematoma
Concussion
Meningitis

Gastroenteritis ⑧
Pyloric stenosis ⑨
Food poisoning
UTI/pyelonephritis
Acute sinusitis ⑩
Toxic ingestion ⑪
Meningitis
Ureteropelvic junction
    obstruction ⑫
Acute hydronephrosis
    due to ureteral stenosis
Renal stones
Diabetic ketoacidosis
Hepatitis
Cholecystitis
Pancreatitis
Pregnancy
Adrenal hemorrhage
Metabolic disorders ⑬
  Urea cycle disorder
  Organic acidemia
  Fatty acid oxidation disorder
  Congenital adrenal
      hyperplasia

Nelson Textbook of Pediatrics, 19e. Chapters 92, 96, 316, 321, 343, 491, 588
Nelsons Essentials, 6e. Chapter 126

(14) In infants, GER appears as a near effortless regurgitation. Infants may be irritable and demonstrate poor weight gain, apnea, or Sandifer syndrome (arching). Older children may complain of effortless vomiting, substernal pain, dysphagia, exacerbation with certain foods, and relief with liquid antacids. When clinical suspicion is present without life-threatening symptoms (i.e., apnea), a trial of an H_2 blocker or proton pump inhibitor may be diagnostic. The occurrence of apnea often prompts additional study.

(15) The presentation of peptic ulcer disease (gastritis, duodenitis, and gastric and duodenal ulcers) may be classic, including epigastric pain, nocturnal awakening, evidence of GI bleeding, relief or exacerbation with meals, or nonspecific, especially in young children. A history of peptic ulcer disease or similar symptoms in family members should prompt a urea breath test or stool antigen assay to look for *Helicobacter pylori*. *H. pylori* antibodies can be tested for but are less useful than the urea breath test for diagnosis. Endoscopy should be considered if symptoms are atypical or there is no response to therapy.

(16) Eosinophilic esophagitis presents with vomiting, feeding problems, pain, and dysphagia. Many patients have other associated atopic diseases.

(17) Vomiting may be a sign of food hypersensitivity (e.g., food protein enterocolitis syndrome, food protein enteropathy). It is commonly due to cow's milk or soy protein. Immunoglobulin (Ig)E-mediated food allergies may also present with vomiting. It may also occur as a sign of a specific disorder (e.g., hereditary fructose intolerance, celiac disease) that becomes evident after the introduction of certain foods.

(18) Gastric stasis and paralytic ileus may be postsurgical or due to a neuropathy or drugs, electrolyte disturbances, endocrinopathies, or injuries. Pseudo-obstruction is a rare chronic disorder of intermittent episodes of ileus. Causes are primarily neuropathic or myopathic. There is often a family history. Manometer and biopsy may be necessary for definitive diagnosis.

(19) Psychogenic vomiting should only be diagnosed after organic causes have been ruled out. Diagnostic advances (e.g., endoscopy with biopsy, motility studies) are responsible for a declining number of diagnoses of psychogenic causes. Patients are often anxious, affected by familial conflict, and not bothered by the vomiting.

(20) Nausea, dizziness, vertigo, and nystagmus characterize vestibular disorders, including motion sickness.

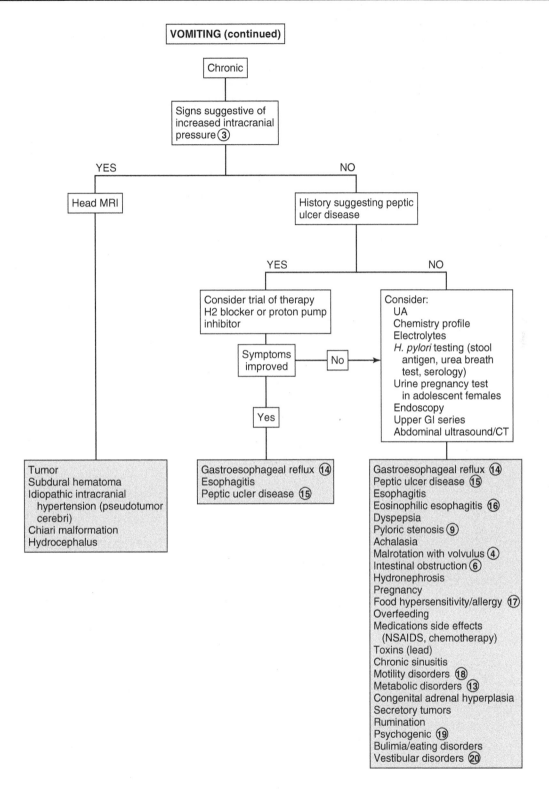

VOMITING (continued)

Chronic

Signs suggestive of
increased intracranial
pressure ③

YES — Head MRI

NO — History suggesting peptic
ulcer disease

YES — Consider trial of therapy
H2 blocker or proton pump
inhibitor

Symptoms
improved

No → Consider:
    UA
    Chemistry profile
    Electrolytes
    H. pylori testing (stool
        antigen, urea breath
        test, serology)
    Urine pregnancy test
        in adolescent females
    Endoscopy
    Upper GI series
    Abdominal ultrasound/CT

Yes

Tumor
Subdural hematoma
Idiopathic intracranial
    hypertension (pseudotumor
    cerebri)
Chiari malformation
Hydrocephalus

Gastroesophageal reflux ⑭
Esophagitis
Peptic ucler disease ⑮

Gastroesophageal reflux ⑭
Peptic ulcer disease ⑮
Esophagitis
Eosinophilic esophagitis ⑯
Dyspepsia
Pyloric stenosis ⑨
Achalasia
Malrotation with volvulus ④
Intestinal obstruction ⑥
Hydronephrosis
Pregnancy
Food hypersensitivity/allergy ⑰
Overfeeding
Medications side effects
    (NSAIDS, chemotherapy)
Toxins (lead)
Chronic sinusitis
Motility disorders ⑱
Metabolic disorders ⑬
Congenital adrenal hyperplasia
Secretory tumors
Rumination
Psychogenic ⑲
Bulimia/eating disorders
Vestibular disorders ⑳

Nelson Textbook of Pediatrics, 19e. Chapters 92, 96, 316, 321, 343, 491, 588
Nelsons Essentials, 6e. Chapter 126

21 In abdominal migraines, pain is the predominant symptom, and in cyclic vomiting syndrome, the vomiting is predominant. In reality, abdominal migraine and cyclic vomiting syndrome often have overlapping symptoms. Characteristics of abdominal migraine include recurrent stereotypical episodes of midline abdominal pain lasting more than 6 hours, associated pallor, lethargy, anorexia, nausea, and normal laboratory values, as well as radiographic and endoscopic studies. The typical migraine symptoms of headache and photophobia only occur in 30% to 40% of children with the abdominal symptoms. The vomiting pattern is replaced by the more typical headaches as the child gets older.

22 Cyclic vomiting syndrome is characterized by recurrent stereotypical episodes of prolonged vomiting accompanied by pallor, lethargy, anorexia, nausea, retching, and abdominal pain. These children present with a recurrent history of these episodes, with normal health in between. A family history of migraine may be absent, and results of laboratory, radiographic, and endoscopic studies are normal.

Criteria for cyclic vomiting syndrome include: (1) at least 5 attacks in any interval, or a minimum of 3 attacks during a 6-month period, (2) episodic attacks of intense nausea and vomiting lasting 1 hour to 10 days and occurring at least 1 week apart, (2) stereotypical pattern and symptoms in the individual patient, (3) vomiting during attacks occurs at least 4 times per hour for at least 1 hour, (4) return to baseline health between episodes, (5) not attributed to another disorder.

Bibliography

Li BUK, Sunku BK: Vomiting and nausea. In Wyllie R, Hyams J, editors: *Pediatric gastrointestinal and liver disease,* ed 4, Philadelphia, 2010, WB Saunders, 2010, pp 64.

Li BUK, Lefevre F, Chelimsky GG, et al: North American Society for Pediatric Gastroenterology, Hepatology, and Nutrition consensus statement on the diagnosis and management of cyclic vomiting syndrome, *J Pediatr Gastroenterol Nutr* 43:379–393, 2008.

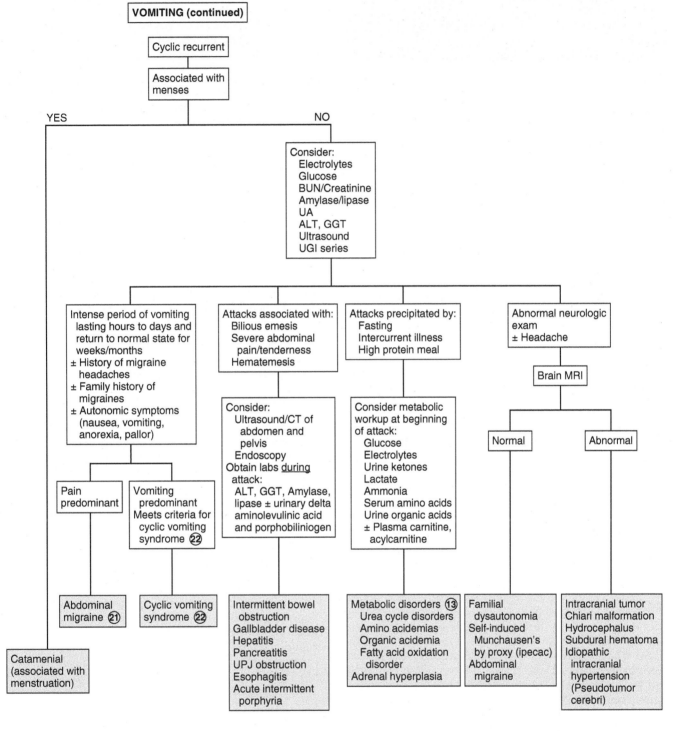

VOMITING (continued)

Cyclic recurrent

Associated with menses

YES — NO

Consider:
Electrolytes
Glucose
BUN/Creatinine
Amylase/lipase
UA
ALT, GGT
Ultrasound
UGI series

Intense period of vomiting lasting hours to days and return to normal state for weeks/months
± History of migraine headaches
± Family history of migraines
± Autonomic symptoms (nausea, vomiting, anorexia, pallor)

Attacks associated with:
Bilious emesis
Severe abdominal pain/tenderness
Hematemesis

Attacks precipitated by:
Fasting
Intercurrent illness
High protein meal

Abnormal neurologic exam
± Headache

Brain MRI

Pain predominant

Vomiting predominant
Meets criteria for cyclic vomiting syndrome ㉒

Consider:
Ultrasound/CT of abdomen and pelvis
Endoscopy
Obtain labs during attack:
ALT, GGT, Amylase, lipase ± urinary delta aminolevulinic acid and porphobiliniogen

Consider metabolic workup at beginning of attack:
Glucose
Electrolytes
Urine ketones
Lactate
Ammonia
Serum amino acids
Urine organic acids
± Plasma carnitine, acylcarnitine

Normal

Abnormal

Abdominal migraine ㉑

Cyclic vomiting syndrome ㉒

Intermittent bowel obstruction
Gallbladder disease
Hepatitis
Pancreatitis
UPJ obstruction
Esophagitis
Acute intermittent porphyria

Metabolic disorders ⑬
Urea cycle disorders
Amino acidemias
Organic acidemia
Fatty acid oxidation disorder
Adrenal hyperplasia

Familial dysautonomia
Self-induced Munchausen's by proxy (ipecac)
Abdominal migraine

Intracranial tumor
Chiari malformation
Hydrocephalus
Subdural hematoma
Idiopathic intracranial hypertension (Pseudotumor cerebri)

Catamenial (associated with menstruation)

Nelson Textbook of Pediatrics, 19e. Chapters 92, 96, 316, 321, 343, 491, 588
Nelsons Essentials, 6e. Chapter 126

Chapter 23
DIARRHEA

Diarrhea is defined as stools of increased frequency, fluidity, and volume. In young children most acute diarrhea is of infectious etiology and is self-limited. Diarrhea lasting longer than 2 weeks may be considered chronic.

1 The history should include associated symptoms as well as the child's growth pattern. A description of the diarrheal stool may help indicate the diagnosis. Watery diarrhea may be osmotic due to carbohydrate malabsorption or secretory due to toxins, gastrointestinal peptides, bile acids, or laxatives. Steatorrhea (greasy stools) indicates fat malabsorption (e.g., pancreatic insufficiency). Mucus and blood in stools indicate intestinal inflammation (e.g., infection, inflammatory bowel disease). In toddlers the presence of undigested food may indicate a normal variation or chronic nonspecific diarrhea ("toddler's diarrhea"). Overflow incontinence secondary to constipation and rectal impaction may be mistaken for diarrhea. Hematuria and abnormal renal function suggest an enterohemorrhagic strain of *Escherichia coli* (E. coli); an associated severe dermatitis (e.g., perioral, acral, perineal) should suggest acrodermatitis enteropathica. The social history should inquire about recent travel, exposure to unsanitary conditions, daycare attendance, risk factors for HIV, and sick contacts.

A diet history that includes seafood, unwashed vegetables, unpasteurized milk, contaminated water, or uncooked meats may suggest a foodborne or waterborne agent in acute cases of diarrhea. In chronic cases, assessing type and quantity of oral intake, especially fluid selection, is helpful because certain selections may exacerbate diarrhea symptoms by an osmotic load. Inquire whether the onset of symptoms coincided with a change in diet (e.g., discontinuation of breast milk or formula, addition of jar foods or cereals, addition of sugar-free or other sorbitol containing compounds).

2 Sudden vomiting and explosive diarrhea within several hours of ingestion of a contaminated food suggests food poisoning from pre-formed toxins produced by *Staphylococcus aureus* or *Bacillus cereus*. Other causes of foodborne illness include other bacteria (*Salmonella, Campylobacter, E. coli, Shigella*) and viruses. Heavy metals, fish or shellfish poisoning, and mushrooms may cause paresthesias, paralysis, or mental status changes in addition to diarrhea.

3 High fevers and seizures have been associated with *Shigella*. *E. coli* 0157:H7 (an enterohemorrhagic strain) causes a hemorrhagic colitis that is followed by hemolytic-uremic syndrome in approximately 10% of cases. Enteroinvasive *E. coli* may also cause bloody diarrhea. In hemolytic-uremic syndrome, watery diarrhea precedes the grossly bloody stools; abdominal cramping with minimal or absent fevers is characteristic. Undercooked beef is the most commonly identified source of outbreaks. Specific testing must be requested when the *E. coli* 0157:H7 strain is suspected. *Yersinia* and *Campylobacter* may be associated with a prolonged course of diarrhea. Bloody diarrhea is often seen with bacteria listed here, but diarrhea may also occur without blood.

4 Infection with *Clostridium difficile (C. difficile)* should be considered whenever diarrhea develops within several weeks of antibiotic treatment. It is uncommon in children less than one year. It may manifest as mild or severe illness with or without grossly bloody diarrhea, abdominal pain, fever, or systemic toxicity. Definitive diagnosis is detection of the *C. difficile* toxin in the stool. Caution is advised in interpretation of the test in infants less than 1 year old because the test may be positive in asymptomatic infants.

5 Food protein-induced enterocolitis syndrome due to cow and/or soy milk allergy or intolerance may present with bloody diarrhea in the first few months of life. Clinical improvement with a trial of a casein or whey hydrolysate formula or elimination of cow's milk from a breast-feeding mother's diet may be therapeutic and eliminate the need for any further evaluation. Early in infancy, food protein-induced enteropathy may present with diarrhea, occult blood loss, and hypoproteinemia.

6 Rotavirus is primarily a wintertime virus that affects infants and small children most often. Vomiting and diarrhea occur abruptly after a 2- to 3-day incubation period; the vomiting generally lasts 1 to 2 days, and loose watery stools last from 2 to 8 days. Fever commonly occurs; gross or occult blood is uncommon.

7 Giardiasis (from infection with *Giardia lamblia*) often results from contaminated food or water, but person-to-person spread is common, especially in daycare centers and other crowded institutions. It should be considered as an etiology in acute cases of diarrhea, although it is most frequently considered a pathogen in chronic diarrhea (i.e., watery, without blood or mucus) with associated weight loss and abdominal pain. Symptoms may also be intermittent and may even include constipation. Diagnosis may be difficult. Sensitivity of stool examination for ova and parasites increases with a greater number of samples. Examination of a single specimen is approximately 70% sensitive. Antigen tests are more sensitive but will not aid in identifying other protozoans. Small intestinal biopsy or aspiration of duodenal or jejunal contents for examination are other more sensitive means of diagnosis. *Cryptosporidium* may cause an acute diarrheal illness, including large watery stools, flatulence, malaise, and abdominal pain, lasting 3 to 30 days in a normal host. It causes a severe, chronic diarrheal illness in immunocompromised patients. It is associated with contact with farm animals or contaminated water but is also spread through person-to-person contact. The organism may be identified in the stool, by microscopy, or enzyme immunoassay.

8 Parenteral diarrhea refers to diarrhea accompanying an infection outside the GI tract. Diarrhea is frequently associated with upper respiratory infections, otitis media, and urinary tract infections. The mechanism is not clear.

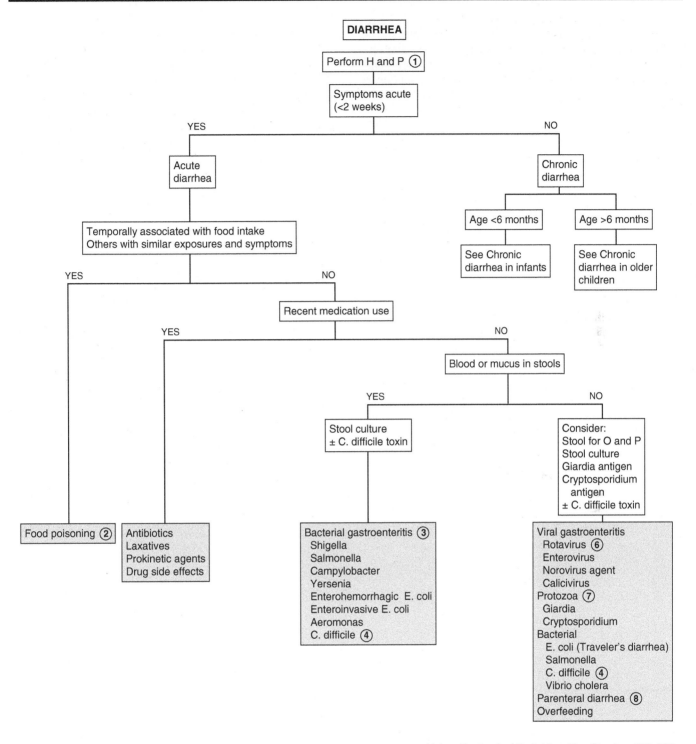

DIARRHEA

Perform H and P ①

Symptoms acute (<2 weeks)

YES → Acute diarrhea

NO → Chronic diarrhea

Chronic diarrhea:
- Age <6 months → See Chronic diarrhea in infants
- Age >6 months → See Chronic diarrhea in older children

Acute diarrhea → Temporally associated with food intake / Others with similar exposures and symptoms

YES → Food poisoning ②

NO → Recent medication use

YES → Antibiotics / Laxatives / Prokinetic agents / Drug side effects

NO → Blood or mucus in stools

YES → Stool culture ± C. difficile toxin

NO → Consider: Stool for O and P / Stool culture / Giardia antigen / Cryptosporidium antigen / ± C. difficile toxin

Bacterial gastroenteritis ③
Shigella
Salmonella
Campylobacter
Yersenia
Enterohemorrhagic E. coli
Enteroinvasive E. coli
Aeromonas
C. difficile ④

Viral gastroenteritis
Rotavirus ⑥
Enterovirus
Norovirus agent
Calicivirus
Protozoa ⑦
Giardia
Cryptosporidium
Bacterial
E. coli (Traveler's diarrhea)
Salmonella
C. difficile ④
Vibrio cholera
Parenteral diarrhea ⑧
Overfeeding

Nelson Textbook of Pediatrics, 19e. Chapters 332, 333
Nelsons Essentials, 6e. Chapter 126

9 Commercial reagents (Clinitest) are available to test for reducing substances; pH testing with Nitrazine paper should be performed on a fresh stool specimen. Positive reducing substances or a pH less than 5.5 suggests carbohydrate malabsorption. Be aware of two caveats: (1) the test for reducing substances is only reliable when the child is being fed adequate amounts of carbohydrates, and (2) sucrose is not a reducing sugar and must be digested or split by bacteria to produce a positive test. Adding hydrochloric acid before the analysis should have the same result.

10 Postinfectious enteritis after acute enteritis is a common cause of prolonged diarrhea. Low-grade mucosal injury is responsible for the malabsorption. In young infants, a secondary lactase deficiency may be a contributing factor; in older infants and children a hypocaloric, high-carbohydrate diet is often responsible for the persistent malabsorption.

11 Approximately 10% of children with Hirschsprung disease develop enterocolitis. Historical "red flags" include a history of delayed passage of meconium, preceding constipation, Down syndrome, and a positive family history. Absent stool on rectal examination and immediate passage of stool after the rectal examination are suggestive. A rectal suction biopsy demonstrating absent ganglion cells is necessary for diagnosis.

12 In chronic diarrhea a finding of leukocytes or occult blood is more suggestive of inflammatory bowel disease than bacterial infection. A Sudan stain for fat will confirm steatorrhea but does not specify whether the abnormality is of bowel, pancreatic, or biliary origin. Stool elastase-1 can help evaluate for pancreatic exocrine function. Many causes of chronic diarrhea demonstrate an acidic pH or positive reducing substances consistent with some element of carbohydrate malabsorption.

13 Cystic fibrosis is characterized by frequent large, foul-smelling fatty stools not classic loose, watery diarrheal stools. When accompanied by a history of recurrent respiratory infections and failure to thrive, a sweat chloride test should be done. Infants younger than 6 months tend to present with failure to thrive; diarrhea (steatorrhea) is more common in older infants and toddlers.

14 Pancreatic insufficiency, chronic neutropenia, and short stature characterize Shwachman-Diamond syndrome.

15 Congenital chloride-losing diarrhea is a rare congenital disorder diagnosed by abnormally high levels of stool chloride.

16 Immune-mediated damage of the small intestine in response to gluten occurs in celiac disease (gluten-sensitive enteropathy). Symptoms of malabsorption and failure to thrive classically develop between 6 months and 3 years; symptom onset follows the addition of cereal grains (e.g., wheat, oat, barley, rye) to the diet. Diarrhea is often a late manifestation of the disorder, which may also include failure to thrive, anorexia, digital clubbing, anemia, abdominal distention, apathy, frequent fatty stools, and symptoms suggestive of specific nutrient deficiencies. IgA anti-tissue transglutaminase immunoassay (TTG) is a sensitive screening test. Biopsy is considered necessary for definitive diagnosis. Variable presentation has resulted in cases being diagnosed in older children.

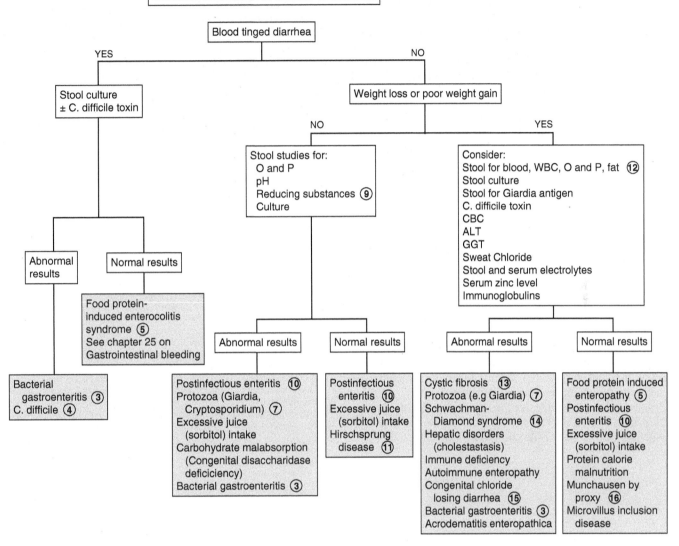

17 Inflammatory bowel disease (e.g., Crohn disease, ulcerative colitis) is very important in the differential diagnosis of chronic diarrhea in the school-aged child. Although rare, inflammatory bowel disease may present in younger children. Ulcerative colitis is more common than Crohn disease in the toddler age group. Weight loss and growth retardation are the cardinal symptoms. Gastrointestinal manifestations include diarrhea, abdominal pain, bloody stools, perianal disease, and malabsorption. Multiple extra intestinal manifestations (e.g., fever, oral ulcers, uveitis, rash, arthralgias) may also occur. Laboratory evaluation usually reveals anemia, an elevated sedimentation rate, leukocytosis, and some degree of hypoalbuminemia, thrombocytosis, and elevated acute phase-reactive proteins depending on the severity of the disease. Stool calprotectin levels may also be helpful in evaluation for IBD. Radiologic studies (e.g., barium enema, upper gastrointestinal series) aid in determining the extent of the disease. Colonoscopy and biopsy are necessary for definitive diagnosis.

18 Chronic nonspecific diarrhea or "toddler's diarrhea" is a frustrating but benign disorder most often affecting normally nourished children between 1 and 5 years of age. Children have up to 6 to 10 loose, watery, foul-smelling stools per day, often with food particles present. The pattern and consistency of the stools may vary considerably from day to day. In some cases they may be well formed in the morning and become looser throughout the day. In others the diarrhea may alternate with periods of constipation. Normal growth and an absence of stool passage at night suggest the diagnosis; stool examination is negative for blood, mucus, and excessive fat.

Previously, most of these cases were probably due to excessive fruit juice intake. As the role of fruit juices has been increasingly recognized, the disorder is diagnosed less frequently today.

19 Lactase levels gradually decrease between 3 and 5 years of age in children with primary adult-type hypolactasia. Subtle increases in malabsorptive symptoms (e.g., flatulence, abdominal pain, loose stools) occur after milk ingestion. Breath hydrogen testing after an oral lactose load may make the diagnosis, although resolution of symptoms after dietary restriction of lactose is strongly suggestive. Postinfectious secondary lactase deficiency can occur in older children but is not as common or as severe as in younger children.

20 Irritable bowel syndrome is a functional GI disorder that is being increasingly recognized in older children and adolescents. Patients report a variable pattern of diarrhea and constipation plus abdominal pain, bloating, urgency, a sense of incomplete stool evacuation, or passage of mucus.

21 Soiling associated with chronic constipation (i.e., encopresis) may be described as diarrhea by parents. The history and rectal examination usually make a rapid diagnosis.

Bibliography

Branski D, Lerner A, Lebenthal E: Chronic diarrhea and malabsorption, *Pediatr Clin North Am* 43:307–331, 1996.

Veereman-Wauters G, Taminiau J: Diarrhea. In Wyllie R, Hyams J, editors: *Pediatric gastrointestinal and liver disease,* ed 4, Philadelphia, 2010, WB Saunders, pp 64.

Steffen R, Wyllie R: Constipation. In Kliegman, Greenbaum L, Lye P, editors: *Practical strategies in pediatric diagnosis and therapy,* ed 2, Philadelphia, 2004, WB Saunders.

Constipation Guideline Committee of the North American Society of Pediatric Gastroenterology, Hepatology and Nutrition: Evaluation and treatment of constipation in infants and children: Recommendations of the North American Society for Pediatric Gastroenterology, Hepatology and Nutrition. *J Pediatr Gastroenterol Nutr,* 43(3) 43:e1-e13, 2006.

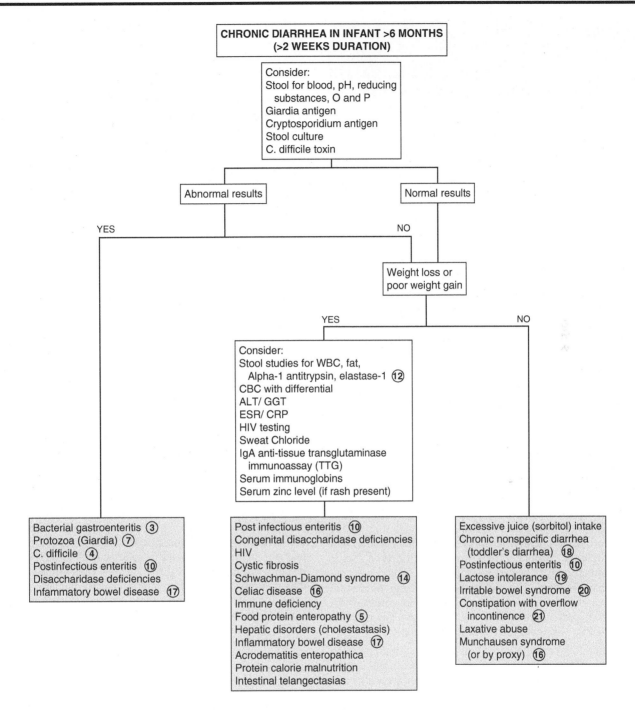

CHRONIC DIARRHEA IN INFANT >6 MONTHS
(>2 WEEKS DURATION)

Consider:
Stool for blood, pH, reducing
   substances, O and P
Giardia antigen
Cryptosporidium antigen
Stool culture
C. difficile toxin

Abnormal results   Normal results

YES   NO

Weight loss or
poor weight gain

YES   NO

Consider:
Stool studies for WBC, fat,
   Alpha-1 antitrypsin, elastase-1 ⑫
CBC with differential
ALT/ GGT
ESR/ CRP
HIV testing
Sweat Chloride
IgA anti-tissue transglutaminase
   immunoassay (TTG)
Serum immunoglobins
Serum zinc level (if rash present)

Bacterial gastroenteritis ③
Protozoa (Giardia) ⑦
C. difficile ④
Postinfectious enteritis ⑩
Disaccharidase deficiencies
Inflammatory bowel disease ⑰

Post infectious enteritis ⑩
Congenital disaccharidase deficiencies
HIV
Cystic fibrosis
Schwachman-Diamond syndrome ⑭
Celiac disease ⑯
Immune deficiency
Food protein enteropathy ⑤
Hepatic disorders (cholestastasis)
Inflammatory bowel disease ⑰
Acrodematitis enteropathica
Protein calorie malnutrition
Intestinal telangectasias

Excessive juice (sorbitol) intake
Chronic nonspecific diarrhea
   (toddler's diarrhea) ⑱
Postinfectious enteritis ⑩
Lactose intolerance ⑲
Irritable bowel syndrome ⑳
Constipation with overflow
   incontinence ㉑
Laxative abuse
Munchausen syndrome
   (or by proxy) ⑯

Chapter 24
CONSTIPATION

Constipation is a very common pediatric problem. It can be defined as delay or difficulty in passage of stools for more than 2 weeks, resulting in distress to the patient. Stools are often painful or hard to pass. Functional constipation that is not due to organic or anatomic causes is encountered most commonly. Encopresis, also known as fecal incontinence, is fecal soiling that occurs in the presence of chronic functional constipation.

1. When the constipation is severe and if it has been a long-standing problem since early infancy, it is necessary to rule out an underlying organic disorder. Inquire specifically about intermittent large stools, because some children with constipation will have a daily bowel movement but with incomplete emptying and retention of a large stool mass. Parents may describe stool withholding maneuvers of gluteal tightening and posturing, which are sometimes interpreted as attempts to strain or defecate. Occasionally, a parent will misinterpret the signs of encopresis as diarrhea.

A diet history for fluid and fiber intake may be helpful. In some infants, ingestion of large amounts of cow's milk is associated with constipation. Concerns about possible abuse should be addressed in the social history. Recent psychosocial changes and stressors should also be explored. The family history may reveal risk factors for Hirschsprung disease, such as the disorder itself or certain syndromes (e.g., trisomy 21, Waardenburg, Williams).

A careful spine and neurologic examination should be done to rule out spinal disorders that could be contributing to the constipation. An anal wink elicited by stroking the perianal skin with a sharp edge ensures normal sacral innervation. A digital rectal examination may be helpful. Children with chronic constipation have a dilated rectal ampulla and a large, hard stool mass unless they had a recent large bowel movement. Most children with Hirschsprung disease will not have any palpable stool in the first few centimeters of the anal canal.

2. If functional constipation is suspected, it is reasonable to presumptively treat the patient with education, dietary changes, and medication. Treatment of constipation consists of a "clean out" of retained stool and a maintenance regimen of stool softening and toileting practices to sustain evacuation and restore normal rectal and colon tone. Attention to family dynamics and the response of both the parents and child to the problem should be addressed. If there is inadequate response or there is concern for organic etiology, further investigation is suggested.

3. Situational constipation is usually short-lived and situational in response to a recent change or stress, such as starting daycare, travel, or the birth of a sibling. For some children, the transition to all-day school and the associated loss of privacy will contribute to withholding behaviors. Any condition causing a decrease in the child's normal activity level (e.g., illness, injury, surgery) is also a risk factor for constipation. A change in diet, especially starting cow's milk, is constipating for some children. Psychological factors or constitutional factors such as intrinsically slow motility can also exacerbate any cause of constipation. In chronic cases, stool retention results in a vicious cycle of retained stool, painful defecation, resisting the urge to defecate, further retaining of stool, and so on. These children are at risk for encopresis (fecal incontinence).

4. Irritable bowel syndrome can be associated with constipation and diarrhea. Pain is often associated with change in appearance or frequency of stooling. A response usually occurs with improved dietary fiber.

5. Constipation can occur because of multiple classes of drugs, including anticonvulsants, anticholinergics, antacids, iron-containing medications, calcium channel blockers, psychotherapeutic drugs, and narcotic-containing medications. Toxins may include metal intoxication (e.g., lead, arsenic, mercury) and botulinum.

6. Laboratory studies are not normally contributory on a routine basis unless there is some suggestion in the history or physical examin ation of a metabolic disturbance. Congenital hypothyroidism is generally diagnosed through newborn screening programs, but the acquired form can occur at any age.

7. Abdominal x-rays are not usually useful in the initial evaluation of constipation. They may be considered in determining if constipation is present at all. Rectal motility studies (manometry) will demonstrate physiologic abnormalities related to defecation that may be primary (Hirschsprung disease) or secondary (chronic constipation). The findings in Hirschsprung disease are so characteristic that many centers are now using manometry to establish the diagnosis. Manometry is useful in children with constipation starting very early in life. It may also be helpful in cases in which constipation has failed to respond to a treatment regimen. In very young infants, a biopsy may be preferred over manometry because the latter is technically difficult at very young ages. Further evaluation by a specialist is necessary to arrive at the remaining possible diagnoses.

8. Chronic intestinal pseudo-obstruction (or neuronal intestinal dysplasia) is a rare disorder of GI motility. It may be congenital or acquired and may be due to a neuropathy or myopathy or be idiopathic.

9. Hirschsprung disease (i.e., congenital aganglionic megacolon) typically occurs as delayed passage of meconium in 40% of affected infants, followed by lower intestinal obstruction in young infants. Milder presentations include severe constipation since birth, narrow-caliber stools, abdominal distention, and failure to thrive. Fecal soiling is almost unheard of in Hirschsprung cases. Patients with short segment disease may not present until older childhood, adolescence, or even adulthood. A rectal mucosal suction biopsy revealing an absence of ganglion cells is often necessary for diagnosis of Hirschsprung disease.

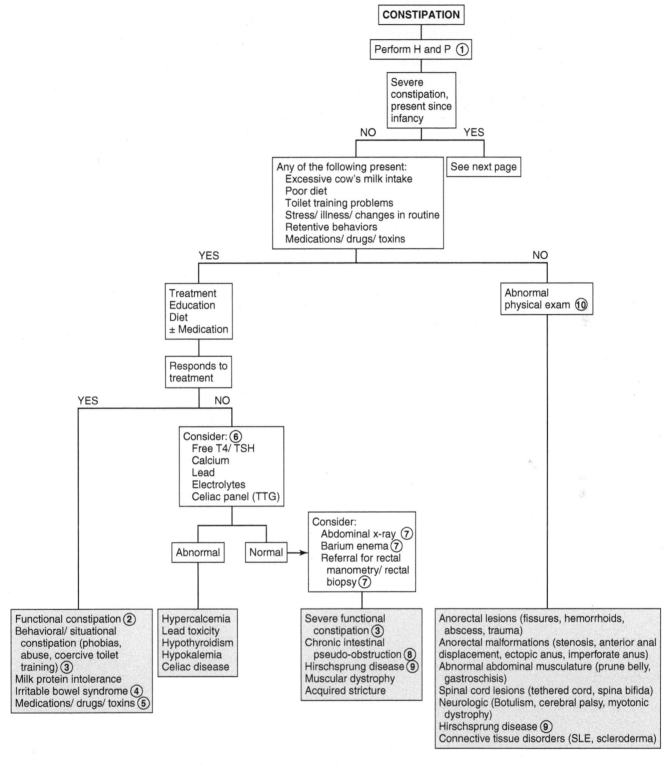

CONSTIPATION

Perform H and P ①

Severe constipation, present since infancy

— NO → / YES →

YES: Any of the following present:
- Excessive cow's milk intake
- Poor diet
- Toilet training problems
- Stress/ illness/ changes in routine
- Retentive behaviors
- Medications/ drugs/ toxins

YES (right branch): See next page

YES ← / → NO

Treatment
Education
Diet
± Medication

Responds to treatment

YES ← / NO →

Consider: ⑥
- Free T4/ TSH
- Calcium
- Lead
- Electrolytes
- Celiac panel (TTG)

Abnormal / Normal →

Consider:
- Abdominal x-ray ⑦
- Barium enema ⑦
- Referral for rectal manometry/ rectal biopsy ⑦

Abnormal physical exam ⑩

Functional constipation ②
Behavioral/ situational constipation (phobias, abuse, coercive toilet training) ③
Milk protein intolerance
Irritable bowel syndrome ④
Medications/ drugs/ toxins ⑤

Hypercalcemia
Lead toxicity
Hypothyroidism
Hypokalemia
Celiac disease

Severe functional constipation ③
Chronic intestinal pseudo-obstruction ⑧
Hirschsprung disease ⑨
Muscular dystrophy
Acquired stricture

Anorectal lesions (fissures, hemorrhoids, abscess, trauma)
Anorectal malformations (stenosis, anterior anal displacement, ectopic anus, imperforate anus)
Abnormal abdominal musculature (prune belly, gastroschisis)
Spinal cord lesions (tethered cord, spina bifida)
Neurologic (Botulism, cerebral palsy, myotonic dystrophy)
Hirschsprung disease ⑨
Connective tissue disorders (SLE, scleroderma)

Nelson Textbook of Pediatrics, 19e. Chapters 96, 298, 324, 536
Nelsons Essentials, 6e. Chapter 126

(10) Physical examination can help identify anatomic abnormalities as well as underlying conditions associated with constipation. Simple anterior displacement of the anus may contribute to constipation because of the anterior angle of the canal that stool must be expelled through, although this concept is not universally accepted. An anteriorly located anus must be distinguished from an ectopic anus, in which the anal canal and internal anal sphincter are displaced anteriorly; the external anal sphincter remains in its normal posterior position. An ectopic anus should be suspected if an anal wink can be elicited posterior to the opening of the anal canal. Children with neurologic impairment of any cause (e.g., cerebral palsy, polyneuritis, spina bifida, muscular dystrophy) are at risk for constipation from poor intestinal motility, inadequate dietary fiber, and impaired sensation. Children with a primary myopathy, collagen vascular disease, or amyloidosis develop progressively more severe constipation.

(11) Newborn screening programs in the United States test for hypothyroidism. Repeat testing should be done as indicated by the state laboratory.

(12) In very young infants, an unprepared barium enema may be helpful in the evaluation of severe constipation. The test will help identify Hirschsprung disease as well as congenital anomalies. If not done diagnostically, the barium enema should be performed after manometry or biopsy to assist in surgical planning, because it demarcates the transition zone.

(13) Meconium ileus (i.e., small bowel obstruction) appears in the newborn period in approximately 10% of infants with cystic fibrosis.

(14) In contrast to meconium ileus, meconium plug syndrome is an obstruction of the colon with inspissated plugs. The condition may occur in the infant of a diabetic mother and in cystic fibrosis, rectal aganglionosis, maternal drug abuse, and after maternal magnesium sulfate therapy for preeclampsia. A Gastrografin enema is usually diagnostic and therapeutic. Many cases are benign, but a sweat chloride test is recommended.

Bibliography

Abi-Hanna A, Lake AM: Constipation and encopresis in childhood, *Pediatr Rev* 19:23, 1998.

Constipation Guideline Committee of the North American Society for Pediatric Gastroenterology, Hepatology and Nutrition: Evaluation and treatment of constipation in infants and children: Recommendations of the North American Society for Pediatric Gastroenterology, Hepatology and Nutrition, *J Pediatr Gastroenterol Nutr* 43:e1–e13, 2006.

Daher S, Tahan S, Solé D, et al: Cow's milk protein intolerance and chronic constipation in children, *Pediatr Allergy Immunol* 12:339–342, 2001.

Steffen R, Wyllie R: Constipation. In Kliegman RM, Lye PS, Greenbaum LA, editors: *Practical strategies in pediatric diagnosis and therapy,* ed 2, Philadelphia, 2004, Elsevier Saunders.

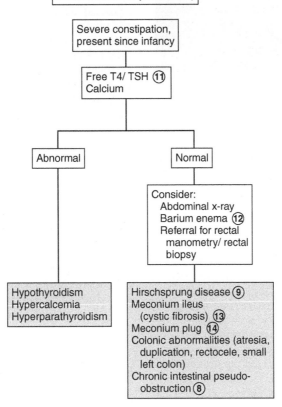

CONSTIPATION (continued)

Severe constipation, present since infancy

Free T4/ TSH ⑪
Calcium

Abnormal

Normal

Consider:
  Abdominal x-ray
  Barium enema ⑫
  Referral for rectal
    manometry/ rectal
    biopsy

Hypothyroidism
Hypercalcemia
Hyperparathyroidism

Hirschsprung disease ⑨
Meconium ileus
  (cystic fibrosis) ⑬
Meconium plug ⑭
Colonic abnormalities (atresia,
  duplication, rectocele, small
  left colon)
Chronic intestinal pseudo-
  obstruction ⑧

Chapter 25
GASTROINTESTINAL BLEEDING

1 The history should include any previous GI problems (e.g., jaundice, liver disease, ulcers, GER, other GI hemorrhages), blood transfusions, coagulopathies, and iron deficiency. A neonatal history of total parenteral nutrition, omphalitis, or umbilical vein catheterization is a risk factor for portal vein thrombosis. For infants, inquire about maternal idiopathic thrombocytopenic purpura. Aspirin, nonsteroidal antiinflammatory drugs (NSAIDs), and probably corticosteroids may play a contributing role in the development of gastritis.

A family history may be helpful in cases of suspected peptic ulcer disease, inflammatory bowel disease (IBD), liver disease, Meckel diverticulum, polyps, or milk allergy. Inquire about a family history of coagulopathies and Hirschsprung disease. A history of nosebleeds raises the possibility of swallowed blood presenting as hematemesis. Hemoptysis may need to be ruled out in cases in which severe coughing is present. Ask about ingestion of undercooked meat, recent medications, and the possibility of other ingestions (e.g., toxins, foreign bodies). Kool-Aid, gelatin, food coloring, antibiotics, bismuth, beets, licorice, cranberries, spinach, and blueberries can all mimic GI bleeding. Large iron ingestions can cause hematemesis due to mucosal injury. Therapeutic doses of iron will cause black stools, but they will remain negative for occult blood.

Examination of vital signs (heart rate, BP, orthostatics) is important to ensure that bleeding does not require emergent treatment for circulatory compromise. The growth curve may reveal failure to thrive, suggestive of IBD. A thorough physical exam is important to identify possible causes of bleeding. A careful abdominal exam may note tenderness (seen with abdominal inflammatory processes), splenomegaly or ascites (seen in portal hypertension), and a right lower quadrant mass may suggest intussusception. A careful skin exam may reveal a diagnosis; for example, hyperpigmented oral lesions (Peutz-Jeghers), petechiae (bleeding abnormality or disseminated intravascular coagulation), purpura (Henoch-Schönlein purpura, hemolytic uremic syndrome), and jaundice or spider nevi (liver disease). A rectal examination may reveal tags, fissures and fistulae (Crohn disease), or erythema with tenderness (group A β-hemolytic streptococcal infection).

2 Confirming the presence of blood is important to avoid an unnecessary evaluation. A stool test for occult blood must be part of the initial evaluation. False-positive test results can occur in young women around the time of their menses and after recent ingestion of rare red meat or fresh peroxidase-containing foodstuffs such as broccoli, radishes, cauliflower, cantaloupe, or turnips. Munchausen by proxy should be considered if a history of significant bleeding is not supported by any documentation of actual blood loss. With a breast-fed infant, if swallowed maternal blood is suspected, definitive diagnosis can be made by an Apt-Downey test. Fecal leukocytes are consistent with an invasive infectious organism or an inflammatory condition.

3 Hematemesis (i.e., vomiting of bright red blood or "coffee grounds") is generally associated with UGI hemorrhage proximal to the ligament of Treitz. Consider passing a nasogastric tube to help in evaluation and management in case of persistent or severe UGI bleeding. Hematochezia (rectal passage of bright red or maroon-colored blood mixed in with the stool) is usually associated with lower GI or colonic bleeding, although brisk UGI hemorrhages may also present in this way. Melena (i.e., dark, tarry-appearing stool) represents bleeding from any site above the ileocecal valve. Occult blood may originate from upper or lower GI sources. Blood originating in the rectum generally maintains a bright red color.

4 Significant GI bleeding warrants a CBC with platelet count, differential, and reticulocyte count to assess for anemia. Microcytosis suggests chronic bleeding, and serial CBCs may help assess severity of bleeding. If bleeding is significant or the history is suggestive of a bleeding disorder, obtain at minimum a PT and activated PTT. LFTs, electrolytes, Cr, and BUN may identify hepatic, renal, and metabolic problems. Hypoalbuminemia is consistent with long-standing liver dysfunction with portal hypertension, IBD, or protein-losing enteropathies. In cases in which there was a limited amount of bleeding and a clinical picture consistent with a benign, self-limited condition (swallowed blood, Mallory-Weiss tear), laboratory tests may not be indicated.

Upper endoscopy is successful in identifying UGI bleeding sites in 80% to 90% of cases. Radiographic contrast studies are less sensitive but may be used if endoscopy is not available. They are contraindicated in cases of active bleeding. Small bowel follow-through examinations may be helpful in identifying atretic lesions, strictures, and rotation abnormalities. Newer endoscopic methods to image the small bowel include balloon enteroscopy and capsule endoscopy. Bleeding scans can help locate bleeding sites not accessible with endoscopy. Angiography is most useful when bleeding is moderately brisk, but it is of limited value for lower GI hemorrhages.

5 Mallory-Weiss tears are common. Forceful recurrent vomiting causes a tear in the distal esophageal mucosa that results in a limited amount of bright red hematemesis. In light of a stable clinical picture consistent with a self-limited vomiting illness and no evidence of obstruction, a diagnostic workup is not indicated.

6 Esophagitis as a complication of GER is a common cause of GI bleeding in children. GER maybe present even in the absence of regurgitation.

7 Gastritis may be due to caustic ingestions, viral infections, *Helicobacter pylori* infection, radiation exposure, or bile reflux. Frequent NSAID, cocaine, or alcohol use may cause gastritis in adolescents.

8 Peptic ulcer disease includes gastric and duodenal ulcers, gastritis, and duodenitis. Gastritis and peptic ulcers are common causes of UGI bleeding in sick or stressed neonates or infants. In this young age group, they are more likely to present acutely as perforation or hemorrhage. Less severe cases may present as irritability, vomiting, and regurgitation. Ulcers in older children and adolescents are more likely to have a history of long-standing intermittent abdominal pain. Epigastric pain, especially if nocturnal or relieved with meals, is suggestive of peptic ulcer disease, although for children this "classic" constellation of symptoms is less reliable than for adults.

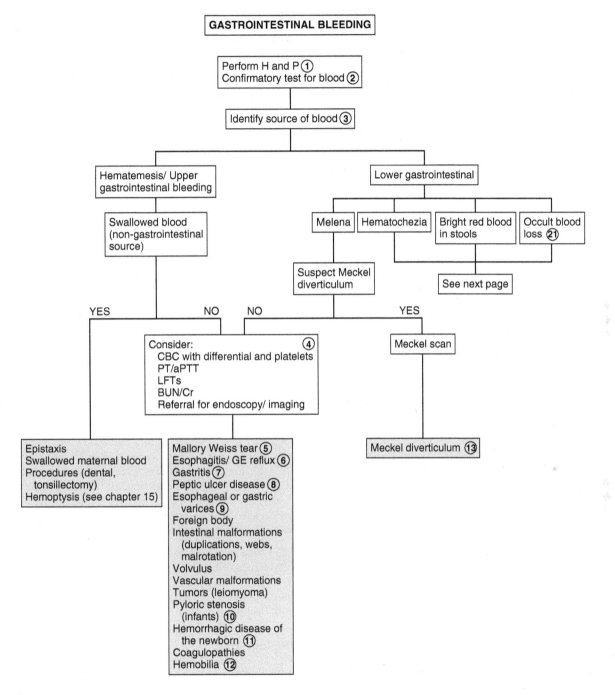

GASTROINTESTINAL BLEEDING

Perform H and P ① / Confirmatory test for blood ②

Identify source of blood ③

Hematemesis/ Upper gastrointestinal bleeding

Lower gastrointestinal

Swallowed blood (non-gastrointestinal source)

Melena | Hematochezia | Bright red blood in stools | Occult blood loss ㉑

Suspect Meckel diverticulum

See next page

YES   NO   NO   YES

Consider: ④
CBC with differential and platelets
PT/aPTT
LFTs
BUN/Cr
Referral for endoscopy/ imaging

Meckel scan

Epistaxis
Swallowed maternal blood
Procedures (dental, tonsillectomy)
Hemoptysis (see chapter 15)

Mallory Weiss tear ⑤
Esophagitis/ GE reflux ⑥
Gastritis ⑦
Peptic ulcer disease ⑧
Esophageal or gastric varices ⑨
Foreign body
Intestinal malformations (duplications, webs, malrotation)
Volvulus
Vascular malformations
Tumors (leiomyoma)
Pyloric stenosis (infants) ⑩
Hemorrhagic disease of the newborn ⑪
Coagulopathies
Hemobilia ⑫

Meckel diverticulum ⑬

Nelson Textbook of Pediatrics, 19e. Chapters 298, 321, 323, 324, 326, 328, 330, 332, 337
Nelsons Essentials, 6e. Chapter 126

9   Varices are commonly due to portal vein hypertension secondary to intrinsic liver disease. Portal vein thrombosis is the next most likely etiology. Thrombus formation can occur as the result of sepsis, pancreatitis, omphalitis, or umbilical vein catheterization. A series of tortuous collateral veins develop to bypass the obstructing thrombus and may appear years later as bleeding esophageal varices. US or endoscopy may be used to assess for varices when the patient is not actively bleeding.

10   Pyloric stenosis classically presents between 3 and 6 weeks of age as nonbilious vomiting that rapidly progresses to frequent projectile vomiting, often complicated by dehydration, weight loss, and metabolic alkalosis. The emesis may develop a coffee-ground appearance and may test positive for blood. US is the preferred diagnostic test.

11   An unsuspected coagulopathy is more likely to occur in the newborn period than at older ages. Be aware of increased risk in breast-fed infants, especially those who did not receive vitamin K at birth.

12   Hemobilia is hemorrhage into the biliary tract.

13   Approximately two thirds of Meckel diverticula occur as a painless but significant lower GI bleeding before 2 years of age. The bleeding is due to ulceration from gastric mucosa contained in the diverticulum. Radioisotope technetium scanning (Meckel scan) can localize ectopic gastric mucosa.

14   Juvenile polyps are a common cause of painless rectal bleeding; most are in the distal colon. Inherited syndromes associated with polyps and increased risk of developing malignancy are familial adenomatous polyposis, Gardner syndrome, Peutz-Jeghers syndrome, and juvenile polyposis. Peutz-Jeghers syndrome is characterized by diffuse intestinal hamartomas and hyperpigmented macules of the oral mucosa.

15   Intussusception is the "telescoping" of one segment of the intestine into a distal segment. It can occur between 3 months and 6 years of age, but most cases occur before age 36 months. Severe episodes of abdominal pain (due to obstruction or ischemia) and crying occur, accompanied initially by periods of normal behavior between paroxysms. Progression to vomiting (sometimes bilious or bloody), lethargy, and shock may occur. "Currant jelly" stools are observed in approximately 60% of cases.

The barium enema, the traditional diagnostic and therapeutic modality, has been replaced in many centers by US for diagnosis and fluoroscopy-guided reduction with hydrostatic or pneumatic pressure ("air enema"). Any method of reduction should always be performed with surgical backup. Nonsurgical reduction should not be attempted if there is any evidence of shock or intestinal perforation (e.g., peritonitis). Barium enemas with air contrast can reveal mucosal abnormalities but overall are not very specific.

16   Although neonates are susceptible to most of the same problems as older age groups, some conditions tend to present almost exclusively in the neonatal period. Necrotizing enterocolitis should always be considered in the presence of prematurity and occasionally can have a late presentation.

17   Bloody diarrhea is a common manifestation of bacterial pathogens (*Yersinia*, *Salmonella*, *Shigella*, and *Campylobacter*) and parasites (ameba). Colitis accompanied by anemia, thrombocytopenia, or renal insufficiency (consistent with hemolytic-uremic syndrome) should prompt a specific investigation for *Escherichia coli* serotype 0157:H7. Recent antibiotic use should raise suspicions for *Clostridium difficile*. Infectious colitis is a rare cause of bleeding in neonates. Be aware of positive tests for *C. difficile* toxin; *C. difficile* may not be a pathogen in the newborn. Occult blood may occur with acute diarrhea due to any cause as a result of minor anal or perineal irritation.

18   Hirschsprung disease typically occurs as an obstruction, but it may appear as an enterocolitis with bleeding.

19   Food protein–induced enterocolitis syndrome and food protein–induced proctitis (milk protein sensitivity) typically present as a history of bloody mucous stools and increasing stool frequency. The family history is often positive. Some infants fed soy-based formula can develop an identical clinical picture. Breast-fed infants can develop allergic symptoms from cow's milk ingested by the mother. In infants with a clinical presentation for milk allergy or intolerance, a trial of a casein or whey hydrolysate formula or elimination of cow's milk from a breastfeeding mother's diet may be therapeutic and eliminate the need for any further evaluation.

20   Fissures are a common cause of bright red streaks coating the stool. They can occur even in the absence of constipation. If the perianal region is erythematous, obtain a culture for group A *Streptococcus* to rule out a perianal cellulitis, which can predispose patients to fissures and bleeding. Hemorrhoids involving veins above the anorectal line may not be visible on examination.

21   Most causes of upper and lower GI bleeding can manifest as occult bleeding. Careful history-taking may narrow the differential diagnosis and guide the appropriate workup. The diagnoses listed are among the most common that may present with occult blood loss.

Bibliography

Boyle JT: Gastrointestinal bleeding in infants and children, *Pediatr Rev* 29: 39–51, 2008.

Friedlander J, Mamula P: Gastrointestinal hemorrhage. In Wyllie R, Hyams J, editors: *Pediatric gastrointestinal and liver disease*, ed 4, Philadelphia, 2010, WB Saunders, pp 64.

Sylvester FA, Hyams JS: Gastrointestinal bleeding. In Kliegman RM, Lye PS, Greenbaum LA, editors: *Practical strategies in pediatric diagnosis and therapy*, ed 2, Philadelphia, 2004, Elsevier Saunders.

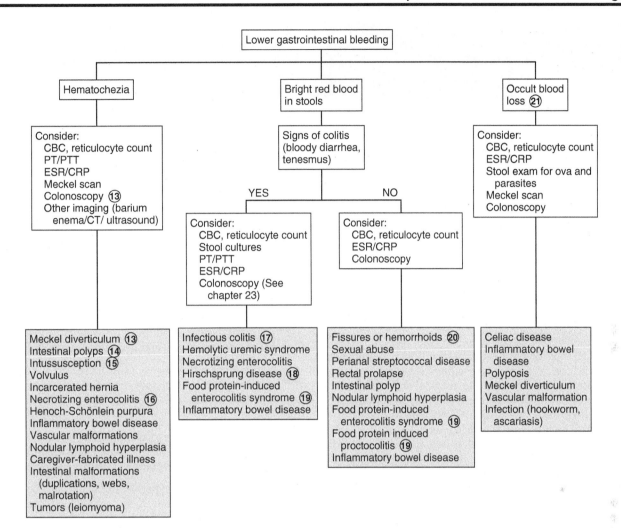

Lower gastrointestinal bleeding

Hematochezia

Consider:
 CBC, reticulocyte count
 PT/PTT
 ESR/CRP
 Meckel scan
 Colonoscopy ⑬
 Other imaging (barium
  enema/CT/ ultrasound)

Meckel diverticulum ⑬
Intestinal polyps ⑭
Intussusception ⑮
Volvulus
Incarcerated hernia
Necrotizing enterocolitis ⑯
Henoch-Schönlein purpura
Inflammatory bowel disease
Vascular malformations
Nodular lymphoid hyperplasia
Caregiver-fabricated illness
Intestinal malformations
 (duplications, webs,
 malrotation)
Tumors (leiomyoma)

Bright red blood in stools

Signs of colitis
(bloody diarrhea,
tenesmus)

YES   NO

Consider:
 CBC, reticulocyte count
 Stool cultures
 PT/PTT
 ESR/CRP
 Colonoscopy (See
  chapter 23)

Infectious colitis ⑰
Hemolytic uremic syndrome
Necrotizing enterocolitis
Hirschsprung disease ⑱
Food protein-induced
 enterocolitis syndrome ⑲
Inflammatory bowel disease

Consider:
 CBC, reticulocyte count
 ESR/CRP
 Colonoscopy

Fissures or hemorrhoids ⑳
Sexual abuse
Perianal streptococcal disease
Rectal prolapse
Intestinal polyp
Nodular lymphoid hyperplasia
Food protein-induced
 enterocolitis syndrome ⑲
Food protein induced
 proctocolitis ⑲
Inflammatory bowel disease

Occult blood loss ㉑

Consider:
 CBC, reticulocyte count
 ESR/CRP
 Stool exam for ova and
  parasites
 Meckel scan
 Colonoscopy

Celiac disease
Inflammatory bowel
 disease
Polyposis
Meckel diverticulum
Vascular malformation
Infection (hookworm,
 ascariasis)

Chapter 26
JAUNDICE

Jaundice is the yellow discoloration of skin, sclerae, and other tissues caused by the deposition of bilirubin. The degree of jaundice is related to the serum level of bilirubin and the degree of its deposition into the extravascular tissues. The most common source of bilirubin is the increased breakdown of hemoglobin. Jaundice may lead to kernicterus, which is a neurologic syndrome resulting from the deposition of unconjugated (indirect) bilirubin in the basal ganglia and brainstem nuclei. The toxic blood level for an individual infant is unpredictable, but in general, kernicterus typically occurrs only in infants with a bilirubin >20 mg/dL.

In older infants jaundice should be distinguished from carotenemia, a diffuse yellowish-orange skin discoloration caused by ingestion of large amounts of carotene-containing foods (e.g., carrots, squash).

1 Although most cases of neonatal jaundice are physiologic, a careful history and physical examination are necessary to rule out more serious disorders. The prenatal and birth history should inquire about delivery complications, maternal infection, diabetes mellitus, and drug use. Oxytocin during labor is associated with an increased risk of jaundice. A history of polyhydramnios suggests an intestinal obstruction. Other conditions resulting in a delayed passage of meconium (Hirschsprung disease, cystic fibrosis) will also contribute to hyperbilirubinemia. Prematurity is a risk factor for hyperbilirubinemia that is often compounded by delayed enteral feeds, parenteral nutrition, and perinatal insults due to hypoxia and acidosis. Vomiting, lethargy, poor feeding, and failure to thrive may suggest an inborn error of metabolism. Breast-fed infants tend to have higher and more prolonged unconjugated bilirubin levels. A family history of jaundice, anemia, splenectomy, or cholecystectomy suggests a hereditary hemolytic disorder.

2 Detailed investigation is warranted in children with conjugated hyperbilirubinemia, defined as a conjugated bilirubin level >2.0 mg/dl or a conjugated fraction >20% of the total bilirubin level. The evaluation should be directed at ruling out infection, metabolic disorders, anatomic abnormalities, and familial cholestatic syndromes.

3 Some risk factors for development of severe hyperbilirubinemia include prematurity, jaundice observed in first 24 hours of life, known blood group incompatibility or hemolytic disease, sibling who required phototherapy, cephalohematoma, bruising, poor breastfeeding, and East Asian race.

4 Nearly all newborns experience some rise in serum bilirubin levels owing to the relative immaturity of their hepatic excretory function. The frequent occurrence of hyperbilirubinemia and jaundice—approximately one third of all newborns develop jaundice—has resulted in the term physiologic jaundice. Levels higher than those used in the definition may occur (i.e., exaggerated physiologic jaundice), but some evaluation must be done to rule out more serious disorders before making the diagnosis. A well-accepted AAP practice parameter exists for the management of hyperbilirubinemia in the healthy term newborn. (See Bibliography.)

5 Breast-fed infants have an exaggerated physiologic jaundice in the first week of life, with significantly higher bilirubin levels than formula-fed infants in the first 5 days of life. This is due to decreased caloric intake until adequate breast milk supply is established with resulting increase in enterohepatic circulation.

6 "Breast milk" jaundice is jaundice occurring after the first week of life. The mechanism is not clearly understood. To confirm the diagnosis, breastfeeding may be discontinued for 24-48 hours to observe whether a decrease in bilirubin level occurs.

7 Isoimmune hemolytic disease occurs when maternal antibodies to the erythrocytes of the fetus cross the placenta and cause destruction of the fetal red blood cells. Incompatibility of the Rh factor causes the most severe disease in progressive pregnancies. ABO incompatibility causes less severe hemolysis. On occasion, infants in the latter group will demonstrate a negative or weakly positive direct Coombs test but the indirect Coombs will be positive.

8 Red blood cell membrane defects include hereditary spherocytosis, hereditary elliptocytosis, infantile pyknocytosis, hereditary stomatocytosis, and hereditary pyropoikilocytosis.

9 Extravascular blood results in increased bilirubin production. Examples include cephalohematoma, ecchymoses, occult hemorrhage as well as swallowed maternal blood.

10 Any condition causing obstruction or delayed passage of meconium (e.g., Hirschsprung disease, meconium plug syndrome) will increase enterohepatic circulation of bilirubin, contributing to indirect hyperbilirubinemia and jaundice.

11 Prolonged indirect hyperbilirubinemia may be the earliest clinical manifestation of congenital hypothyroidism as well as hypopituitarism. These may also cause conjugated hyperbilirubinemia.

12 Oxytocin, excess vitamin K in premature infants, some antibiotics (e.g., sulfonamides, ceftriaxone), and phenol disinfectants are examples of drugs and toxins that may contribute to unconjugated hyperbilirubinemia.

13 Normal liver enzymes indicate that hepatic injury or biliary tract disease is less likely. A significant elevation in elevated gammaglutamyl transpeptidase (GGT) suggests biliary obstruction or intrahepatic cholestasis. Serum alkaline phosphatase is also increased in relation to aminotransferases (i.e., AST and ALT). In obstructive jaundice there is often prolonged prothrombin time that corrects with vitamin K administration due to decreased absorption of fat-soluble vitamins. History of acholic (clay colored) stools supports an obstructive cause. Elevation of serum transaminases is caused by intrinsic hepatocellular disease. With severe disease there may be impaired synthetic function causing hypoalbuminemia and a prolonged prothrombin time that does not correct with vitamin K. Hypoglycemia reflects hepatocellular damage; it indicates more severe disease and mandates an urgent workup.

14 A congenital infection is suggested by intrauterine growth retardation, microcephaly, and ophthalmologic abnormalities (e.g., cataracts, chorioretinitis, posterior embryotoxon). Characteristic facies may suggest syndromes associated with hyperbilirubinemia. Any of the "TORCH infections" (e.g., toxoplasmosis, rubella, cytomegalovirus, herpes virus, syphilis) may cause growth retardation and cholestasis.

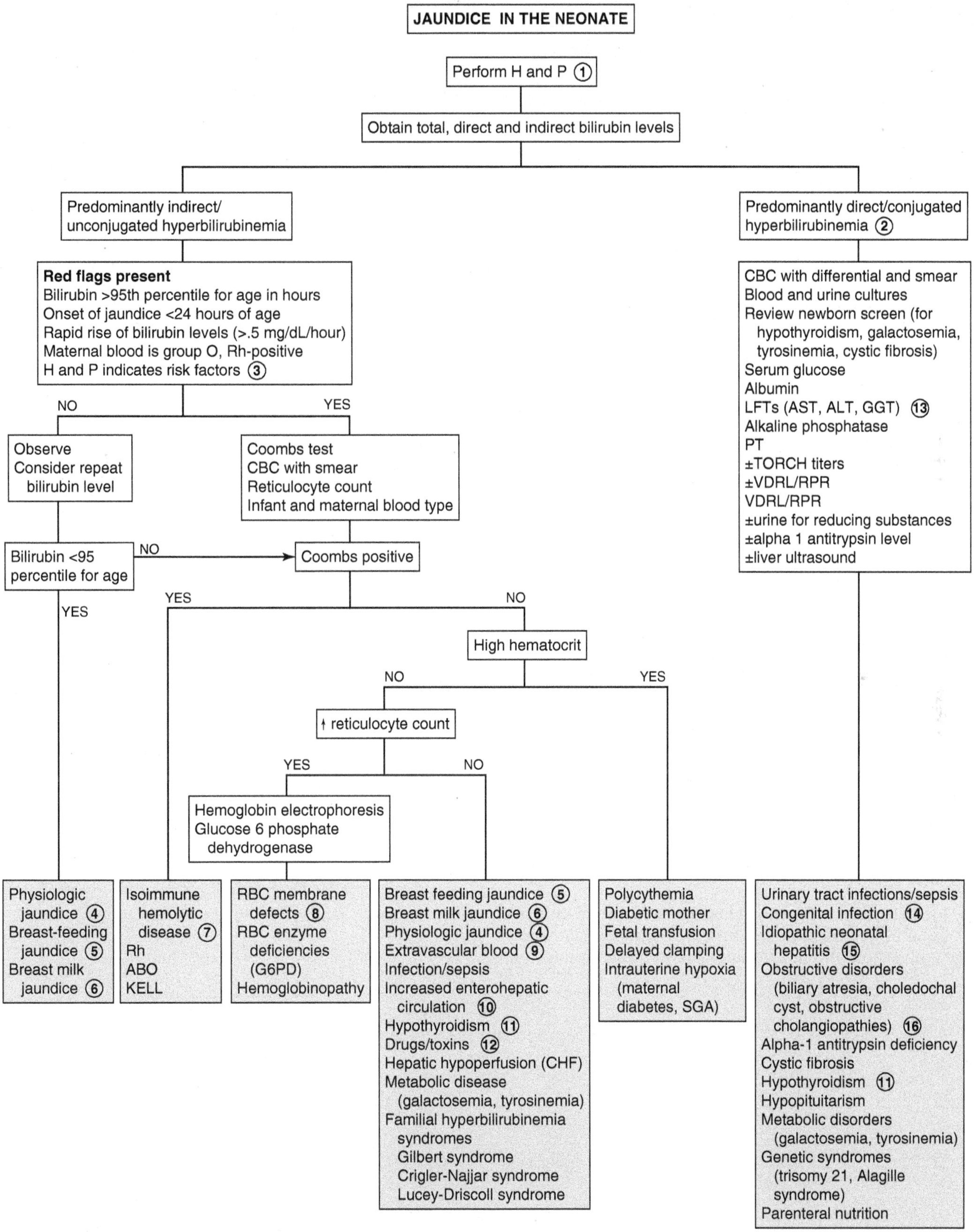

JAUNDICE IN THE NEONATE

Perform H and P ①

Obtain total, direct and indirect bilirubin levels

Predominantly indirect/unconjugated hyperbilirubinemia

Predominantly direct/conjugated hyperbilirubinemia ②

Red flags present
Bilirubin >95th percentile for age in hours
Onset of jaundice <24 hours of age
Rapid rise of bilirubin levels (>.5 mg/dL/hour)
Maternal blood is group O, Rh-positive
H and P indicates risk factors ③

CBC with differential and smear
Blood and urine cultures
Review newborn screen (for hypothyroidism, galactosemia, tyrosinemia, cystic fibrosis)
Serum glucose
Albumin
LFTs (AST, ALT, GGT) ⑬
Alkaline phosphatase
PT
±TORCH titers
±VDRL/RPR
VDRL/RPR
±urine for reducing substances
±alpha 1 antitrypsin level
±liver ultrasound

NO

YES

Observe
Consider repeat bilirubin level

Coombs test
CBC with smear
Reticulocyte count
Infant and maternal blood type

Bilirubin <95 percentile for age   NO →

Coombs positive

YES

YES   NO

High hematocrit

NO   YES

↑ reticulocyte count

YES   NO

Hemoglobin electrophoresis
Glucose 6 phosphate dehydrogenase

Physiologic jaundice ④
Breast-feeding jaundice ⑤
Breast milk jaundice ⑥

Isoimmune hemolytic disease ⑦
Rh
ABO
KELL

RBC membrane defects ⑧
RBC enzyme deficiencies (G6PD)
Hemoglobinopathy

Breast feeding jaundice ⑤
Breast milk jaundice ⑥
Physiologic jaundice ④
Extravascular blood ⑨
Infection/sepsis
Increased enterohepatic circulation ⑩
Hypothyroidism ⑪
Drugs/toxins ⑫
Hepatic hypoperfusion (CHF)
Metabolic disease (galactosemia, tyrosinemia)
Familial hyperbilirubinemia syndromes
  Gilbert syndrome
  Crigler-Najjar syndrome
  Lucey-Driscoll syndrome

Polycythemia
Diabetic mother
Fetal transfusion
Delayed clamping
Intrauterine hypoxia (maternal diabetes, SGA)

Urinary tract infections/sepsis
Congenital infection ⑭
Idiopathic neonatal hepatitis ⑮
Obstructive disorders (biliary atresia, choledochal cyst, obstructive cholangiopathies) ⑯
Alpha-1 antitrypsin deficiency
Cystic fibrosis
Hypothyroidism ⑪
Hypopituitarism
Metabolic disorders (galactosemia, tyrosinemia)
Genetic syndromes (trisomy 21, Alagille syndrome)
Parenteral nutrition

Nelson Textbook of Pediatrics, 19e. Chapters 96, 341, 347-350, 354
Nelsons Essentials, 6e. Chapters 130, 248

15 Idiopathic neonatal hepatitis is defined as prolonged conjugated hyperbilirubinemia without an obvious etiology after known infectious and metabolic and genetic causes have been excluded.

16 Biliary atresia is the most common cause of neonatal cholestasis and should be considered in children with conjugated hyperbilirubinemia and elevated GGT. Children are initially asymptomatic at birth and become jaundiced after a few weeks. There may be acholic stools. Evaluation should include an ultrasound to exclude other anatomic abnormalities including choledochal cyst.

17 Review the medical history in the older child who presents with jaundice because certain illnesses are associated with specific liver complications. Examples include AIDS, cystic fibrosis, hemolytic disorders, hemoglobinopathies, and inflammatory bowel disease. Include a travel history, sexual activity, tattoos, drug and alcohol use, and potential exposure to a hepatitis outbreak. A family history of jaundice, anemia, liver disease, splenectomy, or cholecystectomy suggests a hereditary disorder. A small liver on examination is consistent with a chronic liver disorder (hepatitis or cirrhosis). A large tender liver suggests acute hepatitis or congestive heart failure. Splenomegaly occurs in hemolytic disorders and in some oncologic disorders. Neurologic findings such as tremor, fine motor incoordination, clumsy gait, and chore form movements suggest Wilson disease. Eye examination may reveal Kayser-Fleischer rings (Wilson disease) or posterior embryotoxon (Alagille syndrome). A workup specifically for jaundice may not be necessary when an underlying diagnosis such as congestive heart failure or sepsis is evident.

18 Autoimmune hemolytic anemias often demonstrate a direct or indirect positive Coombs test or rouleaux formation on the smear. Mycoplasma pneumonia, Epstein-Barr virus, and lymphoproliferative disorders are associated with cold antibodies. Most cases of hemolytic anemia associated with warm antibodies are idiopathic. Other causes include lymphoproliferative disorders, systemic lupus erythematosus, malignancy, infection, immunodeficiency, and medications (e.g., penicillins, cephalosporins, tetracycline, erythromycin, ibuprofen, and tylenol).

19 Mechanical damage causing fragmentation hemolysis may occur in systemic disorders such as disseminated intravascular coagulation, thrombotic thrombocytopenic purport, or hemolytic-uremic syndrome. Extracorporeal membrane oxygenation, prosthetic heart valves, and burns may cause hemolysis by a mechanical mechanism.

20 Wilson disease, an autosomal recessive disorder of copper metabolism, presents in the preadolescent or adolescent age group. It may present as acute liver disease, neurologic symptoms (e.g., dysarthria, clumsiness, tremor), or both. Kayser-Fleischer rings in the cornea reflect deposited copper and are pathognomonic. Diagnosis is by low serum ceruloplasmin level, high urinary copper excretion, and increased hepatic copper level on liver biopsy.

21 Some drugs that may cause hyperbilirubinemia in older children include antibiotics (e.g., erythromycin, tetracycline), anticonvulsants (e.g., valproate, phenytoin), acetaminophen, aspirin, alcohol, chlorpromazine, hormones (e.g., estrogens, androgens), isoniazid, pemoline, and antineoplastics. Children on total parenteral nutrition are also at risk.

22 Autoimmune hepatitis may occur acutely (with symptoms such as malaise, anorexia, nausea, vomiting, jaundice) or with chronic liver disease. Other autoimmune problems (e.g., hemolytic anemia, immune thrombocytopenia [ITP], arthritis, thyroiditis, vasculitides, nephritis, diabetes mellitus, or inflammatory bowel disease) may be present. Laboratory evaluation reveals elevated transaminase levels, mild hyperbilirubinemia, hypergammaglobulinemia, and auto-antibodies (antinuclear antibodies, antinuclear anti-smooth muscle and liver-kidney microsomal [LKM] antibodies). Antimitochodrial antibodies may also be elevated, although it is usually associated with primary biliary cirrhosis.

Bibliography

AAP Practice Parameter: Management of hyperbilirubinemia in the newborn infant 35 or more weeks of gestation, *Pediatrics* 114(1):297–316, 2004.

Bhutani VK, Johnson L, Sivieri EM: Predictive ability of a predischarge hour-specific serum bilirubin for subsequent significant hyperbilirubinemia in healthy term and near-term newborns, *Pediatrics* 103:6–14, 1999.

Brumbaugh D, Mack C: Conjugated hyperbilirubinemia in children, *Pediatr Rev* 33:291–302, 2012.

Lauer BJ, Spector ND: Hyperbilirubinemia in the newborn, *Pediatr Rev* 32:341–349, 2011.

Sullivan KM, Gourley GR: Jaundice. In Wyllie R, Hyams J, editors: *Pediatric gastrointestinal and liver disease*, ed 4, Philadelphia, 2010, WB Saunders.

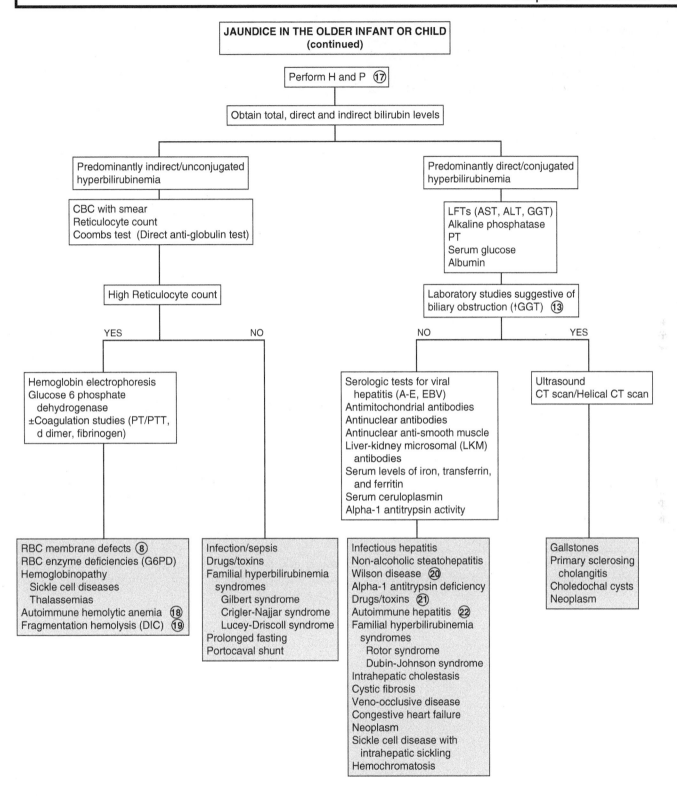

JAUNDICE IN THE OLDER INFANT OR CHILD
(continued)

Perform H and P ⑰

Obtain total, direct and indirect bilirubin levels

Predominantly indirect/unconjugated
hyperbilirubinemia

CBC with smear
Reticulocyte count
Coombs test (Direct anti-globulin test)

High Reticulocyte count

YES   NO

Hemoglobin electrophoresis
Glucose 6 phosphate
   dehydrogenase
±Coagulation studies (PT/PTT,
   d dimer, fibrinogen)

RBC membrane defects ⑧
RBC enzyme deficiencies (G6PD)
Hemoglobinopathy
   Sickle cell diseases
   Thalassemias
Autoimmune hemolytic anemia ⑱
Fragmentation hemolysis (DIC) ⑲

Infection/sepsis
Drugs/toxins
Familial hyperbilirubinemia
   syndromes
      Gilbert syndrome
      Crigler-Najjar syndrome
      Lucey-Driscoll syndrome
Prolonged fasting
Portocaval shunt

Predominantly direct/conjugated
hyperbilirubinemia

LFTs (AST, ALT, GGT)
Alkaline phosphatase
PT
Serum glucose
Albumin

Laboratory studies suggestive of
biliary obstruction (↑GGT) ⑬

NO   YES

Serologic tests for viral
   hepatitis (A-E, EBV)
Antimitochondrial antibodies
Antinuclear antibodies
Antinuclear anti-smooth muscle
Liver-kidney microsomal (LKM)
   antibodies
Serum levels of iron, transferrin,
   and ferritin
Serum ceruloplasmin
Alpha-1 antitrypsin activity

Ultrasound
CT scan/Helical CT scan

Infectious hepatitis
Non-alcoholic steatohepatitis
Wilson disease ⑳
Alpha-1 antitrypsin deficiency
Drugs/toxins ㉑
Autoimmune hepatitis ㉒
Familial hyperbilirubinemia
   syndromes
      Rotor syndrome
      Dubin-Johnson syndrome
Intrahepatic cholestasis
Cystic fibrosis
Veno-occlusive disease
Congestive heart failure
Neoplasm
Sickle cell disease with
   intrahepatic sickling
Hemochromatosis

Gallstones
Primary sclerosing
   cholangitis
Choledochal cysts
Neoplasm

Chapter 27
HEPATOMEGALY

The presence of a palpable liver does not always indicate hepatomegaly. Liver size varies with age. It may be measured by the extension of the liver edge below the costal margin, the span of dullness to percussion, or by imaging. In children, palpation of the liver edge more than 2 cm (>3.5 cm in newborns) below the right costal margin suggests liver enlargement. Liver span may be measured by percussing the upper margin of dullness and by palpating the lower edge in the right midclavicular line.

1 Inquire about a history of prolonged hyperbilirubinemia, as well as underlying conditions that may contribute to liver disease (e.g., blood transfusions). Ask about episodic vomiting, associated neurologic changes, travel, and drug or toxin ingestion. Metabolic disease is suggested by symptoms of failure to thrive, vomiting, loss of developmental milestones, new seizures, or hypotonia. The social history should include sexual activity, medication and drug use, and exposure to possible hepatitis outbreaks or jaundiced persons. A family history of hepatic, neurologic, and psychiatric symptoms should be elicited, as well as a history of neonatal deaths. Birth history may identify perinatally transmitted infections (hepatitis B, toxoplasmosis, syphilis, CMV, rubella, herpes simplex, HIV).

Cutaneous findings suggestive of liver disease include a prominent abdominal venous pattern, palmar erythema, and spider angiomas. Hepatomegaly is often associated with jaundice. (See Chapter 26 for additional diagnoses to consider.) When splenomegaly is present as well, other diagnoses may be considered. (See Chapter 28.) Specific signs may indicate syndromes. Coarse facial features may be seen with mucopolysaccharoidosis. Kayser-Fleischer rings are seen in Wilson disease.

2 Elevated transaminase levels provide nonspecific information about hepatocellular injury. Liver function is better assessed by serum albumin and prothrombin time because they rely on the synthetic function of the liver. Increased levels of alkaline phosphatase and GGT usually indicate cholestasis. Abdominal US will aid in determining whether hepatomegaly is present.

3 Inflammatory bowel disease can be associated with hepatobiliary disease through a variety of mechanisms. These include autoimmune (autoimmune hepatitis), inflammatory (sclerosing cholangitis), medication toxicity (e.g., methotrexate), and related infections (hepatic abscess).

4 Nonalcoholic fatty liver disease is associated with obesity. It may cause fatty liver and ultimately inflammation and fibrosis (nonalcoholic steatohepatitis). It used to be an adult disease but is increasingly described in children.

5 Patients with HIV/AIDS are prone to a variety of hepatobiliary disorders. Other infections that cause hepatosplenomegaly and anicteric hepatitis include cat-scratch disease, typhoid, brucellosis, tularemia, syphilis, Lyme disease, leptospirosis, Rocky Mountain spotted fever, Q fever, tuberculosis, and actinomycosis. Fitz-Hugh–Curtis syndrome is a perihepatitis associated with pelvic inflammatory disease due to *Neisseria gonorrhoeae* or *Chlamydia trachomatis*.

6 Metabolic storage disorders and peroxisomal disorders should be suspected in infants with hepatomegaly, hypotonia, and loss of developmental milestones. These include amino acid defects (e.g., tyrosinemia), glycogen storage disorders, galactosemia, mucopolysaccharidoses, and disorders of lipid metabolism. In addition to the screening tests listed, consider referral for further testing, liver biopsy, specific lymphocyte or urine assay, or bone marrow examination, which may be necessary to diagnose certain metabolic disorders. (See Chapter 22.)

7 Fulminant hepatic failure is the development of advanced liver disease in the absence of previous liver disease. The etiology includes infection, drug reactions, Reye syndrome, and Wilson disease. Fulminant hepatic failure is unlikely in the absence of jaundice.

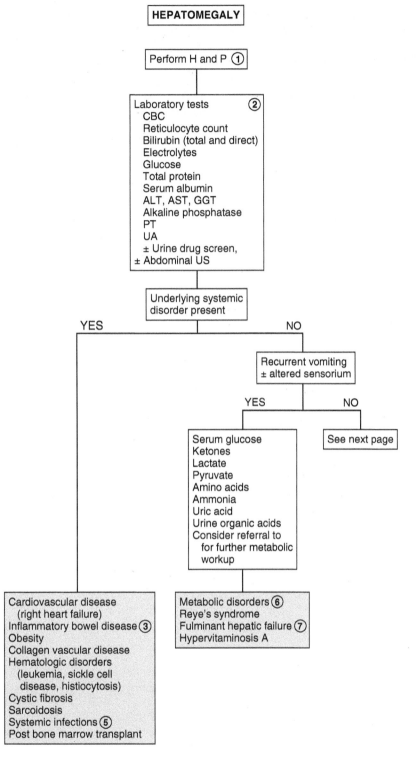

HEPATOMEGALY

Perform H and P ①

Laboratory tests ②
CBC
Reticulocyte count
Bilirubin (total and direct)
Electrolytes
Glucose
Total protein
Serum albumin
ALT, AST, GGT
Alkaline phosphatase
PT
UA
± Urine drug screen,
± Abdominal US

Underlying systemic disorder present

YES — NO

Recurrent vomiting ± altered sensorium

YES — NO

Serum glucose
Ketones
Lactate
Pyruvate
Amino acids
Ammonia
Uric acid
Urine organic acids
Consider referral to for further metabolic workup

See next page

Cardiovascular disease
(right heart failure)
Inflammatory bowel disease ③
Obesity
Collagen vascular disease
Hematologic disorders
(leukemia, sickle cell
disease, histiocytosis)
Cystic fibrosis
Sarcoidosis
Systemic infections ⑤
Post bone marrow transplant

Metabolic disorders ⑥
Reye's syndrome
Fulminant hepatic failure ⑦
Hypervitaminosis A

Nelson Textbook of Pediatrics, 19e. Chapters 79-82, 347-359
Nelsons Essentials, 6e. Chapter 347

8 Zellweger syndrome is the only disorder of peroxisomal metabolism associated with hepatomegaly. Diagnosis is typically made early in life owing to a characteristic phenotype, severe hypotonia, and hepatomegaly.

9 Wilson disease is in the differential diagnosis of acute hepatitis in all children older than 5 years. Kayser-Fleischer rings and neurologic symptoms (e.g., tremor, choreiform movements) are suggestive. Diagnosis is by low serum ceruloplasmin levels, high urinary copper excretion, and increased hepatic copper levels on liver biopsy.

10 Acute hepatitis may present as a mild or severe illness. Most cases resemble a mild flulike nonicteric illness with only tender hepatomegaly on examination. Mild splenomegaly may also occur. Consider serology for CMV and EBV when a high fever and adenopathy are present. Liver biopsy may occasionally be necessary to diagnose certain forms of chronic hepatitis.

11 A nonspecific fatty infiltration of the liver occurs in response to a variety of disorders (e.g., diabetes, cystic fibrosis, inflammatory bowel disease, metabolic disorders). Chemotherapy, other medication and toxins, malnutrition, and obesity are also risk factors.

12 Ascites and tender hepatomegaly are common presenting symptoms of hepatic venous outflow obstruction. Serum transaminases and bilirubin levels are minimally affected acutely. Budd-Chiari syndrome is a noncardiogenic hepatic venous outflow obstruction occurring in conditions predisposing to thrombosis.

Bibliography

Kliegman RM, Stanton B, St. Geme J, Schor N, Behrman RE, editors: *Nelson textbook of pediatrics,* ed 19, Philadelphia, 2011, Elsevier/Saunders, Chapters 79-82, 347-359.

Ross H, Hight DW, Weiss RG: Abdominal masses in pediatric patients. In Wyllie R, Hyams J, editors: *Pediatric gastrointestinal disease: Pathophysiology, diagnosis, management,* ed 2, Philadelphia, 1999, WB Saunders, p 126.

Suchy FJ: Hepatomegaly. In Kliegman RM, Greenbaum, LA, Lye PS, editors: *Practical strategies in pediatric diagnosis and therapy,* ed 2, Philadelphia, 2004, Saunders, pp 333–344.

Wolf AD, Lavine JE: Hepatomegaly in neonates and children, *Pediatr Rev* 21:303–310, 2000.

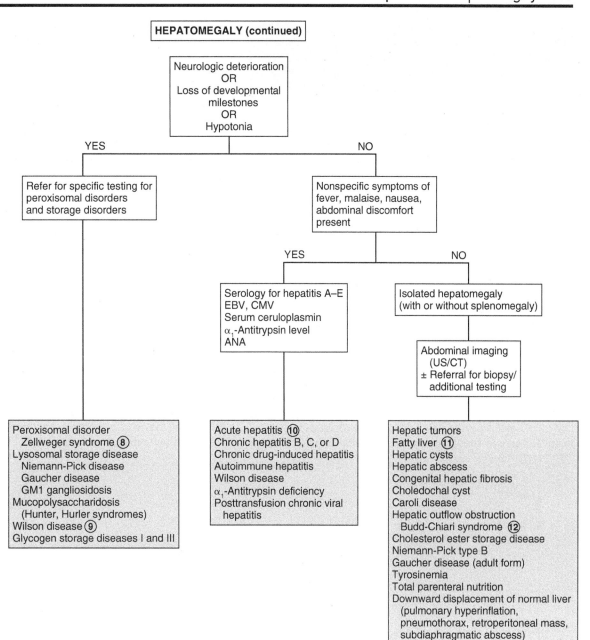

Chapter 28
SPLENOMEGALY

In children, a palpable spleen may or may not be enlarged, because the volume of the spleen may be relatively larger compared with the volume of the abdomen. As a child grows, the absolute and relative size of the spleen decreases. Up to 15% of newborns, 10% of children, and 5% of adolescents have palpable spleens. A splenic edge felt more than 2 cm below the left costal margin is usually abnormal. A persistently palpable spleen may be normal, but some workup is necessary before making this conclusion. A careful H and P will usually suggest the most likely diagnosis and guide the workup.

1. A neonatal history of an umbilical catheter is a risk factor for portal vein thrombosis and subsequent venous obstruction. A history of surgery or blood transfusions may be a risk factor for certain bloodborne infections or thrombosis. Hepatic disease of any cause that results in portal hypertension can result in splenomegaly. Certain ethnic backgrounds suggest a risk of certain disorders, mostly hemolytic or storage disorders. People of Mediterranean or South Asian descent are at risk for thalassemia and glucose-6-phosphate dehydrogenase (G6PD) deficiency. An African ethnicity is a risk factor for sickle cell disease and G6PD deficiency, and an Ashkenazi Jewish ancestry is a risk factor for certain storage disorders, including Gaucher disease.

A family history of jaundice, anemia, cholecystectomy, or splenectomy is suggestive of a hemolytic disorder.

A review of systems positive for anemia, failure to thrive or weight loss, night sweats, lethargy, bruising, bony abnormalities, or respiratory symptoms may suggest an underlying systemic disorder. A travel history should be obtained. Sudden splenomegaly in a child with sickle cell disease suggests acute splenic sequestration, a life-threatening condition. The abdominal examination should include attention to the liver and the possibility of ascites and other abdominal masses. Attention to the characteristic notch on the medial or inferior border of the spleen may help identify it, although other nodular masses may be present. Pain occurs secondary to stretching of the splenic capsule and may occur as left upper quadrant pain or referred pain to the left shoulder. Pain on palpation suggests the capsule has been stretched acutely, such as in an acute infection or hemolysis.

2. Examples of other infections that may cause splenomegaly include spirochetal, rickettsial, parasitic, fungal, mycobacterial, and protozoal (i.e., malaria). Congenital infections (e.g., CMV infection, herpes simplex virus infection, toxoplasmosis, rubella) also result in splenomegaly.

3. Viral infection is the most common cause of splenomegaly in children. In the absence of hemolysis and other worrisome symptoms, a period of observation is acceptable, with additional workup recommended if the splenomegaly persists for 4 to 6 weeks. In the presence of a mononucleosis syndrome, identifying the cause may be reassuring to the physician or family but will not affect the management of the disorder.

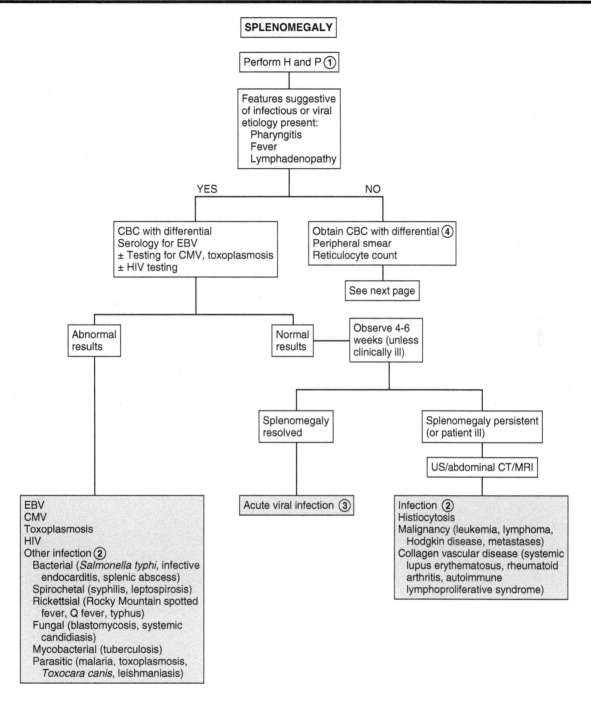

SPLENOMEGALY

Perform H and P ①

Features suggestive
of infectious or viral
etiology present:
  Pharyngitis
  Fever
  Lymphadenopathy

YES   NO

CBC with differential   Obtain CBC with differential ④
Serology for EBV   Peripheral smear
± Testing for CMV, toxoplasmosis   Reticulocyte count
± HIV testing

                                         See next page

Abnormal   Normal   Observe 4-6
results   results   weeks (unless
                                    clinically ill)

                    Splenomegaly   Splenomegaly persistent
                    resolved   (or patient ill)

                                          US/abdominal CT/MRI

EBV   Acute viral infection ③   Infection ②
CMV   Histiocytosis
Toxoplasmosis   Malignancy (leukemia, lymphoma,
HIV   Hodgkin disease, metastases)
Other infection ②   Collagen vascular disease (systemic
  Bacterial (*Salmonella typhi*, infective   lupus erythematosus, rheumatoid
    endocarditis, splenic abscess)   arthritis, autoimmune
  Spirochetal (syphilis, leptospirosis)   lymphoproliferative syndrome)
  Rickettsial (Rocky Mountain spotted
    fever, Q fever, typhus)
  Fungal (blastomycosis, systemic
    candidiasis)
  Mycobacterial (tuberculosis)
  Parasitic (malaria, toxoplasmosis,
    Toxocara canis, leishmaniasis)

Nelson Textbook of Pediatrics, 19e. Chapter 480
Nelsons Essentials, 6e. Chapter 150

4 A CBC, blood smear, and reticulocyte count may indicate hemolytic disease, chronic anemia, or leukemia. In a child up to 3 years of age with a normal CBC, a spleen that is palpable 2 cm below the costal margin may be normal.

5 Laboratory findings suggesting hemolysis include abnormal cell morphology; increased reticulocyte count, RBC distribution width (RDW), indirect bilirubin, urine urobilinogen, and lactate dehydrogenase; decreased serum haptoglobin; and hemoglobinuria.

6 When blasts are seen on peripheral smear, it indicates leukemia requiring referral for bone marrow examination.

7 Sequestration of RBCs may cause rapid splenic enlargement. It may be seen in congenital spherocytosis or other congenital or acquired hemolytic anemias (e.g., sickle cell disease).

8 Mechanical damage causing fragmentation hemolysis may occur in systemic disorders such as disseminated intravascular coagulation, thrombotic thrombocytopenic purpura, and hemolytic-uremic syndrome. Extracorporeal membrane oxygenation, prosthetic heart valves, and burns may cause hemolysis by a similar mechanism.

9 Obstruction of venous drainage at a prehepatic or intrahepatic level or in the portal vein can cause a congestive splenomegaly.

Congestive heart failure, Budd-Chiari syndrome, and hepatic disorders leading to cirrhosis are causes. Pancytopenia frequently results from excessive pooling (i.e., hypersplenism).

10 Storage disorders (e.g., Gaucher disease, glycogen storage disease, mucopolysaccharidosis) are usually diagnosed early in life with abnormal growth, skeletal abnormalities, and developmental delay.

11 Osteopetrosis refers to disorders of increased skeletal density. Hepatosplenomegaly occurs secondary to extramedullary hematopoiesis in severe forms. Milder variants of the disease may have only a mild anemia and no significant hepatosplenomegaly.

12 Pulmonary hyperinflation due to asthma, bronchiolitis, or a pneumothorax may cause splenic displacement.

Bibliography

Kliegman RM, Stanton B, St. Geme J, Schor N, Behrman RE, editors: *Nelson textbook of pediatrics*, ed 19, Philadelphia, 2011, Elsevier/Saunders, Chapter 480.

Maloney KW: Splenomegaly. In Kliegman RM, Greenbaum LA, Lye PS, editors: *Practical strategies in pediatric diagnosis and therapy*, ed 2, Philadelphia, 2004, Elsevier, pp 345–352.

Reznik M, Ozuah PO: Splenomegaly. In McInerny TK, Adam HM, Campbell DE, et al, editors: *American Academy of Pediatrics textbook of pediatric care*, ed 1, Elk Grove Village, Ill, 2008, AAP, pp 1730.

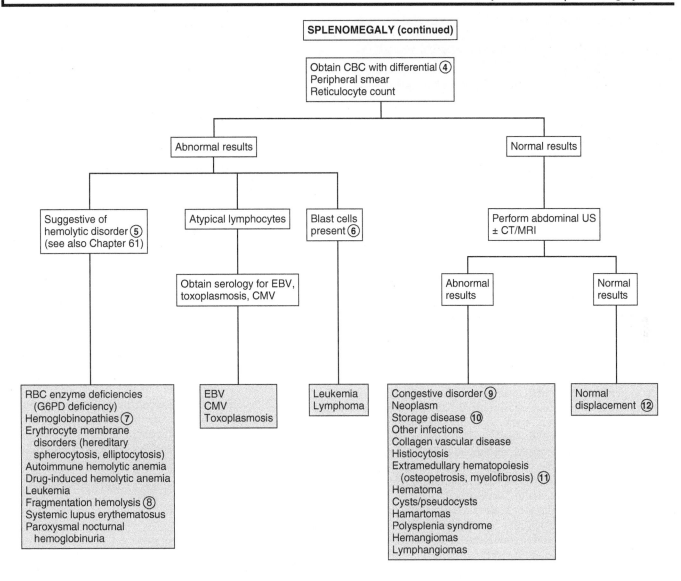

Chapter 29
ABDOMINAL MASSES

Abdominal masses represent a varied group of entities, many of which are age and gender specific. Because the abdominal cavity allows considerable room for growth, there may be few or nonspecific symptoms.

1. For infants, a perinatal and birth history may reveal risk factors for certain disorders. Results of a prenatal US may provide a diagnosis before postnatal imaging. A thorough review of symptoms and social history, including a sexual history, recent travel, and infectious contacts, should be obtained.

The abdominal examination should note the location, size, shape, texture, mobility, and tenderness of the mass. The location will aid in determining which organ is most likely affected. Hepatosplenomegaly is the cause of more than half of childhood abdominal masses. (See Chapters 27 and 28.) A normal liver is nontender with a sharp edge and is palpated in the right upper quadrant 1 to 2 cm below the right costal margin. The normal spleen is usually nonpalpable, although it may be felt in the left upper quadrant with a round edge. The liver and spleen move with respirations. Renal masses usually extend downward from the kidney location, do not tend to cross the midline, and do not move with respiration. Abdominal distention due to ascites must be distinguished from abdominal distention due to a mass. Ascites generally causes bulging flanks and dullness to percussion in the flanks. The fluid shifts with movement of the patient and causes a percussion wave or shifting dullness. In males the external genitalia should be assessed, particularly for a left-sided varicocele, which may be associated with a Wilms tumor. In females with a lower abdominal mass, an assessment should be made to rule out an imperforate hymen.

Although imaging studies have the highest yield in the evaluation of abdominal masses, laboratory evaluation should be considered in certain cases. A urine pregnancy test should be obtained in all adolescent females with a lower abdominal mass. A CBC, LFTs, BUN/Cr, serum electrolytes, serum amylase and lipase, as well as UA may screen for other abdominal problems. LDH and alkaline phosphatase may be clues to malignancy.

2. Abdominal US is a safe, noninvasive method for determining whether a mass is cystic or solid. It is the preferred diagnostic test in neonates and is also appropriate in older children.

3. Hydronephrosis is the most common cause of an abdominal mass in the neonate. It is due to obstruction of the urinary outflow tract. In male infants, posterior urethral valves are the most common cause of hydronephrosis.

4. In infants, a history of polycythemia, dehydration, diabetic mother, asphyxia, sepsis, or coagulopathy are risk factors for renal vein thrombosis. Hematuria, hypertension, and thrombocytopenia are often present.

5. Neuroblastoma is one of the most common malignancies in infants.

6. Ovarian lesions may appear as a mass or pain due to torsion, adhesions, hemorrhage, or rupture. Some ovarian tumors occur as precocious puberty owing to the production of estrogen.

7. The etiology of a hepatic mass includes tumors, hemangiomas, cysts, and abscesses. Adenoma, focal nodular hyperplasia, and hamartomas can occur as solitary lesions. Malignant hepatic tumors include hepatoblastoma and hepatocellular carcinoma.

8. Wilms tumor is the second most common malignancy in childhood.

Bibliography

Gauderer MWL, Chandler JC: Abdominal masses. In Kliegman RM, Greenbaum LA, Lye PS, editors: *Practical strategies in pediatric diagnosis and therapy*, ed 2, Philadelphia, 2004, Elsevier, pp 383–394.

Kliegman RM, Stanton B, St. Geme J, Schor N, Behrman RE, editors: *Nelson textbook of pediatrics*, ed 19, Philadelphia, 2011, Elsevier/Saunders, Chapters 298, 487.

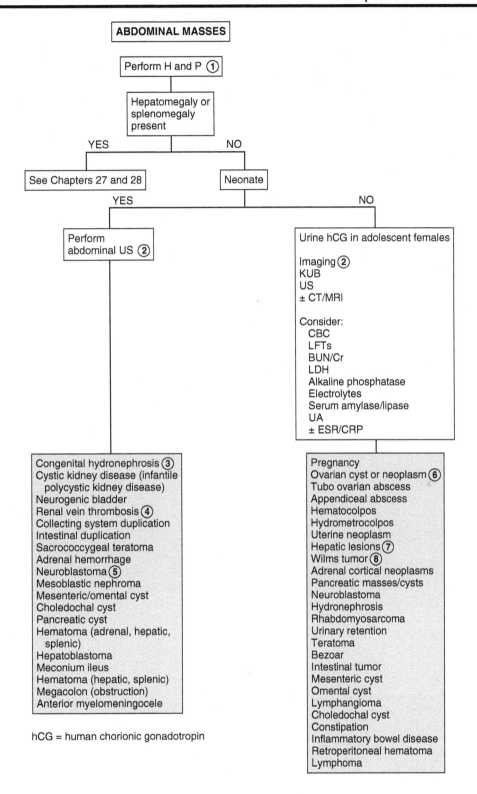

ABDOMINAL MASSES

Perform H and P ①

Hepatomegaly or splenomegaly present

YES — See Chapters 27 and 28

NO — Neonate

YES — Perform abdominal US ②

NO — Urine hCG in adolescent females

Imaging ②
KUB
US
± CT/MRI

Consider:
  CBC
  LFTs
  BUN/Cr
  LDH
  Alkaline phosphatase
  Electrolytes
  Serum amylase/lipase
  UA
  ± ESR/CRP

Congenital hydronephrosis ③
Cystic kidney disease (infantile polycystic kidney disease)
Neurogenic bladder
Renal vein thrombosis ④
Collecting system duplication
Intestinal duplication
Sacrococcygeal teratoma
Adrenal hemorrhage
Neuroblastoma ⑤
Mesoblastic nephroma
Mesenteric/omental cyst
Choledochal cyst
Pancreatic cyst
Hematoma (adrenal, hepatic, splenic)
Hepatoblastoma
Meconium ileus
Hematoma (hepatic, splenic)
Megacolon (obstruction)
Anterior myelomeningocele

Pregnancy
Ovarian cyst or neoplasm ⑥
Tubo ovarian abscess
Appendiceal abscess
Hematocolpos
Hydrometrocolpos
Uterine neoplasm
Hepatic lesions ⑦
Wilms tumor ⑧
Adrenal cortical neoplasms
Pancreatic masses/cysts
Neuroblastoma
Hydronephrosis
Rhabdomyosarcoma
Urinary retention
Teratoma
Bezoar
Intestinal tumor
Mesenteric cyst
Omental cyst
Lymphangioma
Choledochal cyst
Constipation
Inflammatory bowel disease
Retroperitoneal hematoma
Lymphoma

hCG = human chorionic gonadotropin

Nelson Textbook of Pediatrics, 19e. Chapters 198, 487
Nelsons Essentials, 6e. Chapters 153, 159

Genitourinary System

Chapter 30

DYSURIA

Dysuria is pain or burning occurring with urination. It is often associated with urinary symptoms such as frequency, urgency, incontinence, and refusal to void. Dysuria is not specific for UTIs and often occurs in young children.

1 Toddlers may present with secondary enuresis, dribbling, and frequent squatting. Constipation, not being circumcised, female gender, contraceptive diaphragms, and sexual intercourse may predispose to a UTI. Chemical irritants (e.g., detergents, bubble bath) and mechanical irritation (e.g., masturbation, foreign body) may cause dysuria. Dark or tea-colored urine may indicate hematuria. A history of penile or vaginal discharge as well as sexual abuse should be elicited.

Physical examination should include BP, genitalia, abdominal palpation of the kidneys, pelvic exam when indicated, and a careful neurologic exam in children with voiding dysfunction to exclude spinal cord pathology.

2 Urine for UA and culture must be properly obtained. UA, which includes microscopic examination and dipstick method, correlates with infection, particularly in an older child. Dipstick methods test for leukocyte esterase (an enzyme present in WBCs) and nitrites. Microscopic analysis of unspun urine for WBCs (10/mm³) or bacteria on Gram stain is more predictive than spun urine ($\geq$5 WBCs/high-power field), which is commonly used. RBCs are common with a bacterial UTI. WBC casts, when present, are associated with upper tract infections.

Urine culture remains the standard for diagnosis. Any growth in urine collected by suprapubic tap, more than 50,000 colonies by catheterization, or more than 10^5 colonies by clean-catch midstream urine indicate infection. "Bagged" specimens may have skin or fecal contaminants and are not recommended. *Escherichia coli* is the most common pathogen; others include *Proteus*, *Klebsiella*, *Staphylococcus saprophyticus*, and enterococcus.

3 In older children, pyelonephritis may be clinically differentiated from cystitis by the presence of systemic features (fever, vomiting) and signs (flank pain, costovertebral angle tenderness). In infants and young children, the clinical picture may be nonspecific, with fever and other symptoms present in upper or lower tract disease. If necessary, the diagnosis of pyelonephritis may be confirmed by renal scan, the most sensitive being ^{99m}Tc-dimercaptosuccinic acid (DMSA). Renal US may also show pyelonephritis but is not as sensitive; however, it is adequate to detect obstructive uropathy or high-grade reflux that may be associated with pyelonephritis.

The occurrence of the first episode of febrile UTIs in a child aged 2 to 24 months may be a marker for congenital anatomic abnormalities—in particular, vesicourethral reflux (VUR). According to recent guidelines, US of the kidneys and bladder should be performed to detect anatomic abnormalities. A voiding cystourethrogram (VCUG) is indicated if renal and bladder US reveals hydronephrosis, scarring, or other findings that would suggest either high-grade VUR or obstructive uropathy. VCUG

should also be performed if there is a recurrence of a febrile UTI. For males, a UTI at any age requires further evaluation.

4 Nucleic acid amplification tests (NAAT) for *Neisseria gonorrhoeae and Chlamydia trachomatis can be* performed on urine as well as genital specimens (urethral or cervical). Tests based on nucleic acid hybridization are also available. Penile, vaginal, or cervical cultures may be used as well. Wet saline mount of vaginal secretions with microscopy, including use of potassium hydroxide, and Gram stain can be used to detect *Trichomonas*, as well as bacterial vaginosis and vaginal candidiasis. Tests to detect *Trichomonas* antigen are also used.

5 The presence of leukocytes on UA may indicate vaginitis due to sexually transmitted infections (*N. gonorrhoeae, Chlamydia*, herpes simplex, *Trichomonas vaginalis*). They may also indicate *Candida albicans*, enteric pathogens, or group A streptococci. Urethritis is caused by *N. gonorrhoeae, Chlamydia, Mycoplasma genitalium*, and *Ureaplasma urealyticum*. (See Chapter 41.)

6 Nonspecific urethritis is often seen in premenarchal girls and is associated with poor hygiene, tight "nonbreathing" clothes, and chemical irritants (bubble bath, harsh soaps). There may be erythema in the periurethral area. Anal pruritus may indicate pinworms, which can cause urethral irritation and can be confirmed by examination with a tape slide test.

7 Labial adhesions are common in prepubertal girls and are due to recurrent irritation, trauma, or infection of the hypoestrogenized epithelium of the labia minora. Urethral prolapse is an eversion of the urethral mucosa through the meatus. Bleeding and dysuria are common. Lichen sclerosus causes an hourglass-shaped area of atrophy and scarring with depigmentation. Herpes simplex causes ulcers and vesicles. It may be detected by a scraping for direct fluorescent antibody (DFA) testing, PCR, or viral culture. Sexual abuse is often associated with rectal or vaginal bleeding and vaginitis. Appropriate studies should be obtained.

8 Microscopic hematuria may be seen with UTI. Gross hematuria is seen with hemorrhagic cystitis (adenovirus, cyclophosphamide), renal calculi, hypercalcuria, and trauma and is rarely tumor related (clots from Wilms tumor). (See Chapter 32.)

9 Meatal stenosis may occur for a number of reasons. In circumcised boys, it may result from recurrent meatal inflammation from moist diapers. Trauma, hypospadias repair, catheterization, and balanitis xerotica obliterans are other causes. It most often appears as an abnormal urine stream, intermittent dysuria, and occasional bleeding. Phimosis is when the foreskin cannot be retracted because of scarring or narrowing of the preputial opening. It must be distinguished from physiologic phimosis when the foreskin has not completed the normal separation from the glans, usually by 3 to 5 years of age. Paraphimosis is the incarceration of the prepuce behind the glans, often after forcible retraction of the foreskin. Balanitis is an inflammation of the prepuce, which is usually due to urine, but infection may be involved.

Bibliography

Subcommittee on Urinary Tract Infection, Steering Committee on Quality Improvement and Management, Roberts KB: Urinary tract infection: Clinical practice guideline for the diagnosis and management of the initial UTI in febrile infants and children 2 to 24 months, *Pediatrics* 128:595–610, 2011.

Kliegman RM, Stanton B, St. Geme J, Schor N, Behrman RE, editors: *Nelson textbook of pediatrics*, ed 19, Philadelphia, 2011, Elsevier/Saunders, Chapters 114, 185, 254, 276, 513, 532, 538.

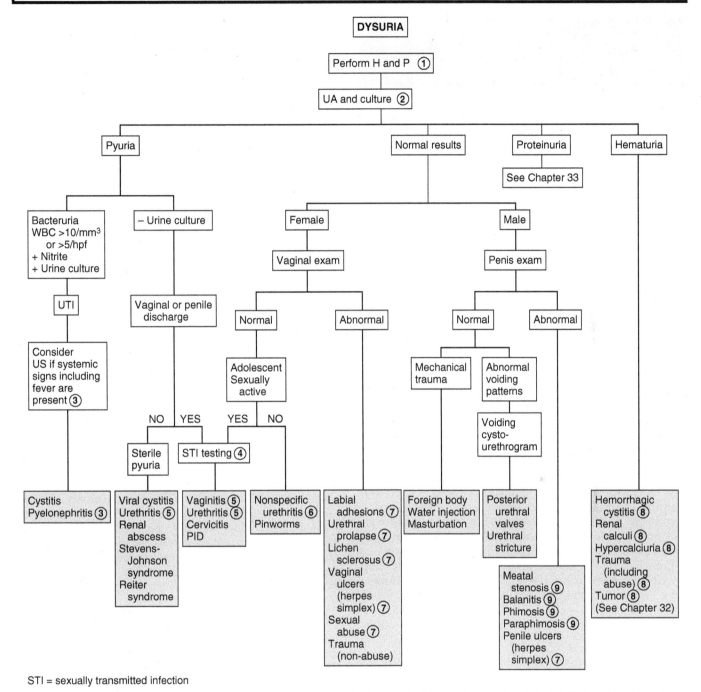

DYSURIA

Perform H and P ①

UA and culture ②

Pyuria | Normal results | Proteinuria | Hematuria

See Chapter 33

Bacteruria
WBC >10/mm³
or >5/hpf
+ Nitrite
+ Urine culture

− Urine culture

UTI

Vaginal or penile
discharge

Consider
US if systemic
signs including
fever are
present ③

Female

Vaginal exam

Normal | Abnormal

Adolescent
Sexually
active

Male

Penis exam

Normal | Abnormal

Mechanical
trauma

Abnormal
voiding
patterns

Voiding
cysto-
urethrogram

NO | YES | YES | NO

Sterile
pyuria

STI testing ④

Cystitis
Pyelonephritis ③

Viral cystitis
Urethritis ⑤
Renal
   abscess
Stevens-
Johnson
syndrome
Reiter
syndrome

Vaginitis ⑤
Urethritis ⑤
Cervicitis
PID

Nonspecific
urethritis ⑥
Pinworms

Labial
   adhesions ⑦
Urethral
   prolapse ⑦
Lichen
   sclerosus ⑦
Vaginal
   ulcers
   (herpes
   simplex) ⑦
Sexual
   abuse ⑦
Trauma
   (non-abuse)

Foreign body
Water injection
Masturbation

Posterior
urethral
valves
Urethral
stricture

Meatal
   stenosis ⑨
Balanitis ⑨
Phimosis ⑨
Paraphimosis ⑨
Penile ulcers
   (herpes
   simplex) ⑦

Hemorrhagic
   cystitis ⑧
Renal
   calculi ⑧
Hypercalciuria ⑧
Trauma
   (including
   abuse) ⑧
Tumor ⑧
(See Chapter 32)

STI = sexually transmitted infection

Nelson Textbook of Pediatrics, 19e. Chapters 114, 185, 254, 276, 513, 532, 538
Nelsons Essentials, 6e. Chapters 114, 116

Chapter 31
ENURESIS

Enuresis is urinary incontinence at an age when most children are continent. Nocturnal enuresis, the most common form, is the involuntary passage of urine during sleep. Diurnal enuresis is the unintended leakage of urine when awake in a child old enough to maintain bladder control. Primary nocturnal enuresis refers to a child who has never been continent at night and is older than age 5 years. Secondary enuresis refers to a child who was successfully toilet trained for at least 3 to 6 months and becomes incontinent once again. It is often related to stress (new sibling, school trauma, physical or sexual abuse).

Monosymptomatic nocturnal enuresis with no associated daytime symptoms of urgency, frequency, or daytime enuresis is usually physiologic and occurs at least monthly in approximately 20% of 5-year-olds and in 10% of 6-year-olds.

1 It is most important to distinguish between monosymptomatic nocturnal enuresis (which is usually benign) and diurnal enuresis (which may have an organic cause). UTI is often associated with enuresis, as well as constipation and encopresis. The timing of the wetting should be determined. Children with overactive bladder (pediatric unstable bladder) may have "squatting," urinary frequency, and urgency and may also have symptoms of attention deficit hyperactivity disorder (ADHD). A history of holding urine until the last minute or enuresis associated with giggling, laughing, coughing, straining, or physical activity may indicate the cause. Polyuria and polydipsia may indicate diabetes mellitus or diabetes insipidus. Neurologic symptoms or signs, as well as midline abnormalities, may indicate an underlying neurologic disorder associated with a neurogenic bladder. In children with nocturnal enuresis, a history of snoring and mouth breathing may indicate sleep apnea. Hypertension or growth failure may indicate chronic renal disease. A careful GU examination should be done to look for meatal stenosis, labial fusion, or other abnormalities. In patients with urethral obstruction, the bladder and kidneys may be enlarged.

2 All children with enuresis should also have a complete UA with microscopic examination and culture when indicated. (See Chapter 30.) Glucosuria may indicate diabetes mellitus. A first morning urine sample with specific gravity above 1.015 to 1.020 excludes diabetes insipidus. In children with incontinence associated with dysuria, frequency, urgency, and foul-smelling urine, the UA and culture may indicate a UTI. (See Chapter 30.) RBCs may be seen with urethral obstruction or hydronephrosis, and glucosuria may be due to diabetes mellitus. Hematuria may be noted in children with hypercalcuria or sickle cell disease or trait.

3 Constipation is often associated with bladder dysfunction, because anorectal and lower urinary tract function are interrelated. This relationship between abnormal bowel and bladder function is known as dysfunctional elimination syndrome.

4 Neurogenic bladder may develop secondary to a lesion of the central or peripheral nervous system. A careful neurologic examination should be included, assessing strength, tone, sensation and reflexes of the lower extremities, and anal wink. The lumbosacral spine should be examined for hair tufts, dimples, masses, or other skin findings that might reveal spinal dysraphism. The voiding cystourethrogram demonstrates a trabeculated bladder with a "Christmas tree" or "pine cone" appearance. MRI should be done to look for spinal cord abnormalities when the cause of the neurogenic bladder has not been determined.

5 In children who have leakage of urine after voiding, a careful examination may indicate labial fusion in which there is retention of urine behind the fused labia. In some girls, especially obese or preschool-aged girls who do not open the labia when voiding, there may be "reflux" of the urine into the vagina, which later leaks out. Some girls who have postvoid dribble syndrome may feel a sense of wetness after voiding lasting for a few minutes, although there is no evidence of urine. This is believed to be due to detrusor "after contractions."

6 Urethral obstruction may appear as abnormal urinary symptoms such as dribbling, poor stream, needing to push, or weak thin stream. It may be congenital (e.g., posterior urethral valves, stricture, urethral diverticula) or acquired, owing to development of a stricture due to infection (*Neisseria gonorrhoeae* urethritis) or trauma (traumatic catheterization, urethral foreign body).

7 In dysfunctional voiding, there is inability of the urethral sphincter and pelvic floor musculature to relax during voiding. Hinman syndrome (detrusor-sphincter dyssynergia) is an extreme form of this in a child without neurologic abnormalities. It is also known as nonneurogenic neurogenic bladder. Children with this syndrome have a staccato stream and a decreased urinary flow rate, day and night wetting, recurrent UTIs, constipation, and encopresis. Imaging shows a trabeculated bladder, a significant amount of residual urine after voiding, and may show vesicourethral reflux, upper urinary tract dilation, and renal scarring.

8 Overactive bladder (urge syndrome, pediatric unstable bladder) is a common cause of daytime wetting. Affected children may have daytime and nighttime wetting, frequency, and urgency, as well as squatting behavior, which is a characteristic symptom. The squatting is an attempt to suppress detrusor contractions, which can last more than a minute.

9 Giggle incontinence is associated with laughing and is common in girls. The entire bladder empties, in contrast to stress incontinence, in which a small amount of urine leaks owing to increased intraabdominal pressure. Common causes of stress incontinence are coughing, straining, or physical activity. Another common cause of wetting is micturition deferral. It is common in preschool-aged children who are engrossed in activities. This may increase the risk for UTI as well.

10 Ectopic ureter is a rare congenital anomaly. Incontinence occurs when the ureter is inserted distal to the external sphincter. It is more common in girls, and there is constant dripping of urine.

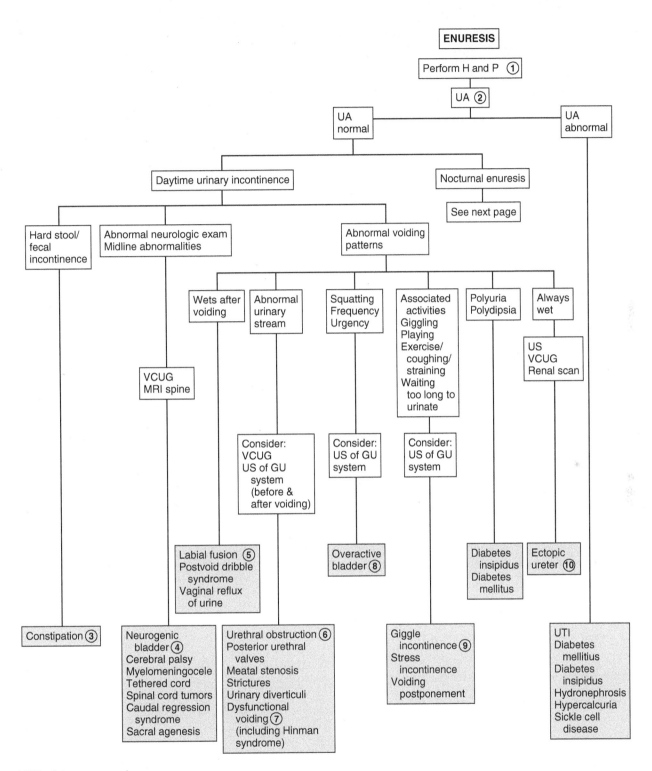

ENURESIS

Perform H and P ①

UA ②

UA normal — UA abnormal

Daytime urinary incontinence — Nocturnal enuresis → See next page

Hard stool/fecal incontinence

Abnormal neurologic exam Midline abnormalities

Abnormal voiding patterns

Wets after voiding

Abnormal urinary stream

Squatting Frequency Urgency

Associated activities Giggling Playing Exercise/coughing/straining Waiting too long to urinate

Polyuria Polydipsia

Always wet

US VCUG Renal scan

VCUG MRI spine

Consider: VCUG US of GU system (before & after voiding)

Consider: US of GU system

Consider: US of GU system

Labial fusion ⑤ Postvoid dribble syndrome Vaginal reflux of urine

Overactive bladder ⑧

Diabetes insipidus Diabetes mellitus

Ectopic ureter ⑩

Constipation ③

Neurogenic bladder ④ Cerebral palsy Myelomeningocele Tethered cord Spinal cord tumors Caudal regression syndrome Sacral agenesis

Urethral obstruction ⑥ Posterior urethral valves Meatal stenosis Strictures Urinary diverticuli Dysfunctional voiding ⑦ (including Hinman syndrome)

Giggle incontinence ⑨ Stress incontinence Voiding postponement

UTI Diabetes mellitus Diabetes insipidus Hydronephrosis Hypercalcuria Sickle cell disease

IVP = Intravenous pyelogram
VCUG = Voiding cystourethrogram

Nelson Textbook of Pediatrics, 19e. Chapters 21, 537
Nelsons Essentials, 6e. Chapter 14

11 A history of dysuria, frequency, urgency, daytime enuresis, polydipsia, polyuria, CNS injury, constipation or encopresis, constant wetness, neurologic signs or symptoms, or abnormal urine stream may indicate an organic cause and prompt further evaluation, as in the case of diurnal enuresis. Nocturnal enuresis is rarely due to an organic etiology.

12 In children with sleep apnea, suggested by severe snoring and obligatory mouth breathing, wetting may occur during sleep apnea. A lateral neck x-ray may be helpful to document large adenoids, and a sleep study to evaluate for obstructive sleep apnea. Referral to an ENT specialist is recommended.

13 Monosymptomatic primary nocturnal enuresis is a common problem. It is more common in boys and often shows a familial pattern. These children have a normal examination (including careful neurologic exam), no associated daytime symptoms, and have normal findings on UA.

Bibliography

Graham KM, Levy JB: Enuresis, *Pediatr Rev* 30:165–173, 2009.

Kliegman RM, Stanton B, St. Geme J, Schor N, Behrman RE, editors: *Nelson textbook of pediatrics*, ed 19, Philadelphia, 2011, Saunders, Chapters 21, 537.

Neveus T, Eggert P, Evans J, et al: Evaluation of and treatment for monosymptomatic enuresis: A standardization document from the International Children's Continence Society, *J Urol* 183:441–447, 2010.

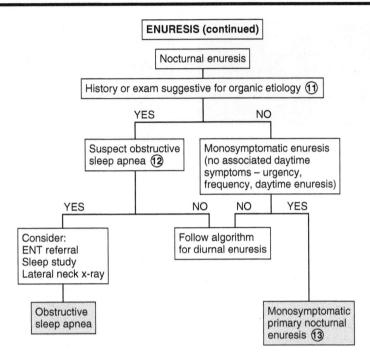

ENURESIS (continued)

Nocturnal enuresis

History or exam suggestive for organic etiology ⑪

YES — NO

Suspect obstructive sleep apnea ⑫

Monosymptomatic enuresis (no associated daytime symptoms – urgency, frequency, daytime enuresis)

YES — NO — NO — YES

Consider:
ENT referral
Sleep study
Lateral neck x-ray

Follow algorithm for diurnal enuresis

Obstructive sleep apnea

Monosymptomatic primary nocturnal enuresis ⑬

Chapter 32
RED URINE AND HEMATURIA

Red or brown urine may indicate hematuria and possible renal disease. Hematuria is a common finding on UA. Microscopic hematuria is defined as more than 5 RBCs per high-power field in the sediment of freshly voided urine. Gross hematuria is visible to the naked eye. The presence of RBCs in the urine must be confirmed because there are many conditions other than hematuria causing red or brown discoloration of the urine.

1. History should include urinary symptoms such as dysuria, frequency, and urgency, as well as flank or abdominal pain. A history of exercise or trauma, including a foreign body, catheterization, or sexual/physical abuse, may indicate the cause of the hematuria. A medication, drug, and dietary history should be obtained. The history should include oliguria and hypertension, as well as systemic illnesses often associated with renal disease (e.g., arthritis, respiratory illness). Family history should include renal abnormalities, hematuria, deafness, renal failure, hypertension, nephrolithiasis, sickle cell disease or trait, dialysis, or renal transplant. BP must be obtained. Physical examination should focus on the GU system and joints and on identifying any abdominal mass or a rash.

2. A positive reagent strip (dipstick) in the absence of RBCs indicates the presence of Hgb or myoglobin. Hemoglobinuria occurs with hemolysis. It may occur in hemolytic anemias, hemolytic-uremic syndrome, mismatched transfusions, freshwater drowning, septicemia, and paroxysmal nocturnal hemoglobinuria. It is also associated with carbon monoxide, fava beans, venoms, mushrooms, naphthalene, quinine, and many other substances. A CBC with smear will often show fragmented cells, and the reticulocyte count may be elevated.

Myoglobinuria occurs with rhabdomyolysis after viral myositis and in children with inborn errors of energy metabolism, often after exercise. The clinical picture as well as elevated muscle enzyme levels may aid in distinguishing myoglobinuria from hematuria. If needed, Hgb and myoglobin may be measured in the urine.

3. Microscopic hematuria is often found on routine screening. If the child is asymptomatic, with normal BP and no proteinuria, the UA should be repeated at least 2 to 3 times over 2 to 3 months. If followup UA is normal, a diagnosis of isolated asymptomatic hematuria is made. If proteinuria is present, the evaluation is the same as for gross hematuria (see algorithm). If the child is symptomatic (hypertension, edema) and has proteinuria and a family history of deafness or kidney disease, a nephrologist should be consulted.

4. Gross hematuria can be localized to the upper or lower urinary tract. Upper tract bleeding causes brown, smoky, or tea-colored urine. Proteinuria suggests glomerular involvement. (See Chapter 33.) Dysmorphic RBCs due to passage through the glomerular basement membrane also indicate upper tract involvement. Lower tract bleeding is bright red, may have clots, rarely contains significant amounts of protein, and shows isomorphic RBC morphology.

5. Symptomatic gross hematuria may be due to renal disease. UTIs commonly cause gross hematuria and can be diagnosed by a positive urine culture when bacterial in origin. Hemorrhagic cystitis is often caused by adenovirus. Nephrolithiasis is associated with renal colic, positive family history, and UA that may show crystals as well as hematuria. Premature infants who received furosemide may have nephrocalcinosis. Stones can be diagnosed by using IV pyelography, spiral CT, or US. X-rays may not detect radiolucent stones. Hypercalciuria, even without the presence of a stone, may cause abdominal or flank pain, dysuria, and hematuria. Meatal stenosis with ulceration, trauma due to catheterization, and sexual abuse may cause hematuria. Abdominal and renal traumas are also causes and require abdominal CT scan with IV contrast medium enhancement. Injury to the bladder and posterior urethra may be associated with pelvic fractures and may be diagnosed by retrograde urethrography.

6. Idiopathic hypercalciuria most often occurs as persistent microscopic hematuria or as recurrent gross hematuria or dysuria. A calcium-to-Cr ratio above 0.2 is suggestive. If this is present, a 24-hour urine collection for calcium should be obtained. Autosomal dominant polycystic kidney disease often appears as gross hematuria. Symptoms may begin in childhood but more often occur in adulthood. Renal and bladder tumors may rarely occur as hematuria. Arteriovenous malformations of the kidney may present as gross hematuria because of rapid transit of blood down the ureter; localization of bleeding may require cystoscopy or angiography. Stress hematuria occurs after exercise. It is painless and of short duration; there is no proteinuria. Patients with benign familial hematuria (thin basement membrane nephropathy) have an excellent prognosis but must be followed. It has an autosomal dominant inheritance. Renal biopsy shows thinning of the glomerular basement membrane on electron microscopy. Nutcracker syndrome is due to the compression of the distal segment of the left renal vein between the superior mesenteric artery and the aorta. Papillary necrosis may result in hematuria in patients with sickle cell disease or trait.

7. Acute postinfectious glomerulonephritis occurs 4 days to 3 weeks after a febrile illness just with hematuria, but also with oliguria, edema, and hypertension. Group A streptococcal infection causing either pharyngitis or impetigo is the most common cause. Laboratory findings include a decrease in C3 and C4 levels and laboratory evidence of a preceding group A streptococcal infection (Streptozyme, antistreptolysin, antihyaluronidase, anti–DNase B titers). Hematuria from immunoglobulin (Ig)A nephropathy appears within 48 hours of a URI. Microscopic hematuria may be present between episodes. Alport syndrome is associated with a family history of renal disease, deafness, and hematuria.

Henoch-Schönlein purpura (HSP) may appear as abdominal pain, joint pain, and lower extremity rash (palpable purpura). In addition to hematuria, proteinuria may also be present. There is no specific laboratory test for HSP; however, serum IgA levels may be elevated. In tuberous sclerosis, hematuria may be due to associated renal cysts and angiomyolipomas. Systemic infections such as bacterial endocarditis and shunt infections may be associated with hematuria and proteinuria. Nephrotic syndrome may be associated with hematuria,

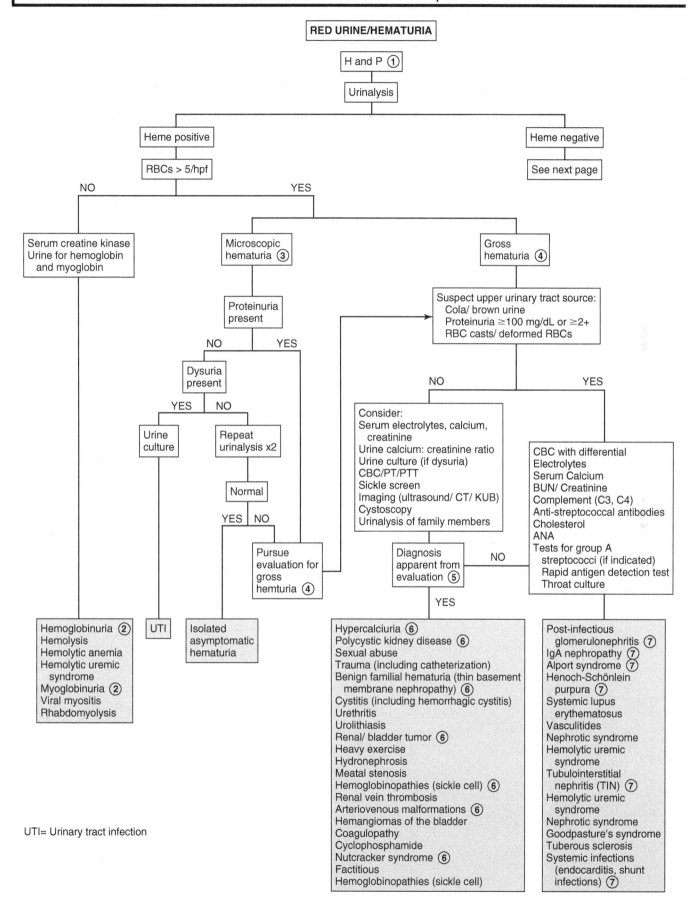

RED URINE/HEMATURIA

H and P ①

Urinalysis

Heme positive | Heme negative

RBCs > 5/hpf | See next page

NO | YES

Serum creatine kinase
Urine for hemoglobin
and myoglobin

Microscopic
hematuria ③

Gross
hematuria ④

Proteinuria
present

Suspect upper urinary tract source:
Cola/ brown urine
Proteinuria ≥100 mg/dL or ≥2+
RBC casts/ deformed RBCs

NO | YES

NO | YES

Dysuria
present

YES | NO

Consider:
Serum electrolytes, calcium,
creatinine
Urine calcium: creatinine ratio
Urine culture (if dysuria)
CBC/PT/PTT
Sickle screen
Imaging (ultrasound/ CT/ KUB)
Cystoscopy
Urinalysis of family members

Urine
culture

Repeat
urinalysis x2

CBC with differential
Electrolytes
Serum Calcium
BUN/ Creatinine
Complement (C3, C4)
Anti-streptococcal antibodies
Cholesterol
ANA
Tests for group A
streptococci (if indicated)
Rapid antigen detection test
Throat culture

Normal

YES | NO

Pursue
evaluation for
gross
hemturia ④

Diagnosis
apparent from
evaluation ⑤

NO

YES

Hemoglobinuria ②
Hemolysis
Hemolytic anemia
Hemolytic uremic
syndrome
Myoglobinuria ②
Viral myositis
Rhabdomyolysis

UTI

Isolated
asymptomatic
hematuria

Hypercalciuria ⑥
Polycystic kidney disease ⑥
Sexual abuse
Trauma (including catheterization)
Benign familial hematuria (thin basement
membrane nephropathy) ⑥
Cystitis (including hemorrhagic cystitis)
Urethritis
Urolithiasis
Renal/ bladder tumor ⑥
Heavy exercise
Hydronephrosis
Meatal stenosis
Hemoglobinopathies (sickle cell) ⑥
Renal vein thrombosis
Arteriovenous malformations ⑥
Hemangiomas of the bladder
Coagulopathy
Cyclophosphamide
Nutcracker syndrome ⑥
Factitious
Hemoglobinopathies (sickle cell)

Post-infectious
glomerulonephritis ⑦
IgA nephropathy ⑦
Alport syndrome ⑦
Henoch-Schönlein
purpura ⑦
Systemic lupus
erythematosus
Vasculitides
Nephrotic syndrome
Hemolytic uremic
syndrome
Tubulointerstitial
nephritis (TIN) ⑦
Hemolytic uremic
syndrome
Nephrotic syndrome
Goodpasture's syndrome
Tuberous sclerosis
Systemic infections
(endocarditis, shunt
infections) ⑦

UTI= Urinary tract infection

particularly in focal segmental sclerosis and membranoproliferative glomerulonephritis. Tubulointerstitial nephritis is often associated with penicillins, cephalosporins, sulfonamides, rifampin, tetracyclines, nonsteroidal antiinflammatory drugs, furosemide, thiazides, heavy metals, and others. It may also be associated with other diseases, such as systemic lupus erythematosus.

Bibliography

Kliegman RM, Stanton BF, St. Geme J, Schor N, Behrman RE, editors: *Nelson textbook of pediatrics*, ed 19, Philadelphia, 2011, Elsevier Saunders. Chapters 503–516.

McInerny TK, Adam HM, Campbell DE, et al, editors: *American Academy of Pediatrics textbook of pediatric care*, Elk Grove Village, Ill, 2009, American Academy of Pediatrics, pp 1566–1569.

Pan CG: Evaluation of gross hematuria, *Pediatr Clin North Am* 53:401–412, 2006

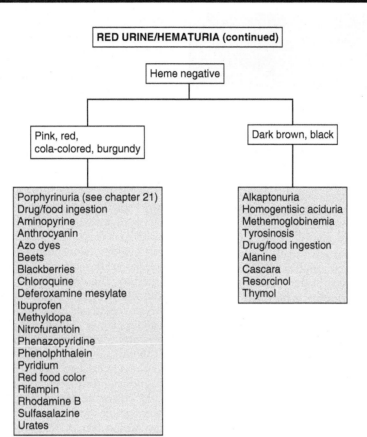

RED URINE/HEMATURIA (continued)

Heme negative

Pink, red, cola-colored, burgundy

Porphyrinuria (see chapter 21)
Drug/food ingestion
Aminopyrine
Anthrocyanin
Azo dyes
Beets
Blackberries
Chloroquine
Deferoxamine mesylate
Ibuprofen
Methyldopa
Nitrofurantoin
Phenazopyridine
Phenolphthalein
Pyridium
Red food color
Rifampin
Rhodamine B
Sulfasalazine
Urates

Dark brown, black

Alkaptonuria
Homogentisic aciduria
Methemoglobinemia
Tyrosinosis
Drug/food ingestion
Alanine
Cascara
Resorcinol
Thymol

Proteinuria is a common laboratory finding that is often a symptom of renal disease. It may also be found in normal, healthy children. It is therefore important to distinguish between pathologic and nonpathologic causes of proteinuria. As many as 10% of children will have 1+ proteinuria at some time in their lives. Because this is a transient finding in a majority of children, it is important to retest the urine before making a diagnosis.

Proteinuria may be defined qualitatively using a urine dipstick examination. Trace proteinuria is usually not significant; 1+ proteinuria (30 mg/dl) may be significant. This should be repeated and viewed in the context of the urine Sp gr. False-negative results may occur with urine that is too dilute (<1.005), and false-positive results may occur with overlong dipstick immersion, alkaline urine, pyuria, bacteriuria, mucoprotein and quaternary ammonium compounds, and detergents.

Quantitative testing for proteinuria is done by a timed 12- to 24-hour urine collection for protein: less than 4 mg/m^2/h is normal, 4-40 mg/m^2/h is abnormal, and over 40 mg/m^2/h is in the nephrotic range. An early morning spot testing of urine protein/Cr ratio (in mg/dL) correlates well with 24-hour urine protein excretion. A value above 0.2 is abnormal in children older than 2 years; for children 6 months to 2 years, over 0.5 is abnormal, and over 2 suggests nephrotic-range proteinuria. This test is not valid in children with decreased muscle mass (i.e., those with nutritional problems).

1 History should include questions about recent exercise, red or tea-colored urine, and respiratory or other febrile illness. History indicative of edema, such as puffiness around the eyes on awakening, increased abdominal girth, and difficulty putting on shoes, may indicate nephrotic syndrome and should be investigated. Family history related to renal disease, hematuria, or hypertension should be pursued. Systemic complaints (e.g., arthralgia, rash, fever) may be symptoms of diseases such as systemic lupus erythematosus (SLE) or Henoch-Schönlein purpura (HSP). On physical examination, BP must be evaluated, as well as evidence of edema. Characteristic rashes may indicate the cause (e.g., a malar rash in SLE or purpuric rash with HSP).

2 Transient proteinuria may occur with fever (usually resolves within 10 to 14 days of the illness), with strenuous exercise (abates within 48 hours), and with stress, cold exposure, dehydration, heart failure, and seizures.

3 Children who have proteinuria on repeat UA, especially those older than 4 years, should be tested for orthostatic proteinuria. This is an increased protein excretion in the upright position only and is less common in younger children. It may account for as much as 60% of all proteinuria in children and has a benign clinical course.

Any of the following tests may be performed to test for orthostatic proteinuria. Spot urine protein/Cr ratio of less than 0.2 in the first morning urine sample for 3 consecutive days confirms the diagnosis. Testing may be done by comparing ambulatory and recumbent (first void) urine samples for protein/Cr ratio. It may also be done by quantitative assessment of proteinuria in ambulatory and recumbent urine specimens. The recumbent specimen should have less than 4 mg/m^2/h of protein. The amount in the ambulatory specimen may vary but is usually 2 to 4 times that of the recumbent specimen.

4 In patients who have persistent asymptomatic proteinuria, further evaluation may proceed as in symptomatic patients. It is reasonable to refer even the patient with normal test results to a nephrologist, because there are different opinions regarding the need for biopsy.

5 Patients with proteinuria who are symptomatic (edema, hypertension) or have hematuria, associated systemic complaints (rash, fever, arthralgia), or a significant family history of glomerulonephritis or renal failure should have further evaluation. In most cases, referral to the nephrologist may be necessary. This evaluation includes assessment of renal function with BUN, Cr, and electrolyte determinations. Nephrotic syndrome consists of proteinuria, hypoalbuminemia, edema, and hyperlipidemia. Total serum protein, albumin, as well as cholesterol and triglycerides are checked. Tests for antistreptococcal antibodies (Streptozyme) as well as complement levels (C3, C4) are done to exclude poststreptococcal glomerulonephritis. The diagnosis of poststreptococcal glomerulonephritis is made in a child with acute nephritic syndrome, evidence of recent streptococcal infection, and a low C3 level. In SLE, C3 and C4 are low. Antinuclear antibody testing may be considered, especially with hypertension or hematuria, to exclude SLE. Hepatitis B and C and HIV may also be associated with glomerulonephritis. A renal US should be considered to examine anatomy.

6 Minimal change nephrotic syndrome is more common in boys and usually appears between ages 2 and 6 years. UA shows 3+ to 4+ proteinuria, and there may be microscopic hematuria. Renal function may be reduced, cholesterol and triglycerides are elevated, and serum albumin is decreased. The C3 level is normal.

7 Nephrotic syndrome may develop with any type of glomerulonephritis, especially membranous, membranoproliferative, postinfectious, SLE, chronic infection, and HSP glomerulonephritis. With poststreptococcal glomerulonephritis, antistreptococcal antibody levels are elevated and complement (C3) is decreased. (See Chapter 32 for conditions causing hematuria with proteinuria.)

8 Nephrotic syndromes may occur with extrarenal neoplasms such as carcinomas and lymphomas (Hodgkin disease).

9 Drugs or chemicals, such as penicillamine, gold, mercury compounds, probenecid, ethosuximide, methimazole, lithium, phenytoin, and many others, may be associated with nephrotic syndrome.

10 Children younger than age 1 with nephrotic syndrome have a poor prognosis. Congenital nephrotic syndrome (Finnish type) is the most common cause. It is an autosomal recessive condition and may occur as failure to thrive due to massive proteinuria. Nephrotic syndrome in infants may be secondary to infections such as syphilis, toxoplasmosis, CMV, rubella, hepatitis B, HIV, or malaria. Drugs, toxins

(e.g., mercury), or SLE may also be causes. Syndromes associated with nephrotic syndrome in infants include nail patella syndrome, Lowe syndrome, congenital brain malformations, and Drash syndrome (e.g., Wilms tumor, nephropathy, and genital abnormalities).

Bibliography
Kliegman RM, Stanton BF, St. Geme J, et al, editors: *Nelson textbook of pediatrics,* ed 19, Philadelphia, 2011, Elsevier Saunders. Chapters 517–521.
Mahesh S, Woroniecki RP: Proteinuria. In McInerny TK, Adam HM, Campbell DE, et al, editors: *American Academy of Pediatrics textbook of pediatric care,* Elk Grove Village, Ill, 2008, AAP. Chapter 210.

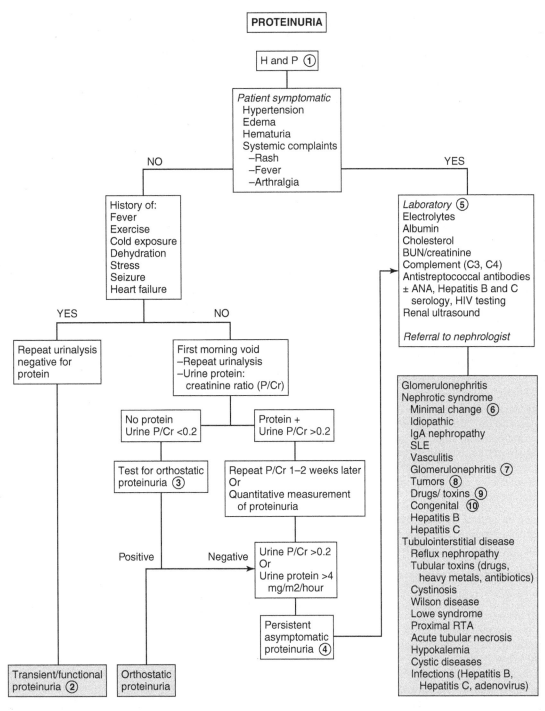

RTA= Renal tubular acidosis
ANA= Antinuclear antibody

Nelson Textbook of Pediatrics, 19e. Chapters 517–521
Nelsons Essentials, 6e. Chapter 162

Chapter 34
EDEMA

Edema is the excess accumulation of interstitial fluid. It can be localized (ascites, pleural effusions) or generalized (anasarca). It may occur as a result of increased capillary pressure (congestive heart failure [CHF]) or decreased plasma protein concentration. Decreased plasma protein may be due to increased losses (nephrotic syndrome, burns), decreased intake (malnutrition), or impaired lymphatic flow.

1 The history and physical examination are very important in limiting the differential diagnosis to specific organ systems. Signs and symptoms specific to heart failure, liver failure, and renal disease should be obtained. History of burns and the presence of severe and extensive burns reveal the etiology. For patients with no clinically obvious etiology, workup should begin by excluding cardiac and renal causes.

The child's growth parameters should be evaluated because growth failure occurs with chronic renal failure. Vital signs may indicate a diagnosis; with heart failure there is tachycardia and tachypnea. Hypertension may indicate renal failure or glomerulonephritis. Pitting in dependent areas (sacrum, lower extremities) is usually present with peripheral edema. Nonpitting edema may be seen with lymphedema or thyroid disease (pretibial myxedema).

2 Angioedema is a form of urticaria affecting deeper tissue planes, including the skin and subcutaneous tissues. It often involves the lips, dorsum of the hands and feet, scalp, scrotum, and periorbital tissues. There are many causes, including foods, drugs, contactants (skin products), inhalants (pollen, dander), bug bites, and infections. A history of recurrent angioedema may indicate episodic angioedema, which is associated with fever and eosinophilia. Hereditary angioedema, which results from a decreased synthesis of C1 esterase inhibitor, occurs as sudden attacks of edema often precipitated by minor trauma, strenuous exercise, or any stressors.

3 Lymphedema is caused by the obstruction of lymphatic flow. Congenital lymphedema may occur in Turner syndrome, Noonan syndrome, and Milroy disease. Acquired obstruction may be due to tumors, lymphoma, filariasis, postirradiation fibrosis, and postinflammatory or postsurgical scarring. Injury to major lymphatic vessels may result in chylous ascites.

4 Heart failure occurs when the heart cannot deliver adequate output to meet the metabolic needs of the body. Signs and symptoms include tachycardia, tachypnea, systemic venous congestion (hepatomegaly), and cardiomegaly. Other features may include feeding difficulties, excessive sweating, and failure to thrive in infants. Respiratory symptoms such as wheezing, rales, and cough may be present, owing to pulmonary congestion. Jugular venous distention or a gallop rhythm may be present. An older child may have orthopnea or may experience syncopal symptoms. Poor peripheral perfusion may result in cool extremities, prolonged capillary refill time, and weaker peripheral pulses as compared with central pulses.

5 Features of hyperthyroidism include goiter and eye findings, including proptosis, exophthalmos, and lid lag. Symptoms due to increased catecholamines include palpitations, tachycardia, hypertension, tremor, and brisk reflexes. A hypermetabolic state results in increased sweating, heat intolerance, and weight loss despite an increased appetite. An associated myopathy may cause weakness, periodic paralysis, and heart failure.

6 Severe anemia, particularly in a newborn, may cause edema. Causes include hemolysis due to ABO or Rh incompatibility or glucose-6-phosphate dehydrogenase (G6PD) deficiency. Kasabach-Merritt syndrome occurs in children with large cavernous hemangiomas of the trunk, extremities, or abdominal organs, where platelets are trapped in the vascular bed. Thrombocytopenia, a microangiopathic hemolytic anemia, and often a consumptive coagulopathy are present. The severe anemia may cause heart failure. Arteriovenous malformations may also be present within the anomalies, resulting in heart failure.

7 CXRs, electrocardiography, and echocardiography are useful in identification of an intrinsic cardiac defect. In congestive heart failure (CHF) the CXR shows cardiac enlargement; evidence of pulmonary edema may be present. In cardiomyopathies there may be left or right ventricular ischemic changes on the electrocardiogram. In myocarditis and pericarditis there may be low-voltage QRS morphology with ST-T wave abnormalities. Electrocardiography is also useful in determining rhythm abnormalities. Echocardiography is most useful in assessing ventricular function as well as underlying structural causes of the heart failure.

8 Congenital heart defects are the most common cause of heart failure in infants and children. Cyanotic lesions with CHF include hypoplastic heart syndromes, transposition of the great vessels, and truncus arteriosus. Ventricular septal defects and patent ductus arteriosus are more common causes of CHF.

9 Cardiomyopathy may occur as a result of a number of diseases. Dilated cardiomyopathy is characterized by massive cardiomegaly and ventricular dilation. The cause is usually unknown (i.e., idiopathic dilated cardiomyopathy). Other causes include genetic (many X-linked), neuromuscular diseases (Friedreich ataxia, Duchenne muscular dystrophy), Kawasaki disease, autoimmune disease (rheumatoid arthritis, systemic lupus erythematosus), hyperthyroidism, and metabolic (mitochondrial disorders) and nutritional disease (beriberi, deficiency of selenium, taurine, and carnitine). Other causes include disorders of coronary arteries (anomalous origin of left coronary), and cardiotoxic drugs (doxorubicin, chronic ipecac abuse). Hypertrophic cardiomyopathy may be secondary to obstructive congenital heart disease, glycogen storage disease, or idiopathic hypertrophic cardiomyopathy. Restrictive cardiomyopathies result in poor ventricular compliance and inadequate ventricular filling; causes include Hurler syndrome and Löffler hypereosinophilic syndrome.

10 Viral myocarditis is most commonly caused by adenovirus and coxsackievirus B. It often results in acute or chronic heart failure. Other infectious causes include diphtheria, systemic bacterial infections (sepsis), and Rocky Mountain spotted fever. Parasites and fungal infections are rarely involved.

11 Arteriovenous malformations may occur within the cranium as well as in the liver, lungs, extremities, and thoracic

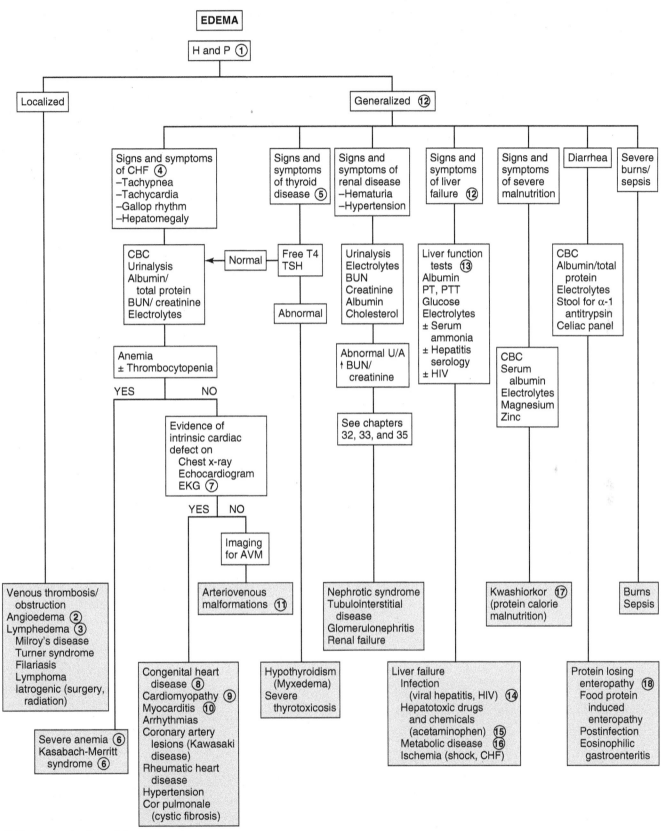

CHF= Congestive heart failure
AVM= Arteriovenous malformations

Nelson Textbook of Pediatrics, 19e. Chapters 517-521
Nelsons Essentials, 6e. Chapter 162

wall. Heart failure is more likely with large intracranial arteriovenous fistulas (e.g., vein of Galen malformation) and hepatic malformations. They are less likely with peripheral arteriovenous fistulas. Physical examination may reveal a bruit, but definitive diagnosis is made by imaging, usually by MRI.

12 Liver failure may be a complication of known liver disease or may be the presenting feature. Features include progressive jaundice, fetor hepaticus, fever, anorexia, vomiting, and abdominal pain. There may be a rapid decrease in liver size without clinical improvement, hemorrhagic diathesis, and ascites. Infants may present with irritability, lethargy, poor feeding, and sleep disturbances. Mental status changes are noted with progression of symptoms. Older children may demonstrate asterixis.

13 In liver failure, hypoalbuminemia results in edema, and bilirubin levels (direct and indirect) are elevated. Serum aminotransferase levels are elevated early but may decrease as the patient's condition deteriorates. PT is prolonged and often does not correct with vitamin K administration. The serum ammonia level is usually elevated, and there may be hypoglycemia, hypokalemia, hyponatremia, metabolic acidosis, or respiratory alkalosis.

14 Viral hepatitis is a common cause of liver failure. It is more likely in children with a combined infection with hepatitis B and D. Other viruses that may result in liver failure include EBV, herpes simplex virus, adenovirus, enterovirus, parvovirus B19, and varicella-zoster virus.

15 Known hepatotoxins include acetaminophen overdose, carbon tetrachloride, and *Amanita phalloides* mushrooms. Idiosyncratic damage may occur with halothane, phenytoin, carbamazepine, or sodium valproate.

16 Metabolic disorders associated with liver failure include Wilson disease, galactosemia, hereditary tyrosinemia, hereditary fructose intolerance, and urea cycle defects.

17 Kwashiorkor is a clinical syndrome resulting from severe protein deficiency and inadequate caloric intake (protein-calorie malnutrition). Early in the disease, symptoms include anorexia, lethargy, apathy, and irritability. Later there is decreased growth, decreased stamina, muscle loss, increased susceptibility to infections, and edema. The edema may mask poor weight gain. Skin changes may be present, and the hair becomes coarse and discolored, resulting in streaky red or gray hair. Laboratory findings include decreased serum albumin, hypoglycemia, hypophosphatemia, and deficiency of potassium and magnesium. Anemia may be normocytic, microcytic, or macrocytic. Signs of vitamin (especially vitamin A) and mineral (zinc) deficiencies may be present.

18 Protein-losing enteropathy may result in edema secondary to hypoalbuminemia. α_1-Antitrypsin, unlike albumin, is resistant to digestion. Measurement of levels in the stool is helpful in the diagnosis of protein-losing enteropathy. Causes include food protein–induced enteropathy and postinfectious enteropathy. Eosinophilic gastroenteritis is another cause; it may be associated with dietary protein hypersensitivity as well as other food allergies. There is often eosinophilia and an elevated serum immunoglobulin (Ig)E. Celiac disease producing severe malnutrition may also present with edema.

Bibliography

Levy PA: Edema. In McInerny TK, Adam HM, Campbell DE, et al, editors: *American Academy of Pediatrics textbook of pediatric care,* Elk Grove Village, Ill, 2008, AAP. Chapter 175.

Paller AS, Mancini AJ: *Hurwitz clinical pediatric dermatology,* ed 4, Philadelphia, 2011, WB Saunders.

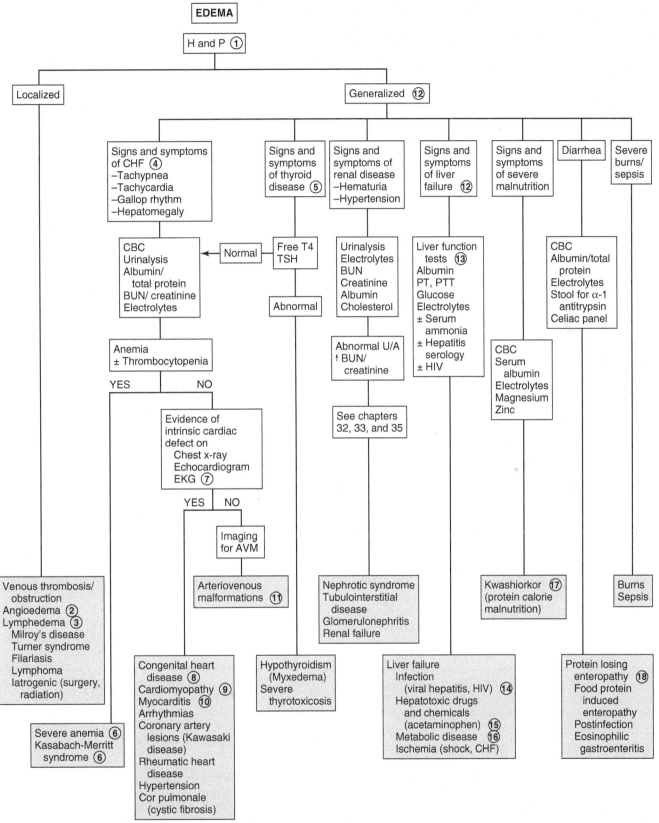

EDEMA

H and P ①

Localized

Generalized ⑫

Signs and symptoms of CHF ④
–Tachypnea
–Tachycardia
–Gallop rhythm
–Hepatomegaly

Signs and symptoms of thyroid disease ⑤

Signs and symptoms of renal disease
–Hematuria
–Hypertension

Signs and symptoms of liver failure ⑫

Signs and symptoms of severe malnutrition

Diarrhea

Severe burns/sepsis

CBC
Urinalysis
Albumin/ total protein
BUN/ creatinine
Electrolytes

Normal ← Free T4 TSH

Abnormal

Urinalysis
Electrolytes
BUN
Creatinine
Albumin
Cholesterol

Liver function tests ⑬
Albumin
PT, PTT
Glucose
Electrolytes
± Serum ammonia
± Hepatitis serology
± HIV

CBC
Albumin/total protein
Electrolytes
Stool for α-1 antitrypsin
Celiac panel

Anemia
± Thrombocytopenia

YES   NO

Abnormal U/A
↑ BUN/ creatinine

CBC
Serum albumin
Electrolytes
Magnesium
Zinc

Evidence of intrinsic cardiac defect on
Chest x-ray
Echocardiogram
EKG ⑦

See chapters 32, 33, and 35

YES   NO

Imaging for AVM

Venous thrombosis/ obstruction
Angioedema ②
Lymphedema ③
Milroy's disease
Turner syndrome
Filariasis
Lymphoma
Iatrogenic (surgery, radiation)

Arteriovenous malformations ⑪

Nephrotic syndrome
Tubulointerstitial disease
Glomerulonephritis
Renal failure

Kwashiorkor ⑰
(protein calorie malnutrition)

Burns
Sepsis

Severe anemia ⑥
Kasabach-Merritt syndrome ⑥

Congenital heart disease ⑧
Cardiomyopathy ⑨
Myocarditis ⑩
Arrhythmias
Coronary artery lesions (Kawasaki disease)
Rheumatic heart disease
Hypertension
Cor pulmonale (cystic fibrosis)

Hypothyroidism (Myxedema)
Severe thyrotoxicosis

Liver failure
Infection (viral hepatitis, HIV) ⑭
Hepatotoxic drugs and chemicals (acetaminophen) ⑮
Metabolic disease ⑯
Ischemia (shock, CHF)

Protein losing enteropathy ⑱
Food protein induced enteropathy
Postinfection
Eosinophilic gastroenteritis

CHF= Congestive heart failure
AVM= Arteriovenous malformations

Nelson Textbook of Pediatrics, 19e. Chapters 517-521
Nelsons Essentials, 6e. Chapter 162

Chapter 35
HYPERTENSION

It is currently recommended that all children older than age 3 have routine BP screening. Children younger than 3 with other medical conditions should also have their BP checked. These include those with a history of prematurity, congenital heart disease, renal disease, solid organ transplant, cancer, medications known to raise BP, other illnesses associated with hypertension (HTN), or evidence of increased ICP. It is important to use an appropriate-size cuff whose width measures 40% of the circumference of the arm, and the cuff bladder length should cover 80% to 100% of the arm circumference. It is also important to use standardized methods of determining systolic (onset of Korotkoff sounds) and diastolic BPs (disappearance of sounds) on auscultation. Use of automated devices is acceptable in newborns and infants when auscultation may be difficult and in settings that require continuous monitoring, such as an intensive care unit. Abnormal BPs from automated devices should be confirmed by auscultation.

BP measurement is complicated by the fact that there is wide fluctuation of BP through the day, as well as with activity, stress, and other factors. BP tables that are adjusted for height should be used to assess for HTN. Guidelines in this chapter are based on the report from the National High Blood Pressure Education Program Working Group on High Blood Pressure in Children and Adolescents. Normal BP is when both systolic and diastolic pressures are less than the 90th percentile for age and sex. Pre-HTN is defined as average systolic or diastolic pressures between the 90th and 95th percentiles. HTN is defined as average systolic or diastolic BP that is above the 95th percentile for age and sex, measured on 3 or more occasions. Stage 1 HTN is when BP is between the 95th and 99th percentiles plus 5 mmHg; in stage 2 HTN the BP is above the 99th percentile plus 5 mmHg. If Stage 1 HTN is asymptomatic and without target organ damage, this allows time for evaluation before starting treatment; in stage 2 HTN, prompt evaluation and pharmacologic therapy is necessary.

Although there are ethnic differences in BP, they are not believed to be clinically relevant. A patient with BP above the 95th percentile in a physician's office or clinic but who is normotensive outside a clinical setting has "white-coat hypertension." Ambulatory BP monitoring (ABPM) is usually required to make this diagnosis.

(1) History should include ingestion of medications and toxins, as well as tobacco use. Symptoms such as abdominal pain, dysuria, frequency, nocturia, enuresis, hematuria, and edema may indicate a renal cause. In infants, growth failure, irritability, and feeding problems may be symptoms of HTN. Joint pain or swelling may be due to collagen vascular diseases. Weight loss, sweating, and pallor may be due to a catecholamine-secreting tumor. Muscle cramps or weakness and constipation may be seen with the hypokalemia associated with hyperaldosteronism. Menstrual disorders, hirsutism, and virilization may indicate forms of congenital adrenal hyperplasia (CAH) associated with HTN. A neonatal history of umbilical artery line

placement can result in renal artery embolization, leading to HTN. History of prolonged loud snoring may identify sleep-related causes of HTN.

On physical examination, pallor and edema may indicate a renal cause. A careful skin examination should identify characteristic findings such as cafe-au-lait spots (neurofibromatosis); tubers, ash leaf spots (tuberous sclerosis); hirsutism (congenital adrenal hyperplasia); malar rash (lupus); and purpura (Henoch-Schönlein purpura). Retinal examination may show changes secondary to chronic HTN. Thyromegaly may be found with hyperthyroidism. There may be a heart murmur with absent or decreased femoral pulses in aortic coarctation, and tachyarrhythmias with pheochromocytomas. It is therefore important to always measure BP in all four extremities. Signs of heart failure may be present with chronic or severe HTN. Bruits may indicate aortic or renal arterial disease. Abdominal examination may identify enlarged kidneys. There may be neurologic deficits or Bell palsy with chronic HTN. Stigmata of syndromes such as Cushing syndrome (buffalo hump, striae, moon face, truncal obesity, hirsutism), Turner syndrome (short stature, webbed neck, shield chest, low hairline), and Williams syndrome (elfin facies, poor growth, retardation) should be identified. A complete family history may be helpful in identifying primary or secondary (e.g., polycystic kidney disease) HTN.

(2) Coarctation of the aorta may occur at any point from the arch to the bifurcation. It is more common in males but is also associated with Turner syndrome. The classic features include decreased or absent lower extremity pulses and lower extremity BP less than upper extremity BP; a short systolic murmur may be heard along the left sternal border, as well as an interscapular systolic murmur over the region of the coarctation.

(3) Malignant HTN is a marked elevation of BP, which may be associated with retinal changes on funduscopy, congestive heart failure, or facial palsy. Hypertensive encephalopathy may occur as nausea, vomiting, altered mental status, visual disturbances, seizures, or stroke. The patient requires emergent diagnosis and management.

(4) The initial evaluation includes measurement of serum BUN, Cr, electrolytes, CBC, UA and renal US. From 75% to 80% of secondary HTN in children is due to renal disease; therefore, initial workup is directed toward detection of renal problems. UTIs may be associated with an obstructive lesion. Hematuria and/or proteinuria may indicate an underlying renal disease. (See Chapters 32 and 33.) A CBC may reveal anemia, which is often associated with chronic renal disease, or a microangiopathic hemolytic anemia associated with hemolytic-uremic syndrome. Determination of BUN and Cr levels may provide evidence of chronicity of HTN and renal involvement. Electrolytes may be helpful in the diagnosis of hyperaldosteronism (i.e., low potassium).

(5) Consider further evaluation for comorbidities (lipid profile, fasting glucose, polysomnography when indicated). A fasting lipid profile should be considered as part of the assessment, because elevated BP in adults is known to accelerate the development of coronary artery disease. Polysomnography is indicated when there is snoring and obstructive sleep apnea is suspected. Evaluation of HTN should also include assessment of target organs. This includes funduscopic examination of the retina and echocardiography. Retinal examination may show arteriolar narrowing and arteriovenous nicking. Hemorrhages

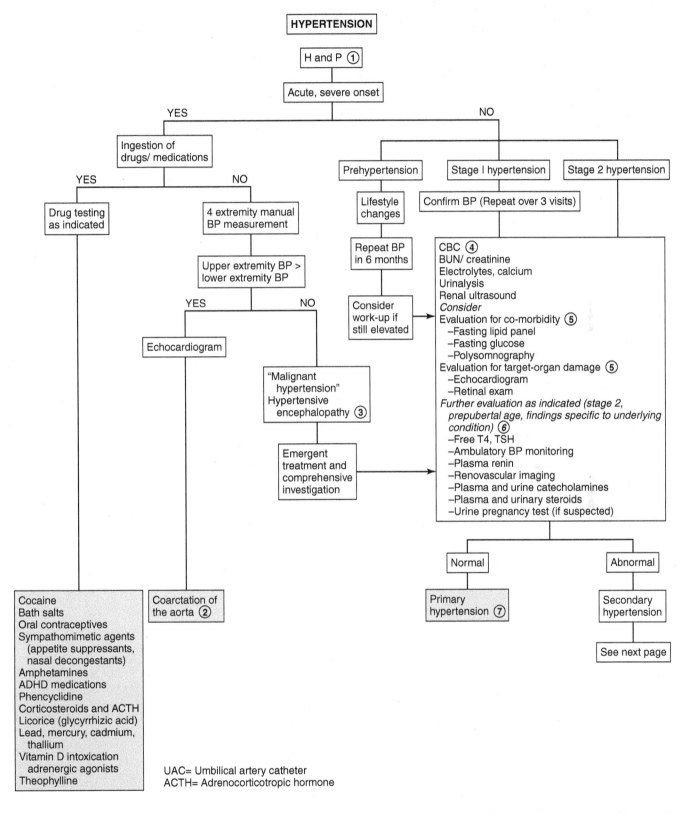

HYPERTENSION

H and P ①

Acute, severe onset

YES — NO

YES branch:

Ingestion of drugs/ medications

YES — NO

Drug testing as indicated

4 extremity manual BP measurement

Upper extremity BP > lower extremity BP

YES — NO

Echocardiogram

"Malignant hypertension" Hypertensive encephalopathy ③

Emergent treatment and comprehensive investigation

Cocaine
Bath salts
Oral contraceptives
Sympathomimetic agents
  (appetite suppressants,
  nasal decongestants)
Amphetamines
ADHD medications
Phencyclidine
Corticosteroids and ACTH
Licorice (glycyrrhizic acid)
Lead, mercury, cadmium,
  thallium
Vitamin D intoxication
  adrenergic agonists
Theophylline

Coarctation of the aorta ②

UAC= Umbilical artery catheter
ACTH= Adrenocorticotropic hormone

NO branch:

Prehypertension | Stage I hypertension | Stage 2 hypertension

Lifestyle changes

Confirm BP (Repeat over 3 visits)

Repeat BP in 6 months

Consider work-up if still elevated

CBC ④
BUN/ creatinine
Electrolytes, calcium
Urinalysis
Renal ultrasound
Consider
Evaluation for co-morbidity ⑤
  –Fasting lipid panel
  –Fasting glucose
  –Polysomnography
Evaluation for target-organ damage ⑤
  –Echocardiogram
  –Retinal exam
*Further evaluation as indicated (stage 2,
prepubertal age, findings specific to underlying
condition)* ⑥
  –Free T4, TSH
  –Ambulatory BP monitoring
  –Plasma renin
  –Renovascular imaging
  –Plasma and urine catecholamines
  –Plasma and urinary steroids
  –Urine pregnancy test (if suspected)

Normal | Abnormal

Primary hypertension ⑦

Secondary hypertension

See next page

Nelson Textbook of Pediatrics, 19e. Chapter 439
Nelsons Essentials, 6e. Chapter 166

and exudates are more likely in adults. Echocardiography is used to detect left ventricular hypertrophy.

6 Other studies are performed if secondary HTN is suspected. A more extensive evaluation is suggested for prepubertal children (usually <10 years of age), those with stage 2 HTN, and those with H and P suggesting a specific underlying cause. Plasma renin is low in mineralocorticoid-related disease (with hypokalemia); renin levels may be elevated in renal artery stenosis. Plasma and urine catecholamines should be obtained in patients with symptoms of catecholamine excess (headache, sweating, tachycardia) or those who are at risk of pheochromocytoma (patients with neurofibromatosis). Screening for renovascular disease is performed in patients with stage 2 HTN if no other cause is identified or if there are predisposing risk factors (history of umbilical artery catheterization, neurofibromatosis, or abdominal bruit). A renal scan may be helpful in determining renal scars (from recurrent UTIs) and ischemic areas secondary to renovascular disease. In young children with HTN, renovascular disease is a common cause and further testing may be needed. Other imaging methods include MR angiography, Doppler flow studies, 3-dimensional CT, or renal angiography. Appropriate referral of children with renal or renovascular disease should be considered for further evaluation. Voiding cystourethrography is used in diagnosis of reflux nephropathy.

7 In older children and adolescents with mild HTN, normal screening laboratory tests, and no evidence of end-organ damage, essential or primary HTN may be considered. This is especially the case in children with a positive family history.

8 In children with features of Cushing syndrome and a negative history of exogenous corticosteroids, further hormonal and imaging studies may be considered. In children with symptoms of hyperthyroidism and systolic HTN, thyroxine and thyroid-stimulating hormone may be measured. Hypercalcemia, which may be associated with hyperparathyroidism, may cause HTN.

CAH due to 11-hydroxylase deficiency or 17-hydroxlase deficiency may both result in HTN. 11-Hydroxylase deficiency is characterized by virilization in females and early puberty in males. In 17-hydroxylase deficiency, there is hypokalemia and suppression of renin and aldosterone. Affected males are unvirilized and may appear phenotypically female with female external genitalia and a blind vagina; affected females have failure of pubertal sexual development and primary amenorrhea.

Low plasma renin activity and elevated aldosterone levels may indicate mineralocorticoid excess.

It is important to note that random plasma renin activity that is not profiled against urine sodium ("spot" or 24-hour urinary excretion) may not be specific or sensitive. Primary hyperaldosteronism is characterized by HTN, hypokalemia, and suppressed plasma renin activity. Elevated plasma renin activity may indicate renovascular disease and should prompt renal referral for further evaluation. Children with catecholamine-secreting tumors (pheochromocytoma) usually have sustained HTN. If plasma or urine catecholamine levels are increased, imaging of the adrenal glands should be considered in the diagnosis of pheochromocytoma. Neuroblastomas and ganglioneuromas may also produce catecholamines.

9 Intermittent HTN may be present in patients with autonomic instability (e.g., Guillain-Barré syndrome, burns, poliomyelitis, Stevens-Johnson syndrome, porphyria). There maybe episodic increases in urinary catecholamine excretion.

10 In children with H and P indicating raised ICP (e.g., headache, vomiting, papilledema, neurologic changes), cranial imaging should be considered to rule out an intracranial mass. Other conditions associated with raised ICP are intracranial hemorrhage and brain injury.

11 Liddle syndrome is an autosomal dominant condition characterized by HTN and hypokalemia. Renin is suppressed and aldosterone levels are low.

Bibliography

Brady TM: Hypertension, *Pediatr Rev* 33:541–552, 2012.
National High Blood Pressure Education Program Working Group on High Blood Pressure in Children and Adolescents: The fourth report on the diagnosis, evaluation, and treatment of high blood pressure in children and adolescents, *Pediatrics* 114:555–576, 2004.

HYPERTENSION (continued)

Secondary hypertension

Renal
Pyelonephritis
Glomerulonephritis
Henoch-Schönlein purpura
Hemolytic uremic syndrome
Hydronephrosis
Renal anomalies
Renal tumors
Renal trauma
Systemic lupus erythematosus
Reflux nephropathy
Ureteral obstruction
Renovascular
Renal artery stenosis
Renal artery thrombosis (UAC)
Renal vein thrombosis
Vasculitis
Endocrine causes (8)
Diabetes
Hyperthyroidism
Cushing syndrome
Hyperparathyroidism
Congenital adrenal hyperplasia
1° hyperaldosteronism
Catecholamine secreting tumors
Other
White coat hypertension
Pregnancy (preeclamsia)
Autonomic instability (9)
Intracranial mass (10)
Arteriovenous shunt
Liddle syndrome (11)
Hypercalcemia
 —Hyperparathyroidism
 —William syndrome

Chapter 36
SCROTAL PAIN

Painful scrotal swelling requires urgent evaluation to rule out conditions such as testicular torsion or incarcerated inguinal hernias, which require immediate surgical management.

(1) To determine the cause of the painful scrotum, the history should include the duration of pain (acute, chronic, or intermittent), radiation of pain to other areas, any other associated pain symptoms, and whether the pain is associated with exercise or trauma (suggesting testicular torsion). GU (dysuria, frequency, hematuria, penile discharge), abdominal, and systemic symptoms may be helpful in diagnosis. Inquire about sexual activity, UTIs, sexually transmitted diseases, and renal stones.

On examination, pubertal development should be assessed. Careful examination of the GU area should include the inguinal canals and spermatic cord, testis and epididymis, and position of testis within the scrotum. Changes in the scrotal skin and presence or absence of the cremasteric reflex should be noted.

(2) Imaging studies are helpful in the diagnosis of painful scrotal swelling. Color Doppler US allows differentiation of torsion from inflammation and can differentiate testicular blood flow from scrotal wall flow. In torsion of the testicular appendix, as opposed to testicular torsion, testicular blood flow will be normal or increased. In prepubertal boys, Doppler signal may not be demonstrated, owing to small testicular size. The ^{99mc}Tc-pertechnetate testicular flow scan is also used to differentiate ischemia (as in testicular torsion), which appears as a "cold spot," from inflammation of the testis, which causes normal or increased uptake of the radionuclide dye. Neither test is 100% accurate. Both require clinical correlation and depend on the skill of the radiologist.

(3) Testicular torsion is the cause in one third of cases of painful scrotum. It is a surgical emergency because of risk of gonadal loss. It usually occurs between the ages of 10 and 18 years and is most often associated with a predisposing anatomic abnormality ("bell-clapper" deformity). It also may be associated with trauma. It occurs rarely in the neonatal period. Testicular torsion usually presents with sudden onset of pain, swelling, and tender enlargement of the testis, which may be high-riding with an abnormal transverse lie. The cremasteric reflex is usually absent. There may be referred pain to the groin or abdomen and associated nausea or vomiting. In most cases, H and P can help to make the diagnosis. Imaging studies show reduced blood flow.

(4) Epididymitis is most common in sexually active adolescents and is due to retrograde spread of a urethral infection, most often due to *Chlamydia*, *Mycoplasma*, and *Neisseria gonorrhoeae*. In prepubertal boys, it is usually associated with a UTI secondary to a structural abnormality of the lower GU tract and involves *Escherichia coli* and other gram-negative organisms. In addition to gradual onset of testicular pain, there may be symptoms of a UTI and urethral discharge. On examination there is scrotal edema, erythema, warmth, and tenderness. The cremasteric reflex is usually preserved, and there may be a reactive hydrocele. When the inflammation involves the testis it is known as epididymoorchitis. The Prehn sign, which is the relief of pain with elevation of the testis, may be suggestive of epididymitis or orchitis. UA often shows pyuria or bacteriuria. A urine culture should be obtained and Gram stain and culture of a urethral discharge. If diagnosis is not definitive, imaging may be used to show increased blood flow to the testis and rule out torsion.

(5) Torsion of the testicular appendix is most common between ages 7 and 12 years. There is gradual onset of testicular pain and swelling with a 3- to 5-mm, tender, indurated mass on the upper pole of the testis. If the mass is visible through the scrotal skin, this is known as the "blue dot" sign. Imaging may show increased flow due to hyperemia of the testis.

(6) Orchitis is rarely an isolated infection. It is usually associated with viral infection: mumps, coxsackievirus, varicella, or dengue.

(7) Incarcerated hernias occur as painful irreducible swellings in the groin or scrotum. Strangulation results from compromised vascular supply.

(8) Henoch-Schönlein purpura is a systemic vasculitis that may present as a purpuric rash or tense edema over the scrotum. There may be swelling and tenderness of the testis.

(9) Idiopathic fat necrosis involves acute painful swelling of the scrotum due to necrosis of intrascrotal fat, the etiology of which is unknown.

(10) Fournier gangrene of the scrotum is a form of necrotizing fasciitis, occurs rarely in children, and when present is usually associated with severe diaper rash, insect bites, circumcision, or perianal skin abscess. Organisms involved are *Staphylococcus aureus*, *Streptococcus*, *Bacteroides fragilis*, *E. coli*, and *Clostridium welchii*. There is acute scrotal swelling with redness and tenderness, as well as systemic symptoms of fever, chills, and septicemia.

Bibliography

Kass EJ, Lundak B: The acute scrotum, *Pediatr Clin North Am* 44:1251, 1997.

Palmer LS: Scrotal pain and swelling. In McInerny TK, Adam HM, Campbell DE, et al, editors: *American Academy of Pediatrics textbook of pediatric care*, Elk Grove Village, Ill, 2008, AAP. Chapter 216.

Kliegman RM, Stanton BF, St. Geme J, et al, editors: *Nelson textbook of pediatrics*, ed 19, Philadelphia, 2011, Elsevier Saunders. Chapter 539.

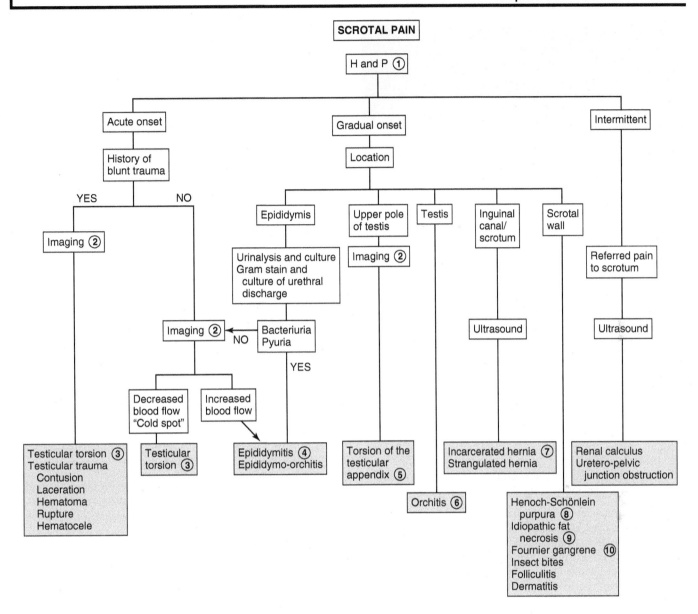

SCROTAL PAIN

H and P ①

Acute onset

History of blunt trauma

YES   NO

Imaging ②

Testicular torsion ③
Testicular trauma
  Contusion
  Laceration
  Hematoma
  Rupture
  Hematocele

Decreased blood flow "Cold spot"

Increased blood flow

Testicular torsion ③

Epididymitis ④
Epididymo-orchitis

Imaging ②

NO

Bacteriuria Pyuria

YES

Urinalysis and culture Gram stain and culture of urethral discharge

Gradual onset

Location

Epididymis

Upper pole of testis

Imaging ②

Torsion of the testicular appendix ⑤

Orchitis ⑥

Testis

Inguinal canal/scrotum

Ultrasound

Incarcerated hernia ⑦
Strangulated hernia

Scrotal wall

Henoch-Schönlein purpura ⑧
Idiopathic fat necrosis ⑨
Fournier gangrene ⑩
Insect bites
Folliculitis
Dermatitis

Intermittent

Referred pain to scrotum

Ultrasound

Renal calculus
Uretero-pelvic junction obstruction

Nelson Textbook of Pediatrics, 19e. Chapter 539
Nelsons Essentials, 6e. Chapter 169

Chapter 37
SCROTAL SWELLING (PAINLESS)

Hernias, hydroceles, varicoceles, and spermatoceles are the most common causes of painless scrotal swelling. A testicular mass may be malignant; therefore, the swelling should be carefully localized by examination and, if necessary, by ultrasound (US).

1. Physical examination should be done with the patient in the upright and supine positions. Communicating hydroceles, hernias, and varicoceles are accentuated in the upright position and the Valsalva maneuver. Transillumination of the scrotum is used to distinguish solid from cystic lesions. When swelling cannot be adequately assessed on physical examination, or if the testis is not palpable within a cystic mass, US evaluation is necessary.

2. Acute idiopathic scrotal wall edema is a rare cause of acute scrotal swelling in boys between 4 and 7 years old. There may be minimal itching and a waddling gait. There is unilateral or bilateral scrotal wall edema; however, the testicles are not affected. The etiology is unknown but suspected to be allergic.

3. Henoch-Schönlein purpura is a systemic vasculitis that may present as a purpuric rash or tense edema over the scrotum. There may be swelling of the testis.

4. Solid extratesticular masses may arise from the epididymis, spermatic cord, and scrotal wall. The most common benign lesion is spermatic cord lipoma. Fibromas, leiomyomas, lymphangiomas, adrenal rest tumors, and dermoid cysts are rare. Tumors of the epididymis are usually benign, the most common being the adenomatoid tumor. Paratesticular rhabdomyosarcoma is the most common paratesticular malignancy, with peak incidence between ages 2 and 5 years; metastasis occurs early.

5. Hernias and hydroceles are the most common scrotal/inguinal masses. Hernias are most common in premature infants and low-birth-weight infants. A hydrocele is a smooth and nontender collection of fluid in the tunica vaginalis. Transillumination confirms the presence of fluid. Noncommunicating hydroceles are present in 1% to 2% of male neonates. Communicating hydroceles often persist. There is increasing scrotal swelling during the day, with decrease in size overnight. Hernias may be associated. Hydroceles may also be reactive secondary to torsion, epididymitis, or tumor. If the testis is abnormal on palpation or if it is not adequately palpated, US is needed to rule out an underlying condition. Hematoceles are filled with blood; they are rare and may indicate intraabdominal bleeding. Varicoceles are dilated, elongated veins of the pampiniform plexus, located posterosuperior to the testis, usually on the left side. They resemble a "bag of worms" and are most common in adolescents. They may cause hypotrophy of the testicle and impaired fertility. Spermatoceles and epididymal cysts occur in the rete testis, efferent ductule, or epididymis and contain sperm. On occasion, US may be necessary for definitive diagnosis.

6. Testicular tumors occur as a painless scrotal mass, with secondary hydrocele in 10% to 15%. Pain may occur with torsion or hemorrhage into the tumor. Germ cell tumors are most common. Tumor marker α fetoprotein is elevated in 80% of yolk sac tumors, whereas β-human chorionic gonadotropin is elevated in teratocarcinomas. Gonadal stromal tumors may produce hormones causing signs and symptoms of precocious puberty and gynecomastia. Lymphomas and leukemia may metastasize to the testis.

7. Testicular microlithiasis may rarely occur as testicular enlargement. This is diagnosed on US and may be associated with subsequent development of testicular malignancies.

Bibliography
Kaplan GW: Scrotal swelling in children, *Pediatr Rev* 21:311–314, 2000.
Palmer LS: Scrotal pain and swelling. In McInerny TK, Adam HM, Campbell DE, et al, editors: *American Academy of Pediatrics textbook of pediatric care*, Elk Grove Village, Ill, 2008, AAP. Chapter 216.

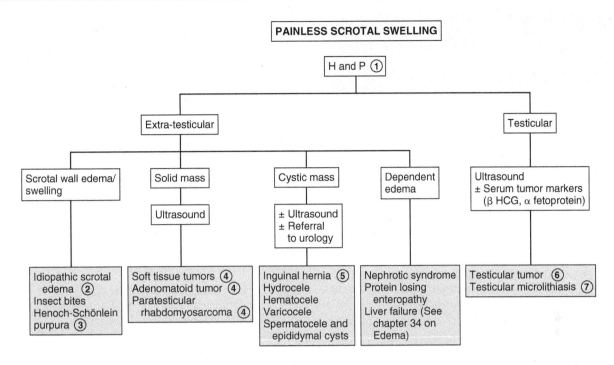

PAINLESS SCROTAL SWELLING

H and P ①

Extra-testicular

Testicular

Scrotal wall edema/ swelling

Solid mass

Cystic mass

Dependent edema

Ultrasound
± Serum tumor markers
(β HCG, α fetoprotein)

Ultrasound

± Ultrasound
± Referral
to urology

Idiopathic scrotal edema ②
Insect bites
Henoch-Schönlein purpura ③

Soft tissue tumors ④
Adenomatoid tumor ④
Paratesticular rhabdomyosarcoma ④

Inguinal hernia ⑤
Hydrocele
Hematocele
Varicocele
Spermatocele and epididymal cysts

Nephrotic syndrome
Protein losing enteropathy
Liver failure (See chapter 34 on Edema)

Testicular tumor ⑥
Testicular microlithiasis ⑦

Nelson Textbook of Pediatrics, 19e. Chapter 539

Chapter 38
DYSMENORRHEA

Dysmenorrhea is defined as crampy lower abdominal or low back pain associated with menstruation. It is characterized into primary dysmenorrhea and secondary dysmenorrhea.

1　History should include onset of symptoms and whether dysmenorrhea started with menarche. Timing of pain during periods, history of sexual activity, and presence of vaginal discharge should be noted. It is important to obtain a history of disruption of daily activity and response to medications to determine the extent of investigation and treatment required. An abdominopelvic examination may reveal the cause in an older or sexually active adolescent. In a younger virginal adolescent, a rectoabdominal examination or US may be adequate. A rectal examination should also be done.

2　Primary dysmenorrhea has no clinically detected pelvic pathology. It is due to uterine contractions caused by prostaglandins produced by the premenstrual secretory endometrium and occurs only with ovulatory cycles. It begins with the onset of the menstrual period and lasts from a few hours to days. Cramping may be associated with nausea, vomiting, diarrhea, and headache. The pelvic examination is normal but is usually not clinically indicated.

If the clinical presentation is consistent with primary dysmenorrhea, it is reasonable to do a trial of therapy. Prostaglandin synthetase inhibitors are effective when given before a menstrual period (or shortly after it begins). Hormonal contraceptives (oral, vaginal ring, contraceptive patch) may also be helpful and may be considered, particularly for girls who need contraception.

3　Secondary dysmenorrhea is associated with underlying pathology. New onset of symptoms in a sexually active teen may be due to a complication of pregnancy or pelvic inflammatory disease (PID). (For further discussion on cervicitis and PID, see Chapter 41.) If there is a positive pregnancy test finding, US evaluation may be needed to exclude an ectopic pregnancy or miscarriage.

4　Onset of symptoms with menarche when cycles are usually anovulatory may be due to müllerian tract abnormalities with partial outflow obstruction. Pelvic examination, US, or laparoscopy may be needed to evaluate outlet obstruction. There may be partial obstruction of menstrual flow, causing cyclic dysmenorrhea with accumulation of menstrual fluid, resulting in hematocolpos, hematometra, or hematosalpinx, depending on the level of the obstruction.

5　Chronic pelvic pain that is worse during a period may be due to endometriosis and may be diagnosed using laparoscopy. Endometriosis is the presence of endometrial tissue outside the normal intrauterine cavity. Unlike in adults, in adolescents the pelvic examination may be normal or there may be minimal tenderness.

6　Psychogenic dysmenorrhea may be related to negative sexual experiences, such as child abuse or rape.

Bibliography

Dinerman LM, Joffe A: Dysmenorrhea. In McInerny TK, Adam HM, Campbell DE, et al, editors: *American Academy of Pediatrics textbook of pediatric care,* ed 1, Elk Grove Village, Ill, 2009, AAP, p 1461.

Kliegman RM, Stanton BF, St. Geme J, Schor N, Behrman RE, editors: *Nelson textbook of pediatrics,* ed 19, Philadelphia, 2011, Elsevier/Saunders. Chapter 110.

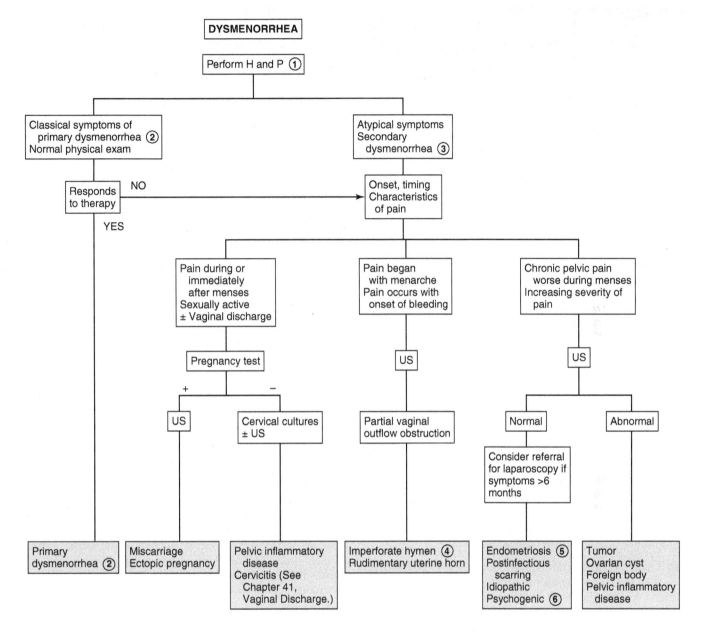

DYSMENORRHEA

Perform H and P ①

Classical symptoms of primary dysmenorrhea ② Normal physical exam

Atypical symptoms Secondary dysmenorrhea ③

Responds to therapy

NO

YES

Onset, timing Characteristics of pain

Pain during or immediately after menses Sexually active ± Vaginal discharge

Pain began with menarche Pain occurs with onset of bleeding

Chronic pelvic pain worse during menses Increasing severity of pain

Pregnancy test

US

US

+

−

US

Cervical cultures ± US

Partial vaginal outflow obstruction

Normal

Abnormal

Consider referral for laparoscopy if symptoms >6 months

Primary dysmenorrhea ②

Miscarriage Ectopic pregnancy

Pelvic inflammatory disease Cervicitis (See Chapter 41, Vaginal Discharge.)

Imperforate hymen ④ Rudimentary uterine horn

Endometriosis ⑤ Postinfectious scarring Idiopathic Psychogenic ⑥

Tumor Ovarian cyst Foreign body Pelvic inflammatory disease

Nelson Textbook of Pediatrics, 19e. Chapter 110
Nelsons Essentials, 6e. Chapter 69

Chapter 39
AMENORRHEA

Amenorrhea is the absence of menstrual periods. Primary amenorrhea occurs when there is no menstrual period by age 15 years, or no signs of puberty as well as menses by age 13 years. Secondary amenorrhea occurs when a previously menstruating female has no menstrual bleeding for at least 3 to 6 months. Oligomenorrhea is when there is more than 6 weeks between menstrual cycles or fewer than 9 periods annually.

1 History should include pubertal development and menstrual patterns in secondary amenorrhea. Pregnancy is the first consideration in an adolescent with secondary amenorrhea, but should always be considered as a possible cause even in primary amenorrhea. Information on sexual history including sexual abuse and use of hormonal contraceptives should be carefully elicited. Obtaining a history of weight change, anorexia, stress, athletic participation, and abnormal eating patterns (anorexia, bulimia) is important to the diagnosis of amenorrhea. History should also include chronic illness, infections, medications, and substance abuse. Family history should include gynecologic problems, age at the onset of puberty and menses, and fertility history of the mother and other female relatives. On physical examination, it is important to assess BP, nutritional status (body mass index [BMI]), and growth parameters. The presence of congenital anomalies may identify syndromes associated with amenorrhea (e.g., Turner syndrome). Galactorrhea is often associated with amenorrhea; acne, hirsutism, and other signs of possible virilization should be identified. Features suggestive of CNS disease (e.g., headache, visual disturbances, and midline facial defects) should also be noted. A careful examination of the reproductive tract is useful in identifying anatomic defects and assessing sexual maturity.

2 Congenital structural abnormalities such as imperforate hymen and transverse vaginal septum may obstruct menstrual outflow. A history of cyclic pain may be present, and a midline lower abdominal mass (hematocolpos/hematometra) may be palpated. Müllerian agenesis (Mayer-Rokitansky-Küster-Hauser syndrome) is characterized by an absent or shallow vagina with an absent cervix and uterus. Gonadal function and secondary sexual development are normal, but urinary tract and skeletal anomalies may be present. Although US is very useful, MRI or laparoscopy may be necessary to define anatomic abnormalities.

3 46,XY disorder of sex development (androgen insensitivity syndrome), previously known as testicular feminization, occurs in phenotypic females who are chromosomally XY but lack androgen receptors. External genitalia appear female, but the vagina is shallow and testes are intraabdominal. At puberty, breasts develop owing to gonadal estrogens; axillary and pubic hair is absent. LH is increased, FSH is usually normal.

4 Hypothalamic dysfunction leading to amenorrhea is a diagnosis of exclusion. It is caused by suppression of gonadotropin-releasing hormone pulsatile secretion and is most commonly associated with chronic illness associated with undernutrition (Crohn disease, celiac disease), stress, excessive exercise, or weight loss and with eating disorders. The female athlete triad consists of disordered eating, amenorrhea, and low bone mass. Withdrawal bleeding may occur with a progestin challenge (see note 9).

5 Polycystic ovary syndrome is characterized by oligomenorrhea or amenorrhea and evidence of hyperandrogenism, either clinical or laboratory. Laboratory evidence may include increased free testosterone and dehydroepiandrosterone sulfate (DHEAS) levels, as well as increased ratio of LH to FSH. Diagnostic criteria vary among experts. In chronic anovulation, withdrawal bleeding occurs with a progestin challenge (prolactin and TSH levels are normal). Polycystic ovary syndrome is a common cause (see note 9).

6 Primary ovarian insufficiency (premature ovarian failure) is also known as hypergonadotropic hypogonadism. FSH is elevated and estradiol is low. Patients with possible Turner syndrome need a karyotype determination. Stigmata of Turner syndrome include short stature, pigmented nevi, high-arched palate, low hairline, shield chest, ptosis, cutis laxa, pterygium colli, shortened fourth metacarpals, cubitus valgus, heart murmurs, nail changes, and deformed ears.

Autoimmune disease may cause primary ovarian insufficiency. Other associated conditions include myasthenia gravis, idiopathic thrombocytopenic purpura, rheumatoid arthritis, vitiligo, and autoimmune hemolytic anemia. Ovarian failure may result from chemotherapy or from irradiation. Gonadotropin-secreting adenomas are not associated with amenorrhea.

7 If there is history of contraceptive use (birth control pills or long-acting implantable or injectable progestins), amenorrhea may be attributed to the suppression of ovulation in the progestin-dominated hormonal environment. Menstrual cycles should revert to normal within 6 months of stopping birth control pills and by 12 months after the last injection of medroxyprogesterone (Depo-Provera).

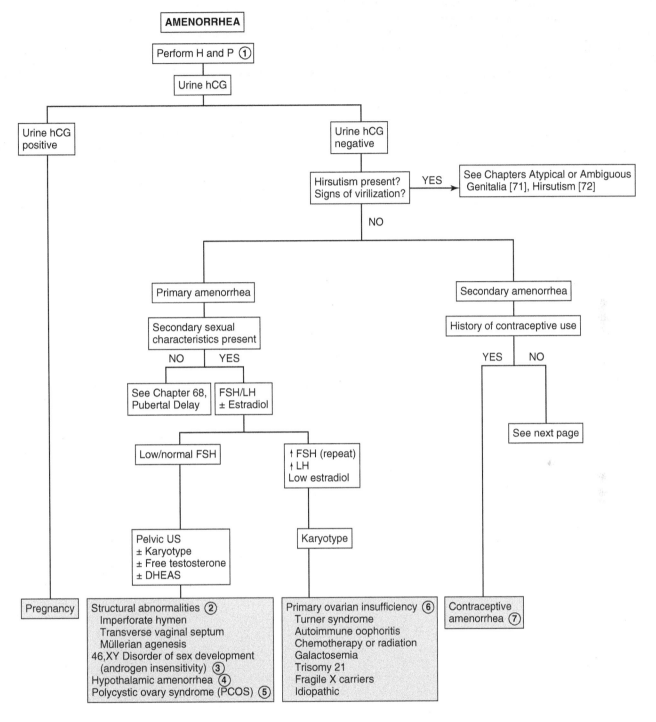

DHEAS = dehydroepiandrosterone sulfate

Nelson Textbook of Pediatrics, 19e. Chapters 110, 546, 580
Nelsons Essentials, 6e. Chapter 69

8 Adolescent girls with hyperprolactinemia may present with amenorrhea or delayed puberty and often with galactorrhea. Cranial imaging (MRI) is recommended to evaluate for pituitary or hypothalamic tumors or disease (craniopharyngioma, prolactinoma, sarcoidosis). Galactorrhea with normal or mildly elevated prolactin levels may be secondary to nipple stimulation and chest wall irritation or trauma. Hyperprolactinemia may be due to drugs including antipsychotics, methyldopa, amitriptyline, benzodiazepines, cocaine, and metoclopramide.

9 Estrogen status may be evaluated by progestin challenge, because estrogen levels are not always reliable. Estrogen status may also be confirmed by vaginal smear or the presence of abundant watery cervical mucus. For a progestin challenge, a 5- to 10-day course of oral medroxyprogesterone acetate or a single dose of intramuscular progesterone is given. If bleeding occurs within 2 weeks of treatment, it implies a functional uterus and outflow tract and an endometrium that has been exposed to estrogen. The amount of bleeding is roughly proportional to the amount and duration of prior estrogen exposure.

10 If there is no bleeding, it usually implies a low-estrogen state or hypoestrogenic amenorrhea. Rarely, it may be that the uterus cannot bleed secondary to uterine scarring caused by prior dilatation and curettage or severe uterine infections (Asherman syndrome). This is rare in teenagers. It is important to rule out pregnancy. If there is any question, the pregnancy test must be repeated.

Bibliography

Emans SJH, Laufer MR: Amenorrhea in the adolescent. In Emans SJ, Laufer MR, editors: *Emans, Laufer, Goldstein's pediatric & adolescent gynecology,* ed 6, Philadelphia, 2012, Lippincott Williams & Wilkins, pp 138–158.

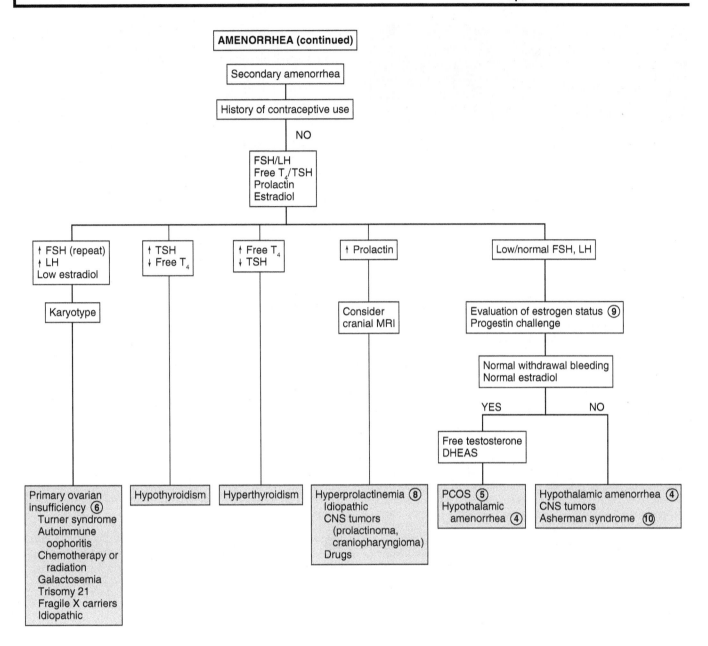

Chapter 40
ABNORMAL VAGINAL BLEEDING

Normal menstrual cycles range from 3 to 7 days. Periodic menstrual bleeding occurring more frequently than every 21 days, greater than every 45 days, or lasting longer than 7 days requires evaluation. With excessive blood loss, iron deficiency anemia may develop. Variations in menstrual cycles may include menorrhagia (normal intervals, excessive flow and duration of bleeding), metrorrhagia (irregular intervals), polymenorrhea (intervals ≤ 21 days), oligomenorrhea (<6 menses/yr), and intermenstrual bleeding.

1. The age of the patient is important, as well as any history of abuse or trauma, including sexual abuse. A history of any foreign body, including intrauterine devices (IUDs) and tampons in older girls, should be elicited. In girls who have reached menarche, a detailed menstrual history including date of menarche and menstrual pattern should be obtained. Increased clots may signify an abnormality. A sexual history (sexually transmitted disease, sexual partners) is important, as well as any use of hormonal contraception. Exposure to medications, including exogenous estrogens, anticoagulants, and platelet inhibitors, may be a cause of bleeding. Abdominal pain or vaginal discharge may indicate infections. Review of systems should include stress, weight change, and chronic diseases. On examination, the site of bleeding should be carefully assessed. An examination of external genitalia must be done (vaginal digital exam if possible) to identify anatomic abnormalities, and a pelvic examination performed when indicated for sexually active patients. Orthostatic BPs may be helpful in cases of heavy bleeding.

2. In the newborn, a small amount of endometrial bleeding may occur secondary to withdrawal from relatively high fetal estrogen levels.

3. In prepubertal-age girls without cyclic bleeding and with no signs of puberty, a vulvovaginal source is most common. Vaginal bleeding is more predictive of a foreign body than a vaginal discharge. The possibility of sexual abuse must be considered. The foreign object may be visualized in the knee-chest position, but if not, examination using anesthesia may be required.

4. Infectious vulvovaginitis usually appears as a discharge, but bleeding may be present. The most common organisms obtained on culture are group A streptococci, *Shigella*, and mixed organisms. The presence of gonococci, *Chlamydia*, or *Trichomonas* should prompt evaluation for sexual abuse.

5. Vulvovaginal trauma is usually caused by straddle injuries and less commonly by vaginal penetration and tearing from forced leg abduction; always consider the possibility of sexual abuse.

6. If a mass is visualized, consider urethral prolapse, which appears as red, friable, often necrotic tissue at the urethra.

7. In lichen sclerosus, the vulvar skin becomes thin and parchment-like (classically in an hourglass pattern around the introitus and anus) and therefore susceptible to bleeding from minor trauma. The diagnosis may be confirmed by biopsy.

8. Neoplasms include hemangiomas, polyps, and sarcoma botryoides (a grapelike mass protruding from the vagina). Malignancies are uncommon (adenocarcinoma and rhabdomyosarcoma).

9. Exogenous exposures to estrogens may occur from ingestion of birth control pills, foods, and beauty products. It has been hypothesized that plastics may contain estrogen-like components.

10. Precocious menarche is a rare form of incomplete precocious puberty with cyclic menstruation but no other secondary sexual characteristics. There may be a slight increase in serum estrogen levels; gonadotropin levels are prepubertal.

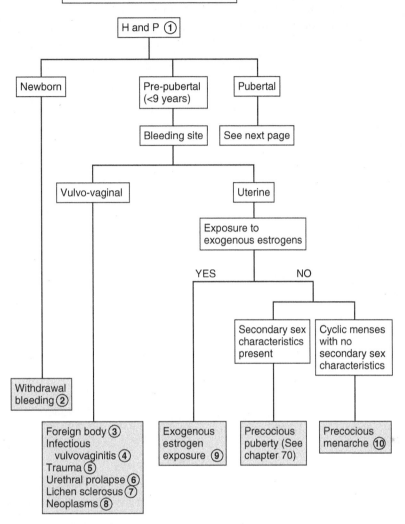

HCG= Human chorionic gonadotropin
IUD= Intrauterine device

Nelson Textbook of Pediatrics, 19e. Chapters 110, 114, 185, 542, 544, 545, 556
Nelsons Essentials, 6e. Chapter 69

11 In pubertal-age girls, first exclude pregnancy. Complications of pregnancy such as miscarriage or ectopic pregnancy may appear as abnormal bleeding. If this is suggested, pelvic examination, quantitative serum human chorionic gonadotropin (hCG) levels, and US are helpful. If the US shows no ectopic pregnancy or there is low suspicion of an ectopic pregnancy, serial hCG testing is needed to document complete abortion or to determine if repeat US or culdocentesis is needed.

12 If the bleeding site is the vagina, the cause may be injury or laceration, abuse, or foreign body (e.g., retained tampon, contraceptive sponge). Foul discharge may be present. Cancer is uncommon. Localization of the bleeding site may require anesthesia and possible referral to a gynecologist.

13 Infections causing vaginitis and cervicitis include chlamydia, gonorrhea, and trichomoniasis, herpes simplex, and human papillomavirus. (See Chapter 41.)

14 Menstrual cycles in adolescents are often "normally" anovulatory in the early years. This is believed to be due to the immaturity of the hypothalamic-pituitary axis. Problems occur when the negative feedback of estrogen does not occur, producing a steady state of estrogen, FSH, and LH, as in chronic anovulation. Constant levels of estrogen result in persistent endometrial stimulation and irregular heavy bleeding when the endometrium cannot be sustained (i.e., abnormal uterine bleeding).

15 Bleeding disorders may be due to thrombocytopenia. Causes include idiopathic thrombocytopenic purpura (ITP), hypersplenism, aplastic anemia, and (rarely) systemic diseases such as leukemia. (See Chapter 62.)

16 Coagulation disorders often cause abnormal uterine bleeding, especially the more severe bleeding that results in anemias requiring transfusions. PT, PTT, platelet function tests, and von Willebrand factor screening should be obtained to test for von Willebrand disease (a common etiology), platelet function disorders, factor deficiencies, liver dysfunction, and vitamin K deficiency. Consultation with a hematologist may be needed for further testing. (See Chapter 62.)

17 Oral contraceptive pills and injectable or implantable progestin contraceptives may be associated with abnormal bleeding.

18 Medications include those with hormonal effects (e.g., estrogens, progestins, androgens, prolactin, antipsychotics, spironolactone) and those with anticoagulant effects (e.g., warfarin, heparin, aspirin).

19 Infections such as pelvic inflammatory disease (PID) may cause uterine bleeding. PID includes diseases of the upper genital tract such as endometritis, salpingitis, tuboovarian abscess, and pelvic peritonitis involving multiple organisms. Causes include *Neisseria gonorrhoeae*, *Chlamydia* trachomatis, and endogenous flora (streptococci, anaerobes, gram-negative bacilli). In addition, *Gardnerella vaginalis*, *Haemophilus influenzae*, enteric gram-negative rods, and *Streptococcus agalactiae*, CMV, *Mycoplasma hominis*, *Ureaplasma urealyticum*, and *Mycoplasma genitalium* may also be associated.

20 Congenital partial obstruction of the hemivagina or uterine horn can result in uterine bleeding.

21 Neoplasms include fibroids (submucous myoma), endometrial polyps, malignant tumors, or estrogen-producing ovarian tumors.

22 Chronic diseases include diabetes, renal disease, and systemic lupus erythematosus. They may affect menstruation by affecting ovulation or normal coagulation. Tuberculosis can rarely cause a local endometrial infection.

Bibliography

Emans SJH, Laufer MR: Abnormal vaginal bleeding in the adolescent. In Emans SJ, Laufer MR, editors: *Emans, Laufer, Goldstein's pediatric & adolescent gynecology*, ed 6, Philadelphia, 2012, Lippincott Williams & Wilkins.

Gray SH: Menstrual disorders, *Pediatr Rev* 34:6–18, 2013.

ABNORMAL VAGINAL BLEEDING (continued)

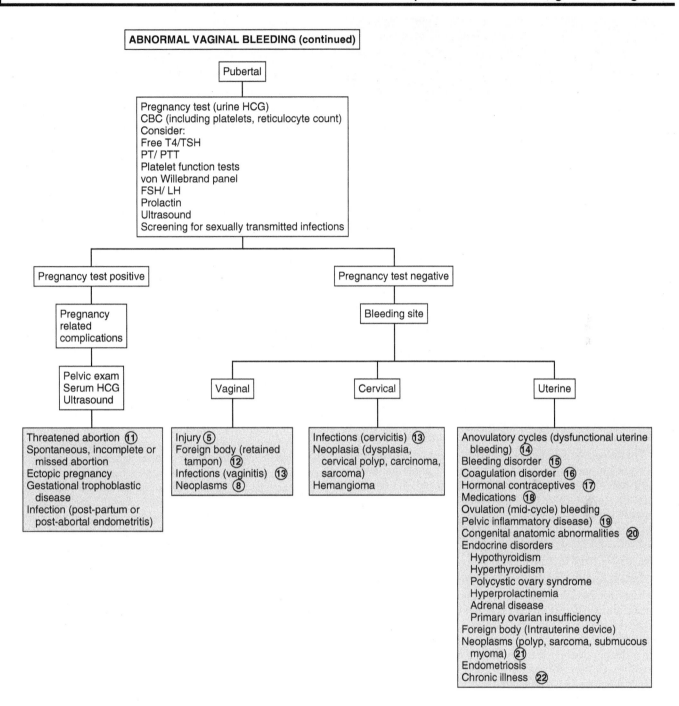

Pubertal

Pregnancy test (urine HCG)
CBC (including platelets, reticulocyte count)
Consider:
Free T4/TSH
PT/ PTT
Platelet function tests
von Willebrand panel
FSH/ LH
Prolactin
Ultrasound
Screening for sexually transmitted infections

Pregnancy test positive | Pregnancy test negative

Pregnancy test positive

Pregnancy related complications

Pelvic exam
Serum HCG
Ultrasound

Threatened abortion ⑪
Spontaneous, incomplete or missed abortion
Ectopic pregnancy
Gestational trophoblastic disease
Infection (post-partum or post-abortal endometritis)

Pregnancy test negative

Bleeding site

Vaginal | Cervical | Uterine

Vaginal

Injury ⑤
Foreign body (retained tampon) ⑫
Infections (vaginitis) ⑬
Neoplasms ⑧

Cervical

Infections (cervicitis) ⑬
Neoplasia (dysplasia, cervical polyp, carcinoma, sarcoma)
Hemangioma

Uterine

Anovulatory cycles (dysfunctional uterine bleeding) ⑭
Bleeding disorder ⑮
Coagulation disorder ⑯
Hormonal contraceptives ⑰
Medications ⑱
Ovulation (mid-cycle) bleeding
Pelvic inflammatory disease) ⑲
Congenital anatomic abnormalities ⑳
Endocrine disorders
   Hypothyroidism
   Hyperthyroidism
   Polycystic ovary syndrome
   Hyperprolactinemia
   Adrenal disease
   Primary ovarian insufficiency
Foreign body (Intrauterine device)
Neoplasms (polyp, sarcoma, submucous myoma) ㉑
Endometriosis
Chronic illness ㉒

Chapter 41
VAGINAL DISCHARGE

Vaginal discharge is a common but nonspecific sign in female adolescents. It should prompt consideration of sexually transmitted disease in sexually active girls.

1. Menstrual history, including changes in cycle or new onset of dysmenorrhea, may be helpful. A history of symptoms including odor, color, amount of discharge, and pruritus should be obtained. Associated illnesses (HIV, diabetes) and medications such as antibiotics and oral contraceptives may be contributing factors. Sexual history should include recent sexual encounters, number of partners, contraceptive and condom use, dyspareunia, history of sexually transmitted infection (STI), and pregnancies if any. Sexual abuse should be considered, particularly in prepubertal girls with vaginal discharge. Most discharge in this age group is not sexually acquired.

Examination includes careful inspection of the vulva, vagina, and introitus for any abnormalities, including bruises, lacerations, excoriations, and vesicles, as well as character of the vaginal discharge. Pelvic examination (if necessary) in prepubertal girls may be done using a Huffman speculum. The Pederson speculum is slightly larger and may be used in an adolescent. Rashes may be seen with STIs, as well as joint and other constitutional symptoms.

2. Physiologic leukorrhea is a whitish mucoid discharge that occurs in newborns and adolescents. In pubertal adolescents it starts before menarche and may decrease with onset of menses or may continue for a few years. During the middle of the menstrual cycle, it is copious and clear; it is scant and sticky during the second half of the cycle. Wet preparation shows epithelial cells and no abnormal findings. If the patient is sexually active, an STI must be ruled out.

3. All cases with suspected sexual abuse require direct cultures for *Neisseria gonorrhoeae* and *Chlamydia*, because results of antigen detection tests may not be admissible in court. Referral to persons with expertise in evaluation of sexually abused children (sexual assault team) is indicated. It is preferable that the physical exam be performed by a sexual abuse team if possible. Culture for gonorrhea and chlamydia should be obtained because it is considered the gold standard. Nucleic acid antigen tests should also be obtained because of increased yield; also, some state laws will accept them as evidence. Wet mount needs to be done, looking for *Trichomonas* and bacterial vaginosis. Any lesion suspicious for herpes should be cultured. Also test for HIV and syphilis.

4. In the prepubertal girl, the vulvar mucosa is thin and more susceptible to irritation and inflammation. Poor hygiene, use of irritant soaps, bubble baths, and "nonbreathing" underwear may be associated with nonspecific or irritant vulvovaginitis.

5. Infectious vulvovaginitis may be due to fecal or respiratory pathogens, including *Escherichia coli*, group A *Streptococcus*, *Staphylococcus aureus*, *Haemophilus influenzae*, *Shigella*, and *Yersinia enterocolitica*. A bloody vaginal discharge may be seen with *Shigella* or group A streptococcal infections.

If there is possible sexual abuse, vaginal secretions must be cultured to exclude an STI.

6. Candidal vulvovaginitis in a prepubertal girl is uncommon but may occur after use of oral antibiotics.

7. Foreign bodies (often retained toilet tissue) in the vagina cause a foul-smelling brown or bloody discharge. If the foreign body cannot be visualized, examination using anesthesia may be needed.

8. Anal pruritus may indicate pinworms and can be diagnosed using a tape test. Pinworms are more common in younger children.

9. Neoplasms are a rare cause of discharge. Examples include rhabdomyosarcoma, as well as adenosis and adenocarcinoma in girls whose mothers were exposed to diethylstilbestrol during pregnancy.

10. In girls, an ectopic ureter may drain into the vagina (25%) and rarely into the cervix or uterus.

11. Müllerian anomalies may also present with vaginal discharge—for example, in a patient with a transverse vaginal septum with a small opening.

12. The appearance of secretions may help in diagnosis; *Candida* causes a thick, whitish, curdy discharge, and *Trichomonas* has a yellow frothy discharge. A mucopurulent discharge with evidence of cervicitis may be seen with *Chlamydia trachomatis*, *N. gonorrhoeae*, and herpes.

Microscopic examination of secretions may help provide the diagnosis. Trichomonads are motile flagellated organisms. Clue cells (i.e., epithelial cells coated with refractile bacteria) are seen with bacterial vaginosis. Potassium hydroxide (KOH) reveals pseudohyphae in *Candida*. A positive "whiff" test, due to release of amine odor, is present with bacterial vaginosis and sometimes with *Trichomonas*. A nucleic acid amplification test (NAAT) is the preferred test for detection of *N. gonorrhoeae* and *C. trachomatis* and can be performed on urethral or cervical specimens as well as urine. Other methods for detection of *C. trachomatis* include enzyme immunoassay, ligase chain reaction, PCR, and culture. HIV and syphilis testing should be considered in all sexually active girls. If herpes simplex virus (HSV) is suspected, cell culture and PCR testing are preferred for a patient presenting with active lesions. HSV serologic tests can be used to diagnose a patient with a history of vesicular genital lesions, and to diagnose a past HSV infection or current infection in a patient with an atypical lesions.

13. Gonorrheal infections may also involve the pharynx, rectum, and joints; disseminated infection may occur.

14. Chlamydial infections usually cause vaginal discharge, dysuria, or frequency. Endometritis with menorrhagia or metrorrhagia may be present. Perihepatitis (Fitz-Hugh–Curtis syndrome) may occur with gonorrhea or chlamydial infection; these are also responsible for most pelvic inflammatory disease (PID).

15. Bacterial vaginosis occurs secondary to replacement of the normal hydrogen peroxide–producing vaginal flora (*Lactobacillus*) by overgrowth of anaerobic microorganisms, as well as *Gardnerella vaginalis*, *Ureaplasma*, and *Mycoplasma*. Although bacterial vaginosis is not categorized as an STI, sexual activity is associated with increased frequency of vaginosis.

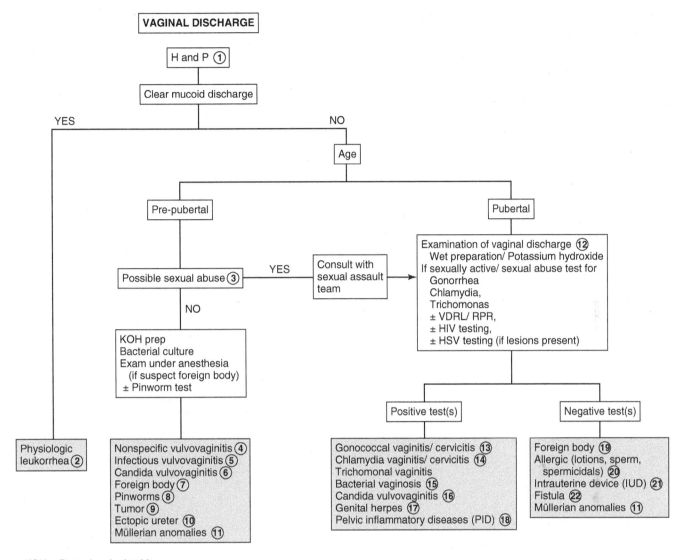

KOH = Potassium hydroxide
VDRL = Venereal Disease Research Laboratory
RPR = Rapid plasma reagin
PAP = Papanicolaou's stain
HSV = Herpes simplex virus
LGV = Lymphogranuloma venereum
HPV = Human papillomavirus
IUD = Intrauterine device

Nelson Textbook of Pediatrics, 19e. Chapters 114, 176, 543
Nelsons Essentials, 6e. Chapter 116

16 *Candida albicans* is the most common fungal infection of the vagina; other *Candida* species may be involved. Diabetes mellitus, pregnancy, and use of antibiotics are predisposing factors.

17 Herpes appears initially as vesicles and pustules associated with vaginal discharge and dysuria, followed by ulceration of the lesions, with associated constitutional symptoms. Tender inguinal lymphadenopathy may be present.

18 PID includes inflammatory disorders of the female upper genital tract. These may include endometritis, salpingitis, tuboovarian abscess, and pelvic peritonitis, often in combination. *C. trachomatis* and *N. gonorrhoeae* are most commonly involved. However, other pathogens may also be associated, such as anaerobes, *G. vaginalis*, *H. influenzae*, enteric gram-negative rods, *Streptococcus agalactiae*, CMV, *Mycoplasma hominis*, *Ureaplasma urealyticum*, and *Mycoplasma genitalium*.

PID is difficult to diagnose because of the wide variation in the symptoms and signs. Many females with PID have subtle or mild symptoms, resulting in many unrecognized cases. Healthcare providers should consider the possibility of PID in young sexually active females presenting with vaginal discharge and/ or abdominal pain.

19 Foreign bodies may also cause discharge in pubertal-age girls. Often it is a retained tampon.

20 Other causes of vaginitis include allergic vulvovaginitis caused by soaps, douches, contraceptive gels or creams, and (rarely) sperm.

21 Chronic discharge may be due to an intrauterine device string.

22 Rectovaginal and anovaginal fistulae may be seen with Crohn disease and rarely with obstetric trauma (more often seen in developing countries with inadequate obstetric care). Vesicovaginal fistula may also be due to obstetric trauma.

Bibliography

Emans SJH, Laufer MR: Vulvovaginal complaints in the adolescent. In Emans SJ, Laufer MR, editors: *Emans, Laufer, Goldstein's pediatric & adolescent gynecology*, ed 6, Philadelphia, 2012, Lippincott Williams & Wilkins, pp 305–324.

Emans SJH, Laufer MR: Sexually transmitted infections: Chlamydia, gonorrhea, pelvic inflammatory disease, and syphilis. In Emans SJ, Laufer MR, editors: *Emans, Laufer, Goldstein's pediatric & adolescent gynecology*, ed 6, Philadelphia, 2012, Lippincott Williams & Wilkins, pp 325–348.

Sugar NF, Graham EA: Common gynecologic problems in prepubertal girls, *Pediatr Rev* 27:213–222, 2006.

Musculoskeletal System

Chapter 42
LIMP

An abnormal gait in a child may be due to pain, weakness, torsional deformity, or a musculoskeletal disorder.

1   A birth history and developmental history are particularly important for problems noticed early or around the time a child begins walking. Prematurity and birth complications are risk factors for hypoxic brain damage (e.g., cerebral palsy). For older children, inquire about a history of trauma and systemic signs and symptoms (fever, rash, generalized weakness, weight loss) that may suggest infections or rheumatic disorders. Always be conscious of the possibility of child abuse (nonaccidental trauma).

The musculoskeletal examination should include careful attention to all joints and the spine. The hip exam is particularly important because hip problems are a common cause of limping, plus hip pathology frequently causes referred pain to the knee. Careful observation of the gait, ideally over a distance such as a long hallway, is critical. Having the child adequately undressed is also necessary for a good evaluation. In a painful gait, the child's stance phase on the affected limb is shortened; trauma, infection, and rheumatic disorders are the most likely etiologies in these cases. Congenital and neuromuscular disorders are more likely to present with a painless (Trendelenburg) gait, which indicates proximal muscle weakness or hip instability. The stance phase is equal from side to side in these cases, but the child tends to shift their weight over the involved side for balance. Bilateral involvement produces a waddling gait.

2   Children are more at risk for epiphyseal fractures than ligamentous sprains because their ligaments are generally stronger than the adjacent growth plates. Because x-rays may be normal or show only physeal widening, the diagnosis is often clinical. Consultation should always be considered when in doubt.

3   Slipped capital femoral epiphysis (SCFE) is the most common hip disorder in adolescents presenting with pain or an abnormal gait. In this condition, a failure of the physis (growth plate) leads to posterior displacement of the metaphysis (femoral neck) relative to the epiphysis (femoral head). In many cases, an undiagnosed chronic slip is diagnosed after it is acutely worsened by trauma. A careful history often elicits chronic complaints of pain, subtle limp, or self-imposed activity restrictions. Examination reveals limited internal rotation of the affected hip and an out-toed, painful gait. AP and frog-leg lateral radiographs are routinely recommended to make the diagnosis; the latter should be performed with caution because of the potential risk for further displacement of the slip. Bilateral views are recommended because the condition is bilateral in 25% of cases at initial presentation. Conditions like hypothyroidism, pituitary disorders, and renal osteodystrophy can impact bone ossification and increase the risk of developing SCFE.

4   When infection or inflammation is suspected, laboratory tests (CBC, ESR, CRP) may be helpful but are nonspecific. Blood cultures yield a positive result in about 50% of cases of osteomyelitis; rates may be higher with specimens from a bone biopsy or abscess aspiration. If the x-ray is negative and clinical suspicion is high, US may aid in detecting joint effusions, especially of the hip. If an effusion is present, joint aspiration is recommended to rule out a septic arthritis. MRI is the preferred diagnostic test when osteomyelitis is suspected.

5   Septic arthritis is an infection confined to the capsule of a joint. Infection within the bone is osteomyelitis; secondary spread to involve the joint may accompany it. Both disorders may present with localized pain and tenderness in an acutely ill child. Osteomyelitis may also occur subacutely with prolonged pain and limp but without fevers or systemic complaints. Bone changes on x-ray may not become evident for 7 to 10 days. Soft tissue changes may be evident earlier, plus films are usually obtained to rule out trauma and tumor initially. MRI is the preferred choice for diagnostic imaging if available. Bone scans are also sensitive and specific early in the clinical course if MRI is not available.

6   Septic arthritis is a medical emergency requiring prompt diagnosis and treatment. Patients typically present with fever, malaise, refusal to walk, and localized joint pain, most commonly knee or hip. Examination reveals erythema, warmth, swelling, and pain with passive motion. US evaluation may suggest the diagnosis by demonstrating an effusion, but joint aspiration is mandated to confirm (or rule out) the diagnosis. (See Chapter 43.)

7   Acute transient synovitis (previously called "toxic synovitis") is one of the most common causes of hip pain and limping in children, usually between 3 and 8 years of age. The etiology is not well defined; it is described as a nonspecific inflammatory condition, although viral, allergic, and traumatic mechanisms have all been suggested. Children present with unilateral hip pain, a painful limp, and slightly restricted abduction and internal rotation. Fevers may be present, but rarely do patients present with the acute toxicity suggestive of septic arthritis. The diagnosis is one of exclusion; the most important diagnosis to exclude is a septic arthritis. Several recent studies have focused on identifying factors that help distinguish a septic joint (which requires emergent treatment) from a transient synovitis (which is managed conservatively). The more of these factors that are present, the greater the likelihood of a septic joint: fever above 38.5 C°, an elevated CRP, an elevated ESR, refusal to bear weight, and an elevated WBC. With transient synovitis, laboratory results are usually normal or suggest a mild inflammatory process. X-rays are usually normal or may show a slightly widened medial joint space or accentuated pericapsular shadow. Rarely, US and aspiration to rule out septic arthritis may be necessary when a child presents acutely with pain and fever; children presenting after 1 or 2 days of symptoms may usually be managed more conservatively.

8   AVN (or Legg-Calvé-Perthes disease) is an ischemic necrosis of the femoral head resulting in a bony deformity of the femoral head. Children between 2 and 12 years of age are affected, with a peak incidence between 4 and 8 years of age; boys are affected more than girls. Children commonly demonstrate a limp before complaining of pain. Pain complaints are usually associated with activity; the pain may be located in the groin or referred to the anteromedial thigh or knee. Common physical findings include slightly restricted abduction and internal rotation; over time, hip flexion contractures, atrophy of the leg muscles, and a leg-length discrepancy may be evident due to disuse.

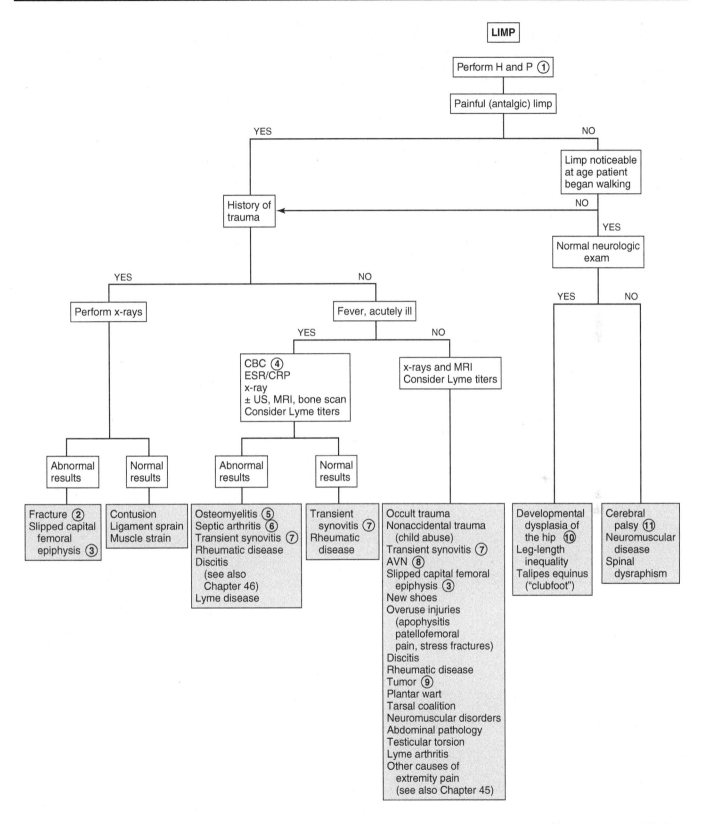

Nelson Textbook of Pediatrics, 19e. Chapters 591, 665, 670, 676
Nelsons Essentials, 6e. Chapter 199

9 Night pain is characteristic of both benign and malignant primary or metastatic tumors. Characteristic x-ray findings usually suggest the diagnosis of benign bone tumors; intervention (biopsy, removal, monitoring) will be required for many of them.

10 If not diagnosed in infancy, developmental dysplasia of the hip (DDH) will usually present as a limp, waddling gait, or leg-length discrepancy after the child starts walking. On physical exam, hip abduction will be limited, a positive Galeazzi sign (knees at different levels with hips flexed when child lying supine) may be evident, and lumbar lordosis may be present (due to altered hip mechanics).

11 Spastic diplegia is the most common type of cerebral palsy. Affected children are delayed in crawling and walking. The condition is characterized by toe-walking and a painless, waddling (Trendelenburg) gait. Examination reveals increased muscle tone, spasticity, hyperactive deep tendon reflexes, tight heel cords, and persistent pathologic reflexes.

Bibliography

Caird MS, Flynn JM, Leung YL, et al: Factors distinguishing septic arthritis from transient synovitis of the hip in children. A prospective study, *J Bone Joint Surg Am* 88:1251–1257, 2006.

Perry DC, Bruce C: Evaluating the child who presents with an acute limp, *BMJ* 341:c4250, 2010.

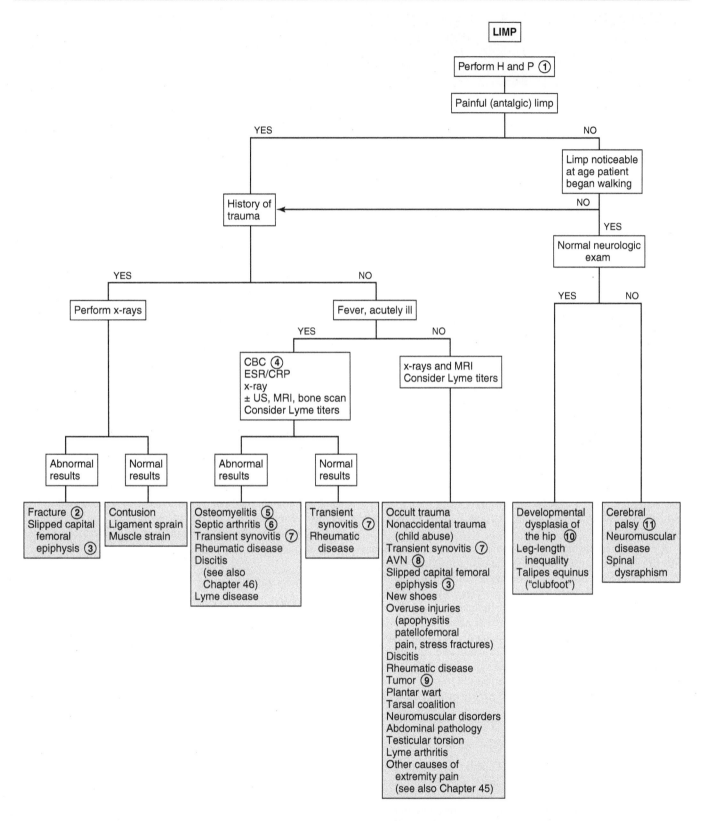

Nelson Textbook of Pediatrics, 19e. Chapters 591, 665, 670, 676
Nelsons Essentials, 6e. Chapter 199

Chapter 43
ARTHRITIS

Arthralgia is joint pain, with or without physical findings. Arthritis is joint swelling or the presence of two or more of the following: joint pain with motion, decreased range of motion, or warmth or erythema overlying a joint. The degree of joint pain and diminished function accompanying arthritis is variable.

1. Although arthritis typically presents with pain and physical findings, occasionally joint findings (swelling, redness, warmth) occur without any associated pain or restricted motion. In the neonate, clinical manifestations of arthritis are nonspecific: poor feeding, irritability, pseudoparalysis of an extremity. In children, morning stiffness or stiffness after prolonged periods of inactivity are common. They may also experience referred pain. Hip disease may be referred to the knees, and pelvic pain may be referred to the back, hip, or anterior thigh. Arthritis may also present as a limp. (See Chapter 42, Limp.)

The history should include a detailed description of joint symptoms, including the affected joints, duration, severity, and pattern of symptoms. Recent illness, travel, trauma, immunizations, and medications are also key history elements. A thorough review of systems is important because rheumatic disorders can affect virtually all organ systems. Inquire specifically about weight loss, anorexia, and fevers, as well as a history of sexual activity. Assess the impact of the complaint on sleep and usual activities. Bone pain severe enough to cause nighttime awakening, especially in association with more constitutional symptoms (fevers, weight loss), should raise suspicion for possible malignancy.

A generalized physical exam should assess for signs of acute infection. Overall growth parameters, ocular findings (uveitis), lymphadenopathy, hepatosplenomegaly, and cutaneous findings could all yield clues to a possible diagnosis. The physical exam should include observation of the gait, a comprehensive joint exam, and a focused exam of each affected joint, ideally using the contralateral side (if unaffected) for comparison. A careful discernment between extraarticular and intraarticular swelling must be made. Adjacent extremities should be assessed for bony tenderness and muscle atrophy.

2. Clinical findings of fever and refusal to bear weight are more predictive of a septic joint than a nonbacterial etiology, as are an increased CRP, ESR, and WBC. The more of these findings that are present, the greater the risk of a septic joint.

3. Acute transient synovitis (see Chapter 42, Limp) usually presents with a less fulminant onset than a septic arthritis. Joint aspiration may rarely be necessary to distinguish between the two conditions if evaluated in the acute period of symptom onset. If performed, synovial fluid analysis will yield a negative Gram stain and culture. (Acute transient synovitis does not typically meet the definition of arthritis, but it does need to be considered in the evaluation of a painful joint or limp.)

4. An acutely inflamed single joint needs to be aspirated if there is any concern about a potential bacterial infection (septic joint). Blood cultures should be obtained if concerned about a septic joint; testing for *Neisseria gonorrhoeae* (urine, rectal, throat) should be performed if the patient is sexually active. Imaging can be at the preference of the consultant performing the aspiration. Synovial fluid should be sent for Gram stain and culture, including inoculation on solid media and in aerobic blood culture bottles. The latter may increase the yield of *Kingella kingae*; if available, PCR testing for that pathogen is even more sensitive. The Gram stain is particularly important, since synovial fluid cultures are often negative. Analysis of synovial fluid for cell count, protein, and glucose will be elevated in both infectious and noninfectious causes of arthritis; very high cell counts ($>$50,000-100,000 cells/mm^3) usually indicate infection.

5. The most common agents of septic arthritis in children and adolescents are *Staphylococcus aureus*, group A streptococcus, and *Streptococcus pneumoniae*. *K. kingae* is being increasingly recognized as an etiology, particularly in children under 4 to 5 years of age. Salmonella is an important cause in patients with sickle cell disease; *N. gonorrhoeae* needs to be considered in sexually active patients; *Neisseria meningitidis*, *Pseudomonas aeruginosa* (as a sequelae to a puncture wound through a tennis shoe), and tuberculosis are rare causes. Group B streptococcus and gram-negative enteric rods can be causative in neonates. *Haemophilus influenzae* type B, once the most common cause of septic joints in young children, is now uncommon owing to immunization.

6. Disseminated gonococcal disease should be considered in sexually active adolescents, although a monoarticular arthritis is a less common presentation of this disease. It more commonly occurs as a tenosynovitis causing polyarthralgia (primarily of the wrists, hands, and fingers) plus fever, chills, and a characteristic rash. A monoarticular arthritis is less likely to be accompanied by systemic symptoms and typically involves the knee. The GU tract, rectum, or pharynx are also usually infected.

7. Careful review of the history is the most important next step in the evaluation. The lab evaluation should be approached thoughtfully; most causes of arthritis in children have no specific laboratory findings, and the risk of slightly abnormal findings with little clinical significance is high. Labs may support a diagnosis but rarely lead to one; referral to a specialist may be a more appropriate and cost-effective diagnostic maneuver than an extensive lab and imaging workup.

8. Lyme disease titers should be obtained in patients with risk factors such as exposure to an endemic area (northeastern, mid-Atlantic, and north-central United States). The clinical presentation of Lyme disease can be highly variable. Early symptoms can include flulike symptoms of variable severity and erythema migrans (an expanding annular rash); less common are facial nerve palsies, meningitis, and cardiac problems. Arthritis is generally a late finding, however, and frequently a history for earlier clinical symptoms is negative. When arthritis occurs, it can be monoarticular or oligoarticular. When clinically suspicious of Lyme disease, obtain an enzyme-linked immunosorbent assay (ELISA) followed by a confirmatory Western blot test if the ELISA is positive or equivocal.

9. Spondyloarthropathy (or spondyloarthritis) traditionally referred to rheumatic diseases that were RF negative, frequently HLA-B27 positive, and involved the spine

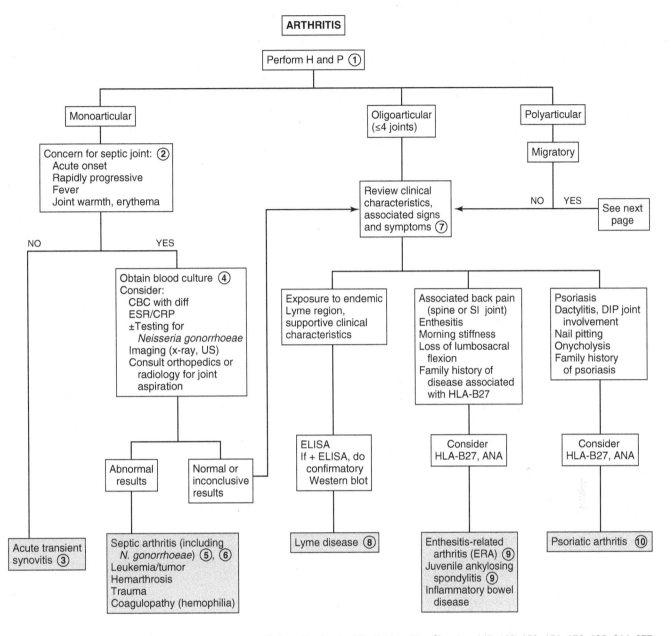

DIP = distal interphalangeal joint
ELISA = enzyme-linked immunosorbent assay
JIA = juvenile idiopathic arthritis
SLE = systemic lupus erythematosus

Nelson Textbook of Pediatrics, 19e. Chapters 147, 149, 150, 151, 176, 185, 214, 677
Nelsons Essentials, 6e. Chapters 89, 118

(especially the SI joints), large joints of the lower extremities, and entheses (where ligaments, tendons and joint capsules insert into bone). The current preferred classification system (per the International Leagues for the Associations for Rheumatology [ILAR]) uses the term enthesitis-related arthritis (ERA) to include patients with both arthritis and enthesitis (the Achilles tendon and plantar fascia are common sites) or with enthesitis and two of the following additional characteristics: SI joint tenderness or lumbosacral pain, the presence of HLA-B27, onset of arthritis in males older than age 6 years, uveitis, or a first-degree relative with an HLA-B27–associated disease. Children meeting ILAR criteria for ERA may ultimately progress to meet criteria for juvenile ankylosing spondylitis or inflammatory bowel disease, although this progression is not predictable. In juvenile ankylosing spondylitis, lower extremity arthritis (commonly including the hip) and severe enthesitis (especially at the foot, ankle, and knee) typically precede axial and SI joint involvement. X-rays can confirm sacroiliitis, but it may take years to get to this point. The arthritis associated with inflammatory bowel disease is polyarticular, affecting both small and large joints; it can also be migratory. Its severity usually reflects the degree of intestinal inflammation.

10 Psoriatic arthritis is included in the ILAR classification. Arthritis may precede the development of psoriasis. It is most commonly an asymmetric oligoarthritis; both large and small joints can be affected, including the distal interphalangeal joints. Dactylitis (swollen "sausage-shaped" digits), nail pitting, and onycholysis are other characteristics. A positive ANA will occur more commonly than a positive HLA-B27 result. RF is negative.

11 Reactive arthritis refers to a monoarthritis or oligoarthritis, usually affecting the lower extremities, following (by weeks or months) a GI or GU infection (*Salmonella, Shigella, Yersinia enterocolitica, Campylobacter jejuni, Cryptosporidium parvum, Giardia intestinalis, Chlamydia trachomatis,* and *Ureaplasma* have all been implicated). Enthesitis, dactylitis, cutaneous manifestations (balanitis, vulvitis, oral lesions, keratoderma blennorrhagica), and systemic symptoms of fever, malaise, and fatigue may occur; the arthritis is usually short-lived. Patients who are HLA-B27 positive have a higher risk of developing a chronic arthritis, especially spondyloarthritis. The arthritis occurring with *Campylobacter* is more likely to be migratory. Reactive arthritis in not included in the ILAR classification system.

12 Arthritis is a frequent component of vasculitis syndromes, including Henoch-Schönlein purpura, polyarteritis nodosa, Wegener's granulomatosis, and Takayasu arteritis. Characteristic skin findings occur with many of the disorders.

13 Arthritis and arthralgias have been associated with many viral infections, including rubella, parvovirus, EBV, CMV, varicella, and influenza. The joint symptoms may occur during the course of the infection or as a postinfectious reaction. Symptoms usually resolve within 6 weeks. The arthritis occurring with mumps is more likely to be migratory.

14 The term juvenile idiopathic arthritis (JIA) encompasses all forms of chronic juvenile arthritis. The current preferred classification system (per ILAR) includes the disorders previously classified as JRA as well as the previously mentioned ERAs and psoriatic arthritis. For all of these disorders, the onset of arthritis must occur before 16 years of age and last a minimum of 6 weeks to meet the diagnostic criteria. (The term "rheumatoid" was removed to eliminate the association with adult seropositive rheumatoid arthritis, which is typically very distinct from childhood arthritis.) If clinical suspicion is high for JIA, labs may support the diagnosis. Hematologic abnormalities reflect the degree of inflammation. RF is present in 5% to 10% of polyarthritis; ANA may be positive in oligoarthritis or polyarthritis. The presence of ANA indicates an increased risk of uveitis. Both RF and ANA may be transiently elevated in the presence of acute infections, so results may be misleading if the clinical diagnosis is not suggestive.

15 Oligoarthritis (≤4 joints) is classified as persistent JIA if no additional joint involvement occurs over time; if additional joint involvement does occur, it is extended oligoarticular JIA. Affected joints are mostly lower large joints (knees and ankles); hip involvement is very rare and should suggest another diagnosis (spondyloarthropathy or nonrheumatologic cause).

16 Polyarthritis includes involvement of 5 or more joints in upper and lower extremities in the first 6 months of symptoms. It is further classified based on the presence or absence of RF.

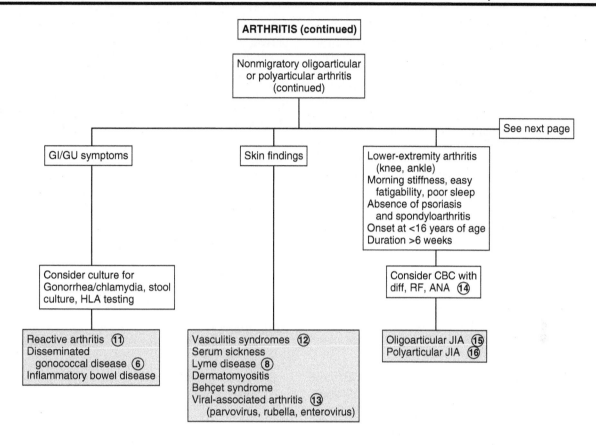

ARTHRITIS (continued)

Nonmigratory oligoarticular
or polyarticular arthritis
(continued)

See next page

GI/GU symptoms

Skin findings

Lower-extremity arthritis
(knee, ankle)
Morning stiffness, easy
fatigability, poor sleep
Absence of psoriasis
and spondyloarthritis
Onset at <16 years of age
Duration >6 weeks

Consider culture for
Gonorrhea/chlamydia, stool
culture, HLA testing

Consider CBC with
diff, RF, ANA ⑭

Reactive arthritis ⑪
Disseminated
   gonococcal disease ⑥
Inflammatory bowel disease

Vasculitis syndromes ⑫
Serum sickness
Lyme disease ⑧
Dermatomyositis
Behçet syndrome
Viral-associated arthritis ⑬
   (parvovirus, rubella, enterovirus)

Oligoarticular JIA ⑮
Polyarticular JIA ⑯

17 Children with systemic-onset JIA (SoJIA) experience short-lived high fevers once to twice daily for a minimum of 2 weeks, often accompanied by a characteristic salmon-colored macular rash. Visceral involvement (hepatosplenomegaly, lymphadenopathy, serositis) is very common and may precede the arthritis, although arthritis (which is usually polyarticular and can involve the hip, cervical spine, and temporomandibular joint) is necessary for the diagnosis. Labs typically reflect an anemia of chronic disease and generally very high inflammatory markers (including ferritin), WBCs, and platelet counts. RF and ANA are typically absent.

18 Arthralgias and arthritis in knees and hands may develop 10 to 28 days after immunization with rubella vaccine. This reaction occurs most commonly in postpubertal females. An associated rash may occur.

19 Poststreptococcal arthritis is an oligoarticular nonmigratory arthritis that affects mostly lower joints after infection with group A streptococcus. These cases do not fulfill the Jones criteria for acute rheumatic fever. Controversy exists over whether poststreptococcal arthritis is a distinct entity or an incomplete form of acute rheumatic fever.

20 In children, systemic lupus erythematosus (SLE) most commonly presents with nonspecific symptoms (malaise, fatigue); small-joint arthralgias and arthritis are frequently present but overlooked in the early phases of the disease. Adults classically experience a migratory arthritis.

21 One of the shortcomings of the ILAR system is that children do experience arthritis that does not fit into one of the classifications (or fits into more than one). The course or progression of these children is still unable to be predicted.

22 The polyarthritis that constitutes one of the Jones criteria for the diagnosis of rheumatic fever is migratory and characterized by extreme tenderness, redness, and swelling of affected joints. It typically affects larger joints (knees, ankles, wrists, elbows) and rarely affects the spine, hands, or hips. This arthritis classically responds very quickly to treatment with aspirin. Arthralgias (in the absence of arthritis) constitute a minor criterion for the diagnosis of rheumatic fever.

23 Hepatitis B arthritis-dermatitis syndrome clinically mimics serum sickness, with an urticarial rash and symmetric migratory polyarthritis.

Bibliography

Berard R: Approach to the child with joint inflammation, *Pediatr Clin North Am* 59:245–262, 2012.

Caird MS, Flynn JM, Leung YL, et al: Factors distinguishing septic arthritis from transient synovitis of the hip in children: A prospective study, *J Bone Joint Surg Am* 88:1251–1257, 2006.

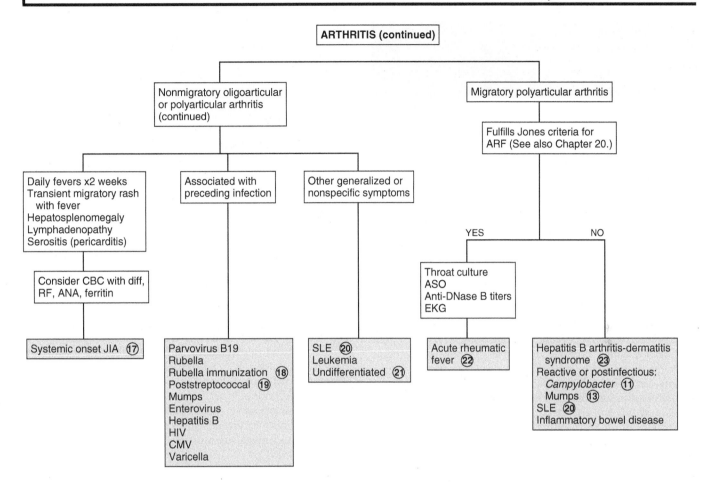

Chapter 44
KNEE PAIN

Knee pain can be an indicator of problems related to the distal femur, proximal tibia, hip, or the knee itself. If arthritis is suspected (warmth or swelling of joint, limited motion, multiple joint involvement, or systemic symptoms), refer to Chapter 43.

1 Knee pain in children can be due to acute problems or chronic processes. A thorough history and examination should include the specific location of the pain, duration of the complaint, and (if relevant) relationship to and mechanism of trauma. It is important to clarify descriptions like "locking," "catching," or "giving out"; have the patient specify whether the knee was truly "stuck" in a position (requiring some type of manipulation by the patient to release it), if the joint was unable to be flexed or extended beyond a certain point, or if they sensed the joint was simply unstable versus if it truly buckled on them.

Range of motion may be affected simply by pain or by intraarticular damage. Forced range of motion should never be attempted on exam. Bilateral knee evaluation allows comparison for symmetry and better detection of subtle findings. Asymmetry of the thigh musculature suggests a chronic problem with resultant muscular atrophy. A careful examination of the hips is critical in the evaluation of knee pain, especially in the absence of trauma; abnormalities could indicate a primary hip disorder.

2 A careful knee exam should include maneuvers (anterior drawer, Lachman, lateral pivot shift, Apley compression, McMurray) that can aid in identifying ligamentous and meniscal problems. Proficiency in performing these maneuvers is essential to doing a reliable exam. Mild injuries are likely to demonstrate pain on ligamentous testing in the absence of laxity or instability. Younger children are at greater risk for fractures than ligament sprains, because the physes (growth plates) are weaker than ligaments.

3 A history of a twisting injury, a "popping" sensation, and rapid development of an effusion (swelling) suggest an anterior cruciate ligament (ACL) injury. Children presenting later may complain of their knee frequently "giving out." Evaluation of a suspected ACL injury should include x-rays to rule out associated avulsion fractures. Because ACL tears are often associated with meniscal injury in children, referral for further evaluation (arthroscopy or MRI) is recommended.

4 A bipartite patella is the result of secondary ossification centers in the patella failing to fuse to the primary ossification center. Most are asymptomatic, but occasionally pain may occur with sports, especially with jumping, or climbing stairs. Symptoms are usually unilateral, and the examination typically reveals pain at the superolateral pole of the patella. X-rays are diagnostic.

5 Patellofemoral stress syndrome (also known as patellofemoral pain syndrome or patellofemoral dysfunction) comprises a spectrum of disorders characterized by anterior knee pain with no clearly definable cause. The term is typically applied to a pain syndrome experienced by adolescents, often after a change in activity level. Pain is vaguely described; it may be around the knee or behind the patella. It is exacerbated by climbing stairs, squatting, running, and after sitting with the knee flexed for an extended period. The pain is frequently bilateral, and examination may be normal or reveal medial patellar tenderness or pain with patellofemoral compression. Diagnosis is usually clinical. Specialty consultation or x-rays may be indicated in atypical or prolonged symptoms that do not respond to therapy. Significant pain or guarding with attempted lateral or medial displacement of the patella (positive apprehension test) suggests a more serious disorder of chronic or recurrent patellar subluxation or dislocation.

6 Certain congenital conditions (high-riding patella, shallow intercondylar notch, genu valgum deformity) may predispose children to patellar misalignment significant enough to produce recurrent subluxation or dislocation. Significant pain or guarding with attempted lateral or medial displacement (positive apprehension sign) suggests subluxation. In patellar dislocation, the knee is usually locked in approximately 45 degrees of flexion.

7 Sinding-Larsen-Johansson syndrome is an apophysitis at the site of insertion of the patellar tendon into the inferior pole of the patella. It is an overuse syndrome that most frequently affects volleyball and basketball players. Pain is localized to the inferior pole of the patella and is aggravated by activity. Diagnosis is usually clinical. Patients with similar complaints and tenderness over the patellar ligament near but not involving the bony attachments are most likely to have patellar tendinitis ("jumper's knee").

8 Osgood-Schlatter disease is an apophysitis at the site of insertion of the patellar tendon into the tibial tuberosity. It is an overuse syndrome common in adolescent athletes who are undergoing a growth spurt. Examination reveals tenderness and swelling at the tibial tubercle and exacerbation of pain with resisted knee extension. Symptoms are commonly bilateral, although one side may be more symptomatic than the other. Patients complain of worsening pain with flexion activities (running, jumping, kneeling, climbing stairs). Typical x-ray findings are soft tissue swelling and occasionally avulsed bony spicules over the tibial tuberosity, although x-rays are not usually indicated when the condition is bilateral. X-rays should be obtained when the pain is unilateral, not located directly over the tibial tuberosity, and when cases are unresponsive to treatment.

9 Meniscal injuries are more common in adolescents than in younger age groups. They are most commonly sports injuries due to a twisting motion that occurs when the knee is flexed and the foot is firmly planted on the ground. Medial meniscal tears are more common than lateral ones. The injury may or may not be evident acutely; sometimes they present later with complaints of vague pain, recurrent effusions, stiffness, "giving out," clicking, and sometimes locking. Examination reveals joint-line tenderness and occasionally a small effusion. X-rays are not helpful; MRIs are the preferred diagnostic entity.

10 Osteochondritis dissecans (OCD) develops after a small area of bone (most commonly in the medial femoral condyle) becomes avascular. The necrotic fragment (with the articular cartilage overlying it) partially or completely separates from the long bone. Patients complain of nonspecific pain, usually located around the patella and associated with activity. Effusion is sometimes present. Locking or popping can occur

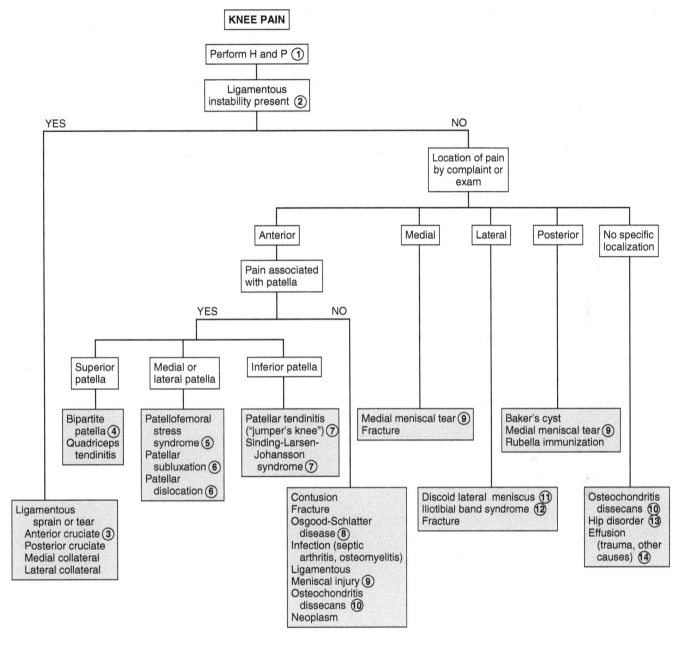

KNEE PAIN

Perform H and P ①

Ligamentous instability present ②

YES

NO

Location of pain by complaint or exam

Anterior — Medial — Lateral — Posterior — No specific localization

Anterior:

Pain associated with patella

YES — NO

Superior patella

Medial or lateral patella

Inferior patella

Bipartite patella ④
Quadriceps tendinitis

Patellofemoral stress syndrome ⑤
Patellar subluxation ⑥
Patellar dislocation ⑥

Patellar tendinitis ("jumper's knee") ⑦
Sinding-Larsen-Johansson syndrome ⑦

Ligamentous sprain or tear
Anterior cruciate ③
Posterior cruciate
Medial collateral
Lateral collateral

Contusion
Fracture
Osgood-Schlatter disease ⑧
Infection (septic arthritis, osteomyelitis)
Ligamentous
Meniscal injury ⑨
Osteochondritis dissecans ⑩
Neoplasm

Medial:
Medial meniscal tear ⑨
Fracture

Lateral:
Discoid lateral meniscus ⑪
Iliotibial band syndrome ⑫
Fracture

Posterior:
Baker's cyst
Medial meniscal tear ⑨
Rubella immunization

No specific localization:
Osteochondritis dissecans ⑩
Hip disorder ⑬
Effusion (trauma, other causes) ⑭

Nelson Textbook of Pediatrics, 19e. Chapters 669, 679
Nelsons Essentials, 6e. Chapters 199, 200

when the bony fragment completely separates into the joint space. X-rays with a notch view are helpful in diagnosis; MRI will better define the cartilaginous involvement.

11 Discoid lateral meniscus is a congenital variant of the lateral meniscus. Patients typically present in late childhood or adolescence with vague complaints of pain and an audible pop or snap with flexion. Examination reveals a palpable bulge at the lateral joint line when the knee is flexed. Standing x-rays may show a widened lateral joint space, flattening of the lateral femoral condyle, or cupping of the lateral aspect of the tibial plateau. MRI or arthroscopy may be necessary for definitive diagnosis.

12 Iliotibial band syndrome is an overuse syndrome that causes lateral knee pain in runners.

13 Poorly localized knee pain accompanied by an abnormal hip examination (restricted or painful internal rotation, abduction or flexion) suggests a primary hip disorder such as AVN or a slipped capital femoral epiphysis (SCFE).

14 Effusions are most likely to occur in association with a traumatic injury. Immediate development of an effusion after an injury usually indicates hemarthrosis. Effusions may develop slowly (2 to 3 days) after an injury or may present intermittently owing to an intracapsular injury (meniscal tear), overuse, or a rheumatoid process. Septic arthritis should be considered when a knee is acutely painful, warm, and swollen, especially if the patient is febrile or toxic; immediate aspiration is essential when septic arthritis is suspected. Aspiration may also be necessary for the diagnosis of chronic or recurrent knee effusions.

Bibliography

Baxter WR: Sports medicine in the growing child. In Morrissy R, Weinstein S, editors: *Lovell & Winter's pediatric orthopaedics*, ed 6, Philadelphia, 2006, Lippincott Williams & Wilkins, pp 1384–1429.

Koh J, section editor: Knee and lower leg. In Sarwark JF, editor: *Essentials of musculoskeletal care*, ed 3, Rosemont, Ill, 2010, American Academy of Orthopaedic Surgeons, pp 976.

Walsh WM, McCarty EC, Madden CC: Knee injuries. In Madden CC, Putukian M, Young CC, editors: *Netter's sports medicine*, Philadelphia, 2010, Saunders Elsevier, pp 417–428.

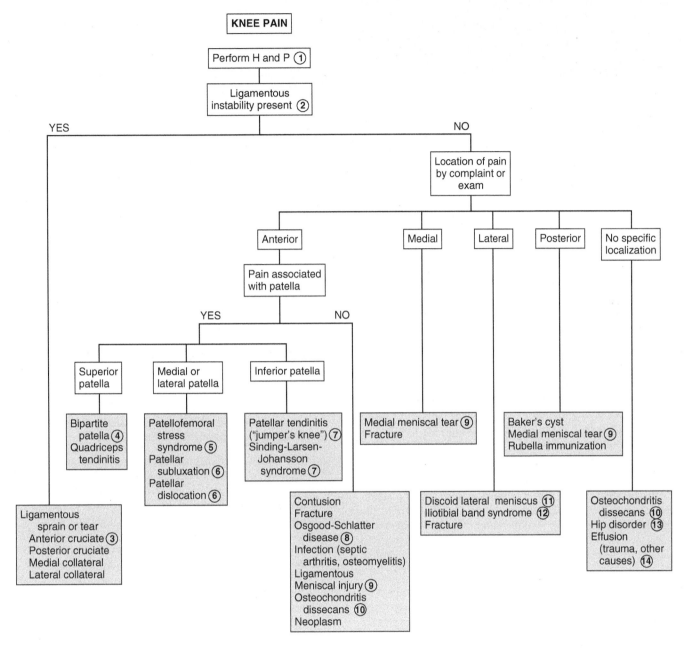

KNEE PAIN

Perform H and P ①

Ligamentous instability present ②

YES — **NO**

Location of pain by complaint or exam

Anterior | Medial | Lateral | Posterior | No specific localization

Pain associated with patella

YES — **NO**

Superior patella | Medial or lateral patella | Inferior patella

Bipartite patella ④
Quadriceps tendinitis

Patellofemoral stress syndrome ⑤
Patellar subluxation ⑥
Patellar dislocation ⑥

Patellar tendinitis ("jumper's knee") ⑦
Sinding-Larsen-Johansson syndrome ⑦

Medial meniscal tear ⑨
Fracture

Baker's cyst
Medial meniscal tear ⑨
Rubella immunization

Ligamentous sprain or tear
Anterior cruciate ③
Posterior cruciate
Medial collateral
Lateral collateral

Contusion
Fracture
Osgood-Schlatter disease ⑧
Infection (septic arthritis, osteomyelitis)
Ligamentous
Meniscal injury ⑨
Osteochondritis dissecans ⑩
Neoplasm

Discoid lateral meniscus ⑪
Iliotibial band syndrome ⑫
Fracture

Osteochondritis dissecans ⑩
Hip disorder ⑬
Effusion (trauma, other causes) ⑭

Nelson Textbook of Pediatrics, 19e. Chapters 669, 679
Nelsons Essentials, 6e. Chapters 199, 200

Chapter 45
EXTREMITY PAIN

This chapter is devoted to extremity pain other than joint problems. (See Chapters 42, 43, 44 for complaints better characterized as limp, arthritis, or knee pain.) Muscle pain (myalgia) is a nonspecific finding in many conditions; evaluation of other aspects of the history and physical (joint pain, weakness, toxin exposure, systemic complaints, or other physical findings) may be more useful in narrowing a differential diagnosis.

1. Be aware of the possibility of unobserved trauma as well as intentional trauma (child abuse), particularly in the preverbal child. Inquire specifically about the lifting of a child by the child's extended arm, which can cause a radial head subluxation.

2. Radial head subluxation ("nursemaid's elbow") is most commonly the result of a preschool-aged child being lifted upward by an extended arm. This upward traction causes the annular ligament to partially slip off the radial head. (Technically, it is a subluxation of the ligament rather than the radius.) The injury is only mildly painful, but the child is reluctant to use the arm. They may prefer holding the arm splinted close to the body, often giving the impression of wrist pain. The history is generally the key to diagnosis; x-ray findings are nonspecific but films should be considered to rule out other injuries when the history is unclear.

3. "Burners" or "stingers" are transient neurologic injuries of the brachial plexus due to compression or traction. Transient severe unilateral pain extends from the shoulder to the fingertips. Accompanying weakness and numbness may occur. These injuries occur most commonly in football players and wrestlers. If bilateral or affecting the lower extremities, spinal cord injury must be considered.

4. Children and adolescents are more susceptible to physeal (growth plate) injury than ligament sprains or diaphyseal (shaft) fractures because physes in growing children are weaker than the surrounding ligaments, tendons, and joint capsule. These injuries may result from excessive force or repetitive microtrauma. Be aware of the possibility of child abuse when unsuspected fractures are detected.

5. Mild to moderate muscle aches (myalgias) are common with many viral infections; lab values (if obtained) are generally normal or consistent with a viral illness. A more severe viral-related myositis presents typically with severe calf pain and difficulty or refusal to walk 5 to 7 days after the acute onset of viral (most commonly influenza type B) symptoms. Labs reveal elevated muscle enzymes and possibly myoglobinuria.

6. Adolescents with juvenile fibromyalgia often experience headaches, fatigue, sleep problems, anxiety, and a subjective sensation of joint swelling in addition to localized areas of muscle tenderness; most experts consider a 3-month duration necessary for diagnosis.

7. Infection within the bone is osteomyelitis; it may present acutely with localized pain and tenderness in an ill-appearing child or subacutely with prolonged pain and limp without fevers or systemic complaints. Bone changes on x-ray may not become evident for 7 to 10 days. MRI is the preferred choice for diagnostic imaging if available. Bone scans are also sensitive and specific early in the clinical course if MRI is not available.

8. Night pain is especially characteristic of both benign and malignant primary bone and metastatic tumors. Pain in the absence of local tenderness is another clue.

9. Shin splints (medial tibial stress syndrome) are the most common overuse injury of the lower leg. They present with diffuse tenderness along the lower third or half of the medial tibia; the pain onset is initially toward the end of a period of exercise but with progression will be present throughout activity. Imaging is not necessary for diagnosis. Consider x-rays only if a stress fracture is suspected; pain due to stress fractures will be localized, more severe, and present throughout activity. Swelling may or may not be associated. Radiographs will be normal in shin splints; they may also be normal until after 3 to 4 weeks of symptoms due to a stress fracture. MRI has replaced bone scan as the preferred imaging for suspected stress fractures in most centers.

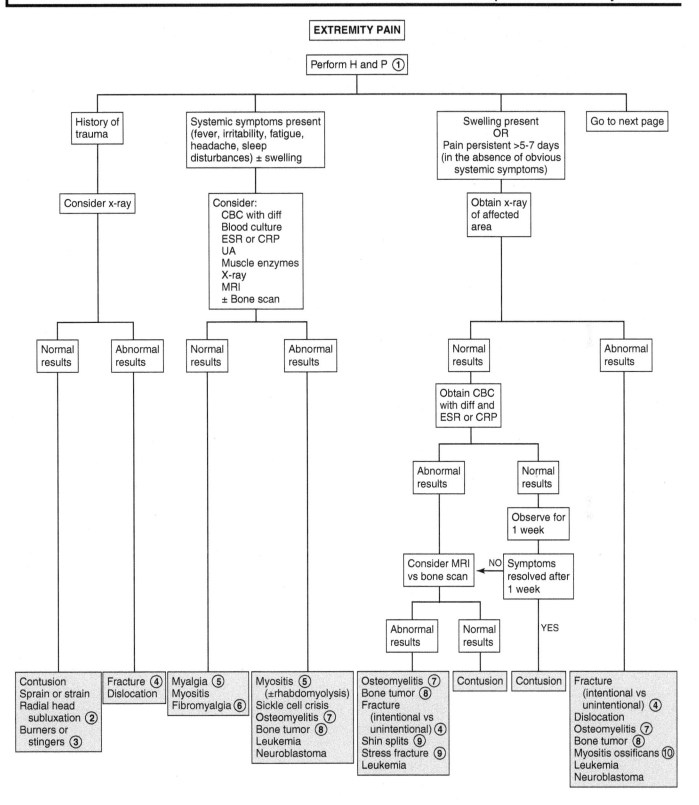

EXTREMITY PAIN

Perform H and P ①

History of trauma

Systemic symptoms present (fever, irritability, fatigue, headache, sleep disturbances) ± swelling

Swelling present
OR
Pain persistent >5-7 days (in the absence of obvious systemic symptoms)

Go to next page

Consider x-ray

Consider:
 CBC with diff
 Blood culture
 ESR or CRP
 UA
 Muscle enzymes
 X-ray
 MRI
 ± Bone scan

Obtain x-ray of affected area

Normal results

Abnormal results

Normal results

Abnormal results

Normal results

Abnormal results

Obtain CBC with diff and ESR or CRP

Abnormal results

Normal results

Observe for 1 week

Consider MRI vs bone scan ← NO — Symptoms resolved after 1 week

Abnormal results

Normal results

YES

Contusion
Sprain or strain
Radial head subluxation ②
Burners or stingers ③

Fracture ④
Dislocation

Myalgia ⑤
Myositis
Fibromyalgia ⑥

Myositis ⑤
 (±rhabdomyolysis)
Sickle cell crisis
Osteomyelitis ⑦
Bone tumor ⑧
Leukemia
Neuroblastoma

Osteomyelitis ⑦
Bone tumor ⑧
Fracture
 (intentional vs unintentional) ④
Shin splits ⑨
Stress fracture ⑨
Leukemia

Contusion

Contusion

Fracture
 (intentional vs unintentional) ④
Dislocation
Osteomyelitis ⑦
Bone tumor ⑧
Myositis ossificans ⑩
Leukemia
Neuroblastoma

Nelson Textbook of Pediatrics, 19e. Chapters 162, 250, 495, 666, 673, 679
Nelsons Essentials, 6e. Chapters 92, 293

10 A contusion of the quadriceps muscle may be complicated by ossification of the hematoma (myositis ossificans), causing pain and stiffness for several months after the injury.

11 Complex regional pain syndrome (previously called reflex sympathetic dystrophy) is a rare condition presenting acutely with intense extremity pain. There is either no history of trauma or one of a very minor injury followed by acute pain, swelling, and color and temperature change of the affected area days to weeks later. Erythema, warmth, and swelling occur initially; chronically, disuse atrophy and cool, clammy skin develop.

12 Growing pains (benign nocturnal pains of childhood) are common. Children complain of bilateral diffuse extremity pain, usually in the legs (thigh or calf). It typically occurs late in the day or at night and does not affect daytime activity. Massaging characteristically produces relief in these children; in contrast, massage would aggravate pain in most serious conditions. The physical examination is normal. Pain that is unilateral, localized to a joint, or persists during the day should never be assumed to be growing pains.

13 Nerve compression manifests with tingling, numbness, and paresthesias ("pins and needles") in addition to pain. Carpal tunnel syndrome classically presents with numbness on the radial (thumb) side of the hand, and ulnar nerve entrapment presents with numbness on the ulnar side of the hand (fourth and fifth fingers). Although rare in children, cervical nerve compression should be considered, especially if there is a history of neck trauma or symptoms are worse with the arm in an overhead position (thoracic outlet syndrome). When arm or shoulder pain accompanies numbness and tingling, MRI or EMG should be considered to rule out cervical nerve compression.

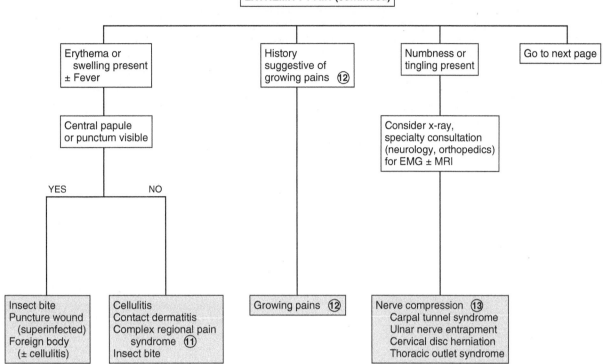

EXTREMITY PAIN (continued)

Erythema or swelling present ± Fever

Central papule or punctum visible

YES | NO

Insect bite
Puncture wound (superinfected)
Foreign body (± cellulitis)

Cellulitis
Contact dermatitis
Complex regional pain syndrome ⑪
Insect bite

History suggestive of growing pains ⑫

Growing pains ⑫

Numbness or tingling present

Consider x-ray, specialty consultation (neurology, orthopedics) for EMG ± MRI

Nerve compression ⑬
Carpal tunnel syndrome
Ulnar nerve entrapment
Cervical disc herniation
Thoracic outlet syndrome

Go to next page

14 Overuse syndromes do not require x-rays for diagnosis. X-rays or consultation with a sports medicine physician should be considered if symptoms do not improve in response to an appropriate course of treatment. X-rays may also aid in the diagnosis of conditions listed here that are not evident by history and physical and those that are not consistent with overuse syndromes.

15 Carpal tunnel syndrome is caused by compression of the median nerve at the wrist and presents with vague pain and numbness in the thenar region.

16 Tenosynovitis of the wrist presents with pain and swelling of the lateral aspect of the wrist. Crepitation or a locking or sticking sensation may occur with movement of the thumb.

17 Ulnar nerve irritation or entrapment causes tingling, numbness, and weakness of the fourth and fifth fingers.

18 Tarsal coalitions may develop in late childhood or adolescence, causing stiff and painful flat feet.

19 Plantar fasciitis is heel pain that may radiate over the entire plantar fascial surface. The pain is typically worse in the morning and improves over the course of the day.

20 Sever's disease is an apophysitis at the site of the heel cord (Achilles tendon) insertion into the calcaneus. It is an overuse syndrome seen in children 6 to 10 years of age; children complain of posterior heel pain with activity. A limp is often present.

21 Accessory navicular bones may become symptomatic in late childhood or early adolescence, with pain and tenderness along the medial aspect of the navicular bone.

22 Freiberg disease (AVN of the head of the second or third metatarsal) causes pain in the forefoot that worsens with activity; it occurs most commonly in 8- to 17-year-old females. Köhler disease (AVN of the tarsal navicular) affects boys more often than girls; it most commonly presents with pain in the midfoot around age 5 to 6 years.

23 The term "Little League elbow" encompasses a variety of disorders in and around the elbow, the most common of which is a traction apophysitis (inflammation at the site of tendon insertion into the bone) of the medial epicondyle.

24 Panner disease, an osteochondrosis of the capitellum (distal humerus), presents acutely with lateral elbow pain in the young (5- to 13-year-old) athlete. In older athletes, the condition is called osteochondritis dissecans capitellum. Its onset is more insidious, and it is more likely to be associated with a loose body.

25 Slipped capital femoral epiphysis (SCFE) and AVN of the hip (Legg-Calvé-Perthes disease) present with a limp, hip pain, or poorly localized medial thigh or knee pain. If either condition is suspected, x-rays should be obtained.

26 Localized tenderness over the anterior iliac crest characterizes iliac apophysitis. It is seen most commonly in adolescent runners, especially during a growth spurt and when they are increasing their mileage.

Bibliography

Benjamin HJ: The pediatric athlete. In Madden CC, Putukian M, Young CC, editors: *Netter's sports medicine*, Philadelphia, 2010, Saunders Elsevier, pp 55–64.

McCarty EC, Walsh WM, Hald RD, et al: Musculoskeletal injuries in sports. In Madden CC, Putukian M, Young CC editors: *Netter's sports medicine*, Philadelphia, 2010, Saunders Elsevier, pp 299–303.

Petron DJ, Crist JC: Neurologic problems in the athlete. In Madden CC, Putukian M, Young CC editors: *Netter's sports medicine*, Philadelphia, 2010, Saunders Elsevier, pp 252–264.

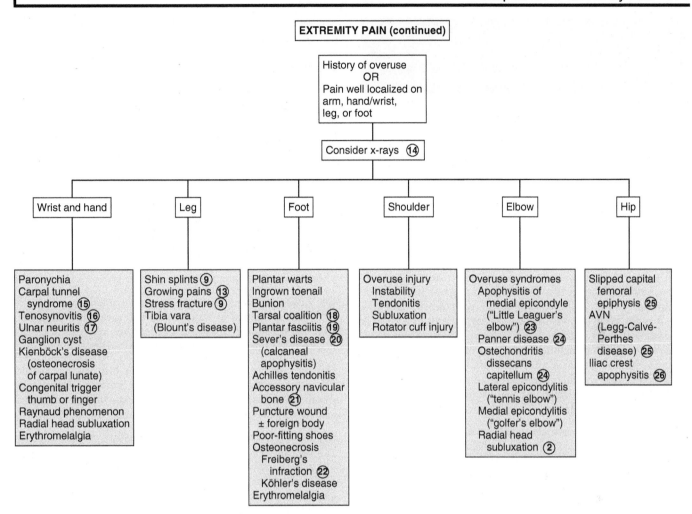

EXTREMITY PAIN (continued)

History of overuse
OR
Pain well localized on arm, hand/wrist, leg, or foot

Consider x-rays ⑭

Wrist and hand

Paronychia
Carpal tunnel
  syndrome ⑮
Tenosynovitis ⑯
Ulnar neuritis ⑰
Ganglion cyst
Kienböck's disease
  (osteonecrosis
  of carpal lunate)
Congenital trigger
  thumb or finger
Raynaud phenomenon
Radial head subluxation
Erythromelalgia

Leg

Shin splints ⑨
Growing pains ⑬
Stress fracture ⑨
Tibia vara
  (Blount's disease)

Foot

Plantar warts
Ingrown toenail
Bunion
Tarsal coalition ⑱
Plantar fasciitis ⑲
Sever's disease ⑳
  (calcaneal
  apophysitis)
Achilles tendonitis
Accessory navicular
  bone ㉑
Puncture wound
  ± foreign body
Poor-fitting shoes
Osteonecrosis
  Freiberg's
    infraction ㉒
  Köhler's disease
Erythromelalgia

Shoulder

Overuse injury
  Instability
  Tendonitis
  Subluxation
  Rotator cuff injury

Elbow

Overuse syndromes
  Apophysitis of
    medial epicondyle
    ("Little Leaguer's
    elbow") ㉓
  Panner disease ㉔
  Ostechondritis
    dissecans
    capitellum ㉔
  Lateral epicondylitis
    ("tennis elbow")
  Medial epicondylitis
    ("golfer's elbow")
  Radial head
    subluxation ②

Hip

Slipped capital
  femoral
  epiphysis ㉕
AVN
  (Legg-Calvé-
  Perthes
  disease) ㉕
Iliac crest
  apophysitis ㉖

Chapter 46
BACK PAIN

Back pain is uncommon in children, especially chronic or severe back pain. Most children who complain of back pain have mild, self-resolving symptoms of limited duration. Symptoms of severe or persistent back pain, as well as any abnormal findings on physical examination, mandate a thorough evaluation. As with adults, however, clear etiologies are not always identified, particularly in older children and adolescents without other associated symptoms.

1. The history should inquire about trauma, associated leg pain, gait abnormalities, weakness, extremity pain or tingling, bowel or bladder incontinence, and any systemic signs or symptoms (fever, malaise, rashes, GI symptoms). Also ask about aggravating or relieving factors (particularly whether it is relieved with rest) and whether it wakes the patient from sleep. The physical should include careful neurologic and abdominal examinations, as well as a complete musculoskeletal exam. The neurologic exam should include assessment of anal tone and (in males) the cremasteric reflex; a pelvic exam may be indicated in older adolescent females.

2. The presence of associated abdominal pain, vomiting, dysuria, hematuria, or vaginal complaints should prompt a specific evaluation for intraabdominal or pelvic problems. Be vigilant for subtle neurologic signs and symptoms that may be overlooked in the presence of an acute illness (especially if bedridden); an MRI would be indicated in the case of any neurologic problems.

3. Discitis is an infection or inflammation of an intervertebral disc space. The most common pathogen is *Staphylococcus aureus*. Children younger than age 7 years are most commonly affected; the peak incidence is at age 3. Common clinical findings are back pain, limping, and a stiff, straight posture due to loss of normal lumbar lordosis. These children often refuse to bend over to pick something up because of the pain related to spinal flexion. The degree of systemic illness is variable. Younger children (<3 years of age) are more likely to present with a toxic picture of fever, refusal to walk, irritability, and decreased appetite. Older children and adolescents may complain of back pain and pain with walking and may or may not be febrile. Spine films will not reveal characteristic disc space narrowing or vertebral end plate irregularities until a few weeks after symptoms begin. MRI or bone scan may be necessary for early diagnosis; MRI is preferred because it will better differentiate conditions with similar presentations (vertebral osteomyelitis, abscesses).

4. Spinal x-rays or a bone scan may suggest the extent of metastatic tumor involvement in the spine, but MRI will be necessary for more specific definition of the disease process. CT scans may be preferred when pathologic fractures are suspected, because of better bony detail.

5. Intraabdominal, retroperitoneal, or pelvic processes can cause referred back pain. More specific signs and symptoms should aid in the diagnosis of problems such as pyelonephritis, pancreatitis, nephrolithiasis, and abscesses (perinephric, pelvic, paraspinal muscle, psoas muscle). A paraspinal abscess will generally present with some neurologic signs; an MRI is recommended if suspected.

6. Primary vertebral osteomyelitis is rare in young children. It typically occurs in children older than 8 years, and an insidious onset is more likely than an acute toxic presentation. Presentation commonly includes a vague or dull backache that may be worse at night; fever may or may not be present. Pott's disease is tuberculosis spondylitis, a rare complication of untreated tuberculosis that is more likely to occur in children than adults.

7. If pain persists, consider repeating x-rays versus obtaining other imaging in 2 weeks. Callus formation may indicate fractures not obvious on initial films. In cases of suspected child abuse, a bone scan should be considered early in the evaluation when initial x-rays are negative.

8. Contusions and abrasions are the most common back injuries sustained in routine play and sports in young children. No additional workup is needed if no other injuries and an otherwise normal physical exam are present.

9. Back pain associated with bowel or bladder deficits, gait abnormalities, lower extremity pain, weakness, or reflex or sensation deficits is suggestive of space-occupying lesions (spinal cord tumors, metastatic lesions) and warrants urgent evaluation.

10. Spondylolysis is a defect (stress fracture) of the bony connection between a vertebral body and its arch (pars interarticularis). Spondylolisthesis is the forward slippage or displacement of one vertebra in relation to another. Classic spondylolisthesis in children and adolescents involves the fifth lumbar and first sacral vertebral bodies. In these cases, fatigue or stress fractures of the pars interarticularis bilaterally allow forward slippage of the superior vertebra on the inferior vertebra. Symptoms vary based on the degree of subsequent nerve compression.

Children participating in sports involving repetitive flexion and hyperextension (gymnasts, football players, weight lifters) are at increased risk for spondylolysis. Symptoms (poorly localized lumbar and lumbosacral pain, hamstring tightness) often do not occur until the adolescent growth spurt; spinal hyperextension typically exacerbates the pain. Defects often remain asymptomatic indefinitely. When symptoms do occur, they are not always consistent with the severity of the spondyolytic defect or the degree of slippage.

11. Consider a urine pregnancy test in adolescent females prior to obtaining x-rays.

12. Kyphosis is an exaggeration of the normal thoracic or thoracolumbar curve in the sagittal plane. In postural or flexible cases, it is fully correctable with voluntary effort, and any associated pain is typically mild. Spine films should be obtained in severe cases and when significant back pain is present to rule out Scheuermann's disease. This is a structural hyperkyphosis; x-rays will show vertebral end plate irregularities and vertebral body wedging. Most cases of scoliosis, regardless of the age at onset, are idiopathic. Idiopathic scoliosis is not painful during childhood and adolescence. If pain is noted with a scoliotic curve, carefully consider infectious, inflammatory, and neoplastic causes.

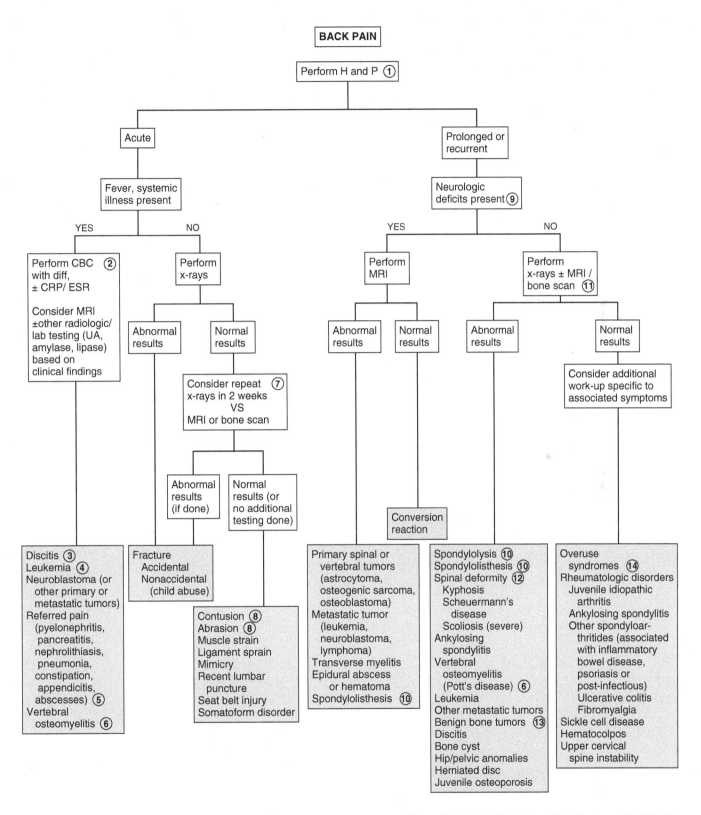

BACK PAIN

Perform H and P ①

Acute

Prolonged or recurrent

Fever, systemic illness present

Neurologic deficits present ⑨

YES — Perform CBC ② with diff, ± CRP/ ESR

Consider MRI ±other radiologic/ lab testing (UA, amylase, lipase) based on clinical findings

NO — Perform x-rays

Abnormal results

Normal results

Consider repeat ⑦ x-rays in 2 weeks VS MRI or bone scan

Abnormal results (if done)

Normal results (or no additional testing done)

YES — Perform MRI

Abnormal results

Normal results

Conversion reaction

NO — Perform x-rays ± MRI / bone scan ⑪

Abnormal results

Normal results

Consider additional work-up specific to associated symptoms

Discitis ③
Leukemia ④
Neuroblastoma (or other primary or metastatic tumors)
Referred pain (pyelonephritis, pancreatitis, nephrolithiasis, pneumonia, constipation, appendicitis, abscesses) ⑤
Vertebral osteomyelitis ⑥

Fracture
  Accidental
  Nonaccidental
  (child abuse)

Contusion ⑧
Abrasion ⑧
Muscle strain
Ligament sprain
Mimicry
Recent lumbar puncture
Seat belt injury
Somatoform disorder

Primary spinal or vertebral tumors (astrocytoma, osteogenic sarcoma, osteoblastoma)
Metastatic tumor (leukemia, neuroblastoma, lymphoma)
Transverse myelitis
Epidural abscess or hematoma
Spondylolisthesis ⑩

Spondylolysis ⑩
Spondylolisthesis ⑩
Spinal deformity ⑫
  Kyphosis
  Scheuermann's disease
  Scoliosis (severe)
Ankylosing spondylitis
Vertebral osteomyelitis (Pott's disease) ⑥
Leukemia
Other metastatic tumors
Benign bone tumors ⑬
Discitis
Bone cyst
Hip/pelvic anomalies
Herniated disc
Juvenile osteoporosis

Overuse syndromes ⑭
Rheumatologic disorders
  Juvenile idiopathic arthritis
  Ankylosing spondylitis
  Other spondyloar-thritides (associated with inflammatory bowel disease, psoriasis or post-infectious)
  Ulcerative colitis
  Fibromyalgia
Sickle cell disease
Hematocolpos
Upper cervical spine instability

Nelson Textbook of Pediatrics, 19e. Chapters 495, 671, 679
Nelsons Essentials, 6e. Chapter 202

13 Benign tumors of the spine are rare. The most common ones are osteoid osteoma, osteoblastoma, and eosinophilic granuloma. Presentation is typically a prolonged period of back pain (especially at night) that eventually evolves to stiffness and (rarely) a painful scoliosis or mild neurologic defects.

14 Overuse syndromes are more common in athletic adolescents than younger children. The stress of normal physiologic activity results in microtrauma, which typically resolves. Overuse injuries result when repetitive activity without adequate conditioning or rest prohibits this resolution. Both bone and soft tissues (muscles, tendons, bursae, cartilage) are susceptible to overuse injuries. Gymnasts, dancers, weight lifters, and football players are particularly prone to overuse injuries of the back. Carrying a heavy book bag or backpack may cause back pain.

Bibliography

Gurd DP: Back pain in the young athlete, *Sports Med Arthrosc* 19:7–16, 2011.

Corneli HN: Pain—back. In Fleisher G, Ludwig S, editors: *Textbook of pediatric emergency medicine,* ed 6, Philadelphia, 2010, Lippincott Williams & Wilkins, pp 429–433.

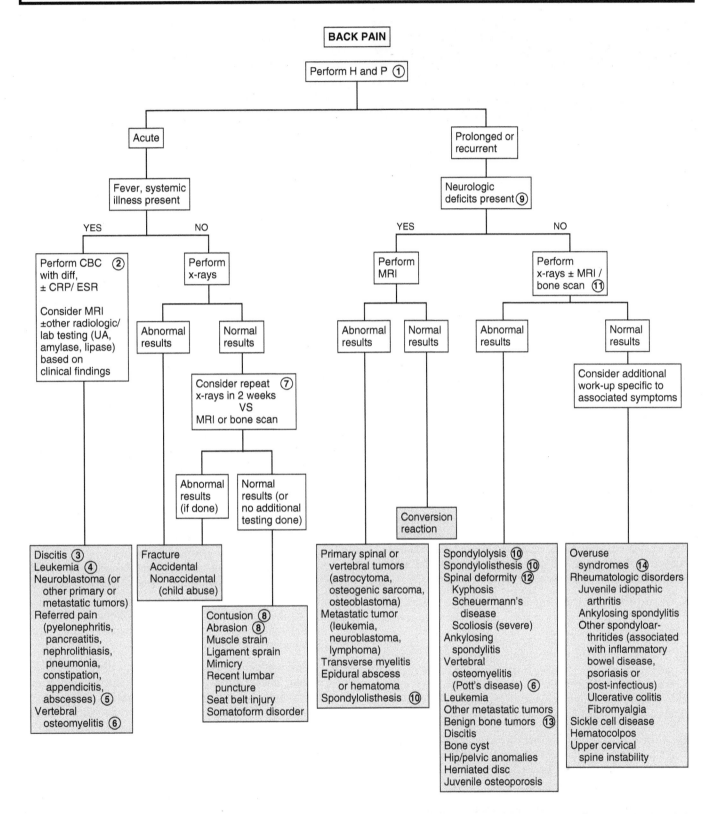

BACK PAIN

Perform H and P ①

Acute

Prolonged or recurrent

Fever, systemic illness present

Neurologic deficits present ⑨

Acute branch:

YES → Perform CBC ② with diff, ± CRP/ESR

Consider MRI ±other radiologic/ lab testing (UA, amylase, lipase) based on clinical findings

NO → Perform x-rays

- Abnormal results
- Normal results → Consider repeat ⑦ x-rays in 2 weeks VS MRI or bone scan
  - Abnormal results (if done)
  - Normal results (or no additional testing done)

Prolonged or recurrent branch:

YES → Perform MRI
- Abnormal results
- Normal results → Conversion reaction

NO → Perform x-rays ± MRI / bone scan ⑪
- Abnormal results
- Normal results → Consider additional work-up specific to associated symptoms

Diagnosis boxes:

Discitis ③
Leukemia ④
Neuroblastoma (or other primary or metastatic tumors)
Referred pain (pyelonephritis, pancreatitis, nephrolithiasis, pneumonia, constipation, appendicitis, abscesses) ⑤
Vertebral osteomyelitis ⑥

Fracture
Accidental
Nonaccidental (child abuse)

Contusion ⑧
Abrasion ⑧
Muscle strain
Ligament sprain
Mimicry
Recent lumbar puncture
Seat belt injury
Somatoform disorder

Primary spinal or vertebral tumors (astrocytoma, osteogenic sarcoma, osteoblastoma)
Metastatic tumor (leukemia, neuroblastoma, lymphoma)
Transverse myelitis
Epidural abscess or hematoma
Spondylolisthesis ⑩

Spondylolysis ⑩
Spondylolisthesis ⑩
Spinal deformity ⑫
Kyphosis
Scheuermann's disease
Scoliosis (severe)
Ankylosing spondylitis
Vertebral osteomyelitis (Pott's disease) ⑥
Leukemia
Other metastatic tumors
Benign bone tumors ⑬
Discitis
Bone cyst
Hip/pelvic anomalies
Herniated disc
Juvenile osteoporosis

Overuse syndromes ⑭
Rheumatologic disorders
Juvenile idiopathic arthritis
Ankylosing spondylitis
Other spondyloar- thritides (associated with inflammatory bowel disease, psoriasis or post-infectious)
Ulcerative colitis
Fibromyalgia
Sickle cell disease
Hematocolpos
Upper cervical spine instability

Nelson Textbook of Pediatrics, 19e. Chapters 495, 671, 679
Nelsons Essentials, 6e. Chapter 202

Chapter 47
STIFF OR PAINFUL NECK

Most causes of neck pain and stiffness in children are benign; however, potentially life-threatening conditions (meningitis, cervical spine fracture) must always be considered in the evaluation.

1. The history should clarify the onset, duration, and nature of the complaint and include a comprehensive review of systems. The physical examination should note stiffness and range of motion of the neck (lateral movement and flexion-extension) and the specific nature and location of the pain (muscle spasm, muscle or bone tenderness). The differential diagnosis for a child who exhibits full mobility of their neck, even if it is painful, differs from that of a child whose range of motion is limited.

Torticollis or "wry neck" describes a condition in which the infant's or child's neck is tilted to one side and rotated to the opposite side. It is the primary manifestation of congenital torticollis, but it can also be a symptom of several other problems (infection, CNS neoplasm, structural abnormalities, neurologic disorders). A thorough neurologic examination including mental status, cranial nerve involvement, upper extremity pain or weakness, and cerebellar function is important.

2. Congenital muscular torticollis appears in the first several weeks of life. The head is tilted toward a shortened sternocleidomastoid muscle; a fibrotic mass is frequently palpable in the muscle belly. Other signs of intrauterine mechanical deformation (plagiocephaly, facial asymmetry, foot deformities, developmental hip dysplasia) are frequently present. Plain x-rays of the cervical spine to rule out congenital vertebral abnormalities should be obtained in the absence of any of these associated clinical findings or if there is no response to a stretching program.

3. A suspected cervical spine injury should be treated in the acute setting with cervical spine immobilization until appropriate x-rays can be taken.

4. The most common cervical spine subluxation involves the atlantoaxial (C1-C2) joint. It may result from mild as well as severe trauma. Symptoms can include neck pain, sternocleidomastoid muscle tenderness, and torticollis. Symptoms of spinal cord compression are rare in children.

5. Although clavicular fractures are usually indicated by localized pain and tenderness, the predominant presenting symptom can occasionally be torticollis due to spasm of the sternocleidomastoid muscle.

6. The ligamentous laxity and hypermobility of the cervical spine and a potentially narrow spinal canal in young children place them at risk for spinal cord injury without radiographic abnormalities (SCIWORA). These injuries are due to stretching or distortion of the spinal cord or nerve roots. Careful history-taking is essential because initial neurologic deficits (weakness, paresthesias) may be transient, resolving shortly after the injury then recurring minutes to days later. MRI is indicated when suspected.

7. In meningitis, meningeal signs (nuchal rigidity, Kernig and Brudzinski signs) are usually accompanied by systemic signs of illness, including fever, altered consciousness, poor feeding, headache, and possibly seizures. Classic meningeal signs are not always present in meningitis, particularly in children younger than 18 to 24 months. With bacterial meningitis, CSF analysis usually reveals a low glucose level of usually less than 40 mg/dL, a high protein level, a neutrophilic leukocytosis, and a positive Gram stain.

8. Tumor of any origin (nerve, muscle, bone) may present acutely with a stiff neck, owing to swelling or nerve compression. Nocturnal pain may indicate an osteoid osteoma. Diagnosis is by x-ray or MRI.

9. Hypermobility or instability of the occipitoatlantal or the atlantoaxial joints due to ligamentous hyperlaxity occurs in up to 60% of children with Down syndrome. These children are at an increased risk for spinal cord injury. Patients may be asymptomatic or have slowly progressive neurologic symptoms including neck pain, clumsiness or increased falling, change in tone, weakness, sensory deficits, or changes in bowel or bladder control. The Special Olympics currently require cervical spine imaging for patients with Down syndrome prior to participation in certain activities that may carry an increased risk of spinal injury. Otherwise, routine cervical spine imaging for asymptomatic patients with Down syndrome is currently not recommended as a routine part of health maintenance by the American Academy of Pediatrics. Families, however, need to be continually educated regarding worrisome signs and symptoms (as above) that are suggestive of spinal cord impingement and would warrant urgent evaluation.

Grisel syndrome is a rare mild atlantoaxial subluxation that occurs in children without other risk factors for subluxation (Down syndrome, connective tissue disorders, rheumatoid arthritis) and in the absence of trauma. It is presumed to be due to inflammation (related to pharyngitis or URI), causing increased laxity of the cervical spinal ligaments.

Other etiologies include rare congenital conditions (Marfan syndrome, Klippel-Feil syndrome, os odontoideum, Morquio syndrome).

10. Eye problems (nystagmus, superior oblique muscle weakness, strabismus) may result in compensatory neck stiffness and torticollis in infants.

11. Neuroimaging may not be indicated if a drug effect is suspected. Several antipsychotic and antiemetic medications (most commonly haloperidol, prochlorperazine, and metoclopramide) can produce acute dystonic reactions within days of exposure. Oculogyric crisis is a dystonic reaction characterized by torticollis and involuntary deviation and fixation of the gaze, usually upward.

12. Benign paroxysmal torticollis is characterized by torticollis of variable duration that may or may not be accompanied by symptoms of pallor, agitation, ataxia, or vomiting. The onset is in the first year of life, and consciousness is not impaired. The family history is usually positive for migraine.

Bibliography

American Academy of Pediatrics: Health supervision for children with Down syndrome, *Pediatrics* 128:393–406, 2011.

Tzimenatos L, Vance C, Kuppermann N: Neck stiffness. In Fleisher G, Ludwig S, editors: *Textbook of pediatric emergency medicine*, ed 6, Philadelphia, 2010, Lippincott Williams & Wilkins, pp 392–401.

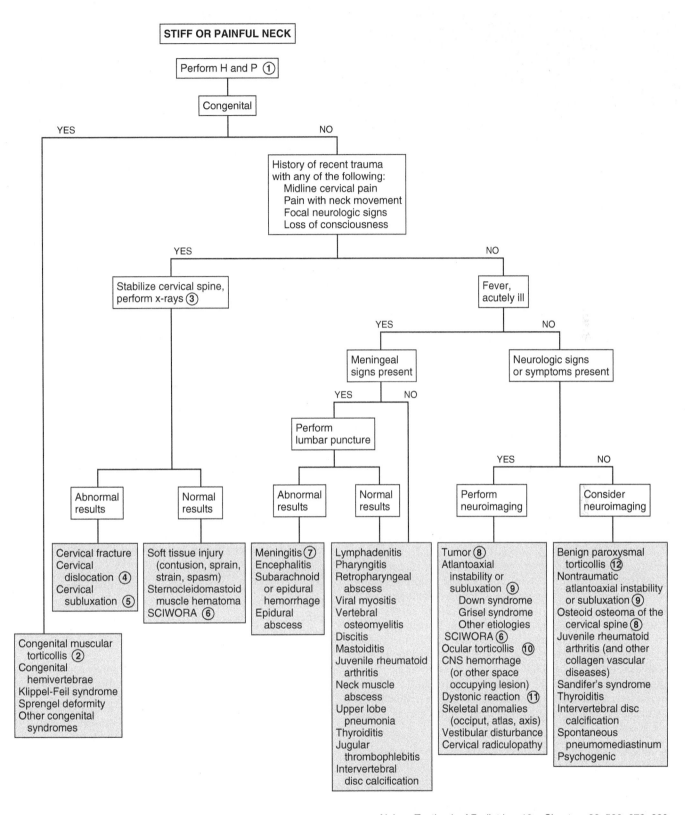

Nelson Textbook of Pediatrics, 19e. Chapters 66, 590, 672, 680
Nelsons Essentials, 6e. Chapters 42, 202

Chapter 48
IN-TOEING, OUT-TOEING, AND TOE-WALKING

In-toeing and out-toeing are common and generally benign rotational deformities in children. Some positional deformities will be noted before walking age. The rotational variation can occur anywhere between the hip and the foot. Toe walking is frequently a benign condition but warrants careful assessment.

Version is the normal degree of rotation or twisting of a limb segment. Femoral anteversion is normal. More specifically, the distal aspect of the femur (femoral condyles) is normally rotated medially (twisted anteriorly) relative to the proximal aspect (the femoral head and neck). Femoral anteversion is greatest at birth and decreases (via normal bony remodeling) gradually until age 8 or 9 years to 15 to 20 degrees of anteversion (which is normal). The term *torsion* is defined as version that is in excess of 2 standard deviations of the norm. The distal aspect of the tibia is normally rotated medially relative to the proximal aspect (tibial torsion), resulting in a bowed or in-toed appearance of the lower extremity. This appearance is usually exaggerated in the infant owing to in utero positioning. (The use of this term *torsion* in the literature is somewhat inconsistent. The term is applied to excess femoral anteversion [internal femoral torsion], yet internal tibial "torsion" is considered normal at birth.)

1 The history for a child presenting with a gait problem should include the age at onset, a birth and developmental history, progression of the problem and any exacerbating factors (fatigue, running). Also inquire about a family history of rotational disorders and skeletal disorders (including vitamin D–resistant rickets). In addition to a careful spine, lower extremity, and neurologic examination, a rotational profile (next page) is very helpful in the evaluation of torsional deformities. The graphs show the mean and 2 standard deviations of the expected degrees of the foot progression angle, thigh foot angle, femoral medial rotation (for boys and girls) and femoral lateral rotation according to age; it can frequently be reassuring to families to see that their child's gait is within normal limits.

2 Internal (medial) tibial torsion is the most common cause of in-toeing in children younger than 3 years. It is usually bilateral; if unilateral and associated with a bowing (varus) deformity, pathologic skeletal abnormalities need to be considered. Normal bony remodeling typically decreases the degree of tibial torsion to the normal expected range by early school age.

3 Internal (medial) femoral torsion (also referred to as excessive femoral anteversion) is the most common cause of in-toeing in children older than 2 years. Females are affected more often than males. In addition to "W" sitting, affected children frequently exhibit generalized ligamentous laxity.

4 An atavistic great toe (or dynamic hallucis abductus) "searches" or "wanders" medially when walking and gives the impression of a dynamic in-toeing process. The abnormality is not evident at rest.

5 Metatarsus adductus is commonly presumed to be an effect of in utero molding (compression) on the developing foot; subtle orthopedic abnormalities (muscle imbalance, subluxation) may also be factors. The forefoot is adducted and occasionally supinated relative to the normal midfoot and hindfoot, making the foot appear C-shaped (with the medial border concave and the lateral border convex). Assessment of the mobility of the deformity is very important; feet that can be manually corrected to neutral (or overcorrected) are mild cases and may be treated with stretching and observed. If the deformity is fixed and does not actively or passively correct, referral for orthopedic consultation is indicated.

6 The exam abnormalities of clubfoot or talipes equinovarus include plantar flexion (cavus), metatarsus adductus of the forefoot and midfoot, and equinus and varus of the hindfoot.

7 External (lateral) femoral torsion is an occasional cause of bilateral out-toeing. Unilateral cases in older children require assessment for a slipped capital femoral epiphysis.

8 External (lateral) tibial torsion is less common than medial tibial torsion. It usually occurs in conjunction with a calcaneovalgus foot, a positional deformity due to intrauterine malposition, characterized by dorsiflexion and mild eversion of the ankle. A more serious underlying problem (posteromedial bow of the tibia, vertical talus) may rarely be associated.

9 Flat feet ("pes planus") may give the impression of out-toeing when the patient is standing. It is important to distinguish flexible (in which the arch reappears when on tiptoes) from rigid flat feet; the latter is more likely to be problematic and require treatment.

10 Habitual (or idiopathic) toe walking may be a normal finding until 3 years of age. Neurologic examination and range of motion (passive dorsiflexion beyond 15 degrees) are normal in these cases. Assessment to rule out other causes is indicated beyond age 3 or if acquired after the patient has been walking normally for a period of time.

11 A small amount of length-leg discrepancy is normal. Most children easily compensate for a discrepancy between 1 and 2 cm.

12 Torsion dystonia (dystonia musculorum deformans) is a movement disorder that begins in childhood. Toe walking is observed owing to intermittent unilateral posturing (extension and rotation) of a lower extremity, followed by progression to generalized involvement.

Bibliography

Lincoln TL, Suen PW: Common rotational variations in children, *J Am Acad Orthop Surg* 11:312–320, 2003.

Scherl SA: Common lower extremity problems in children, *Pediatr Rev* 25:52, 2004.

Smith BG: Lower extremity disorders in children and adolescents, *Pediatr Rev* 30:287, 2009.

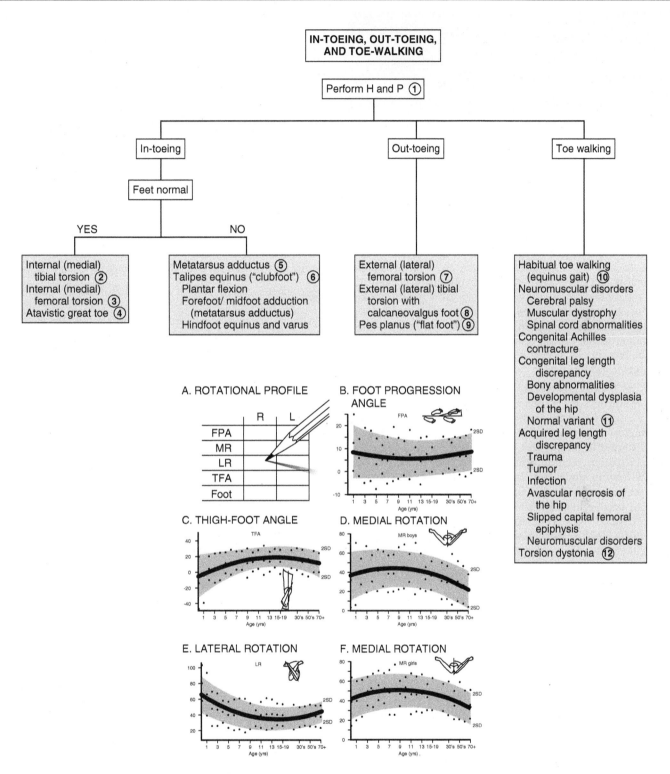

IN-TOEING, OUT-TOEING, AND TOE-WALKING

Perform H and P ①

In-toeing

Feet normal

YES — NO

Internal (medial) tibial torsion ②
Internal (medial) femoral torsion ③
Atavistic great toe ④

Metatarsus adductus ⑤
Talipes equinus ("clubfoot") ⑥
  Plantar flexion
  Forefoot/ midfoot adduction (metatarsus adductus)
  Hindfoot equinus and varus

Out-toeing

External (lateral) femoral torsion ⑦
External (lateral) tibial torsion with calcaneovalgus foot ⑧
Pes planus ("flat foot") ⑨

Toe walking

Habitual toe walking (equinus gait) ⑩
Neuromuscular disorders
  Cerebral palsy
  Muscular dystrophy
  Spinal cord abnormalities
Congenital Achilles contracture
Congenital leg length discrepancy
  Bony abnormalities
  Developmental dysplasia of the hip
  Normal variant ⑪
Acquired leg length discrepancy
  Trauma
  Tumor
  Infection
  Avascular necrosis of the hip
  Slipped capital femoral epiphysis
  Neuromuscular disorders
Torsion dystonia ⑫

A. ROTATIONAL PROFILE

B. FOOT PROGRESSION ANGLE

C. THIGH-FOOT ANGLE

D. MEDIAL ROTATION

E. LATERAL ROTATION

F. MEDIAL ROTATION

Nelson Textbook of Pediatrics, 19e. Chapters 666–668
Nelsons Essentials, 6e. Chapters 197, 200, 201

From Staheli LT: Torsional deformities.
Pediatr Clin North Am 33:1373, 1986.

Chapter 49
BOWLEGS AND KNOCK-KNEES

Angular deformities such as bowlegs and knock-knees are common complaints. Spontaneous resolution is the rule for most cases. It is important to know when to be concerned about a potentially pathologic diagnosis when treating an angular deformity.

Angular alignment of the lower extremities at birth is typically varus (bowlegged) at the knee, although parents often do not comment on this alignment until a child starts standing. Normal bony remodeling occurs over the first 2 years of life, with typical resolution of this physiologic genu varus (bowlegs) to a near-neutral position. Subsequent development between the third and fourth year of life normally results in a valgus alignment at the knees (genu valgus or knock-knees), which gradually neutralizes to the normal adult alignment of mild valgus by age 7 or 8 years.

1. The history should clearly elucidate the nature of the complaint, age at onset, progression, and any previous treatment. A complete medical (including a review of growth parameters), developmental (particularly the age when the child started walking), and family history should be part of the evaluation. Include a birth history and feeding history (breastfeeding, unusual diets) and inquire about medications (some anticonvulsants can impact vitamin D and phosphate). It may also be helpful to ask parents to clarify their exact concerns and fears about the child's appearance and future prognosis, because education and reassurance about the expected course of angular deformities is often all that is needed.

The physical assessment should include careful measurements and observation of the gait. A rotational profile should be done because rotational deformities can contribute to the appearance of genu varum or valgum. (See Chapter 48.) Joints should be assessed for laxity and swelling suggesting arthritis. Extremities should be assessed for asymmetry suggesting bony abnormalities (congenital absence of bones, hypoplasia). Café-au-lait spots or neurofibromas may indicate neurofibromatosis. Any pain or tenderness on exam should be noted.

2. Gentle reassurance of parental concerns and education about the expected course of these conditions are often all that is necessary. Certain indicators, such as short stature and significant asymmetry, do indicate further workup for a cause other than physiologic. If any worrisome prognosticators are present, preliminary x-ray (standing AP) evaluation of the lower extremities should be done to localize the deformity and identify any obvious bony abnormalities. Failure to follow a normal developmental sequence, rapid progression of the deformity, family history of a pathologic condition, and physical findings suggestive of an underlying abnormality (neurofibromatosis, arthritis, infection) all warrant further evaluation.

3. Genu varum (physiologic bowlegs) is usually a combination of a normal varus angulation of the knee and internal tibial torsion that is normal in the infant and toddler. Neutralization by 2 to 3 years of age is the norm. Persistence beyond age 3 or a severe case (>4 to 5 inches intercondylar distance, 16 degrees or greater tibial femoral angle) warrants investigation to rule out a pathologic cause.

4. Physiologic genu valgum (knock-knees) develops as the natural overcorrection of physiologic genu varus and occurs between the third and fourth years of life. Resolution generally occurs between 5 and 8 years of age.

5. Asymmetric growth of the tibial growth plate (due to abnormal ossification) results in tibia vara (Blount's disease), characterized by severe progressive bowing. Infantile onset (age 1 to 3 years) is most common in overweight toddlers, African-Americans, early walkers, and children with a family history of Blount's disease; most (80%) have bilateral involvement. A later juvenile onset (age 4 to 10 years) is more likely to affect overweight African-American males. Bilateral involvement is less frequent in this age group (50%), and pain (rather than deformity) is more likely to be the primary complaint. The condition can also develop in adolescents. X-rays show medial metaphyseal irregularity, "beaking" of the medial tibial epiphysis, and wedging of the proximal epiphysis; specific radiographic criteria exist to characterize the stage of disease.

6. Congenital pseudoarthrosis of the tibia appears early in infancy as an anterolateral bowing of the tibia; 50% of affected children have neurofibromatosis. (The condition affects 10% of all patients with neurofibromatosis.)

7. Rickets may be nutritional (vitamin D or calcium deficiency), genetic (vitamin D resistance) or due to hypophosphatasia (renal disorders, nutritional). A history of prolonged breastfeeding without adequate vitamin D supplementation is common in children with rickets. A widened physis and "frayed" appearance of the metaphysis are common radiologic findings in rickets.

8. Bony dysplasias may be characterized by metaphyseal, diaphyseal, epiphyseal, or physeal plate abnormalities. Children with these conditions are more likely to be small for their age and have a later age of onset of walking.

Bibliography

Schoenecker PL, Rich MM: The lower extremity. In Morrissy R, Weinstein S, editors: *Lovell & Winter's pediatric orthopaedics,* ed 6, Philadelphia, 2006, Lippincott Williams & Wilkins, pp 1158–1211.

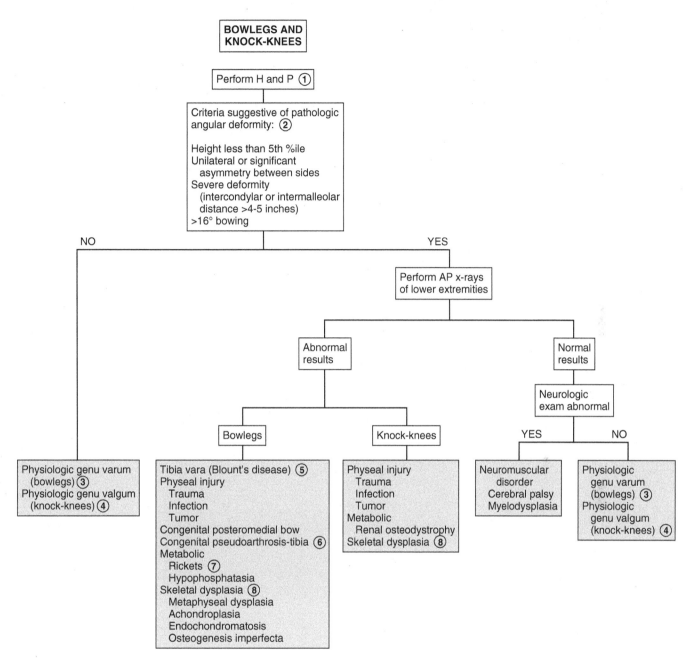

BOWLEGS AND KNOCK-KNEES

Perform H and P ①

Criteria suggestive of pathologic angular deformity: ②

Height less than 5th %ile
Unilateral or significant
    asymmetry between sides
Severe deformity
    (intercondylar or intermalleolar
    distance >4-5 inches)
>16° bowing

NO

YES

Perform AP x-rays of lower extremities

Abnormal results

Normal results

Neurologic exam abnormal

Bowlegs

Knock-knees

YES

NO

Physiologic genu varum
(bowlegs) ③
Physiologic genu valgum
(knock-knees) ④

Tibia vara (Blount's disease) ⑤
Physeal injury
    Trauma
    Infection
    Tumor
Congenital posteromedial bow
Congenital pseudoarthrosis-tibia ⑥
Metabolic
    Rickets ⑦
    Hypophosphatasia
Skeletal dysplasia ⑧
    Metaphyseal dysplasia
    Achondroplasia
    Endochondromatosis
    Osteogenesis imperfecta

Physeal injury
    Trauma
    Infection
    Tumor
Metabolic
    Renal osteodystrophy
Skeletal dysplasia ⑧

Neuromuscular
    disorder
    Cerebral palsy
    Myelodysplasia

Physiologic
    genu varum
    (bowlegs) ③
Physiologic
    genu valgum
    (knock-knees) ④

Nelson Textbook of Pediatrics, 19e. Chapters 48, 667
Nelsons Essentials, 6e. Chapter 200

Neurology

Chapter 50
HEADACHES

Headaches are common and usually benign. Parents often seek medical attention for a child because they are concerned about the potential of a serious or life-threatening cause of the headaches. Most headache complaints will be primary headache disorders; evaluation is essential to rule out more worrisome secondary causes of headache.

1. A thorough history should inquire about the quality, pattern, and progression of the complaint as well as inciting factors, recent trauma, response to medications, and associated visual or sensory (or other neurologic) disturbances. Social and emotional issues should be reviewed; teens should typically be interviewed in private. The impact of the headaches on a child's visual activity should be elicited. A thorough family history should inquire about headaches (particularly migraines), other neurologic problems, and general medical conditions that could cause secondary headaches. A headache diary may be helpful in characterizing headache patterns and identifying associated symptoms and triggers.

Older children are often able to describe their headache; nonverbal young children may become irritable, rock, rub their eyes or head, vomit, or seek a darkened environment.

When intracranial pressure (ICP) is increased (due to hydrocephalus, mass lesions, edema, or hemorrhage), headaches are frequently characterized by "red flags" such as pain that is present in the morning or awakens the patient from sleep and then remits with being upright; increased pain with cough, straining, or position change; altered sensorium or personality, or a patient's description of "the worst headache of my life."

In addition to a thorough neurologic examination, the physical examination should include a blood pressure evaluation, a thorough ENT examination (including dentition), and an assessment of visual acuity. Worrisome physical findings include abnormal neurologic signs, meningeal signs, papilledema, and altered sensorium.

2. Migraines are the most likely recurrent headache disorder to present with a first acute severe headache. Other chronic or recurrent headache disorders will more commonly present for evaluation after repeated episodes (even if they have not quite reached the diagnostic 3 month duration criteria) but may need to be considered in the evaluation of any first severe acute headache.

3. Magnetic resonance imaging is generally preferred for identifying structural lesions, infection, inflammation, and ischemia. Computed tomography (CT) is preferred in acute cases of suspected trauma or fracture. Imaging choice should consider that head CTs carry a higher radiation risk whereas MRIs are more costly, time-consuming, and they require sedation.

4. Headaches developing within 7 days of head trauma with signs or symptoms of concussion are defined as acute post-traumatic headache.

5. Migraines are classically characterized by a positive family history for migraines, associated nausea, vomiting or abdominal pain, sensitivity to light and sound, an aura (scotomata, blurriness, visual distortions, sensory changes) or other transient neurologic disturbances. Relief with sleep is common. Triggers (e.g., stress, fatigue, illness) can often be identified. Migraines can be unilateral or bilateral in children, and the pain is typically characterized by a pounding or pulsing quality. (Auras, a longer headache duration, and a unilateral location become more common with increasing age.) Neurologic deficits (e.g., hemiplegia, vertigo, visual changes) may occur with some of the less common subtypes.

6. Many experts consider the absence of a family history for migraines as a risk factor for a space-occupying intracranial lesion in children with acute headaches. Be conscious that migraine presentations can vary between family members, and headaches are often unrecognized as "migraines" by families; detailed questioning may be required. Most experts recommend neuroimaging for the child who has migrainous headaches with an absolutely negative family history of migraine or its equivalent (e.g., motion sickness, cyclic vomiting).

7. The second edition of the International Classification of Headache Disorders provides detailed diagnostic criteria for several subtypes of migraines. Diagnosis of a migraine disorder requires at least two episodes meeting the diagnostic criteria. The classifications include migraines with and without aura (including hemiplegia and visual disturbances) as well as childhood periodic syndromes.

8. Neuroimaging (MRI is preferable if available) is warranted when the neurologic examination is abnormal or unusual neurologic features occur during the migraine, when a child has headaches that awaken him or her from sleep or that are present on first awakening (then remit with upright posture), or are very brief in duration occurring only with cough or bending over.

9. Brain tumors present with symptoms due to increased intracranial pressure (ICP) or focal destruction or invasion of brain tissue; presentations vary according to tumor type, location and patient age. The increased intracranial pressure typically causes headaches that may wake a child at night, are typically worse in the morning, are aggravated by coughing or bending over, and are frequently accompanied by vomiting; papilledema, sixth nerve palsy, altered level of consciousness, and gait instability may also be noted on examination.

10. An increased risk of brain abscesses is present in children with immunodeficiency disorders, right-to-left cardiac shunts (especially tetralogy of Fallot), chronic ENT infections (ear, sinus, mastoid, dental), penetrating head injuries, soft tissue infections of the face or scalp, and infected VP shunts.

11. Hydrocephalus is most likely to cause headaches in older children (whose cranial sutures are closing). Headaches are generalized; they may be acute or gradual in onset and mild or severe in quality, depending on how rapidly the hydrocephalus is progressing.

12. Third ventricle cysts may function as a ball-valve mechanism causing intermittent severe ("thunderclap") headaches due to transient increases in ICP. Other cysts (e.g., arachnoid, epidermoid, dermoid) may present with progressive headaches or seizures.

13. Neurologic abnormalities, altered mental status, or meningeal signs (e.g., nuchal rigidity, Kernig, and Brudzinski signs) warrant an evaluation to rule out meningitis.

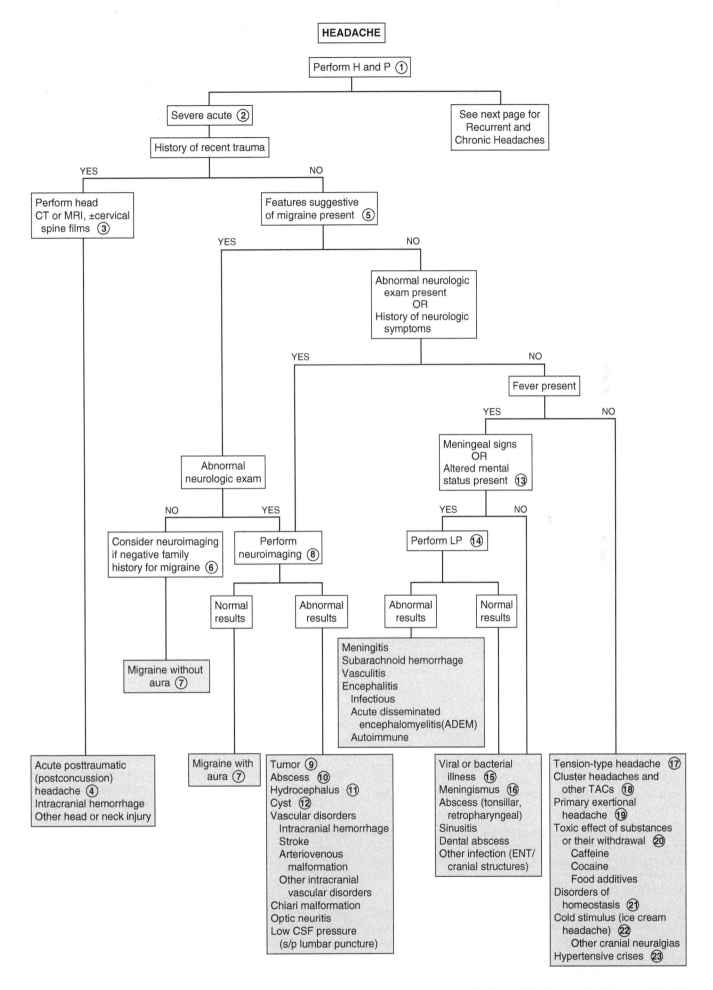

HEADACHE

Perform H and P ①

Severe acute ②

See next page for Recurrent and Chronic Headaches

History of recent trauma

YES

Perform head CT or MRI, ±cervical spine films ③

NO

Features suggestive of migraine present ⑤

YES

NO

Abnormal neurologic exam present OR History of neurologic symptoms

YES

NO

Fever present

YES

NO

Meningeal signs OR Altered mental status present ⑬

YES

NO

Perform LP ⑭

Abnormal neurologic exam

NO

Consider neuroimaging if negative family history for migraine ⑥

YES

Perform neuroimaging ⑧

Normal results

Abnormal results

Abnormal results

Normal results

Migraine without aura ⑦

Meningitis
Subarachnoid hemorrhage
Vasculitis
Encephalitis
    Infectious
    Acute disseminated
        encephalomyelitis(ADEM)
    Autoimmune

Acute posttraumatic (postconcussion) headache ④
Intracranial hemorrhage
Other head or neck injury

Migraine with aura ⑦

Tumor ⑨
Abscess ⑩
Hydrocephalus ⑪
Cyst ⑫
Vascular disorders
    Intracranial hemorrhage
    Stroke
    Arteriovenous
        malformation
    Other intracranial
        vascular disorders
Chiari malformation
Optic neuritis
Low CSF pressure
    (s/p lumbar puncture)

Viral or bacterial illness ⑮
Meningismus ⑯
Abscess (tonsillar, retropharyngeal)
Sinusitis
Dental abscess
Other infection (ENT/ cranial structures)

Tension-type headache ⑰
Cluster headaches and other TACs ⑱
Primary exertional headache ⑲
Toxic effect of substances or their withdrawal ⑳
    Caffeine
    Cocaine
    Food additives
Disorders of homeostasis ㉑
Cold stimulus (ice cream headache) ㉒
    Other cranial neuralgias
Hypertensive crises ㉓

Nelson Textbook of Pediatrics, 19e. Chapters 491, 588
Nelsons Essentials, 6e. Chapter 180

14 The risk of increased ICP must be considered before performing a lumbar punture (LP), although this risk in children is low. There are no specific guidelines regarding imaging before performing an LP in children; clinical judgment should take into consideration factors such as the presence of papilledema, focal neurologic deficits, a history of hydrocephalus, a VP shunt, or history of neurosurgery or cranial space-occupying lesion.

15 Headache often accompanies fever of any cause. Headaches can frequently be caused by systemic infections (e.g., influenza, sepsis) and extracranial infections (e.g., ear, eye, mastoid), as well as cranial infections like meningitis and encephalitis.

16 Meningismus describes symptoms consistent with meningeal irritation but due to infection of other head and neck structures rather than meningitis.

17 Tension-type headaches are the most common headaches experienced by children. They are typically described as having a "squeezing" (as opposed to "pounding") quality and a band-like (nonfocal) distribution. They can be episodic or chronic, they tend to be less severe, and they have a shorter duration than migraines. Triggers (e.g., stressors, fatigue) can frequently be identified. Neurologic examination is always normal, mild sensitivity to sound or light may occur; in chronic cases, mild nausea may occur as well.

18 Trigeminal autonomic cephalagias (TACs) are characterized by headaches and parasympathetic autonomic features and are rare in children. Like all headache classifications, they can be acute or chronic. Cluster headaches are comprised of acute severe attacks of unilateral pain around the temple or eye with associated ipsilateral rhinorrhea, sweating, eye redness, tearing, eyelid swelling, pinpoint pupils, or ptosis. Others in this category (e.g., paroxysmal hemicrania, short-lasting unilateral neuralgiform headache attacks with conjunctival injection and tearing) present with similar, but less severe, symptoms. Neuroimaging is usually recommended in these cases to rule out the possibility of a more serious cause.

19 A primary exertional headache can be triggered by exercise or exertion in people who do not suffer from migraines. It can last from minutes to hours and is clearly precipitated by exercise. Imaging to exclude an intracranial hemorrhage is recommended for the first occurrence of this headache type.

20 The International Headache Classification Disorder-II encompasses headaches attributed to exposure to or withdrawal from a variety of substances within a single classification. Examples include medications, drugs of abuse, carbon monoxide, caffeine, and food additives. Definitive diagnosis cannot be made until significant improvement is documented after the exposure to the substance has ended.

21 Disorders of homeostasis encompass problems with blood gases (hypoxia), volume distributions, blood pressure, and endocrine disorders. Examples include headaches occurring due to altitude change, hypertensive crises, or fasting. Evaluation should be based on clinical presentation.

22 Stimulus or irritation of various branches of the cranial nerves cause pain in the areas that those branches innervate. Cold stimulus (e.g., ice cream) and compression (e.g., tight headgear or helmet) are causes; trigeminal, glossopharyngeal, and occipital neuralgia patterns are recognized.

23 No convincing association between mild and moderate hypertension and headaches has been demonstrated; an acute severe headache may occur with a rare hypertensive crisis.

24 Headache may be a component of childhood periodic syndromes, which include cyclic vomiting, abdominal migraine, and benign paroxysmal vertigo. Neurologic findings noted during episodes (e.g., nystagmus, visual disturbances) are completely absent between episodes. These syndromes are considered childhood precursors of migraine.

25 Migraine-type symptoms during (hemicranias epileptic) and after seizures are a well-recognized entity.

26 Chronic headaches are defined as occurring on more than 15 days per month for a period of at least 3 months.

27 The category of new daily persistent headache (NDPH) encompasses new headaches without an identifiable cause (in particular, medication overuse) that are occurring daily from within 3 days of their onset. This type of headache is usually bilateral with mild to moderate severity; it may have features of either migraine or tension-type headaches, but no more than one of the following characteristics: photophobia, phonophobia, mild nausea. The abrupt onset is critical to making this diagnosis (which can only be applied after 3 months of headache); if a patient cannot describe this type of onset, this term should not be applied.

28 Idiopathic intracranial hypertension (previously pseudotumor cerebri) can present acutely but is more commonly diagnosed as a cause of progressive headache. It is most common in young obese women. There may be a history of an enlarged blind spot and constricted visual fields. Papilledema is usually present, and a sixth nerve palsy is common; otherwise, the physical examination is typically normal. Vomiting is infrequent. Neuroimaging is normal; however, it must precede an LP in order to rule out intracranial processes. The CSF studies are normal except for an increased opening pressure, and the LP typically provides relief of the headache. Intracranial hypertension can also occur secondary to a multitude of etiologies, including metabolic, infectious, hematologic, and drug-related causes.

29 Temporomandibular joint (TMJ) syndrome causes pain localized to the temporomandibular joint. It is aggravated by chewing motions and associated with a clicking sound.

30 Medication-overuse causes headaches in patients taking analgesics daily or on most days; it often complicates other headache types. The headache occurs due to a vicious cycle of pain and analgesic use (sometimes inappropriately dosed) followed by more pain and more analgesic use as the effect wears off. The definitive diagnosis cannot be made until improvement is documented within two months of stopping the medication overuse (the term "probably medication-overuse" headaches is appropriate until then).

31 Posttraumatic or postconcussion headaches are described as chronic when they persist beyond 3 months. Chronic posttraumatic headaches frequently occur as part of a broader posttraumatic syndrome, which includes more problems with balance, sleep, cognitive function, mood, etc. A neck injury (e.g., whiplash) may cause similar chronic symptoms. Cervical spine films with or without neuroimaging should be done acutely in the case of whiplash; subsequent neuroimaging may rarely be indicated to rule out a chronic subdural hematoma.

Bibliography

Akinci A, Guven A, Degerliyurt A, et al: The correlation between headache and refractive errors, *Journal of AAOPS* 12:290–293, 2008.

Blume HK: Pediatric headache: a review, *Pediatr Rev* 33:562–576, 2012.

Headache Classification Subcommittee of the International Headache Society: The international classification of headache disorders: ed 2, *Cephalagia* 24 (suppl 1):9–160, 2004.

Lewis DW, Ashwal S, Dahl G, et al: Practice parameter: evaluation of children and adolescents with recurrent headaches: report of the Quality Standards Subcommittee of the American Academy of Neurology and the Practice Committee of the Child Neurology Society, *Neurology* 59:490–498, 2002.

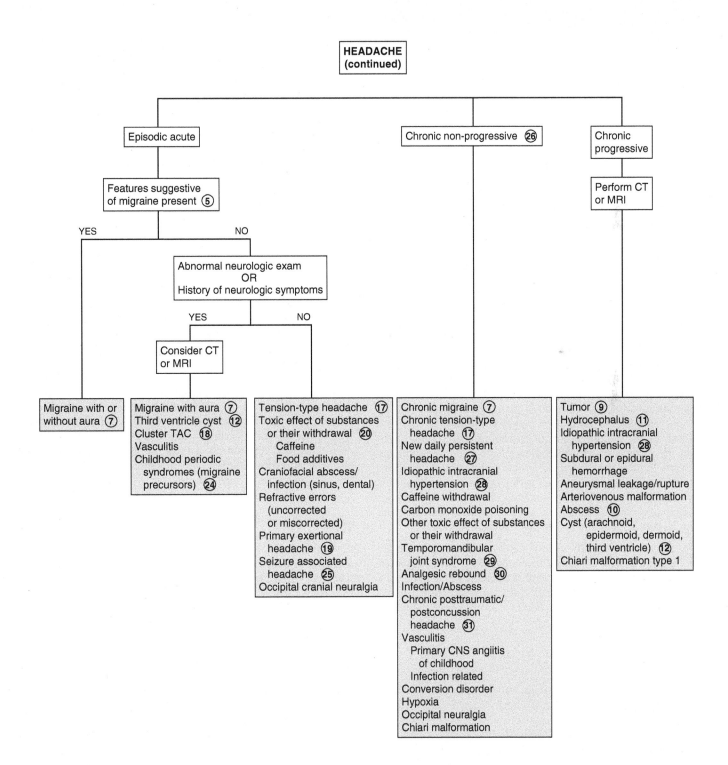

Chapter 51

SEIZURES AND OTHER PAROXYSMAL DISORDERS

A seizure is a paroxysmal disturbance in brain function that manifests as an alteration in motor activity, level of consciousness, or autonomic function. Seizures and seizure disorders were traditionally classified according to whether the manifestations were generalized or focal and whether consciousness was preserved or impaired. Advances in neuroscience that allow specific, objective diagnostic criteria for seizures and seizure disorders have led to revision of the terminology and classification system of these entities; the current system emphasizes diagnosis based on objective, measurable criteria. The traditional definition of status epilepticus is the occurrence of prolonged or recurrent seizures (without a return to consciousness) for 30 minutes or longer. A number of nonepileptic paroxysmal disorders occur in childhood and must be distinguished from epileptic seizures.

1. A description of the event is the most valuable part of the evaluation because physical findings are rare and diagnostic studies may not be conclusive. Indeed, the description of the event is generally going to be the key to discerning whether the event was likely a seizure versus a nonepileptic event; a video recording of the event can be extremely helpful in this regard. Inquire about the occurrence of an aura, preceding mood or behavioral changes, a detailed description of the event including motor, verbal, and autonomic changes (e.g., pupillary dilatation, drooling, incontinence, pallor, vomiting), as well as a history of any inciting events (e.g., trauma, fever, crying). Obtain the medical history, including a birth and developmental history. Inquire about medication use and potential ingestions of toxic substances. In children with a known seizure disorder, specifically ask about medication compliance. Neurocutaneous lesions (e.g., café-au-lait spots, ash leaf macules) and vascular lesions should be noted on the physical examination.

2. Seizures meeting the criteria for simple febrile seizures are generally benign events with excellent long-term prognoses. Two to five percent of the general population will experience a (usually simple) febrile seizure; of those, approximately 30% will have a recurrence. The risk of subsequent epilepsy following a simple febrile seizure is low and affected by various predictors such as age of occurrence, duration of fever, height of fever, family history, etc. Complex febrile seizures are defined as focal or prolonged (longer than 15 minutes) or occurring in a flurry of repetitive episodes during the febrile illness. Genetic factors are being increasingly recognized as contributing factors in complex febrile seizures. (Remember, children younger than 6 months of age do not meet the criteria for a simple febrile seizure and should not be evaluated along this pathway.)

3. The evaluation of complex febrile seizures should be individualized based on the presentation. A very prolonged seizure, a focal seizure (characteristic of herpes simplex virus [HSV] encephalitis), or an abnormal neurologic examination should prompt a thorough evaluation for a CNS infection. The diagnostic test of choice for herpes simplex virus encephalitis is a PCR for HSV performed on a spinal fluid specimen; tests should also be obtained for bacterial and viral etiologies of meningitis. MRI should be obtained for all children with a focal seizure. An EEG should be obtained acutely if concerned about febrile status epilepticus.

4. By definition, the term complex febrile seizure applies to children between 6 months and 60 months of age. Outside of that age group, seizures with fever can be due to multiple other causes (e.g., HHV6, *Shigella,* immunizations).

5. A lumbar puncture is not routinely recommended for a child age 6-12 months (who is well appearing and fully immunized) who has experienced a simple febrile seizure because their risk of having bacterial meningitis is extremely low. Less straightforward is the recommendation for performing an LP on a child who has had antibiotics (by any route) in the days preceding the seizure or whose immunization status is unknown or deficient (particularly for Hib and pneumococcus, which are known pathogens for bacterial meningitis). Most of the studies regarding outcomes of febrile seizures have been done on children with high immunization rates. Because the outcomes of febrile seizures for children with incomplete or unknown immunization status or any pretreatment with antibiotics is unknown, an LP is recommended as an option for these children.

6. Any labs obtained, particularly CBCs, should be directed towards evaluating the source of the fever, not to evaluate the seizure. (Of note, when considering bacteremia as the source of the fever, the incidence of bacteremia is the same in febrile children under 24 months of age, regardless of whether they have a febrile seizure or not.)

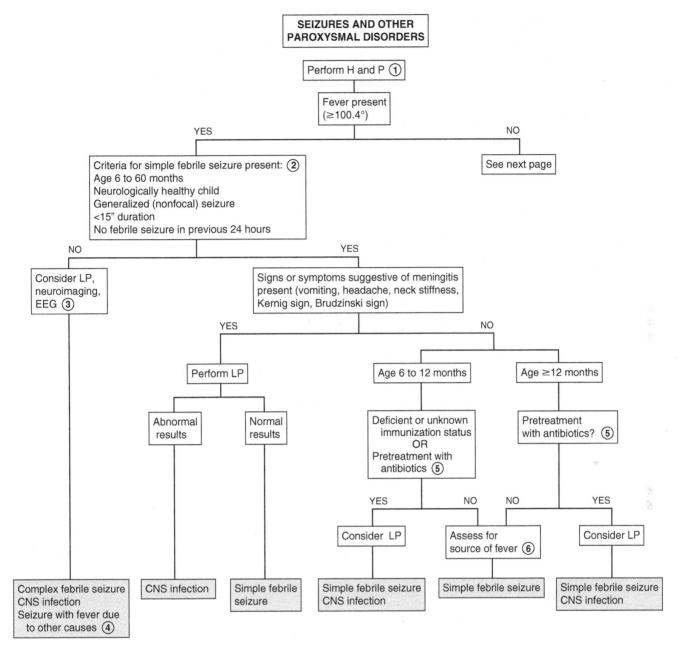

Nelson Textbook of Pediatrics, 19e. Chapters 17, 586, 587, 594
Nelsons Essentials, 6e. Chapter 181

7 Evaluation of infants younger than 2 months of age with seizures requires consideration of causes mostly unique to the neonatal age group; that approach to neonatal seizures is not covered in this chapter.

8 Breath-holding spells should be distinguished from seizures before proceeding with an evaluation for seizures. The term "breath-holding spells" is somewhat of a misnomer as the episodes are not due to intentional breath holding. Cyanotic or "blue" breath-holding spells are described as prolonged expiratory apnea or a sudden lack of inspiratory effort, often during crying. In pallid breath-holding spells, a reflex vagal-bradycardia is responsible for the event, usually following a minor injury. Both can be triggered by injury, anger, or frustration. Apnea, brief loss of consciousness, tonic posturing, and occasionally anoxic seizures can follow. Breath-holding spells typically occur between ages 6 and 18 months, although they may be seen in children up to 6 years. Children recover quickly from these events, and no diagnostic evaluation is indicated. However, affected children should be assessed for iron deficiency, which should be treated if it is present.

9 The presence of autonomic symptoms, altered level of consciousness, lack of suppression with gentle restraint, and a history of CNS insult or injury should raise suspicion of seizures. A nonepileptic event is suggested by abrupt resolution with return to full level of consciousness (LOC) or when the movement ceases abruptly when children can be aroused from sleep. Older children experiencing seizures may additionally manifest abnormal vocalizations, incontinence, or a change in mood or behavior preceding the event; they may subsequently be able to describe an aura or other preictal symptoms.

10 Head banging (jactatio capitis nocturna) is a common behavior of rhythmic to-and-fro movements of the head and body. Children have no memory of this behavior, which typically occurs as they are going to sleep. It typically resolves by 5 years of age.

11 Myoclonus refers to a brief involuntary muscle "jerk"; its clinical significance varies significantly based on whether it is occurring as an isolated involuntary movement or as a component of a more complex epilepsy syndrome or movement disorder. It is common and usually benign in sleeping infants (neonatal sleep myoclonus); random myoclonic jerks can be normal (physiologic) in people of all ages during sleep. In infants, the condition can be distinguished from seizures based on it occurring only during sleep and ceasing when the infant wakes up, as well as the absence of any autonomic symptoms. It resolves by 2 to 3 months of age.

12 Infants with hyperekplexia (stiff baby syndrome or startle disease) may have nocturnal myoclonus, stiffening upon awakening, an exaggerated startle reflex, and occasionally apnea. A few children may continue to experience an exaggerated startle response with stiffening and falling throughout life.

13 The term epilepsy defines a disorder in which there is a persistent underlying abnormality of the brain, which can generate seizure activity; the term applies after the occurrence of two or more unprovoked seizures and is classified based on a number of features, including age at onset, cognitive and developmental antecedents and consequences, neurological examination, EEG characteristics, triggering factors, and sleep patterns. Epilepsy as a diagnosis should be distinguished from an electroclinical (epilepsy) syndrome. Electroclinical syndromes are clinical entities of a specific complex of signs and symptoms comprising a distinct clinical disorder. (This term was proposed by the International League Against Epilepsy [ILAE] in their 2010 report on terminology to reduce the imprecise use of the term "syndrome" in previous classification systems; not all epilepsy meets criteria for an electroclinical syndrome.) Etiologies of epilepsy can be genetic, structural/metabolic, or unknown. (Currently, the advances in neuroscience are making the descriptions and diagnosis of seizures a dynamic work in progress!) Epilepsy syndromes may be attributed to an identifiable problem (cerebral or metabolic abnormality); if not, they are labeled as idiopathic (the term cryptogenic is no longer used) and presumed to have a genetic basis.

14 Neuroimaging should be performed emergently if there is a risk of a serious condition requiring immediate treatment (e.g., intracranial hemorrhage, brain swelling, space occupying lesion); head trauma occurring in close proximity to the seizure, associated with any loss of consciousness or change in mental status, persistent headache, or vomiting would meet this criteria. Imaging should also be considered for children who experience a focal seizure and children with known conditions that predispose them to abnormal neuroimaging studies (e.g., developmental delays of unclear etiology, sickle cell disease, bleeding disorders, hydrocephalus, cerebral vascular disease, malignancy, HIV infection, hemihypertrophy or travel to an area endemic for cysticercosis). Neuroimaging should also be considered when a child is found unconscious and it is not clear whether trauma or seizure caused the loss of consciousness.

15 MRI is the preferred imaging study in the evaluation of seizures because of its increased sensitivity relative to CT. A CT, however, can be adequate to detect emergent treatable conditions; it is the preferred mode of imaging when acute trauma has occurred.

16 Seizures may occur secondary to an acute problem or as a manifestation of epilepsy (genetic cause). The classification of "structural/metabolic" causes includes trauma, infection and metabolic disorders (most commonly abnormalities of sodium, calcium and glucose) as well as drugs or toxins.

17 Isolated seizures (with or without a recognizable cause) with no subsequent sequelae can occur.

18 Focal seizures are presumed to begin in one cerebral hemisphere (in contrast to generalized seizures which are believed to begin in both hemispheres at the same time). In focal seizures, the degree of impairment in the level of consciousness can be variable. Manifestations may include focal motor signs, automatisms (semi-purposeful movements), or autonomic (including somatosensory) symptoms. EEGs reveal focal epileptiform discharges. Neuroimaging is indicated in all children with focal seizures to rule out anatomic lesions. (The terms "partial simple" and "partial complex" seizures have been abandoned by the ILAE due to the imprecise definitions of the terms.)

19 Based on the American Academy of Neurology 2001 statement, no lab tests are indicated in children older than 6 months of age with a first nonfebrile seizure who has returned to baseline and has no clinical history suggesting an etiology (e.g., trauma, dehydration, toxin ingestion, stigmata suggestive of rickets). If the child has not returned to baseline and there is a history suggesting a problem (e.g., vomiting, dehydration), labs pertinent to the evaluation of the suspected problem may be appropriate; a sodium level for children less than 6 months, calcium and blood glucose levels are the most likely to be abnormal (AAN 2000). A careful history for risk of toxic ingestion

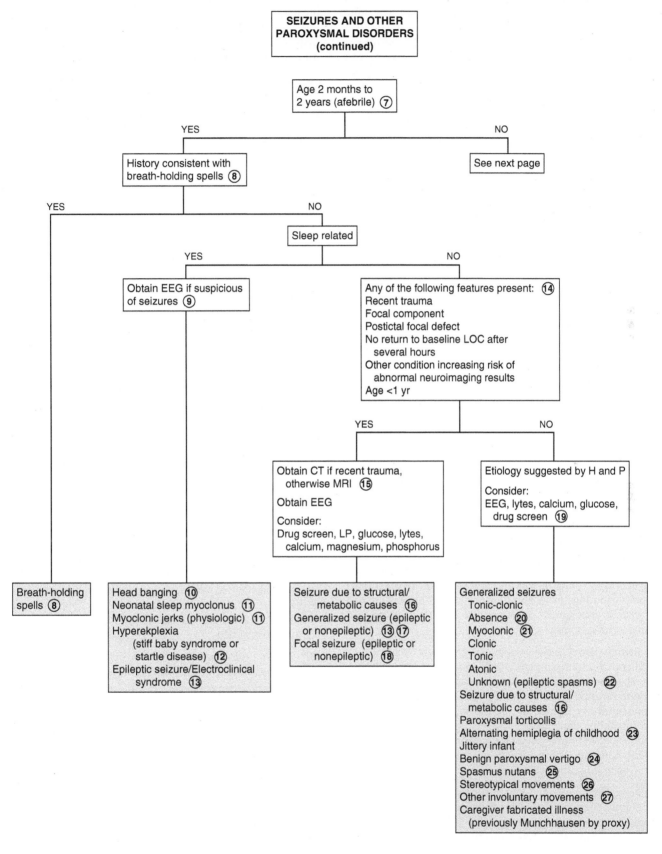

SEIZURES AND OTHER
PAROXYSMAL DISORDERS
(continued)

Age 2 months to
2 years (afebrile) ⑦

YES — History consistent with
breath-holding spells ⑧

NO — See next page

YES — Breath-holding spells ⑧

NO — Sleep related

YES — Obtain EEG if suspicious
of seizures ⑨

Head banging ⑩
Neonatal sleep myoclonus ⑪
Myoclonic jerks (physiologic) ⑪
Hyperekplexia
   (stiff baby syndrome or
   startle disease) ⑫
Epileptic seizure/Electroclinical
   syndrome ⑬

NO — Any of the following features present: ⑭
Recent trauma
Focal component
Postictal focal defect
No return to baseline LOC after
   several hours
Other condition increasing risk of
   abnormal neuroimaging results
Age <1 yr

YES — Obtain CT if recent trauma,
   otherwise MRI ⑮

Obtain EEG

Consider:
Drug screen, LP, glucose, lytes,
   calcium, magnesium, phosphorus

Seizure due to structural/
   metabolic causes ⑯
Generalized seizure (epileptic
   or nonepileptic) ⑬⑰
Focal seizure (epileptic or
   nonepileptic) ⑱

NO — Etiology suggested by H and P

Consider:
EEG, lytes, calcium, glucose,
   drug screen ⑲

Generalized seizures
   Tonic-clonic
   Absence ⑳
   Myoclonic ㉑
   Clonic
   Tonic
   Atonic
   Unknown (epileptic spasms) ㉒
Seizure due to structural/
   metabolic causes ⑯
Paroxysmal torticollis
Alternating hemiplegia of childhood ㉓
Jittery infant
Benign paroxysmal vertigo ㉔
Spasmus nutans ㉕
Stereotypical movements ㉖
Other involuntary movements ㉗
Caregiver fabricated illness
   (previously Munchhausen by proxy)

Nelson Textbook of Pediatrics, 19e. Chapters 17, 586, 587, 594
Nelsons Essentials, 6e. Chapter 181

should always be obtained and investigated if suspicious. A lumbar puncture (LP) is indicated only if age is less than 6 months, if a CNS infection is suspected or if a child (of any age) has not returned to baseline mental status. EEGs are recommended when a seizure is the suspected diagnosis; however, it is not necessary to obtain them urgently.

Routine EEGs are recommended by the American Academy of Neurology as part of the routine work-up of a first nonfocal, nonfebrile seizure; however, the ideal timing of that procedure is not clear. It should not be done acutely because patients may continue to show transient postictal abnormalities for up to 48 hours. The purpose of the EEG is to help predict the risk of recurrence and provide information regarding the child's long-term prognosis. (This recommendation may be controversial because it does not influence treatment recommendations.)

20 Absence seizures are generalized seizures that typically manifest as brief staring spells, sometimes with automatisms. The onset is most commonly between 5 and 8 years of age, although they may be overlooked for prolonged periods due to their very brief duration. Hyperventilation will often reproduce the event. Diagnosis is by characteristic 3 Hz spike-and-slow-wave complexes on the EEG.

21 Myoclonic seizures vary in their prognosis and neurodevelopmental outcome. Infantile spasms are the most serious variant. Symptoms commonly begin between 4 and 7 months of age with clusters of rapid "jackknifing" contractions of the neck, trunk, and limbs followed by a brief sustained tonic contraction. Hypsarrhythmia is the characteristic finding on EEG. An EEG is necessary to distinguish infantile spasms from benign myoclonus of infancy (a benign involuntary movement) and a myoclonic epilepsy (which vary in severity and outcome).

22 Epileptic spasms (which includes infantile spasms) are classified as an unknown seizure type because they do not fit well into the generalized or focal subsets.

23 Intermittent episodes of hemiplegia (which may alternate between sides of the body) characterize alternating hemiplegia of childhood. Onset is in infancy; attacks are more likely to be flaccid in young infants and more dystonic in older ones. Episodes can range from minutes to weeks. Other involuntary movements, nystagmus, or autonomic disturbances may accompany the episodes.

24 Benign paroxysmal vertigo most commonly occurs in toddlers. Children experience brief episodes of sudden imbalance. They are frightened by the episodes and frequently fall to the floor, refusing to stand or walk. Consciousness and speech are preserved. Nystagmus is usually evident. Neurologic evaluation (including imaging and EEG) is typically normal, except for abnormal vestibular function noted on ice water caloric testing. This condition is considered a migraine variant and a likely precursor to migraine headaches.

25 Paroxysmal head-nodding, torticollis (head tilt), and nystagmus characterize spasmus nutans; consciousness is preserved. Onset is in the first few months of life and it resolves by 5 years. Neuroimaging is recommended to rule out tumors.

26 Repetitive purposeless movements are often exhibited by autistic or handicapped children, especially in environments with a low level of stimulation. They may be difficult to

distinguish clinically from seizure activity. Syncopal convulsions may occasionally be self-induced by performing the Valsalva maneuver. Masturbation in young children is also sometimes mistaken as seizures by parents.

27 Involuntary movements may occur as isolated entities or as a component of more complex movement disorders; chorea, dystonia, hypokinesia, myoclonus are examples. Tics and stereotypic movements are described as involuntary movements even though affected individuals may have some ability to suppress those motions. Some electroclinical (epilepsy) syndromes are characterized by both seizures and involuntary movements, but movement disorders alone can be difficult to distinguish from seizures when they manifest as abrupt or paroxysmal involuntary movements. In general, movement disorders do not manifest during sleep, have a more stereotypical appearance than seizures, and are not associated with loss of consciousness or abnormal EEG findings.

28 Benign childhood epilepsy with centrotemporal spikes (previously called benign rolandic epilepsy) typically presents as a brief hemifacial seizure (parents may describe the child's face as "twisted") that awakens the child from sleep. Generalization occurs rarely. Drooling and an inability to speak are common, but consciousness is preserved. The EEG shows characteristic centrotemporal spikes. Onset is between 3 and 13 years of age and resolution occurs in adolescence. The family history is often positive for epilepsy.

29 Narcolepsy is characterized by recurrent short sleep attacks. It is often accompanied by cataplexy (a sudden collapse due to loss of muscle tone but with preserved consciousness) and induced by laughter, excitement, or startle. Vivid hallucinations (e.g., visual, auditory, tactile) may occur with transition to and from sleep; sleep paralysis may accompany them. Disturbed nighttime sleep is very common.

30 Night terrors are a sudden partial arousal from non-REM sleep, occurring about 2 hours after sleep onset, accompanied by inconsolable screaming and crying. They occur most often in preschoolers and early school-aged children. Children appear awake but do not recognize people and have no memory of the event. Confusional arousals are similar, but less extreme events with a more gradual onset, and the child is less likely to try to get out of bed.

31 Rarely, prolonged episodes of hyperventilation may result in loss of consciousness and some seizure activity.

Bibliography

Berg AT, Berkovic SF, Buchhalter J, et al: Report of the commission on classification and terminology: update and recommendations, *Epilepsia* 51:676–685, 2010.

Hirtz D, Ashwal S, Berg A, et al: Practice parameter: Evaluating a first nonfebrile seizure in children: Report of the quality standards subcommittee of the American Academy of Neurology, the Child Neurology Society, and the American Epilepsy Society, *Neurology* 55:616–623, 2000.

Obeid M, Mikati MD: Expanding spectrum of paroxysmal events in children: potential mimickers of epilepsy, *Pediatric Neurology* 37:309–316, 2007.

Piña-Garza JE: Paroxysmal disorders. In Piña-Garza JE, editor: *Fenichel's clinical pediatric neurology*, ed 7, Philadelphia, 2013, Saunders/Elsevier, pp 1–46.

Subcommittee on Febrile Seizures. Febrile seizures: Guideline for the neurodiagnostic evaluation of the child with a simple febrile seizure, *Pediatrics* 127:389–394, 2011.

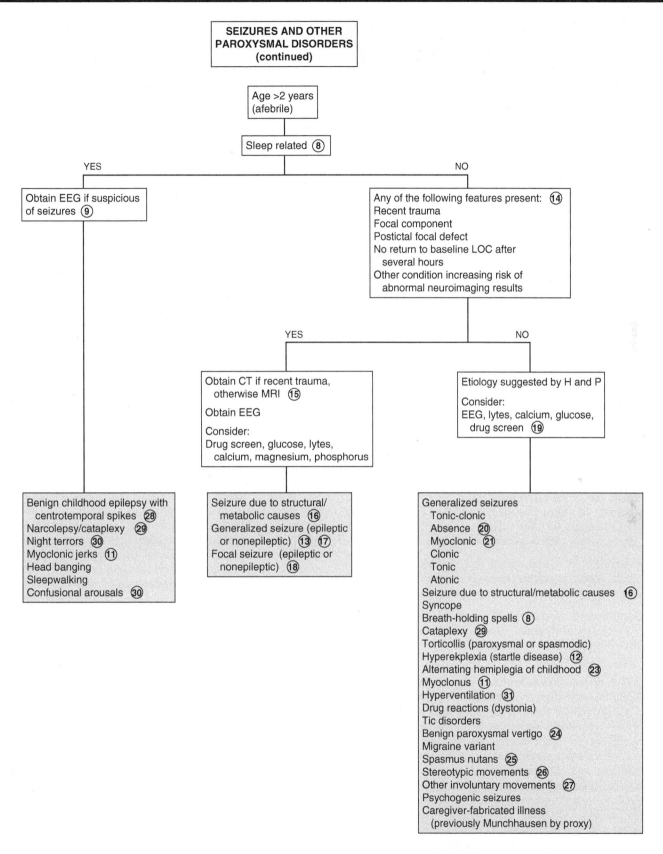

SEIZURES AND OTHER
PAROXYSMAL DISORDERS
(continued)

Age >2 years
(afebrile)

Sleep related ⑧

YES

Obtain EEG if suspicious
of seizures ⑨

NO

Any of the following features present: ⑭
Recent trauma
Focal component
Postictal focal defect
No return to baseline LOC after
    several hours
Other condition increasing risk of
    abnormal neuroimaging results

YES

Obtain CT if recent trauma,
    otherwise MRI ⑮

Obtain EEG

Consider:
Drug screen, glucose, lytes,
    calcium, magnesium, phosphorus

NO

Etiology suggested by H and P

Consider:
EEG, lytes, calcium, glucose,
    drug screen ⑲

Benign childhood epilepsy with
    centrotemporal spikes ㉘
Narcolepsy/cataplexy ㉙
Night terrors ㉚
Myoclonic jerks ⑪
Head banging
Sleepwalking
Confusional arousals ㉚

Seizure due to structural/
    metabolic causes ⑯
Generalized seizure (epileptic
    or nonepileptic) ⑬ ⑰
Focal seizure (epileptic or
    nonepileptic) ⑱

Generalized seizures
    Tonic-clonic
    Absence ⑳
    Myoclonic ㉑
    Clonic
    Tonic
    Atonic
Seizure due to structural/metabolic causes ⑥
Syncope
Breath-holding spells ⑧
Cataplexy ㉙
Torticollis (paroxysmal or spasmodic)
Hyperekplexia (startle disease) ⑫
Alternating hemiplegia of childhood ㉓
Myoclonus ⑪
Hyperventilation ㉛
Drug reactions (dystonia)
Tic disorders
Benign paroxysmal vertigo ㉔
Migraine variant
Spasmus nutans ㉕
Stereotypic movements ㉖
Other involuntary movements ㉗
Psychogenic seizures
Caregiver-fabricated illness
    (previously Munchhausen by proxy)

Nelson Textbook of Pediatrics, 19e. Chapters 17, 586, 587, 594
Nelsons Essentials, 6e. Chapter 181

Chapter 52
INVOLUNTARY MOVEMENTS

Involuntary movements can be the primary or secondary manifestation of numerous neurologic disorders; they can also be benign. Hyperkinetic movements are much more common than hypokinetic movements (parkinsonism) in children. Classification has historically been difficult because of ambiguous or overlapping terminology, plus affected children commonly demonstrate more than one type of disordered movement. The Task Force on Childhood Movement Disorders published a consensus statement in 2010 proposing definitions for hyperkinetic movements recognized in children based on the best available evidence. Hyperkinetic movements are defined as unwanted or excess movements.

1 Distinguishing movement disorders from seizures is often the first diagnostic challenge because many movement disorders are also paroxysmal. Characteristics suggestive of seizures include: (1) symptoms that persist or worsen during sleep, (2) brief, nonstereotypical movements, (3) altered level of consciousness, and (4) accompanying epileptiform activity on EEG. An EEG should be performed whenever a seizure disorder is suspected. If seizures are deemed unlikely, identifying or classifying the type of abnormal movement is the next step in narrowing the differential diagnosis. Videotaping the abnormal movements can be an extremely helpful diagnostic aid. Once the movement has been classified, evaluation is based on the suspected diagnosis for these disorders: imaging, medication trials, electromyography, or genetic testing may be indicated.

2 Hypokinesia or parkinsonism (e.g., bradykinesia, rigidity, tremor, abnormal posture) is rare in childhood. It may occur in children affected by rare genetic or neurodegenerative disorders.

3 Huntington disease in children is more likely to manifest bradykinesia or dystonia rather than chorea (more likely in adults). A juvenile onset occurs often in the Westphal variant of Huntington disease.

4 Wilson disease (hepatolenticular degeneration) is an autosomal recessive disorder characterized by liver failure and neurologic symptoms; children are more likely to present with the former. Neurologic symptoms (e.g., dystonia, dysarthria, chorea, rigidity, postural abnormalities, tremors, drooling) develop with disease progression. Diagnosis is by decreased serum ceruloplasmin and increased urinary copper excretion; liver biopsy determines the extent of the disease. Kayser-Fleischer rings (yellow-brown rings around the cornea due to copper deposition in the Descemet membrane) develop when the disease has progressed to include neurologic symptoms. When present, they are pathognomonic for the disease.

5 Chorea is a sequence of discrete random involuntary movements or fragments of involuntary movements. These movements tend to occur in a jerky flow of rapid ongoing motions that can make distinguishing the distinct start and end point of individual movements difficult. They are not reliably associated with

an intentional movement (but intentional movement can worsen them), and children often try to disguise the movements by incorporating them into a more purposeful movement ("parakinesias"). They are not predictable or stereotypical of any particular body region and cannot be voluntarily suppressed with relaxation; children are frequently described as fidgety or hyperactive. Chorea affecting the shoulder or hip joints is called "ballism" and frequently manifests as large-amplitude flailing motions of the limbs. Affected children frequently are usually unable to maintain a voluntary posture (e.g., tongue protrusion, hand grip).

The movement of athetosis is a slow, smooth, continuous writhing motion that prevents a child from maintaining a stable posture. It tends to affect a particular body region; distal (as opposed to proximal) extremities are more likely to be involved, plus the face, neck, and trunk can be affected. It can be worsened by intentional movement but also appears at rest. In children, athetosis rarely occurs in isolation; it frequently coexists with chorea (choreoathetosis), most commonly in a specific form of cerebral palsy (dyskinetic) in which dystonia is typically a predominant finding as well.

6 A variety of drugs can induce hyperkinetic movements. An acute dystonic reaction typically occurs very early in the course of medication use; later reactions can also occur. The correct classification of tardive dyskinesia is unclear; it may be a subtype of chorea. Other authors classify it as a dystonia or a mimicker of motor tics. It refers to a drug-induced syndrome of orofacial movements (e.g., tongue protrusion, lip smacking, puckering, grimacing). Neuroleptics and antiemetics (dopamine antagonists) are the most common causes. Chorea is more likely to occur with the abrupt discontinuation of a dopamine antagonist.

7 Sydenham chorea is an infrequent neurologic component of acute rheumatic fever. The onset is usually insidious, occurring several weeks to months after an acute group A β-hemolytic streptococcal infection and may be accompanied by emotional lability and hypotonia. The chorea is usually asymmetric, although involvement of bilateral metacarpophalangeal joints producing a "piano-playing" effect is also commonly reported. Acute and convalescent antistreptolysin O titers may confirm a recent strep infection, but the diagnosis of Sydenham chorea is clinical (negative titers do not exclude it). If suspected, a cardiac evaluation is essential to rule out rheumatic carditis.

8 Systemic disorders that may occasionally cause chorea include hyperthyroidism, hypoparathyroidism, systemic lupus erythematosus, and pregnancy. Encephalitis and Lyme disease are other rare causes.

9 Severe choreoathetosis is seen in a small percentage of children after bypass surgery ("post pump") for congenital heart disease. Diagnosis is clinical.

10 Choreoathetosis and ataxia are late findings of alternating hemiplegia of childhood (attacks of flaccid hemiplegia with nystagmus, dystonia, and tonic spells).

11 Benign hereditary (familial) chorea is an autosomal dominant disorder appearing early in childhood with mild but continuous (not episodic or paroxysmal) chorea. Intention tremor, dysarthria, hypotonia, and athetosis may also be present. Development may be delayed, but intelligence is normal. Diagnosis is clinical. The family history may be overlooked if incomplete expression of the disorder occurs in parents.

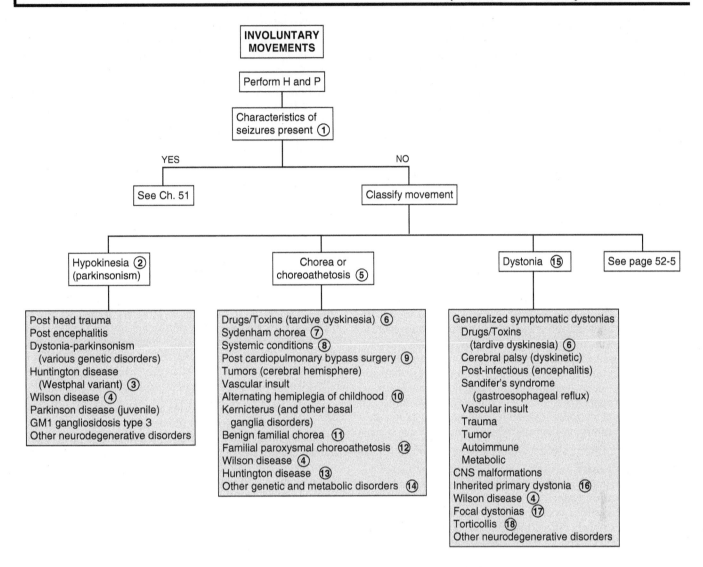

INVOLUNTARY MOVEMENTS

Perform H and P

Characteristics of seizures present ①

YES → See Ch. 51

NO → Classify movement

Hypokinesia ② (parkinsonism)

Post head trauma
Post encephalitis
Dystonia-parkinsonism
  (various genetic disorders)
Huntington disease
  (Westphal variant) ③
Wilson disease ④
Parkinson disease (juvenile)
GM1 gangliosidosis type 3
Other neurodegenerative disorders

Chorea or choreoathetosis ⑤

Drugs/Toxins (tardive dyskinesia) ⑥
Sydenham chorea ⑦
Systemic conditions ⑧
Post cardiopulmonary bypass surgery ⑨
Tumors (cerebral hemisphere)
Vascular insult
Alternating hemiplegia of childhood ⑩
Kernicterus (and other basal
  ganglia disorders)
Benign familial chorea ⑪
Familial paroxysmal choreoathetosis ⑫
Wilson disease ④
Huntington disease ⑬
Other genetic and metabolic disorders ⑭

Dystonia ⑮

See page 52-5

Generalized symptomatic dystonias
  Drugs/Toxins
    (tardive dyskinesia) ⑥
  Cerebral palsy (dyskinetic)
  Post-infectious (encephalitis)
  Sandifer's syndrome
    (gastroesophageal reflux)
  Vascular insult
  Trauma
  Tumor
  Autoimmune
  Metabolic
CNS malformations
Inherited primary dystonia ⑯
Wilson disease ④
Focal dystonias ⑰
Torticollis ⑱
Other neurodegenerative disorders

Nelson Textbook of Pediatrics, 19e. Chapters 587, 590
Nelsons Essentials, 6e. Chapter 183

12 Familial paroxysmal choreoathetosis is characterized by paroxysmal attacks of choreoathetosis, dystonia, or ballismus (flailing extremities). Episodes are short lived and may be triggered by startle or sudden movement or change in position.

13 Huntington disease is an autosomal dominant neurodegenerative disorder of the basal ganglia, which rarely presents in childhood. Rigidity and dystonia are the most common pediatric manifestations, although chorea, mental deterioration, behavioral problems, and seizures may also occur.

14 Other disorders that may include choreoathetosis include ataxia-telangiectasia (which may manifest with chorea without ataxia), Fahr disease, pantothenate kinase-associated neurodegeneration (previously Hallervorden-Spatz disease), neuroacanthocytosis disorders, and Lesch-Nyhan syndrome.

15 The definition of dystonia is "a movement disorder in which involuntary sustained or intermittent muscle contractions cause twisting and repetitive movements, abnormal postures, or both"; the term "torsion spasm" has also been used to describe this movement disorder. The movements can be brief or prolonged, they can be triggered by attempted movements (often only specific ones), they tend to occur in a particular pattern (resulting in identifiable postures) for a given child, and (with the exception of those associated with seizures) they are absent during sleep. Previously cocontraction (simultaneous contracture of agonist and antagonist muscles) was identified as a component of dystonia. Currently cocontraction is not believed to be common in dystonia; when it does occur, it is suspected to be an element (possibly voluntary) of compensation.

16 Several primary inherited dystonias are identified. Primary torsion dystonia (previously dystonia musculorum deformans) is an autosomal dominant disorder in children that typically begins with a focal dystonia (e.g., arm, leg, or larynx) and progresses to generalized involvement; one particular mutation is more common in the Ashkenazi Jewish population. Dopa-responsive dystonia (Segawa syndrome) is an autosomal dominant disorder characterized by dopamine deficiency; symptoms demonstrate a diurnal variation, with worsening over the course of the day and a dramatic response to levodopa.

17 Focal dystonias involve a specific body region; examples include writer's cramp, blepharospasm, torticollis, and opisthotonus. Blepharospasm (spasmodic eye closing) in children is often drug induced, although it occasionally occurs due to other causes of dystonia; it needs to be distinguished from tics.

18 When torticollis is associated with dystonia in the face or limbs, an MRI is indicated to rule out intracranial and cervical spine disorders.

19 Myoclonus describes a series of involuntary, repeated shock-like unidirectional muscle jerks. The sudden muscle contraction (positive myoclonus) may be followed by a period of muscle relaxation (negative myoclonus). The movements may occur in a random (multifocal) or generalized pattern; they may be rhythmic (myoclonus tremor) with fast and slow phases (correlating with contraction and relaxation); they can diminish but do not necessarily disappear during sleep, and movement may induce or worsen them. Myoclonus can be distinguished from tics because there is no preceding urge or suppressibility. It is more likely to signify a more ominous disorder in children than adults, although it can also be benign in children.

20 Physiologic myoclonus can be associated with sleep (at onset, during sleep, and when waking up); this is termed sleep or nocturnal myoclonus. It can also be associated with anxiety.

21 Benign myoclonus of infancy is characterized by clusters of jerks of the head, neck, and arms. These nonepileptic events are distinguished from the more ominous infantile myoclonic spasms by cessation at about 3 months of age, a normal EEG, and subsequent normal development.

22 Essential myoclonus is a chronic condition of jerking (focal, segmental, generalized) that may be sporadic or familial. Facial, trunk, and proximal muscles are typically affected, and no other neurologic problems are associated. Diagnosis is clinical. EEGs and imaging studies are normal.

23 Juvenile myoclonic epilepsy (previously Janz syndrome) is one of the most common epilepsies of childhood. The onset is typically in adolescence, and it is characterized by myoclonic movements, generalized tonic-clonic seizures, and absence seizures. The myoclonic jerks are frequently the first manifestation; they are most prominent in the morning (causing the patient to drop things) but are often ignored and diagnosis is delayed until a generalized seizure occurs. Characteristic EEG findings are bilateral, symmetrical spike and polyspike-and-wave discharges of 3.5 Hz to 6 Hz.

24 Myoclonus and opsoclonus may occur together as a syndrome with or without ataxia. The condition is characterized by opsoclonus (flurries of conjugate eye movements) and severe myoclonic jerking of the trunk and head. It may occur as an idiopathic disorder, due to encephalitis, or as a paraneoplastic disorder, most commonly associated with neuroblastoma.

25 Tremor is an involuntary, rhythmic continuous oscillatory (to-and-fro) movement about a joint axis. The speed and the direction of the movement is the same in both directions. Depending on when it is most noticeable, a tremor may be designated as "rest", "postural", or "action". "Intention tremor" implies a worsening tremor as an intentional movement approaches its target; it is associated with cerebellar dysfunction.

26 A low level physiologic tremor is normal in all people. It may be exacerbated by stress, anxiety, and certain medications.

27 Jitteriness occurs in response to a stimulus and is common in normal full-term infants, lasting for a few weeks. Etiologies that should be considered include hypoxic-ischemic encephalopathy, drug withdrawal, hypoglycemia, hypomagnesemia, hypocalcemia, and intracranial hemorrhage. In contrast to seizures, eye deviations and altered respiratory patterns do not occur with jitteriness. Normal jitteriness can be stopped by gently touching and flexing the moving limb.

28 Essential (familial) tremor is an inherited condition that affects only the limb being used. It may manifest simply as incoordination in young children; with time it is more clearly associated with action. The rhythmicity and the absence of worsening toward the end of an intentional movement distinguish it from cerebellar dysfunction (dysmetria).

29 Motor tics are distinctly recognizable purposeless movements or movement fragments that are characteristically associated with a preceding urge to perform the movement and are suppressible (at least briefly). They may occur as simple brief movements or as part of a more complex series of movements. Phonic tics involve simple vocalizations. Tics tend to vary over time, manifesting with different movements and frequency and typically disappearing after a certain period. They are often triggered by an identifiable stressor (e.g., fatigue, anxiety, excitement). Stereotypical movements (stereotypies) are repeated benign purposeless movements that appear intentional and can be suppressed without tension (examples are foot tapping or hair twisting).

(30) Transient tics, typically eye blinking or facial movements, may last several weeks or up to one year and are often associated with a positive family history.

(31) Tourette syndrome is a life-long condition of vocal and motor tics that begins between 2 and 15 years of age. Attention deficit disorder and obsessive-compulsive behaviors occur in many cases. Symptoms are typically exacerbated by stress. Diagnosis is clinical.

(32) Childhood acute neuropsychiatric symptoms (CANS) is a proposed classification encompassing an acute dramatic onset of neuropsychiatric symptoms in children, including tics and obsessive-compulsive disorder (OCD). It is proposed to replace pediatric autoimmune neuropsychiatric disorder associated with streptococci (PANDAS) because several controversies have developed around that syndrome.

(33) Mirror movements are involuntary movements of one side of the body that mirror intentional movements of the opposite side of the body. They are normal starting in infancy and may persist up to 10 years of age.

Bibliography

Delgado MR, Albright AL: Movement disorders in children: definitions, classifications, and grading systems, *J Child Neurol* 18: S1–S8, 2003.

Piña-Garza JE: Movement disorders. In Piña-Garza JE, editor: *Fenichel's clinical pediatric neurology*, ed 7, Philadelphia, 2013, Saunders/Elsevier, pp 277–294.

Sanger TD, Chen D, Fehlings DL, et al: Definition and classification of hyperkinetic movements in childhood, *Mov Disord* 25:1538–1549, 2010.

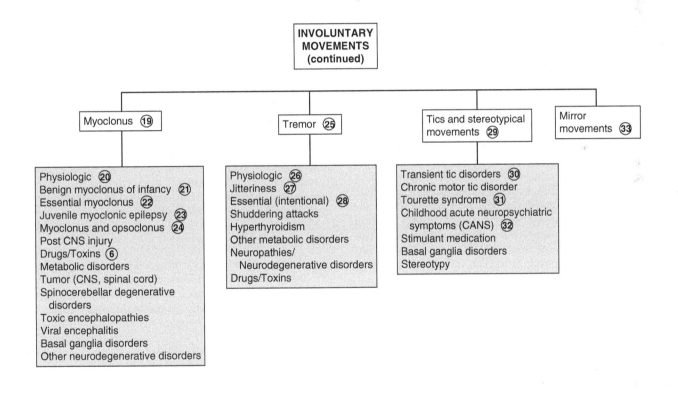

Chapter 53
HYPOTONIA AND WEAKNESS

Weakness is generally a complaint of the older child. Young infants are more likely to present with hypotonia than weakness. Although the two frequently occur together, they are not synonymous. Active tone is physiologic resistance to movement; passive tone is range of motion around joints. Hypotonia is a reduction in joint resistance to passive range of motion. Weakness relates to strength of (or power generated by) muscle. Any component of the nervous system may be responsible. Brain disorders are more common in hypotonic infants, whereas neuromuscular disorders are more likely in older children.

1 When considering a floppy infant, signs or symptoms suggestive of a cerebral disorder include seizures, impaired level of consciousness, poor feeding, jitteriness, dysmorphic features, organ malformations, fisting of hands, brisk deep tendon reflexes, clonus, and autonomic dysfunction. Pertinent history includes perinatal events (including a history of drug or teratogen exposure), intrauterine movements, birth weight, and a family history of infant deaths or neuromuscular disorders. A history of traumatic or precipitous birth may be a risk factor for intracranial hemorrhage. The degree and distribution of the hypotonia and weakness are significant to the diagnosis. Hypotonic infants manifest significant joint hyperextensibility (scarf sign) and abnormal postural reflexes (e.g., traction response, axillary suspension, ventral suspension). They usually have markedly diminished spontaneous movements. The persistence of primitive reflexes (e.g., Moro, tonic neck reflex) in the absence of spontaneous movements is suggestive of a cerebral disorder; the absence of deep tendon reflexes is more suggestive of a peripheral (motor neuron unit) disorder. Occasionally, characteristic facies or physical stigmata will suggest the diagnosis (e.g., Down syndrome, Prader-Willi syndrome).

A feeding and developmental history is relevant in the assessment of older infants and toddlers. For the older child presenting with weakness, inquire about fatigability, falling, school (cognitive) performance, and the possibility of ingestions, as well as a family history. In toddlers and older children, strength can be assessed by observation of various tasks (e.g., standing on one foot, running, climbing stairs, rising to stand from a sitting or lying position [Gower sign]).

2 Hypotonia and weakness are almost universal findings in infants with Down syndrome. The strength improves, but the hypotonia persists as they grow older. Infants with Prader-Willi syndrome present with marked hypotonia, poor suck and feeding difficulties in early infancy. Characteristic phenotypic features (e.g., narrow bifrontal diameter, almond-shaped palpebrae, short stature, small hands and feet), hypogonadism, pathologic food seeking behaviors and obesity become evident later in childhood. Weakness improves in these children, although the hypotonia persists. MECP2 duplication is an x-linked condition causing infantile hypotonia, progressive spasticity, recurrent respiratory infections, and seizures.

3 Myasthenia gravis is a spectrum of disorders characterized by easy fatigability of muscles due to either an immune-mediated neuromuscular blockade or a disorder of the motor endplate. Transient neonatal myasthenia gravis occurs due to transfer of maternal antibodies from an affected mother to her fetus; affected infants can demonstrate hypotonia, poor feeding, and even respiratory insufficiency, which will resolve without further sequelae as the abnormal antibodies disappear. The juvenile form of myasthenia gravis is an acquired autoimmune disorder that occurs due to the presence of anti-acetylcholine receptor antibodies; it may begin in late infancy or childhood. Congenital myasthenia gravis syndromes are rare hereditary deficiencies of motor endplate acetylcholinesterase production or function (including defects of its receptors). Ptosis and extraocular muscle weakness are the most common symptoms. Rapid fatigue of muscles with worsening symptoms as the day progresses is characteristic. Diagnosis is confirmed by characteristic electromyography (EMG) findings. Anti-acetylcholine antibodies are only present in the immune-mediated versions (not in the congenital forms), and their presence is inconsistent in neonates born to mothers affected with myasthenia gravis. Rapid symptomatic improvement with a short-acting cholinesterase inhibitor (edrophonium or prostigmine methylsulfate) is a clinical diagnostic test; it should be performed only in infants and children meeting specific criteria and only in a setting with critical care support available.

4 In congenital myotonic dystrophy, severe hypotonia, weakness, swallowing and sucking difficulties, congenital joint contractures, and sometimes respiratory insufficiency are evident at birth; these are usually infants born to mothers with symptomatic myotonic dystrophy. In childhood-onset myotonic dystrophy, myotonia (a disturbance of muscle relaxation) may be the first symptom. It may precede the distal weakness by several years. Facial weakness is also characteristic. EMG findings are characteristic later in childhood, and genetic testing is available for definitive diagnosis; diagnosis of the neonatal form, however, is usually based on clinical findings (often supported by a family history).

5 Creatine kinase (CK) is released by damaged or degenerating muscle fibers. Electromyography measures the electric potentials during various states of muscle contractions and may identify certain types of muscle diseases. Muscle biopsy can distinguish between neurogenic and myopathic processes, and histochemical studies will identify specific metabolic myopathies. More specialized molecular and biochemical testing may be necessary when metabolic disorders or progressive encephalopathies are suggested. The evaluation for a metabolic disorder should include blood for a CBC, electrolytes, pH, glucose, ammonia, lactate, acylcarnitine profile, and amino acids and urine for ketones, reducing substances, organic acids, and carnitine. Neurologic and/or genetic consultation should be considered for specific recommendations for testing based on clinical suspicions.

6 Systemic disorders may cause hypotonia due to a disturbance of cerebral function. The onset may be acute or insidious. Depending on the clinical picture, laboratory studies to assess serum electrolytes, renal and thyroid function, and to rule out infection should be considered. A lumbar puncture (LP) and cerebral spinal fluid (CSF) evaluation may be necessary to rule out certain suspected infectious causes. If symptoms have been

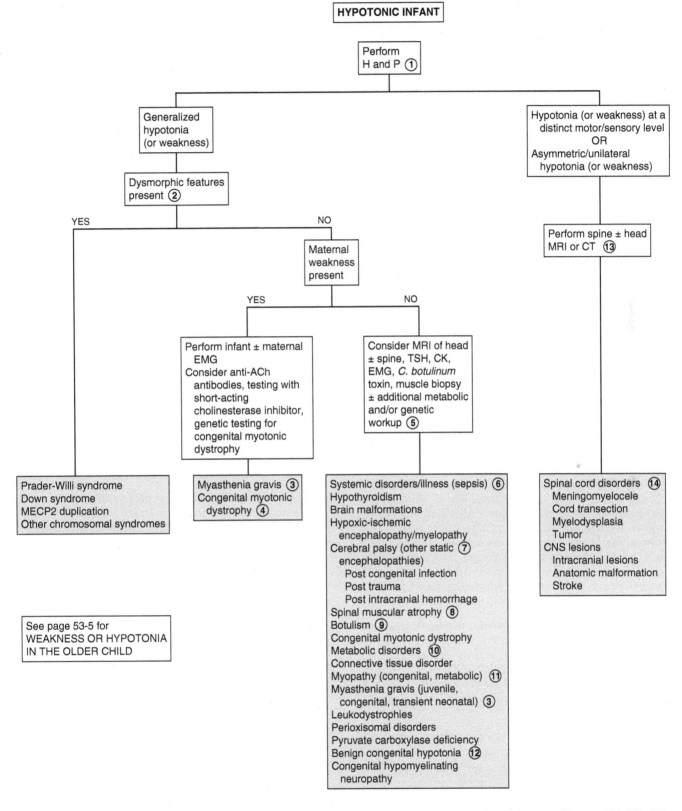

HYPOTONIC INFANT

Perform H and P ①

Generalized hypotonia (or weakness)

Hypotonia (or weakness) at a distinct motor/sensory level OR Asymmetric/unilateral hypotonia (or weakness)

Dysmorphic features present ②

YES   NO

Maternal weakness present

Perform spine ± head MRI or CT ⑬

YES   NO

Perform infant ± maternal EMG
Consider anti-ACh antibodies, testing with short-acting cholinesterase inhibitor, genetic testing for congenital myotonic dystrophy

Consider MRI of head ± spine, TSH, CK, EMG, *C. botulinum* toxin, muscle biopsy ± additional metabolic and/or genetic workup ⑤

Prader-Willi syndrome
Down syndrome
MECP2 duplication
Other chromosomal syndromes

Myasthenia gravis ③
Congenital myotonic dystrophy ④

Systemic disorders/illness (sepsis) ⑥
Hypothyroidism
Brain malformations
Hypoxic-ischemic encephalopathy/myelopathy
Cerebral palsy (other static ⑦ encephalopathies)
    Post congenital infection
    Post trauma
    Post intracranial hemorrhage
Spinal muscular atrophy ⑧
Botulism ⑨
Congenital myotonic dystrophy
Metabolic disorders ⑩
Connective tissue disorder
Myopathy (congenital, metabolic) ⑪
Myasthenia gravis (juvenile, congenital, transient neonatal) ③
Leukodystrophies
Perioxisomal disorders
Pyruvate carboxylase deficiency
Benign congenital hypotonia ⑫
Congenital hypomyelinating neuropathy

Spinal cord disorders ⑭
    Meningomyelocele
    Cord transection
    Myelodysplasia
    Tumor
CNS lesions
    Intracranial lesions
    Anatomic malformation
    Stroke

See page 53-5 for WEAKNESS OR HYPOTONIA IN THE OLDER CHILD

Nelson Textbook of Pediatrics, 19e. Chapters 584, 599–608
Nelsons Essentials, 6e. Chapter 182

chronic or other neurologic abnormalities exist, a metabolic investigation should also be done. If a genetic disorder is suspected, chromosome studies including microarray and consultation with a geneticist may be helpful.

7 Cerebral palsy (CP) is a static encephalopathy, a nonprogressive clinical disorder characterized by varying degrees of mental and motor impairment. Rarely, hypotonia is prominent or persistent. In most cases hypotonia will progress to spasticity and dyskinetic movements. Commonly identified causes of CP include perinatal hypoxia or asphyxia, congenital infection and intracranial hemorrhage or trauma; many cases are likely due to undetected prenatal events.

8 In spinal muscular atrophies, degenerative loss of anterior horn cells in the spinal cord and brainstem motor neurons occurs. Progressive weakness develops in variants presenting in infants; juvenile variants of this disorder present beyond infancy. Diagnosis is by EMG, DNA probes, and muscle biopsy.

9 Infantile botulism most commonly occurs in infants between 2 weeks and 6 months of age. Source of the spores carrying the toxin of *Clostridium botulinum* may be honey, corn syrup, soil or dust. Infants present with a descending flaccid paralysis. Cranial nerve symptoms are typically noted first (manifesting as poor suck, feeble cry, drooling); fever is characteristically absent. A recent history including poor feeding, constipation, weak cry and smile, hypotonia, ptosis, and mydriasis is common. Clinical diagnosis is key to early intervention; diagnosis is confirmed by recovery of the organism or toxin from stool, blood, or food sources. Older children can present with food-borne botulism due to ingestion of preformed toxin in poorly canned foods.

10 Metabolic disorders (particularly inborn errors of metabolism) usually appear in the neonatal period, although partial or incomplete errors may not appear until later. A complaint of hypotonia combined with a history of recurrent bouts of lethargy, vomiting, acidosis, and other neurologic findings should prompt appropriate metabolic screening laboratory studies. Some of the conditions to be considered include amino acid disorders, organic acidemia, urea cycle defects, fatty acid oxidation defects, adrenal insufficiency, and mitochondrial disorders.

11 Developmental disorders of muscle are referred to as congenital myopathies; they are characterized by infantile hypotonia and weakness of variable severity and are generally nonprogressive. Serum CK values are typically normal; diagnosis is usually by muscle biopsy. Metabolic myopathies include errors of glycogen and lipid metabolism as well as disorders of mitochondrial function.

12 Benign congenital hypotonia is a diagnosis of exclusion; it describes a nonprogressive hypotonia affecting infants and children with no clear etiology, little or no developmental delay, and a generally good prognosis.

13 If acute intracranial hemorrhage is suspected (e.g., traumatic birth, depressed skull fracture, other head trama), a head CT is the most appropriate urgent imaging study.

14 Spinal cord disorders often present with hyperreflexia, clonus, a positive Babinski sign, and defined sensory loss in the extremities. Hypotonia may be the prominent acute sign in infants. The diagnosis should be considered in infants with hypotonia after a difficult delivery (particularly breech deliveries).

In older children disorders include traumatic transection, spinal cord tumor, transverse myelitis, and epidural spinal abscesses. Hypotonia is subsequently replaced by hypertonia.

15 Proximal leg weakness, wasting, and cramps are typically the initial manifestations of GM2-gangliosidosis, an autosomal recessive disorder of hexosaminidase A deficiency with several phenotypic variants (including Tay-Sachs disease).

16 Duchenne muscular dystrophy (DMD), an x-linked recessive disorder, is the most common type of muscular dystrophy. Diagnosis is usually in late infancy or early childhood when a child presents with the hyperlordotic posture and Gower sign, typically by age 3 years. A Trendelenburg gait, muscle atrophy, and pseudohypertrophy of the calves subsequently develop. Toe walking and frequent falling are common; a history of delayed motor milestones may be noted retrospectively. Duchenne and Becker muscular dystrophies are both caused by a defect in the muscle protein dystrophin; Becker muscular dystrophy (BMD) has a later onset and less severe course. Genetic testing for the dystrophin gene defect is diagnostic if the CK is elevated and the clinical picture is consistent with DMD. Muscle biopsy may be needed if the genetic testing is normal; it may also be useful in distinguishing between DMD and BMD.

17 Guillain-Barré syndrome is an acute demyelinating polyneuropathy characterized by an ascending motor weakness and areflexia; sensory and autonomic nerves may be affected. Respiratory compromise can occur if respiratory muscles are involved. The syndrome frequently follows an upper respiratory tract infection or *Campylobacter* diarrhea. Elevated CSF protein without pleocytosis is characteristic; EMG results are consistent with acute denervation of muscle.

18 The most common causes of progressive distal weakness are neuropathies, most of which are familial. Dysesthesias (painful tingling and burning sensations) often accompany the weakness. Autonomic symptoms (e.g., orthostatic hypotension, gastrointestinal dysmotility, abnormal sweating) may be present, and deep tendon reflexes are usually markedly diminished relative to the degree of weakness. Diagnosis of these disorders is by nerve conduction velocity studies and EMG. A lumbar puncture and an evaluation of the CSF may be necessary to rule out certain suspected infectious causes. For example, nonpolio enteroviruses may cause poliomyelitis-like disease.

19 Several species of North American ticks carry a toxin that can cause a paralysis clinically similar to Guillain-Barré syndrome. Tendon reflexes are usually diminished. Sensation is preserved, but burning or tingling may occur.

20 Scapulohumeral or scapuloperoneal syndromes have characteristics of both nerve and muscle disease; patients present with proximal arm and distal leg weakness.

21 Transverse myelitis presents acutely with hypotonia and weakness. There is an identifiable motor-sensory level, impaired bowel and bladder function, hyperreflexia, and an abnormal Babinski sign. In children younger than 3 years old, spinal cord dysfunction symptoms develop rapidly (hours to days); in older children the symptoms develop more gradually (days to weeks). Spinal MRI shows abnormal signal intensity of the involved level, and CSF examination shows a mild pleocytosis and elevated protein level (specifically myelin basic protein and immunoglobulins).

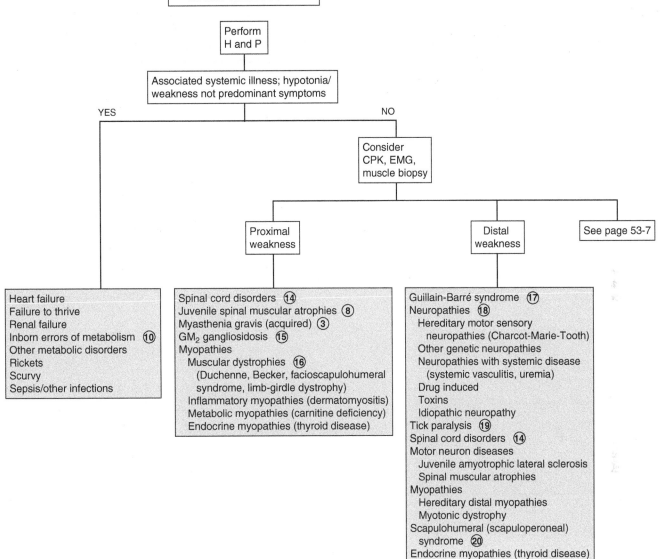

WEAKNESS OR HYPOTONIA IN THE OLDER CHILD

Perform H and P

Associated systemic illness; hypotonia/ weakness not predominant symptoms

YES

NO

Consider CPK, EMG, muscle biopsy

Proximal weakness

Distal weakness

See page 53-7

Heart failure
Failure to thrive
Renal failure
Inborn errors of metabolism ⑩
Other metabolic disorders
Rickets
Scurvy
Sepsis/other infections

Spinal cord disorders ⑭
Juvenile spinal muscular atrophies ⑧
Myasthenia gravis (acquired) ③
GM₂ gangliosidosis ⑮
Myopathies
    Muscular dystrophies ⑯
        (Duchenne, Becker, facioscapulohumeral
        syndrome, limb-girdle dystrophy)
    Inflammatory myopathies (dermatomyositis)
    Metabolic myopathies (carnitine deficiency)
    Endocrine myopathies (thyroid disease)

Guillain-Barré syndrome ⑰
Neuropathies ⑱
    Hereditary motor sensory
        neuropathies (Charcot-Marie-Tooth)
    Other genetic neuropathies
    Neuropathies with systemic disease
        (systemic vasculitis, uremia)
    Drug induced
    Toxins
    Idiopathic neuropathy
Tick paralysis ⑲
Spinal cord disorders ⑭
Motor neuron diseases
    Juvenile amyotrophic lateral sclerosis
    Spinal muscular atrophies
Myopathies
    Hereditary distal myopathies
    Myotonic dystrophy
Scapulohumeral (scapuloperoneal)
    syndrome ⑳
Endocrine myopathies (thyroid disease)

22 In periodic paralysis, patients experience episodes of severe weakness, often followed by partial or complete paralysis. Episodes are usually related to hypokalemia or hyperkalemia and may be primary (genetically transmitted) or secondary due to endocrine, renal, or gastrointestinal causes of hypokalemia or hyperkalemia.

Bibliography

Peredo DE, Hannibal MC: The floppy infant: Evaluation of hypotonia, *Pediatr Rev* 30:e66–76, 2009.

Piña-Garza JE: The hypotonic infant. In Piña-Garza JE, editor: *Fenichel's clinical pediatric neurology*, ed 7, Philadelphia, 2013, Saunders/Elsevier, pp 147–169.

Piña-Garza JE: Flaccid limb weakness in childhood. In Piña-Garza JE, editor: *Fenichel's clinical pediatric neurology*, ed 7, Philadelphia, 2013, Saunders/Elsevier, pp 170–194.

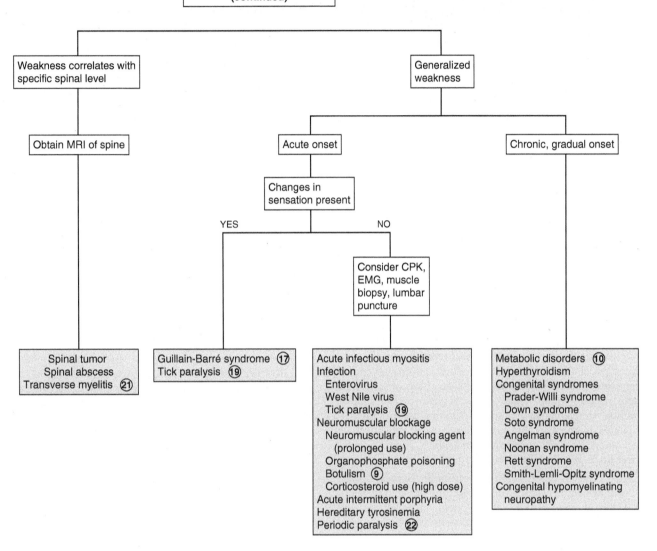

WEAKNESS OR HYPOTONIA
IN THE OLDER CHILD
(continued)

Weakness correlates with specific spinal level

Generalized weakness

Obtain MRI of spine

Acute onset

Chronic, gradual onset

Changes in sensation present

YES

NO

Consider CPK, EMG, muscle biopsy, lumbar puncture

Spinal tumor
Spinal abscess
Transverse myelitis ㉑

Guillain-Barré syndrome ⑰
Tick paralysis ⑲

Acute infectious myositis
Infection
    Enterovirus
    West Nile virus
    Tick paralysis ⑲
Neuromuscular blockage
    Neuromuscular blocking agent
        (prolonged use)
    Organophosphate poisoning
    Botulism ⑨
    Corticosteroid use (high dose)
Acute intermittent porphyria
Hereditary tyrosinemia
Periodic paralysis ㉒

Metabolic disorders ⑩
Hyperthyroidism
Congenital syndromes
    Prader-Willi syndrome
    Down syndrome
    Soto syndrome
    Angelman syndrome
    Noonan syndrome
    Rett syndrome
    Smith-Lemli-Opitz syndrome
Congenital hypomyelinating
    neuropathy

Chapter 54
ATAXIA

Ataxia is a disturbance of the fine control of movement and posture that is normally coordinated by the cerebellum and its input and output pathways; dysfunction of the posterior columns can also be causative. It is often a benign phenomenon in children; however, an acute presentation warrants evaluation to rule out a serious CNS disorder.

1. The approach to an acquired ataxia is based primarily on the temporal course (i.e., acute, episodic, chronic). Acute ataxia typically presents as an unsteady, wide-based gait or refusal to walk; uncoordinated upper extremity movements may also be noted. A careful history is essential to prevent unnecessary testing. Inquire about acutely associated symptoms (e.g., fever, systemic illness, headache, vomiting, nystagmus, diplopia, vertigo), and also about the child's general health or more subtle symptoms that may have occurred over preceding weeks or months. Ask about conditions that may put a child at risk for thromboembolic disease. Recent trauma, a family history of similar episodes and access to potential toxins or ingestions are also important. Consider that any acute ataxia could be the initial presentation of an episodic or recurrent disorder.

The physical examination should include a thorough neurological assessment, including careful observation of gait, tone, strength, reflexes, maintenance of truncal posture, coordination of voluntary movements, and speech. Cranial nerves (particularly related to the eye), the fundoscopic exam, alterations in mental status (including excessive irritability), and any asymmetrical findings should be noted.

2. Ataxia due to posterior fossa tumors develops gradually but may acutely worsen due to bleeding or rapid development of hydrocephalus. Headaches, personality changes, and abnormal neurologic exam findings consistent with increased intracranial pressure are common.

3. Vertebral artery dissection should be suspected when ataxia develops after neck injuries.

4. Vascular disorders (e.g., stroke, transient ischemic attack [TIA], vasculitis) are rare as a cause of ataxia in children; children with a risk of thromboembolic disease (including Kawasaki disease) are at higher risk.

5. Ataxia or an unsteady gait may be prominent after a head injury due to hemorrhage or cerebellar contusion; it can also accompany concussion. Symptoms of postconcussive syndromes may last 1 to 6 months; ataxia in affected children may be significant. Imaging at the time of the injury is recommended to rule out intracranial hemorrhage.

6. Drug ingestion is one of the most common causes of acute ataxia; some level of mental status changes frequently accompanies the ataxia in these cases. Anticonvulsants, benzodiazepines, alcohol, and antihistamines are commonly implicated; thorough questioning may be required to identify ingestion histories. Accidental ingestions are most common prior to school age, but peak again in adolescence with substance abuse. Urine toxicology screens detect a limited number of substances; specific screens for suspected agents should be performed.

7. Ataxia may occur in patients who experience certain subtypes of migraine with aura (i.e., basilar-type, hemiplegic). Occasionally these headache manifestations will occur in school-age children.

8. In benign paroxysmal vertigo, toddlers and preschool children are affected by brief episodes of sudden imbalance. True ataxia does not occur, but the vertigo is so severe that the child collapses on the floor and is often frightened to the point that he or she refuses to stand or walk. Nystagmus may be evident, consciousness is not impaired, and headache is absent. Diagnosis is clinical.

9. Specific genetic defects for many metabolic disorders causing episodic or recurrent ataxia are being increasingly identified. In general, the first episode of such disorders resembles an acute ataxia; developmental delays or regression, family history of similar disorders (or consanguinity), associated symptoms of altered mental status, vomiting and diarrhea, unusual body odors, and (ultimately) a pattern of recurrence associated with illness, dietary changes, or other stressors are consistent with these diagnoses. Examples include Hartnup disease (associated with aminoaciduria and nicotinamide deficiency causing photosensitivity), maple syrup urine disease (the intermittent form causes recurrent attacks of ataxia and encephalopathy during times of stress), and pyruvate dehydrogenase deficiency.

10. Episodic genetic ataxias (not associated with metabolic disorders) are also being increasingly identified through genetic advances. Ion channel mutations have been identified as causative in two autosomal dominant episodic ataxias: episodic ataxia type 1 (paroxysmal ataxia and myokymia) and episodic ataxia type 2 (acetazolamide-responsive ataxia).

11. Multiple sclerosis rarely will present under 6 years of age. Acute ataxia, usually in association with fever is the most common initial presentation. Definitive diagnosis is usually not made until recurrent attacks have occurred, although imaging may suggest the diagnosis after the initial attack.

12. Ataxia-telangiectasia is an autosomal recessive degenerative ataxia with associated immunologic abnormalities. The ataxia manifests at approximately 2 years of age and progresses to an inability to walk by adolescence. Disturbance of voluntary gaze, strabismus and nystagmus are also common. Telangiectasias develop in mid-childhood (commonly affecting bulbar conjunctivae, nose, ears, and exposed extremity surfaces), and diminished immunoglobulin levels predispose children to recurrent sinopulmonary infections.

13. Friedreich ataxia is an autosomal recessive disorder characterized by a slowly progressive ataxia, dysarthric speech, nystagmus, and skeletal abnormalities (flat feet, hammertoes, progressive kyphoscoliosis). Onset is usually before age 10 years. Significant weakness and sensory loss in distal hands and feet are typical. A cardiac evaluation should be performed to rule out an associated cardiomyopathy.

14. Other progressive hereditary ataxias include spinocerebellar degenerations, hypobetalipoproteinemia, abetalipoproteinemia, ataxia with oculomotor apraxia type I, juvenile sulfate lipidosis, juvenile GM2-gangliosidosis, Refsum disease, and Marinesco-Sjögren syndrome. A small number of x-linked disorders featuring

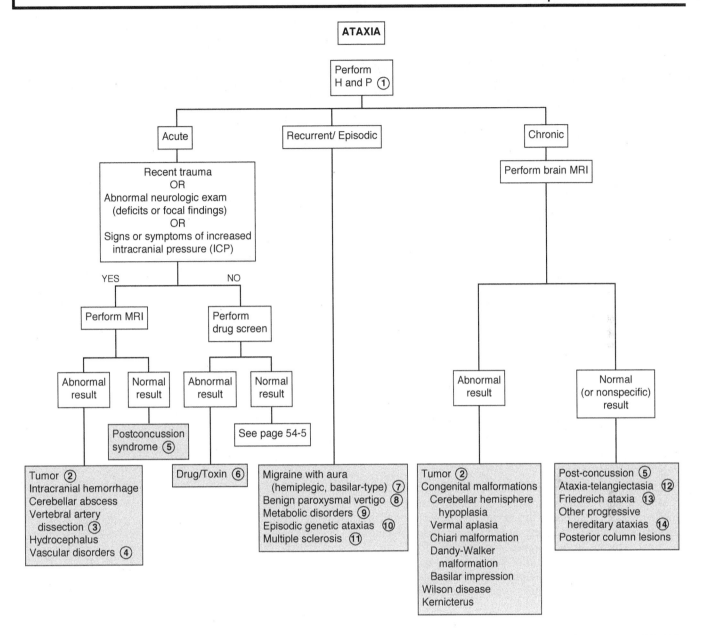

Nelson Textbook of Pediatrics, 19e. Chapters 590, 593, 633
Nelsons Essentials, 6e. Chapter 183

ataxia are also recognized. The majority of these conditions will be diagnosed clinically or via specific blood or genetic tests; neuroimaging is usually not contributory. Any of the acute recurrent ataxias (e.g., Hartnup disease, maple syrup urine disease) may eventually become progressive without return to baseline between attacks.

15 Labryinthitis can complicate acute otitis media, sinusitis, mastoiditis or bacterial meningitis. Severe vertigo, vomiting, nystagmus and hearing loss may also be present.

16 Acute cerebellar ataxia (acute postinfectious cerebellitis) is the most common acute ataxia in children (approximately 40% of all cases). The etiology is generally a postinfectious cerebellar demyelination, which is presumed to be the result of an autoimmune reaction following infection. (Immunization has been suspected of inciting this condition, but evidence does not support this theory.) A preceding illness (5 to 21 days) is identified in most cases; varicella is no longer the most commonly identified infectious trigger due to universal varicella immunization. The onset is acute ataxia and truncal instability with maximal severity at the onset; occasionally a child is unable to walk at all at the onset. Head titubation (bobbing), tremor, dysmetria, and ocular abnormalities may also occur, but mental status is always normal and reflexes are preserved. The diagnosis is one of exclusion. A drug screen is probably the most appropriate test to be done acutely to rule out unsuspected ingestions; other testing serves primarily to rule out other etiologies. As improvement should begin within a few days in acute cerebellar ataxia, imaging should be performed if rapid improvement of the ataxia does not occur. If a lumbar puncture is performed, findings are usually normal or may show mild pleocytosis with an increased CSF protein level. Most children will fully recover.

17 Acute disseminated encephalomyelitis (acute postinfectious demyelinating encephalomyelitis) is another postinfectious, immune-mediated condition with a more severe presentation than acute cerebellar ataxia, including altered mental status, seizures (which may progress to status epilepticus), and multifocal neurologic defects. MRI will show foci of demyelination and an LP, if performed, will reveal normal findings or may show mild pleocytosis with an increased CSF protein level. Repeated episodes may suggest multiple sclerosis.

18 The Miller-Fisher syndrome is considered a variant of Guillain-Barré syndrome, although it is also suspected to be a variant of brainstem encephalitis. The cranial nerves are affected by the immune-mediated demyelination in this condition. Ataxia, ophthalmoplegia, and areflexia occur after an infectious illness (particularly *Campylobacter* gastroenteritis). Vertical gaze is characteristically affected while horizontal gaze is typically preserved. The areflexia aids in distinguishing this from acute postinfectious ataxia. CSF examination results vary based on the timing relative to symptom onset; an elevated protein without an increased cell count is characteristic later in the course.

19 Ataxia and cranial nerve dysfunction characterize brainstem encephalitis; mental status changes, hemiparesis and respiratory irregularities can also occur. Epstein-Barr virus, *Listeria,* and enterovirus (type 71) have been identified as etiologies. MRI will show increased signal intensity in the brainstem. Evaluation of the CSF shows pleocytosis, normal glucose levels, and normal or slightly elevated protein levels. Brainstem auditory evoked response testing indicates abnormalities within the brainstem; EEGs will be normal. Neuroimaging will yield nonspecific findings but will rule out other etiologies.

20 Opsoclonus-myoclonus syndrome is characterized by opsoclonus, myoclonus, ataxia, and encephalopathy. It may occur as a postinfectious entity, but is clearly recognized as a paraneoplastic cerebellar syndrome and should prompt an investigation for neuroblastoma or (rarely) other neoplasms.

21 Acute episodic ataxia ("pseudoataxia") may rarely be the only clinical manifestation of nonconvulsive seizure activity. EEG is diagnostic.

Bibliography

Friday JH: Ataxia. In Fleisher G, Ludwig S, editors: *Textbook of pediatric emergency medicine*, ed 6, Philadelphia, 2010, Lippincott Williams & Wilkins, pp 164–167.

Piña-Garza JE, Ataxia: In Piña-Garza JE, editor: *Fenichel's clinical pediatric neurology*, ed 7, Philadelphia, 2013, Saunders/Elsevier, pp 215–235.

Ryan MM, Engle EC: Topical review: Acute ataxia in childhood, *J Child Neurol* 18:309–316, 2003.

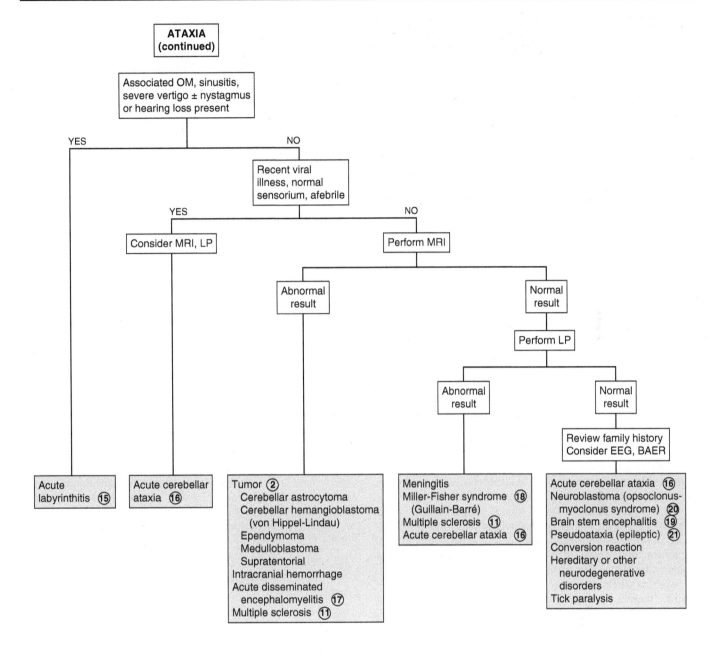

ATAXIA
(continued)

Associated OM, sinusitis,
severe vertigo ± nystagmus
or hearing loss present

YES

NO

Recent viral
illness, normal
sensorium, afebrile

YES

NO

Consider MRI, LP

Perform MRI

Abnormal
result

Normal
result

Perform LP

Abnormal
result

Normal
result

Review family history
Consider EEG, BAER

Acute
labyrinthitis ⑮

Acute cerebellar
ataxia ⑯

Tumor ②
  Cerebellar astrocytoma
  Cerebellar hemangioblastoma
    (von Hippel-Lindau)
  Ependymoma
  Medulloblastoma
  Supratentorial
Intracranial hemorrhage
Acute disseminated
  encephalomyelitis ⑰
Multiple sclerosis ⑪

Meningitis
Miller-Fisher syndrome ⑱
  (Guillain-Barré)
Multiple sclerosis ⑪
Acute cerebellar ataxia ⑯

Acute cerebellar ataxia ⑯
Neuroblastoma (opsoclonus-
  myoclonus syndrome) ⑳
Brain stem encephalitis ⑲
Pseudoataxia (epileptic) ㉑
Conversion reaction
Hereditary or other
  neurodegenerative
  disorders
Tick paralysis

Chapter 55
ALTERED MENTAL STATUS

An alteration in consciousness (awareness of self and environment) may range from delirium (e.g., irritability, confusion, agitation) to coma. A delirious state is often characterized by alternating periods of lucidity and frequently progresses to lethargy or coma.

1 A child presenting with any alteration in consciousness must be emergently stabilized before a search is started for the cause. The patient should then be evaluated to rule out a potentially life-threatening intracranial process that requires urgent treatment. The Glasgow Coma Scale (GCS) is the most widely used tool for assessing and monitoring changes in mental status. The GCS utilizes eye opening, motor responses, and verbal responses and is a more objective means of describing altered levels of consciousness when compared with less specific terms such as stuporous, obtunded, or lethargic. Any focality or asymmetry of the neurologic examination could suggest a problem localized to one cerebral hemisphere.

The history should include a recent review of systems and a history of trauma, medications, and possible toxic ingestions.

Certain components of the physical examination may suggest an underlying systemic disorder. For example, certain skin findings may suggest neurocutaneous disorders, Addison disease, anemia, carbon monoxide poisoning, or infectious conditions; needle track marks and signs of trauma should also be noted. Hepatomegaly can suggest hepatic failure (Reye syndrome) or heart failure. Fractured extremities raise the possibility of a fat embolism. Toxidromes (such as apnea and pinpoint pupils associated with opiates) help identify a possible ingestion.

A patient's breathing pattern may aid in the diagnosis of altered mental status. Hyperventilation occurs with toxic-metabolic encephalopathies, increased intracranial pressure, and metabolic acidosis. Hypoventilation occurs with many drug ingestions. Other breathing patterns (e.g., Cheyne-Stokes, apneustic breathing) may indicate specific sites of CNS dysfunction. The odor of the breath may be helpful. Many disorders and certain ingestions are accompanied by a characteristic odor.

Serum glucose and urine toxicology screens are recommended as first line lab evaluations; subsequent lab work can be obtained based on a suspected cause. Tests to be considered are a CBC, electrolytes, blood urea nitrogen, creatinine, calcium, magnesium, phosphorus, liver function tests, and an arterial blood gas analysis. Blood cultures, thyroid studies, serum ammonia levels, and serum osmolality may be helpful; an osmolal gap and anion gap should be calculated, especially if an ingestion is suspected. An EKG may reveal arrhythmias or characteristics of certain toxidromes.

2 A lumbar puncture is contraindicated in children if they have any of the following: (1) cardiorespiratory compromise, (2) focal neurologic findings or other suspicion of mass lesion, (3) signs of increased intracranial pressure other than a bulging fontanel, (4) skin or soft tissue infection overlying the site of the lumbar puncture or (5) thrombocytopenia.

3 MRI is helpful in the diagnosis of acute disseminated encephalomyelitis (ADEM), a condition in which symptoms related to the encephalopathy predominate (e.g., confusion, irritability, occasionally coma). MRI typically shows white matter lesions. Autoimmune encephalitis is a much more common cause of encephalitis than previously recognized; its presentation is variable and can include behavioral changes, seizures, and sleep disturbances. The presence of specific antibodies and MRI findings are helpful in the diagnosis.

4 Rare infectious causes of encephalopathy include cat scratch disease, Rocky Mountain spotted fever, Lyme disease, toxic shock syndrome, and measles.

5 A history of head trauma should prompt an evaluation for an intracranial injury. Other worrisome signs and symptoms include a bulging fontanel, retinal hemorrhages, focal neurologic findings, and signs of brain stem dysfunction (e.g., abnormal respiratory pattern and abnormal corneal, oculocephalic, or oculovestibular reflexes). Signs of increased intracranial pressure include a unilateral fixed or dilated pupil, ptosis, Cushing triad (i.e., hypertension, bradycardia, periodic breathing or apnea), cranial nerve VI palsy, papilledema, and a history of vomiting, headache, or ataxia.

6 A head CT is a good initial study and is usually readily available; it will reveal hemorrhages, most masses, and hydrocephalus. Subsequent MRI may be needed to identify infratentorial masses, cerebral edema, infarction, or more subtle CNS findings.

7 Abusive head trauma (shaken baby syndrome) usually occurs in children younger than 12 months. Children often have no external signs of trauma, although retinal hemorrhages and a bulging fontanel may be evident on examination. Neuroimaging reveals subdural hematomas. A complete evaluation for other injuries is indicated when abuse is suspected.

8 An intravenous dose of naloxone is recommended to potentially treat this rapidly reversible cause of altered mental status.

9 Overdoses and poisonings are common in children. A sudden onset of altered mental status, seizures, and vomiting, especially with a preceding period of confusion or delirium, should raise suspicion for a possible ingestion. Toxicology screens may be helpful, although they may be of limited value because they are not standardized. If certain agents are suspected, tests for them should be specifically requested. Immunosuppressive agents (including steroids) may cause altered mental status. Prescription drugs commonly reported in overdose cases are benzodiazepines, salicylates, acetaminophen, barbiturates, and tricyclic antidepressants. Poisons (from household products), alcohol, and illegal substance abuse should also always be considered. Many toxins cause a characteristic toxidrome of signs and symptoms (including EKG abnormalities) that may aid in their identification. Level of consciousness, pupillary examination, and vital signs are the most helpful components in identifying a toxidrome.

10 Inborn errors of metabolism usually occur in the neonate with vomiting, lethargy, or seizures, although partial or incomplete errors may not occur until later childhood or adolescence. Initial labs may suggest a metabolic disorder (e.g., acidosis, hypoglycemia), but additional evaluation should be performed if clinically suspicious of an inborn error of metabolism.

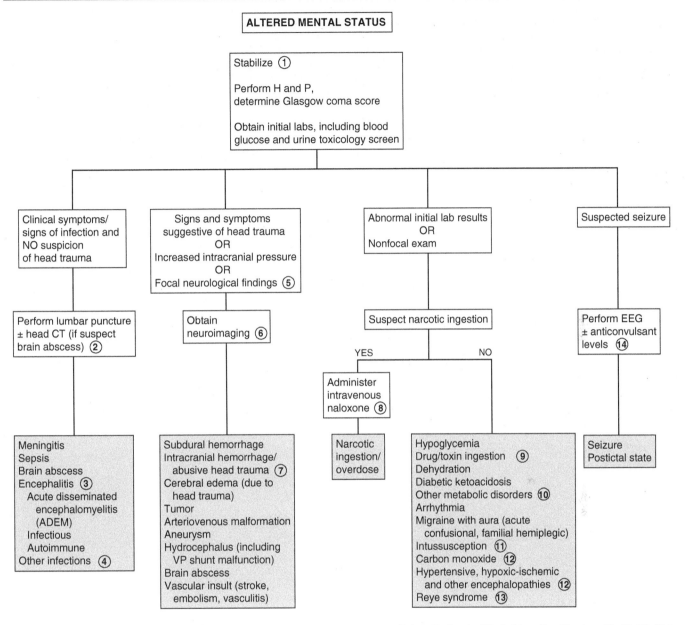

ALTERED MENTAL STATUS

Stabilize ①

Perform H and P,
determine Glasgow coma score

Obtain initial labs, including blood
glucose and urine toxicology screen

Clinical symptoms/
signs of infection and
NO suspicion
of head trauma

Signs and symptoms
suggestive of head trauma
OR
Increased intracranial pressure
OR
Focal neurological findings ⑤

Abnormal initial lab results
OR
Nonfocal exam

Suspected seizure

Perform lumbar puncture
± head CT (if suspect
brain abscess) ②

Obtain
neuroimaging ⑥

Suspect narcotic ingestion

Perform EEG
± anticonvulsant
levels ⑭

YES   NO

Administer
intravenous
naloxone ⑧

Meningitis
Sepsis
Brain abscess
Encephalitis ③
   Acute disseminated
      encephalomyelitis
      (ADEM)
   Infectious
   Autoimmune
Other infections ④

Subdural hemorrhage
Intracranial hemorrhage/
   abusive head trauma ⑦
Cerebral edema (due to
   head trauma)
Tumor
Arteriovenous malformation
Aneurysm
Hydrocephalus (including
   VP shunt malfunction)
Brain abscess
Vascular insult (stroke,
   embolism, vasculitis)

Narcotic
ingestion/
overdose

Hypoglycemia
Drug/toxin ingestion ⑨
Dehydration
Diabetic ketoacidosis
Other metabolic disorders ⑩
Arrhythmia
Migraine with aura (acute
   confusional, familial hemiplegic)
Intussusception ⑪
Carbon monoxide ⑫
Hypertensive, hypoxic-ischemic
   and other encephalopathies ⑫
Reye syndrome ⑬

Seizure
Postictal state

Nelson Textbook of Pediatrics, 19e. Chapters 60, 62, 63, 584
Nelsons Essentials, 6e. Chapter 184

The evaluation for a metabolic disorder should include blood for a CBC, electrolytes, pH, glucose, ammonia, lactate, acylcarnitine profile, and amino acids, plus urine for ketones, reducing substances, and organic acids. A patient or family history of recurrent episodes of lethargy, vomiting, personality changes, or frequent hospitalizations should raise suspicion for a metabolic disorder and prompt an appropriate laboratory evaluation. Neurologic and/or genetic consultation should be considered for specific recommendations for testing based on clinical suspicions.

In older infants and children, altered mental status may be due to electrolyte and other metabolic or endocrine abnormalities (e.g., diabetic ketoacidosis, hypernatremia, hyponatremia, hypocalcemia, hypercalcemia, adrenal disorders, thyroid disorders).

11 Symptoms of apathy and lethargy may initially predominate in children with intussusception before progression to obvious abdominal pain and bloody stools occurs.

12 Hypertensive encephalopathy will be suggested by an elevated blood pressure and possibly elevated renal function tests and proteinuria. Children with chronic cardiopulmonary disorders (e.g., cystic fibrosis, congenital heart disease, neuromuscular disorders) can experience an insidious onset of changes in mental status due to gradually declining arterial oxygen concentrations. Choking, drowning, or suffocation will cause acute anoxia encephalopathy; other causes to consider are severe anemia, severe methemoglobinemia, carbon monoxide poisoning, and hypothermia or hyperthermia due to extreme environmental conditions. Rarer causes of encephalopathy include Hashimoto's encephalopathy (associated with high levels of antithyroid antibodies), acute hepatic failure (due to drugs or viral hepatitis), uremia (acute or chronic, due to renal failure), burn encephalopathy, hypomagnesia, hyperalimentation, thiamine deficiency, and rheumatologic diseases (systemic lupus erythematosus, Behcet's disease). Psychiatric conditions rarely cause coma or stupor in children; adolescents may rarely present with psychosomatic symptoms (feigning unresponsiveness).

13 The incidence of Reye syndrome, a mitochondrial encephalopathy, has significantly declined due to the decreased use of aspirin in children. It is characterized by an acute onset of vomiting, combativeness, and mental status changes ranging from delirium to coma. Hepatic enzyme levels and serum ammonia levels are elevated; hypoglycemia, metabolic acidosis, and cerebral edema may occur. The syndrome typically is associated with a preceding viral infection (e.g., varicella, influenza B, influenza A).

14 In a child with a known seizure disorder, be sure to obtain anticonvulsant levels.

Bibliography

Nelson DS: Coma and altered level of consciousness. In Fleisher G, Ludwig S, editors: *Textbook of pediatric emergency medicine*, ed 6, Philadelphia, 2010, Lippincott Williams & Wilkins, pp 176–186.

Piña-Garza JE: Altered mental status. In Piña-Garza JE, editor: *Fenichel's clinical pediatric neurology*, ed 7, Philadelphia, 2013, Saunders/Elsevier, pp. 47–75.

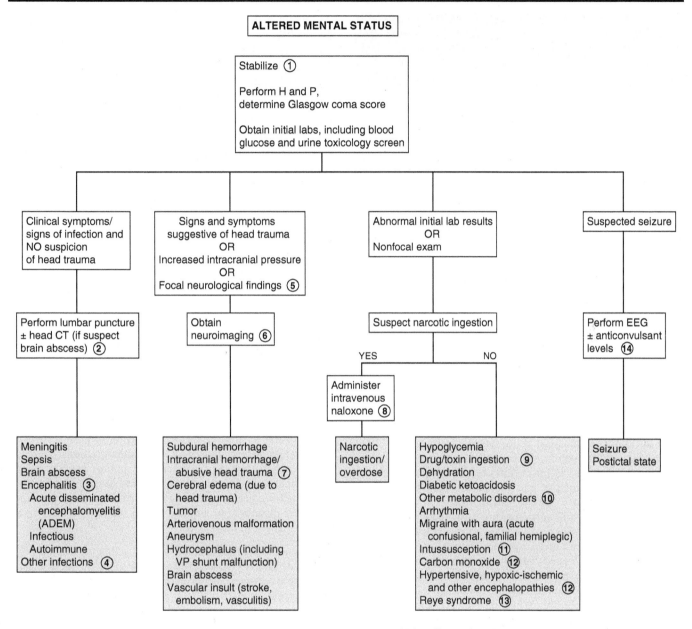

ALTERED MENTAL STATUS

Stabilize ①

Perform H and P,
determine Glasgow coma score

Obtain initial labs, including blood
glucose and urine toxicology screen

Clinical symptoms/
signs of infection and
NO suspicion
of head trauma

Signs and symptoms
suggestive of head trauma
OR
Increased intracranial pressure
OR
Focal neurological findings ⑤

Abnormal initial lab results
OR
Nonfocal exam

Suspected seizure

Perform lumbar puncture
± head CT (if suspect
brain abscess) ②

Obtain
neuroimaging ⑥

Suspect narcotic ingestion

Perform EEG
± anticonvulsant
levels ⑭

YES   NO

Administer
intravenous
naloxone ⑧

Meningitis
Sepsis
Brain abscess
Encephalitis ③
  Acute disseminated
    encephalomyelitis
    (ADEM)
  Infectious
  Autoimmune
Other infections ④

Subdural hemorrhage
Intracranial hemorrhage/
  abusive head trauma ⑦
Cerebral edema (due to
  head trauma)
Tumor
Arteriovenous malformation
Aneurysm
Hydrocephalus (including
  VP shunt malfunction)
Brain abscess
Vascular insult (stroke,
  embolism, vasculitis)

Narcotic
ingestion/
overdose

Hypoglycemia
Drug/toxin ingestion ⑨
Dehydration
Diabetic ketoacidosis
Other metabolic disorders ⑩
Arrhythmia
Migraine with aura (acute
  confusional, familial hemiplegic)
Intussusception ⑪
Carbon monoxide ⑫
Hypertensive, hypoxic-ischemic
  and other encephalopathies ⑫
Reye syndrome ⑬

Seizure
Postictal state

Nelson Textbook of Pediatrics, 19e. Chapters 60, 62, 63, 584
Nelsons Essentials, 6e. Chapter 184

Chapter 56
HEARING LOSS

Hearing loss can be conductive or sensorineural (or mixed) due to problems along the peripheral auditory pathway (i.e., external ear, middle ear, inner ear, and the auditory nerve). Conductive hearing loss is usually due to problems in the external and middle ear; sensorineural hearing loss (SNHL) is usually due to inner ear and auditory nerve problems. Screening of all newborn infants has been recommended by the U.S. Preventive Task Force since 2001 because early detection of and intervention for hearing loss are clearly beneficial to language development, and there has been minimal risk associated with the screening and treatment for the condition. Many cases of hearing loss, however, are progressive and may not be detected at birth. Children with acquired or late-onset hearing loss may present with a more subtle problem, such as poor school performance. Sometimes children with effusion or eustachian tube dysfunction present with a complaint of hearing loss. The role of the primary care practitioner is to identify the hearing loss and make appropriate referrals for comprehensive evaluation and treatment. Identifying hearing loss as early as possible is critical to minimizing the adverse effects on speech and language and school performance.

1. Perinatal risk factors for hearing loss include congenital infections, craniofacial abnormalities, birthweight <1500 grams, hyperbilirubinemia requiring exchange transfusion, low Apgar scores (<4 at 5 minutes and <6 at 10 minutes), ototoxic medications (gentamicin), and mechanical ventilation (especially for more than 5 days) or ECMO. Prenatal exposure to retinoids, cisplatin, and certain toxins (e.g., alcohol, mercury, quinine) have also been associated with hearing loss. For older children, inquire about noise exposure, trauma, and toxic ingestions or exposures. A family history of hearing loss, a history of bacterial meningitis, and characteristics of syndromes associated with hearing loss are risk factors at any age.

A family history positive for hearing loss developing under age 30 years, kidney abnormalities, different colored eyes, a white forelock of hair, night blindness, cardiac arrhythmias, or sudden cardiac death should raise suspicion for hereditary causes of hearing loss.

On the physical examination, carefully assess the head and neck for head shape, abnormal hair findings (white forelock), branchial cleft remnants, and abnormal ear findings. Eye placement and color should be noted; microphthalmia or retinitis could suggest a congenital infection. Skin and neurologic examinations are also important; any characteristics suggestive of genetic syndromes should be noted.

A history of absent or delayed language milestones is significant in the evaluation of hearing loss. Some general "red flags" suggesting language delays include (1) not startling to loud sounds by 3 months, (2) not vocalizing by 6 months, (3) not localizing speech or other sounds by 9 months, (4) not babbling multiple sounds or syllables by 12 months, (5) not saying "mama" or "dada" specifically by 13 months, (6) less than 50% of speech understandable by 24 months and (7) not following a one-step command by 13 to 15 months.

2. Mild conductive hearing loss is common with otitis media and normally improves with the resolution of the effusion. Small tympanic membrane perforations have little effect on hearing, but large perforations may.

3. Tympanometry provides information about tympanic membrane compliance and middle ear pressure. It is most helpful in identifying middle ear effusions and perforations of the tympanic membrane (TM). Before age 4 months, the excessive compliance of the ear canal limits the usefulness of the test. Newborn screening programs rely on otoacoustic emissions (OAE) testing and auditory brainstem evoked response (ABR) tests to evaluate infant hearing. The advantage of ABR testing over OAE is its potential to identify an auditory neuropathy. Once a child can cooperate, pure tone audiometry with bone and air conduction results is recommended; most children can be reliably tested by this method by age 4 years. Referral for testing via other methods (depending on the age of the child) may be indicated if a child is too young to complete pure tone audiometry or if they are unable to cooperate with the testing.

4. A temporary shift in hearing threshold after exposure to potentially injurious sounds can precede permanent noise-induced hearing loss (NIHL). NIHL has been attributed to high levels of continuous noise (e.g., music, recreational vehicles, power tools) and high intensity sounds of short duration (e.g., gunfire, firecrackers).

5. Referral to a multidisciplinary center is ideal to provide evaluation and treatment by audiology, otolaryngology, and speech pathology. Genetics consultation may be helpful since approximately half of sensorineural hearing loss cases are associated with a genetic etiology. Genetics can aid in providing a specific diagnosis, prognostic factors, and counseling on associated risks and conditions.

6. Genetics are estimated to be a factor in approximately 50% of cases of SNHL; two thirds of the cases are not associated with any syndrome. Genetic counseling is becoming an increasingly important part of the evaluation of hearing loss as advances in genetics are identifying mitochondrial disorders and mutations associated with an increased susceptibility to deafness. Approximately 80% of cases of SNHL are inherited as autosomal recessive traits. Hearing impairment associated with some genetic disorders may not develop until later in childhood.

7. Effects of ototoxic drugs may not appear for up to 6 months after exposure to the drug. Aminoglycosides, loop diuretics, and chemotherapy agents (especially cisplatin) are the most common offenders. Quinine, lead, and arsenic have also been identified as causes of hearing loss.

8. Both conductive and sensorineural hearing loss have been reported in children who experience head trauma due to temporal bone fractures or inner ear concussion; spontaneous resolution usually occurs.

9. Hearing loss due to congenital cytomegalovirus (CMV), toxoplasmosis, and syphilis may not appear until months to

years after birth. Some children with congenital CMV suddenly lose residual hearing at age 4 to 5 years. Other infections (e.g., meningitis, Lyme disease, parvovirus, measles, mumps, rubella) are rare causes of SNHL. Perilymph fistulas, vascular insults to the inner ear, and a first episode of Meniere disease should also be considered.

10 The tympanogram in otitis media with effusion is typically rounded or flat.

11 Guidelines for management of the young child (age 2 months to 12 years) with otitis media with effusion are available.

Bibliography

Gifford KA, Holmes MG, Bernstein HH: Hearing loss in children, *Pediatr Rev* 30:207–215, 2009.

Roizen NJ: Etiology of hearing loss in children: Nongenetic causes, *Pediatr Clin North Am* 46:49–64, 1999.

Rosenfeld RM, Culpepper L, Doyle KJ, et al: American Academy of Pediatrics Subcommittee on Otitis Media with Effusion; American Academy of Family Physicians; American Academy of Otolaryngology–Head and Neck Surgery, Clinical practice guideline: otitis media with effusion. *Otolaryngol Head Neck Surg* 130(5)((suppl)):S95–S118, 2004

Tomaski SM, Grundfast KM: A stepwise approach to the diagnosis and treatment of hereditary hearing loss, *Pediatr Clin North Am* 46:35–48, 1999.

US Preventive Services Task Force: Universal screening for hearing loss in newborns: US Preventive Services Task Force Recommendation Statement, *Pediatrics* 122:143–148, 2008.

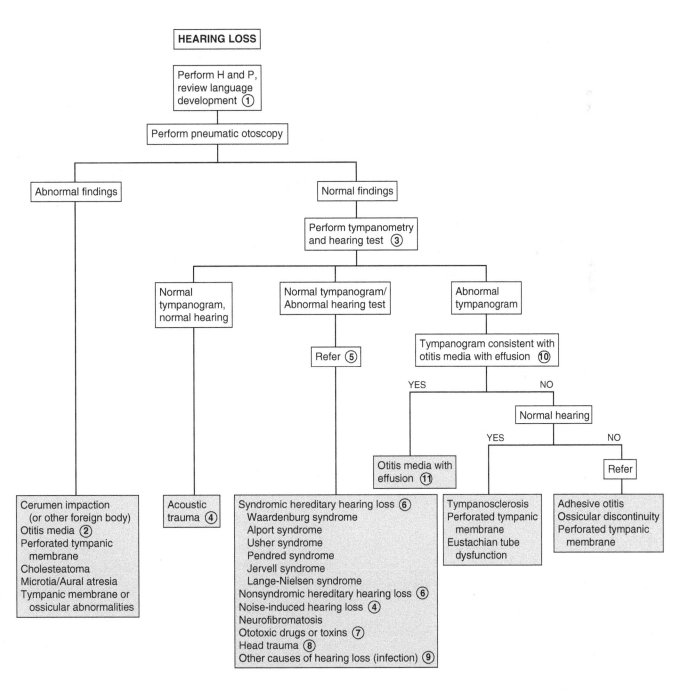

Dermatology

Chapter 57
ALOPECIA

Alopecia is the absence or loss of hair. Hypotrichosis (very sparse or thin hair) accompanies alopecia in many conditions.

1. The H and P often reveal the diagnosis. Key points to ask about include the presence or absence of pruritus, whether the degree of hair loss seems to vary over time or not, and (if appropriate) whether there is a history of hair coming out in clumps. For cases of acquired hair loss, inquire about a history of recent significant illnesses, surgeries, or potentially stressful psychosocial events, as well as the possibility of anxiety, significant stress, or obsessive-compulsive disorder (OCD). Ask about a family history of hair problems as well as other hereditary disorders (which may include hair abnormalities). The examination should note the presence or absence of scarring, "black dot" or "exclamation point" hairs (indicating hairs broken off at the scalp), and whether residual hairs' lengths are consistent or variable. A complete skin exam should also be performed. Most diagnoses can be confirmed by microscopic examination of a hair pull (a tuft of hair gently removed to include the roots), a potassium hydroxide (KOH) examination, culture, or biopsy. Note how much resistance is required to pull hairs from the scalp.

2. Nevus sebaceous (sebaceous nevus of Jadassohn) lesions are small hamartomas of the skin. They appear as well-demarcated, hairless, yellowish-orange plaques on the scalp or neck of newborns. They remain relatively flat through infancy and childhood. Hormonal stimulation during adolescence causes an increase in size, with a potential for malignant changes. These nevi should be removed before adolescence.

3. Aplasia cutis congenita (congenital absence of skin) usually presents as small (1-2 cm) solitary atrophic lesions or ulcerations on the newborn scalp. If surrounded by a rim of dark hair (collar sign), they may be a marker for an underlying neurocutaneous abnormality. They are most commonly isolated findings but are rarely associated with other anomalies or malformation syndromes.

4. Occipital hair loss occurring in a young infant is a form of traction alopecia. Some hair loss occurs normally early in the newborn period. Rubbing the head on a sheet or mattress simply exaggerates this normal phase of hair loss.

5. Pressure on the scalp during a prolonged vaginal birth may result in a (usually) transient annular "halo" pattern of alopecia on the scalp. The same effect may occur around the edge of a caput succedaneum or cephalohematoma.

6. Congenital triangular alopecia overlying the frontotemporal suture may not be noticed until age 2 to 3 years. It is usually unilateral, with the base of the triangular area (3-5 cm) abutting on the anterior hairline.

7. Ectodermal dysplasias are a heterogeneous group of hereditary disorders characterized by a primary defect of the teeth, skin, and appendage structures (hair, nails, eccrine and sebaceous glands). Scalp hair is fine and sparse; eyelashes and eyebrows may be sparse or absent.

8. A variety of congenital structural defects of the hair shaft cause alopecia or hypotrichosis with short, fragile hair that does not appear to grow. The defects may be isolated or associated with rare genetic or metabolic disorders. Trichorrhexis nodosa is the most common brittle hair shaft defect. The genetic form may present at birth; it is more commonly acquired, owing to traumatic hair grooming practices (hot combs, excessive hair dryer use, straightening chemicals) and is reversible when damaging hair care practices are discontinued.

9. Loose anagen syndrome of childhood is a condition of actively growing but loosely anchored hairs. It is most often seen in young (age 2-5 years) blond females, who present with diffuse or patchy alopecia, apparent lack of hair growth, and hairs that are easily pulled from the head.

10. Tinea capitis can occur with patchy or diffuse scaling, localized or "black dot" alopecia, or kerion. Alopecia may be the chief complaint, especially if the patient is regularly using moisturizing hair or scalp preparations. (It may be helpful to ask what the scalp looks like when the family does *not* use oil or grease-based hair products.) *Trichophyton tonsurans* is the causative dermatophyte in the majority of tinea capitis infections. A culture is recommended for diagnosis, although the diagnosis may be suggested by examination of a KOH preparation of scale or involved hairs. Kerions are boggy, pustular plaques that develop as a hypersensitivity reaction to the dermatophyte. The reaction is inflammatory, and cultures of the purulent matter are usually negative for bacteria.

11. Severe cases of cellulitis, impetigo, folliculitis, and varicella may occasionally result in scarring and alopecia.

12. Rare causes of primary cicatricial (localized, scarring) alopecia include discoid lupus, lichen planopilaris, follicular decalvans, incontinentia pigmenti, and folliculitis keloidosis; these disorders are rare in children.

13. Alopecia areata is an immune-mediated disorder characterized by well-circumscribed round or oval patches of hair loss on the scalp and other sites. The affected skin surface usually appears normal. When the condition is diffuse over the scalp, it is called alopecia universalis; when it is diffuse over the body, including eyebrows and eyelashes, it is alopecia totalis.

14. Hair pulling or trichotillomania may be habitual, a response to stress or anxiety, or associated with OCD. It is characterized by an erratic pattern of hair loss and the presence of broken hairs of irregular lengths. Parents and children frequently deny the practice.

15. Hair styling resulting in prolonged or extensive traction can cause nonscarring alopecia along the margins of tightly braided or styled hair. Pustules and folliculitis are often present.

16. Avulsion may be a manifestation of child abuse.

17. *Anagen* describes the growing phase of hairs; *telogen* describes the resting phase. Except for the newborn period, hairs are present in all phases of the growth cycle at any given time. In telogen effluvium, a stressor (illness, surgery) causes an interruption of the normal cycle of hair growth, causing a large proportion of the growing (anagen phase) hairs to switch to resting (telogen phase). The phenomenon becomes evident 3 to 5 months later when growth resumes and pushes out the large number of

resting hairs, causing a sudden diffuse loss of hair. Other inciting stressors are medications, febrile illnesses, crash diets, anesthesia, childbirth, endocrine disorders, and severe stress.

18 Anagen effluvium (toxic alopecia) is acute severe hair loss due to abnormal interruption of the anagen phase. It typically is due to radiation or chemotherapy.

19 Androgenetic (male pattern) baldness typically begins as hair thinning at the anterior scalp line. It can begin in late childhood or adolescence and can affect both males and females.

20 Other nutritional disorders resulting in thin or absent hair include kwashiorkor (severe protein/amino acid deficiency), marasmus (severe caloric malnutrition), iron deficiency, gluten-sensitive enteropathy, essential fatty acid deficiency, and biotinidase deficiency.

Bibliography

Paller AS, Mancini AJ: *Hurwitz clinical pediatric dermatology*, ed 4, Philadelphia, 2011, Elsevier Saunders.
Cohen BA: In Schachner LA, Hansen RC, editors: *Pediatric dermatology: Expert consult*, ed 4, Philadelphia, 2011, Elsevier Saunders.

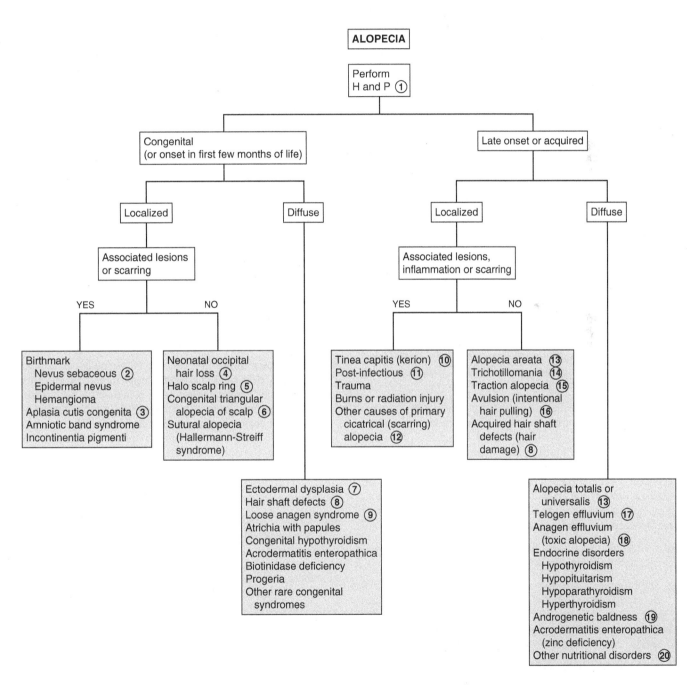

Chapter 58
VESICLES AND BULLAE

Vesicles are small (<0.5 cm) fluid-filled lesions; bullae are larger vesicles (>0.5-1 cm). Fluid may be clear or hemorrhagic. Vesiculobullous lesions (blisters) may be infectious or noninfectious. Noninfectious lesions may be spontaneous or induced by trauma or friction. Most vesiculobullous disorders are rare in children but need to be considered in chronic blistering conditions. Many are clinically indistinguishable from each other; skin biopsy, immunofluorescence, and electron microscopy are often necessary to make the definitive diagnosis.

The usefulness of this algorithm is limited (without photographs) to categorizing potential diagnoses based on some broad clinical criteria. A more specific dermatology reference will often be necessary to confirm suspected diagnoses.

1 Erythema toxicum (ET) is a common, benign, self-limited neonatal rash. Tiny papules, vesicles, or pustules are present on a blotchy erythematous macular base; the rash can be present on any surface except for the palms and soles. The onset generally is in the first few days of life (occasionally later), and remission is usually by 2 weeks. If microscopically examined, the lesions show an accumulation of eosinophils within the pilosebaceous apparatus.

2 Transient neonatal pustular melanosis is another benign, self-limited neonatal rash. Small, fragile vesicles or pustules are noted at birth and can be present on any surface. The lesions rupture quickly, leaving a characteristic rim of scale and hyperpigmented macule that gradually fades. Histologic exam shows primarily neutrophils.

3 A generalized vesicular exanthem can occur in disseminated herpes simplex virus (HSV) infection of the newborn. Lesions associated with localized infections (involving only skin, eyes, and mouth) may be subtle, but diagnosis is critical because localized disease in these infants can progress to encephalitis or disseminated disease. PCR tests and cultures are diagnostic options for HSV; Tzanck smears are of limited usefulness because they are not very sensitive, plus will not distinguish between HSV and varicella.

4 Congenital candidiasis typically manifests as diffuse papules and pustules, rarely bullae.

5 Staphylococcal scalded skin syndrome is an exfoliative dermatitis characterized by diffuse tender erythema, flaccid bullae, sheets of desquamating skin, and a positive Nikolsky sign (blistering elicited by light touch). The face, neck, groin, and axillae are most commonly affected.

6 Epidermolysis bullosa (EB) constitutes a group of inherited blistering disorders. The clinical severity, age of presentation, and level/site of skin cleavage vary. Blistering may be spontaneous or in response to pressure or trauma. Most variants become evident in the neonatal period. The most common variant (EB simplex of the hands and feet [Weber-Cockayne syndrome]) may not manifest until adolescence or young adulthood, with blisters developing on the hands and feet after significant trauma or friction, especially in hot weather conditions.

7 Incontinentia pigmenti is a hereditary disorder with multisystem involvement; it mainly affects females. Cutaneous manifestations develop in the first 2 weeks of life, with red streaks and crops of vesicles or bullae developing on the trunk or in a characteristic linear distribution on the extremities. Evolution to verrucous lesions followed by characteristic pigmentation changes subsequently occurs, usually by 4 months of age. Blisters may recur later with febrile illnesses. The hair, eyes, CNS, and teeth are also affected.

8 Miliaria or heat rash may be characterized by tiny (1-2 mm) clear, thin-walled vesicles without any associated redness (miliaria crystallina) or with larger (2-4 mm) vesicles or papules with associated erythema (miliaria rubra). Areas occluded by heavy clothing or affected by sunburn are most commonly affected.

9 Sucking blisters are presumably due to in utero sucking on the affected area. They may be located on the dorsal surfaces of the forearm, hands, or fingers.

10 The lesions of bullous impetigo are flaccid bullae that rupture easily, leaving superficial erosions. This form of impetigo is much less common than the nonbullous form (crusted lesions). In the newborn, the diaper area is most commonly affected.

11 The skin lesions of acrodermatitis enteropathica can be vesiculobullous or psoriasiform in nature. They are likely to be found in acral, oral, and perineal locations.

12 Vesicles are a more common manifestation of scabies in infants and young children than in older children. They are most likely to be found on the palms and soles and in the axillae and groin. Severe pruritus is characteristic.

13 Erythema multiforme (EM) is a blistering hypersensitivity reaction classically characterized by target lesions. Target lesions are well-demarcated round or oval macules with distinct "rings"—outermost erythema surrounding a whitish ring and then a central dusky blue/gray or blistered center; the typical size ranges from 1 to 3 cm. A self-limited outbreak of target lesions occurs in EM; the outbreak is usually symmetric and involving primarily the upper extremities. Limited involvement of one mucosal surface may occur. Many types of infectious agents have been associated with EM; HSV is the most common.

14 Linear immunoglobulin (Ig)A disease (chronic bullous dermatosis of children) usually occurs in the preschool years. The disorder is characterized by a widespread eruption of large sausage-shaped bullae with a variable degree of pruritus. The inguinal region, lower trunk, buttocks, legs, and tops of the feet are most commonly affected, but the bullae may develop anywhere. Sometimes the bullae develop in an annular or rosette-like configuration surrounding a central crust ("cluster of jewels").

15 In dermatitis herpetiformis, outbreaks of clusters of small papules and vesicles occur in a symmetric distribution on the extensor surfaces, lower trunk, and buttocks. The outbreaks are extremely pruritic and tender. Hemorrhagic bullae on the palms and soles occasionally occur. The disorder is associated with a gluten-sensitive enteropathy.

16 The term *pemphigus* encompasses a group of chronic blistering disorders with variable severity and prognoses.

VESICLES AND BULLAE

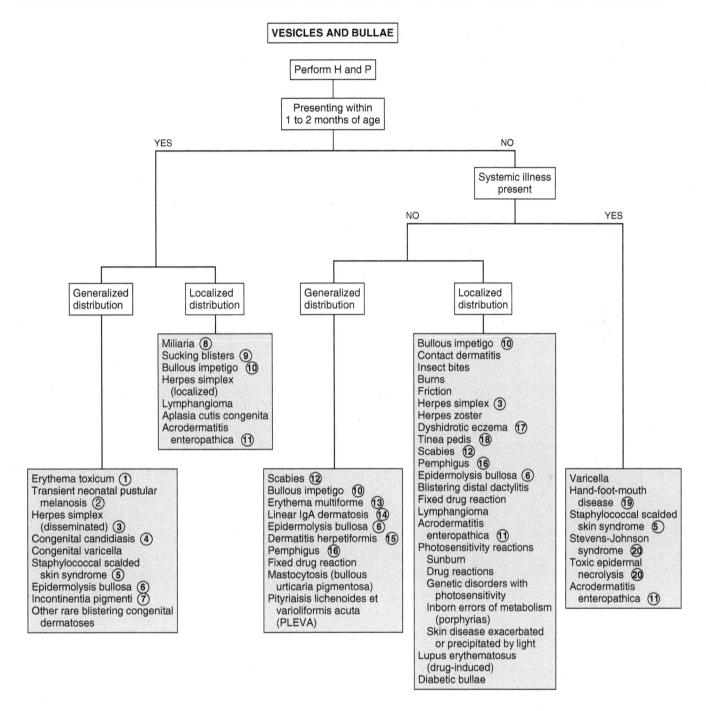

Perform H and P

Presenting within 1 to 2 months of age

YES — NO

Systemic illness present

NO — YES

Generalized distribution | **Localized distribution** | **Generalized distribution** | **Localized distribution**

Localized distribution (YES branch):
Miliaria ⑧
Sucking blisters ⑨
Bullous impetigo ⑩
Herpes simplex (localized)
Lymphangioma
Aplasia cutis congenita
Acrodermatitis enteropathica ⑪

Generalized distribution (YES branch):
Erythema toxicum ①
Transient neonatal pustular melanosis ②
Herpes simplex (disseminated) ③
Congenital candidiasis ④
Congenital varicella
Staphylococcal scalded skin syndrome ⑤
Epidermolysis bullosa ⑥
Incontinentia pigmenti ⑦
Other rare blistering congenital dermatoses

Generalized distribution (NO branch):
Scabies ⑫
Bullous impetigo ⑩
Erythema multiforme ⑬
Linear IgA dermatosis ⑭
Epidermolysis bullosa ⑥
Dermatitis herpetiformis ⑮
Pemphigus ⑯
Fixed drug reaction
Mastocytosis (bullous urticaria pigmentosa)
Pityriaisis lichenoides et varioliformis acuta (PLEVA)

Localized distribution (NO branch):
Bullous impetigo ⑩
Contact dermatitis
Insect bites
Burns
Friction
Herpes simplex ③
Herpes zoster
Dyshidrotic eczema ⑰
Tinea pedis ⑱
Scabies ⑫
Pemphigus ⑯
Epidermolysis bullosa ⑥
Blistering distal dactylitis
Fixed drug reaction
Lymphangioma
Acrodermatitis enteropathica ⑪
Photosensitivity reactions
  Sunburn
  Drug reactions
  Genetic disorders with photosensitivity
  Inborn errors of metabolism (porphyrias)
  Skin disease exacerbated or precipitated by light
Lupus erythematosus (drug-induced)
Diabetic bullae

Localized distribution (YES branch, right):
Varicella
Hand-foot-mouth disease ⑲
Staphylococcal scalded skin syndrome ⑤
Stevens-Johnson syndrome ⑳
Toxic epidermal necrolysis ⑳
Acrodermatitis enteropathica ⑪

Nelson Textbook of Pediatrics, 19e. Chapters 589, 646, 647, 658
Nelsons Essentials, 6e. Chapters 195, 196

The characteristic lesions are flaccid bullae with subsequent shallow erosions. Onset in childhood is rare; there is an infantile subtype with a predilection for acral regions, and a childhood vulvar subtype. In the pemphigus vulgaris variant, painful oral lesions may precede cutaneous involvement by weeks or months.

17 Recurrent outbreaks of small pruritic vesicles on the hands and feet occur in dyshidrotic eczema; larger vesicles and bullae sometimes occur. The palms, soles, and lateral aspects of the fingers and toes are most commonly affected.

18 An inflammatory vesicular reaction may occasionally occur with tinea pedis.

19 Hand-foot-mouth syndrome is a viral (usually due to coxsackie or enteroviruses) illness characterized by a prodrome of fever, anorexia, and sore throat followed by an enanthem of small ulcerating oral vesicles. The characteristic exanthem of oval vesicles (when it occurs) affects primarily the hands and feet (occasionally includes elbows, knees, or buttocks) and develops after the oral lesions. Vesicles can also be seen with other enteroviral infections.

20 Stevens-Johnson syndrome (SJS) is a more severe, potentially life-threatening blistering hypersensitivity reaction. It is often characterized by target lesions (in a more extensive distribution than in EM) and requires involvement of two or more mucosal surfaces (mouth, eye, urogenital, esophageal) for diagnosis. *Mycoplasma pneumoniae* is the most common pathogen associated with SJS; several medications are also recognized precipitants. Drugs are more likely to be associated with SJS than EM. Toxic epidermal necrolysis is identified as a severe form of SJS, with a prodrome of fever and malaise and a subsequent severe dermatitis (including some bullae) with exfoliation of large sheets of full-thickness epidermis. It is most commonly precipitated by drugs.

Bibliography

Cohen BA: In Schachner LA, Hansen RC, editors: *Pediatric dermatology,* ed 4, Philadelphia, 2011, Elsevier Saunders.

Paller AS, Mancini AJ: *Hurwitz clinical pediatric dermatology,* ed 4, Philadelphia, 2011, Elsevier Saunders.

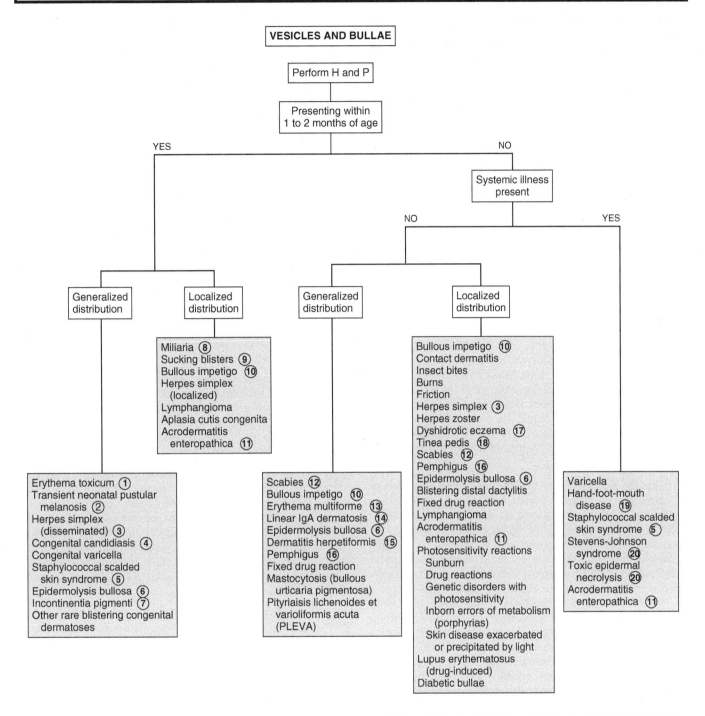

VESICLES AND BULLAE

Perform H and P

Presenting within
1 to 2 months of age

YES

NO

Systemic illness
present

Generalized distribution

Localized distribution

Miliaria ⑧
Sucking blisters ⑨
Bullous impetigo ⑩
Herpes simplex
   (localized)
Lymphangioma
Aplasia cutis congenita
Acrodermatitis
   enteropathica ⑪

Erythema toxicum ①
Transient neonatal pustular
   melanosis ②
Herpes simplex
   (disseminated) ③
Congenital candidiasis ④
Congenital varicella
Staphylococcal scalded
   skin syndrome ⑤
Epidermolysis bullosa ⑥
Incontinentia pigmenti ⑦
Other rare blistering congenital
   dermatoses

NO

YES

Generalized distribution

Localized distribution

Scabies ⑫
Bullous impetigo ⑩
Erythema multiforme ⑬
Linear IgA dermatosis ⑭
Epidermolysis bullosa ⑥
Dermatitis herpetiformis ⑮
Pemphigus ⑯
Fixed drug reaction
Mastocytosis (bullous
   urticaria pigmentosa)
Pityriaisis lichenoides et
   varioliformis acuta
   (PLEVA)

Bullous impetigo ⑩
Contact dermatitis
Insect bites
Burns
Friction
Herpes simplex ③
Herpes zoster
Dyshidrotic eczema ⑰
Tinea pedis ⑱
Scabies ⑫
Pemphigus ⑯
Epidermolysis bullosa ⑥
Blistering distal dactylitis
Fixed drug reaction
Lymphangioma
Acrodermatitis
   enteropathica ⑪
Photosensitivity reactions
   Sunburn
   Drug reactions
   Genetic disorders with
      photosensitivity
   Inborn errors of metabolism
      (porphyrias)
   Skin disease exacerbated
      or precipitated by light
Lupus erythematosus
   (drug-induced)
Diabetic bullae

Varicella
Hand-foot-mouth
   disease ⑲
Staphylococcal scalded
   skin syndrome ⑤
Stevens-Johnson
   syndrome ⑳
Toxic epidermal
   necrolysis ⑳
Acrodermatitis
   enteropathica ⑪

Nelson Textbook of Pediatrics, 19e. Chapters 589, 646, 647, 658
Nelsons Essentials, 6e. Chapters 195, 196

Chapter 59
FEVER AND RASH

Fever and rash are components of many disease processes, most of which are benign self-limited conditions. Rarely, this combination of symptoms may herald a life-threatening illness, so it is essential to narrow the differential diagnosis with a careful history and physical. Causes of fever and rash include infections, vasculitides, and hypersensitivity disorders. Laboratory tests should be ordered according to the presumptive diagnosis based on the history and physical. Many rashes are pathognomonic for certain diseases (varicella), and testing may not be indicated.

1. The history should include the characteristics of the rash, presence of pruritus or pain or tenderness, appearance in relationship to the fever, and the evolution and progression of the rash. A history of ill contacts, recent travel, exposures (pets, wildlife, insects), medications (including the possibility of IV drug use), and sexual activity should be obtained. Past medical history should be reviewed, and a history of any prodromal or associated symptoms (abdominal pain, rash, headaches) obtained. Examination should include a general assessment of the patient to determine the severity of the illness, including vital signs and height of fever. Tachycardia and tachypnea in a patient with fever and rash may indicate sepsis, particularly if there is altered mental status. The development of hypotension may indicate septic shock.

2. Note the distribution of the rash and lesion morphology and color, as well as the presence and characteristics of any enanthems (eruptions on mucosal surfaces). The term *macular* describes flat lesions, *papular* describes raised or palpable lesions, and the term *morbilliform* (classically used to describe the rash of measles) describes coalescence of maculopapular lesions into a diffuse or sheet-like distribution. Another important characteristic is whether a rash blanches with pressure or not. (Reddish lesions that blanch are due to dilated capillaries; nonblanchable lesions imply RBCs have leaked out of the blood vessels [extravasation]). Distribution may be generalized or localized, symmetric or asymmetric, centripetal (more lesions on the trunk, less on the extremities and face), or centrifugal (more lesions on the distal extremities and face, less on the trunk). The characteristics of the rash and associated symptoms frequently suggest a diagnosis.

3. Target lesions are well-demarcated round or oval macules with distinct "rings"—a rim of outer erythema surrounding a whitish ring and then a central dusky blue/gray or bullous center; the typical size ranges from 1 to 3 cm.

4. Fifth disease (also called erythema infectiosum) is caused by human parvovirus B19. The rash starts with a "slapped cheek" appearance with circumoral pallor, followed 1 to 4 days later by a more diffuse maculopapular rash that becomes lacy or reticular in appearance as it fades. A less common manifestation of parvovirus B19 is a petechial rash in a papular-purpuric "gloves and socks" acral distribution.

5. The classic presentation of roseola (also called roseola infantum, exanthema subitum, or sixth disease) is an acute high fever lasting for 3 to 5 days, followed by a short-lived (hours to 1 to 3 days), nonspecific, morbilliform, rose-colored rash that appears as defervescence occurs. The etiology can be human herpesviruses 6 or 7.

6. Enteroviruses are a common cause of petechial rashes. The patients usually do not appear ill and may not require extensive testing. Close followup, however, is essential.

7. Although rarely seen today in countries with good immunization practices, several distinctive clinical findings can aid in the diagnosis of measles. Initial prodromal symptoms are the three "C's"—cough, conjunctivitis, and coryza—which last for a few days before the development of high fever and the characteristic morbilliform exanthem that erupts (and subsequently fades) in a head-to-toe pattern. It affects the trunk more than the extremities and may sometimes be petechial or hemorrhagic. Atypical or modified measles are milder cases that may develop in a child with partial protection (transplacental antibody in young infants, vaccination before 1 year of age, or recipients of immunoglobulin). Koplik spots (a white or bluish-white dot-like enanthem found on the buccal mucosa near the lower molars) are pathognomonic for measles when noted; they develop during the prodromal phase but are present for only a brief period of time (12 to 24 hours).

8. The classic rubella (German measles) rash consists of discrete pink macular lesions that appear initially on the face and spread in a head-to-toe progression. They tend to coalesce in the truncal region and remain as discrete macules on the extremities. The facial rash is typically faded by the time the rash reaches the extremities.

9. Papular acrodermatitis (also called Gianotti-Crosti syndrome) is a characteristic outbreak of discrete, flat-topped, dark or dusky papules, usually 1 to 10 mm in size. Crops of lesions erupt symmetrically on the face, buttocks, and extensor surfaces of limbs; palms and soles can be affected. Low-grade fever may or may not occur. It is a recognized reaction to immunizations and viral infections. EBV is the most commonly associated virus; hepatitis B, coxsackie A16, CMV, and parainfluenza are others.

10. Group A streptococcus (GAS) is associated with several characteristic skin findings. Scarlatina (scarlatiniform rash or scarlet fever) describes a diffuse, fine papular, "ashy" or "sandpaper" rash that tends to develop initially on the neck and upper chest. The rash may be concentrated in creases (axillae, antecubital fossae, inguinal), where it takes on a linear petechial appearance (Pastia's lines). Subsequent desquamation of the rash, particularly on the hands and feet, is characteristic in both treated and untreated GAS infections.

11. A typical erythema migrans rash is pathognomonic for Lyme disease. It begins as a red macule or papule at the site of the tick bite and expands to an average diameter of 15 cm. It may be a uniform erythematous macule or demonstrate central clearing (target lesion).

12. The rash of rickettsial infections is often a late development in the illness course. The typical rash of Rocky Mountain spotted fever (RMSF) due to *Rickettsia rickettsii* begins as a blanchable macular rash that initially develops on the wrists and ankles then spreads centrally and includes the palms, soles, trunk, and face. The macules frequently evolve into petechial (and sometimes purpuric) lesions. Rash may be entirely

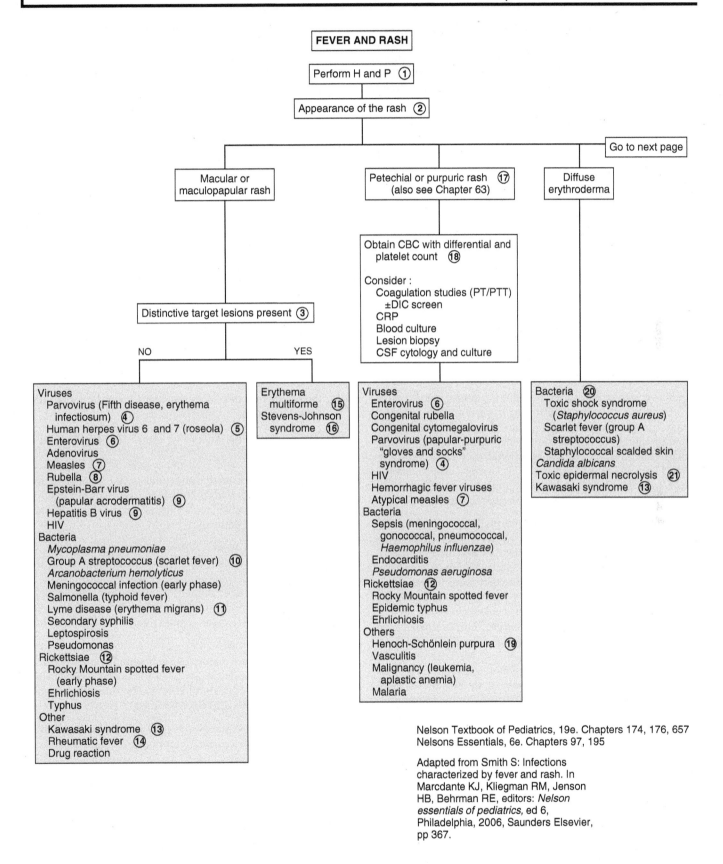

FEVER AND RASH

Perform H and P ①

Appearance of the rash ②

Go to next page

Macular or maculopapular rash

Petechial or purpuric rash ⑰ (also see Chapter 63)

Diffuse erythroderma

Obtain CBC with differential and platelet count ⑱

Consider :
 Coagulation studies (PT/PTT) ±DIC screen
 CRP
 Blood culture
 Lesion biopsy
 CSF cytology and culture

Distinctive target lesions present ③

NO   YES

Viruses
  Parvovirus (Fifth disease, erythema infectiosum) ④
  Human herpes virus 6 and 7 (roseola) ⑤
  Enterovirus ⑥
  Adenovirus
  Measles ⑦
  Rubella ⑧
  Epstein-Barr virus (papular acrodermatitis) ⑨
  Hepatitis B virus ⑨
  HIV
Bacteria
  Mycoplasma pneumoniae
  Group A streptococcus (scarlet fever) ⑩
  Arcanobacterium hemolyticus
  Meningococcal infection (early phase)
  Salmonella (typhoid fever)
  Lyme disease (erythema migrans) ⑪
  Secondary syphilis
  Leptospirosis
  Pseudomonas
Rickettsiae ⑫
  Rocky Mountain spotted fever (early phase)
  Ehrlichiosis
  Typhus
Other
  Kawasaki syndrome ⑬
  Rheumatic fever ⑭
  Drug reaction

Erythema multiforme ⑮
Stevens-Johnson syndrome ⑯

Viruses
  Enterovirus ⑥
  Congenital rubella
  Congenital cytomegalovirus
  Parvovirus (papular-purpuric "gloves and socks" syndrome) ④
  HIV
  Hemorrhagic fever viruses
  Atypical measles ⑦
Bacteria
  Sepsis (meningococcal, gonococcal, pneumococcal, *Haemophilus influenzae*)
  Endocarditis
  Pseudomonas aeruginosa
Rickettsiae ⑫
  Rocky Mountain spotted fever
  Epidemic typhus
  Ehrlichiosis
Others
  Henoch-Schönlein purpura ⑲
  Vasculitis
  Malignancy (leukemia, aplastic anemia)
  Malaria

Bacteria ⑳
  Toxic shock syndrome (*Staphylococcus aureus*)
  Scarlet fever (group A streptococcus)
  Staphylococcal scalded skin
Candida albicans
Toxic epidermal necrolysis ㉑
Kawasaki syndrome ⑬

Nelson Textbook of Pediatrics, 19e. Chapters 174, 176, 657
Nelsons Essentials, 6e. Chapters 97, 195

Adapted from Smith S: Infections characterized by fever and rash. In Marcdante KJ, Kliegman RM, Jenson HB, Behrman RE, editors: *Nelson essentials of pediatrics,* ed 6, Philadelphia, 2006, Saunders Elsevier, pp 367.

absent in 20% of cases. The ehrilichioses (*Ehrlichia chaffeensis, Anaplasma phagocytophilum, Ehrlichia ewingii*) are other zoonoses that are clinically similar to rickettsial infections, although rash development is even more variable with these infections. A history of tick exposure is often, but not always, obtained in these cases.

13 The onset of the rash of Kawasaki syndrome typically occurs 3 to 5 days after fever onset. It typically has a generalized distribution and a morbilliform or scarlatiniform nature. It may, however, be limited to the diaper region in young infants.

14 The Jones criteria must be fulfilled to make a diagnosis of rheumatic fever. (See Chapter 20.) Erythema marginatum is rare but constitutes one of the major criteria; it is classically described as serpiginous, evanescent, macular lesions that are pale in the center. It appears on the trunk and extremities (but not the face), is not pruritic, and will become more evident upon warming of the skin.

15 Erythema multiforme (EM) is a blistering hypersensitivity reaction classically characterized by a limited outbreak of target lesions, usually in a symmetric distribution involving the upper extremities. Limited involvement of one mucosal surface may occur. Herpes simplex virus (HSV) is the infectious agent most commonly associated with EM.

16 Stevens-Johnson syndrome (SJS) is a more severe, potentially life-threatening blistering hypersensitivity reaction. It may also demonstrate target lesions (in a more extensive distribution than in EM) and requires involvement of two or more mucosal surfaces (mouth, eye, urogenital, esophageal) for diagnosis. Fevers are more likely with SJS. *Mycoplasma pneumoniae* is the infectious agent most commonly associated with SJS; several medications are also recognized precipitants.

17 Petechiae are tiny dark (red or purple) pinpoint lesions that do not blanch with pressure. Purpura are larger dark (purple or brown) nonblanchable lesions that may or may not be raised (palpable). These rashes in a febrile child mandate an immediate and careful evaluation because they may indicate potentially life-threatening infections, especially in a child younger than 2 years. Sepsis due to *Neisseria meningitides* (as well as other organisms) is of particular concern. Purpura may be associated with disseminated intravascular coagulation (DIC), severe thrombocytopenia, or vasculitides. Mechanical factors (forceful cough, vomiting, compression due to tourniquet or BP cuff) occasionally lead to petechiae; in these cases the distribution is likely to be localized (to an extremity [owing to compression] or to the face or neck following coughing or vomiting) and the children afebrile and not severely ill-appearing.

18 In a patient with a petechial or purpuric rash, a CBC should be obtained. Other tests may be considered, depending on clinical presentation; remember, fever and petechiae in a child may quickly evolve into a critical illness. Thrombocytopenia may be associated with many infections, including viral ones. Even with a normal platelet count and coagulation studies, a WBC count below 5000/mm^3 or above 15,000/ mm^3, an absolute band count greater than 1,500 cells/mm^3, or abnormal CSF findings suggest an increased risk for bacterial or rickettsial infection. The presence of purpura definitely warrants an urgent evaluation. Of note, petechial rash with fever is most commonly

a benign phenomenon (not associated with thrombocytopenia), usually due to enteroviral infection.

19 In children with Henoch-Schönlein purpura, the rash usually begins as macules or urticarial lesions, later becoming raised and petechial or purpuric. Lesions are usually concentrated on the buttocks and lower extremities (gravity-dependent areas). Involvement of other organ systems (GI, renal, neurologic) suggest the diagnosis.

20 Manifestations of staphylococcal infections range from bullous impetigo (localized skin infections) to staphylococcal scalded skin syndrome (diffuse erythema, exquisite tenderness, extensive blisters, superficial erosions with subsequent desquamation) to toxic shock syndrome (TSS). TSS is a severe multisystem disease with a variable degree of cutaneous manifestations ranging from sunburn-like erythroderma (diffuse, involving non–sun-exposed areas), intraepidermal blistering (Nikolsky sign), and desquamation. Streptococcal infections can cause similar erythroderma and TSS conditions.

21 Toxic epidermal necrolysis is presumed to be a severe form of SJS, with a prodrome of fever and malaise and a subsequent severe dermatitis (including severe erythroderma, some vesicles, and exfoliation of large sheets of full-thickness epidermis). It is most commonly precipitated by drugs.

22 The classic rash of HSV is small vesicles and/or superficial ulcerations on an erythematous base.

23 Primary infections with varicella-zoster virus manifest as chickenpox. Pruritic, clear fluid–filled vesicles develop initially on the scalp and face and spread to the trunk, with minimal involvement of the extremities. The lesions become cloudy then crust over within 24 to 48 hours; lesions in multiple stages are present simultaneously. Recurrent infections (zoster) follow a dermatomal pattern.

24 Erythema nodosum is a hypersensitivity reaction that manifests as discrete, tender, nodular lesions on the extensor surfaces of the extremities. Fever may precede or be coincident with the development of the lesions. The etiology is often unknown; recognized causes include infection, inflammatory bowel disease, connective tissue disease, and medications.

25 Erysipelas is a rare manifestation of group A streptococcus. Infections of the deeper layers of the skin present as well-demarcated, bright red, painful lesions. The skin appears infiltrated, and the borders are raised and firm.

26 Eschars are a rare manifestation of infections due to *Pseudomonas aeruginosa* and certain fungal and rickettsial infections.

27 Fever only rarely precedes pityriasis rosea, but the rash distribution is quite distinctive. A solitary oval herald patch (an annular lesion with raised edges and fine scale) frequently (but not always) precedes the development of a more diffuse eruption of smaller pink or brownish oval lesions with fine scale, sometimes with central clearing evident. These lesions tend to follow the cutaneous cleavage lines, frequently described as a "Christmas tree" pattern on the back.

Bibliography

Bell LM, Newland JG: Fever and rash. In Bergelson JM, Shah SS, Zaoutis TE, editors: *Pediatric infectious diseases: Requisites*, ed 1, Philadelphia, 2008, Mosby-Elsevier, pp 251.

Thompson ED, Herzog KD: Fever and rash. In Zaoutis LB, Chiang VW, editors: *Comprehensive pediatric hospital medicine*, ed 1, Philadelphia, 2007, Elsevier, pp 329.

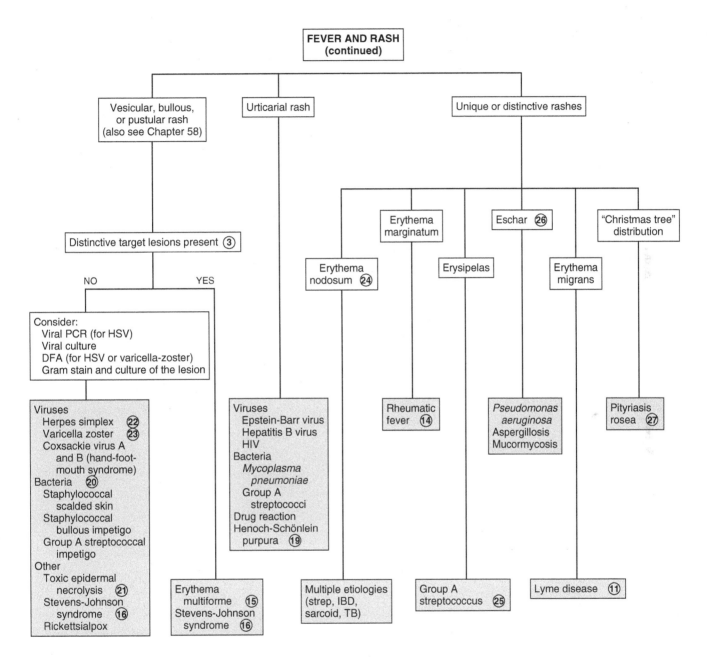

Adapted from Smith S: Infections characterized by fever and rash. In Marcdante KJ, Kliegman RM, Jenson HB, Behrman RE, editors: *Nelson essentials of pediatrics*, ed 6, Philadelphia, 2006, Saunders Elsevier, pp 367.

Hematology

Chapter 60
LYMPHADENOPATHY

Lymphadenopathy is the presence of one or more enlarged lymph nodes measuring >1 cm in diameter for axillary and cervical nodes, >1.5 cm for inguinal nodes and >0.5 cm for epitrochlear lymph nodes. It may be due to (1) reactive lymphadenopathy, a common and normal function of lymph nodes characterized by hyperplasia in response to antigenic stimuli; (2) lymphadenitis, an inflammatory response to bacteria or their products, accompanied by erythema, warmth, and tenderness; (3) malignancy by primary origin in the node or secondary to metastases; and (4) rare lipid storage disorders.

1. A good history is essential. The age of the child may indicate the cause. Adenopathy in neonates may be due to infections *in utero* (e.g., cytomegalovirus, syphilis, toxoplasmosis, human immunodeficiency virus [HIV]). In toddlers, adenopathy is usually due to either focal infections that drain to the affected node or systemic viral infections. Malignancy is more likely to be a cause of lymphadenopathy in older children. Immunodeficiency may predispose children to opportunistic infections or malignancies. Certain medications (e.g., procainamide, sulfasalazine, phenytoin, or tetracycline) may cause adenopathy. Family or exposure history may suggest infections such as HIV, syphilis, tuberculosis, group A β-hemolytic streptococci, or mononucleosis. Birth and travel history may indicate exposure to endemic infections (e.g., tuberculosis, histoplasmosis), as well as consumption of infected foods (e.g., *Brucella, Mycobacterium* from unpasteurized milk products). Diagnostic clues may be revealed by social history (e.g., socioeconomic status or ethnicity), family diet (e.g., consumption of raw meats), and presence of family pets (e.g., cat-scratch disease, toxoplasmosis from kitty litter). Adolescents must be asked about sexual activity, risk factors for HIV, and exposure to sexually transmitted diseases (e.g., syphilis). Lymphogranuloma venereum may cause inguinal lymphadenopathy. An acute onset may suggest infection, whereas an insidious onset accompanied by systemic symptoms (e.g., anorexia, weight loss, fevers, night sweats) suggests Hodgkin disease.

On physical examination, all areas that may be involved must be palpated, including cervical, preauricular and postauricular, axillary, epitrochlear, inguinal, and supraclavicular. Location of the node may be helpful in diagnosis, whether lymphadenopathy is localized or generalized. Localized lymphadenopathy often indicates involvement in the area of lymphatic drainage. Supraclavicular lymphadenopathy is usually a red flag for mediastinal tumors or infections or for metastatic abdominal tumors. Palpation of the nodes is helpful, with erythema, warmth, and tenderness indicating adenitis. Tender, nonerythematous, soft nodes may indicate a viral or a systemic infection. Firm or hard, rubbery, nontender nodes may indicate infiltrating tumors. Hard, matted, fixed, nontender nodes indicate tumor or fibrosis after acute infection.

2. Reactive adenopathy is usually a transient response to infections of the upper respiratory tract or skin. Pharyngeal infections commonly cause cervical lymphadenopathy. Common viral agents include adenovirus, parainfluenza, influenza, rhinovirus, and enterovirus. Cytomegalovirus (CMV) and Epstein-Barr virus (EBV) may cause a localized or generalized lymphadenopathy,

often with hepatosplenomegaly. Bacterial causes include group A β-hemolytic streptococci or oral anaerobes such as *Fusobacterium*. Scalp infections such as tinea capitis may cause occipital lymphadenopathy.

3. If there is pharyngitis associated with cervical adenitis, a throat culture or rapid streptococcal antigen detection test may be done to help diagnose group A β-hemolytic streptococci. Viral causes include EBV, herpes simplex, and enteroviruses.

4. Acute onset, unilateral adenitis is usually bacterial in origin and may form an abscess. Bacterial infections of skin and soft tissue (e.g., abscess, cellulitis, erysipelas, and fasciitis) are primarily caused by group A β-hemolytic streptococci or *Staphylococcus aureus*.

5. Subacute or chronic adenitis may be due to mycobacterial infections. Tuberculosis is increasing in incidence in children and is usually associated with hilar adenopathy, with the lungs as the primary source of the infection. A positive tuberculin skin test and a chest x-ray may confirm tuberculosis. Induration of >15 mm is considered positive in a child older than 4 years with no risk factors. In children with known contacts with tuberculosis, or who are clinically suspected to have tuberculosis, on immunosuppressive therapy, or who have immunosuppressive conditions, including HIV infection, induration >5 mm is considered positive. Children at increased risk of disseminated disease or increased environmental exposure to tuberculosis are considered positive at >10 mm induration. Interferon-gamma release assays may also be used in children ≥5 years.

6. Cervical adenitis is usually due to atypical mycobacteria, primarily *Mycobacterium avium-intracellulare, M. kansasii, M. scrofulaceum,* and *M. marinum.* Diagnosis is determined using acid-fast staining and culture of the excised node or by fine-needle aspiration. An indeterminate tuberculin skin test with 5 to 9 mm of induration suggests infection with atypical mycobacteria. With modern methods of milk pasteurization, *M. bovis,* a previously common cause of cervical adenitis, is rarely seen.

7. Cat-scratch disease, caused by a gram-negative bacillus, *Bartonella henselae,* occurs after exposure to a scratch or bite of a cat, with development of a papule at the site of trauma, followed in 7 to 14 days by regional lymphadenitis, usually axillary. Other symptoms include low-grade fever and malaise. The lymph nodes usually regress spontaneously within several weeks. Some 10% may have a purulent drainage that is culture negative. Serologic tests, such as indirect fluorescent antibody (IFA), enzyme-linked immunosorbent assay (ELISA), IgM tests, or polymerase chain reaction (PCR) testing are useful in making the diagnosis. If needed, diagnosis can be confirmed by biopsy of the node showing granulomas, central necrosis, and organisms seen on Warthin-Starry silver stain.

8. Kawasaki disease is determined clinically in children by noting 5 consecutive days of high fever accompanied by at least four of the following five conditions: cervical lymphadenopathy, oral mucosal erythema, conjunctivitis without exudates, rash, and extremity changes, such as edema and desquamation in the absence of known causes of these signs. The lymph node is typically single and large but is not consistently present.

9. If any of the "red flags" are present, malignancy is suspected and the necessary evaluation should be done. This may include examination of the CBC for anemia, thrombocytopenia,

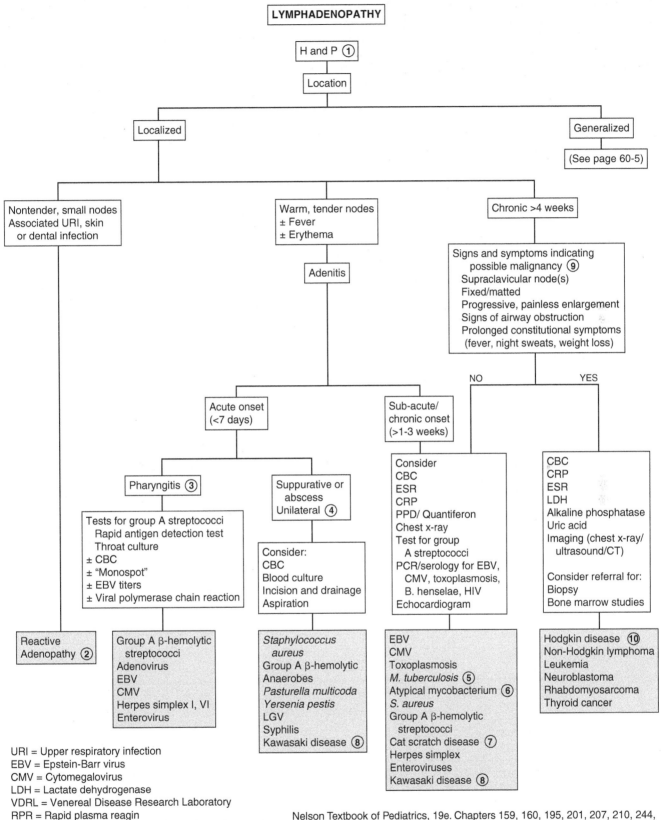

LYMPHADENOPATHY

H and P ①

Location

Localized | Generalized

(See page 60-5)

Nontender, small nodes
Associated URI, skin
or dental infection

Warm, tender nodes
± Fever
± Erythema

Chronic >4 weeks

Signs and symptoms indicating
possible malignancy ⑨
Supraclavicular node(s)
Fixed/matted
Progressive, painless enlargement
Signs of airway obstruction
Prolonged constitutional symptoms
(fever, night sweats, weight loss)

Adenitis

NO   YES

Acute onset
(<7 days)

Sub-acute/
chronic onset
(>1-3 weeks)

Pharyngitis ③

Suppurative or
abscess
Unilateral ④

Consider
CBC
ESR
CRP
PPD/ Quantiferon
Chest x-ray
Test for group
   A streptococci
PCR/serology for EBV,
   CMV, toxoplasmosis,
   B. henselae, HIV
Echocardiogram

CBC
CRP
ESR
LDH
Alkaline phosphatase
Uric acid
Imaging (chest x-ray/
   ultrasound/CT)

Consider referral for:
Biopsy
Bone marrow studies

Tests for group A streptococci
   Rapid antigen detection test
   Throat culture
± CBC
± "Monospot"
± EBV titers
± Viral polymerase chain reaction

Consider:
CBC
Blood culture
Incision and drainage
Aspiration

Reactive
Adenopathy ②

Group A β-hemolytic
   streptococci
Adenovirus
EBV
CMV
Herpes simplex I, VI
Enterovirus

*Staphylococcus
   aureus*
Group A β-hemolytic
Anaerobes
Pasturella multicoda
Yersenia pestis
LGV
Syphilis
Kawasaki disease ⑧

EBV
CMV
Toxoplasmosis
M. tuberculosis ⑤
Atypical mycobacterium ⑥
S. aureus
Group A β-hemolytic
   streptococci
Cat scratch disease ⑦
Herpes simplex
Enteroviruses
Kawasaki disease ⑧

Hodgkin disease ⑩
Non-Hodgkin lymphoma
Leukemia
Neuroblastoma
Rhabdomyosarcoma
Thyroid cancer

URI = Upper respiratory infection
EBV = Epstein-Barr virus
CMV = Cytomegalovirus
LDH = Lactate dehydrogenase
VDRL = Venereal Disease Research Laboratory
RPR = Rapid plasma reagin
PPD = Purified protein derivative (tuberculosis skin test)
PCR = Polymerase chain reaction

Nelson Textbook of Pediatrics, 19e. Chapters 159, 160, 195, 201, 207, 210, 244,
246, 268, 282, 490, 501, 658
Nelsons Essentials, 6e. Chapter 99

leukopenia, or leukocytosis, and for blast cells. Because of a tumor burden or bone involvement, there may be an elevation of lactate dehydrogenase, alkaline phosphatase, and uric acid levels. A chest x-ray may show mediastinal lymphadenopathy, which is suggestive of lymphoma. A CT scan may also be considered. Close clinical follow up should be done to watch for progression of symptoms. If cancer is suspected, a referral should be made to the appropriate specialist for biopsy or for bone marrow studies.

10 Hodgkin disease usually occurs as painless cervical or supraclavicular lymphadenopathy in older children and adolescents. Approximately 30% have systemic symptoms (e.g., fatigue, weight loss, fevers, night sweats). Pruritus, hemolytic anemia, and chest pain after alcohol ingestion are clues. Diagnosis is confirmed by lymph node biopsy and/or bone marrow aspiration. Non-Hodgkin lymphoma usually occurs as supraclavicular, cervical, or axillary adenopathy. In children in the United States, B-cell lymphomas originate in the abdomen with inguinal or iliac lymphadenopathy. About half of children with acute lymphoblastic leukemia present with adenopathy at the time of diagnosis. Systemic signs and symptoms (e.g., fever, malaise, weight loss, pallor, bone pain, petechiae, hepatosplenomegaly) may be present. The CBC may show anemia, thrombocytopenia, leukocytosis or leukopenia, and circulating blast cells. Acute myelogenous leukemia is less common in children but appears similarly. Several other malignancies, including disseminated neuroblastoma, rhabdomyosarcoma, and thyroid cancer, may occur as localized or generalized lymphadenopathy.

11 Generalized lymphadenopathy may be due to infections. HIV-infected children may have systemic symptoms, failure to thrive, and evidence of opportunistic infections. Many viruses including EBV and CMV may cause generalized lymphadenopathy. Syphilis caused by the spirochete *Treponema pallidum* results in both localized and generalized lymphadenopathy. In primary syphilis there is usually localized inguinal adenopathy; in secondary syphilis there is usually generalized lymph node involvement. Epitrochlear involvement is suggestive. Diagnostic tests include rapid plasma reagin (RPR), Venereal Disease Research Laboratory (VDRL), and fluorescent treponemal antibody absorption (FTA-ABS). (See Chapter 41.) *Toxoplasma gondii* is a parasite of cats and can be acquired by humans from contact with cat feces or by eating raw meat. Although the infection may be transmitted to the fetus, lymphadenopathy is uncommon in the newborn and is more common in older children and young adults. Disseminated tuberculosis may present as generalized lymphadenopathy, pulmonary infiltrates, and systemic symptoms. Atypical mycobacteria may cause generalized lymphadenopathy in HIV-infected children.

12 Sinus histiocytosis is a rare disorder with massive cervical lymphadenopathy, fever, elevated erythrocyte sedimentation rate, leukocytosis, and hypergammaglobulinemia. It may be diagnosed using biopsy and tends to resolve spontaneously. Rosai-Dorfman disease is a form of sinus histiocytosis with massive lymphadenopathy.

13 Drug reactions occasionally cause adenopathy. Examples include serum sickness from drugs such as cephalosporins or the drug itself.

Bibliography

Sahai S: Lymphadenopathy, *Pediatr Rev* 34(5):216–27, 2013.

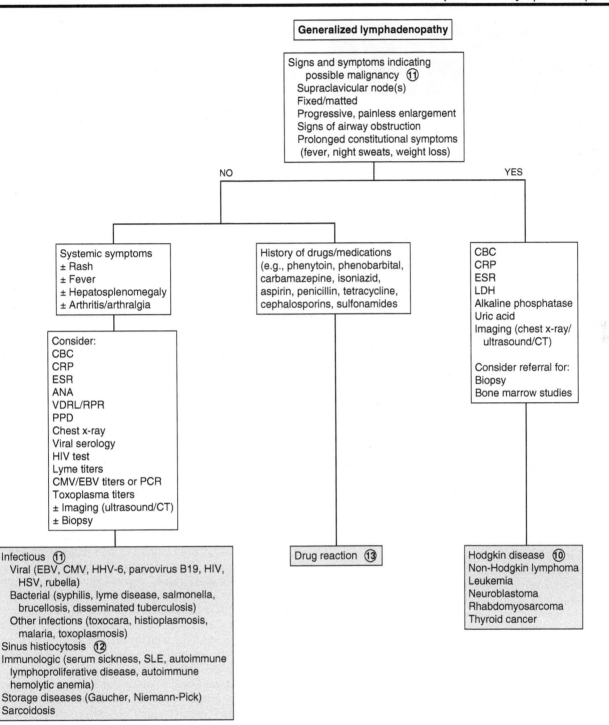

Generalized lymphadenopathy

Signs and symptoms indicating
possible malignancy ⑪
Supraclavicular node(s)
Fixed/matted
Progressive, painless enlargement
Signs of airway obstruction
Prolonged constitutional symptoms
(fever, night sweats, weight loss)

NO — YES

Systemic symptoms
± Rash
± Fever
± Hepatosplenomegaly
± Arthritis/arthralgia

History of drugs/medications
(e.g., phenytoin, phenobarbital,
carbamazepine, isoniazid,
aspirin, penicillin, tetracycline,
cephalosporins, sulfonamides)

CBC
CRP
ESR
LDH
Alkaline phosphatase
Uric acid
Imaging (chest x-ray/
ultrasound/CT)

Consider referral for:
Biopsy
Bone marrow studies

Consider:
CBC
CRP
ESR
ANA
VDRL/RPR
PPD
Chest x-ray
Viral serology
HIV test
Lyme titers
CMV/EBV titers or PCR
Toxoplasma titers
± Imaging (ultrasound/CT)
± Biopsy

Infectious ⑪
  Viral (EBV, CMV, HHV-6, parvovirus B19, HIV,
    HSV, rubella)
  Bacterial (syphilis, lyme disease, salmonella,
    brucellosis, disseminated tuberculosis)
  Other infections (toxocara, histioplasmosis,
    malaria, toxoplasmosis)
Sinus histiocytosis ⑫
Immunologic (serum sickness, SLE, autoimmune
  lymphoproliferative disease, autoimmune
  hemolytic anemia)
Storage diseases (Gaucher, Niemann-Pick)
Sarcoidosis

Drug reaction ⑬

Hodgkin disease ⑩
Non-Hodgkin lymphoma
Leukemia
Neuroblastoma
Rhabdomyosarcoma
Thyroid cancer

Chapter 61
ANEMIA

Anemia is defined as a decrease in hemoglobin concentration of more than 2 standard deviations below the mean. Normal values of hemoglobin and hematocrit vary with age and gender so it is important to use age and sex adjusted norms. Race may also influence norms; African American children have a normal hemoglobin that may be <0.5 g/dl less than white or Asian children. Adolescent females often have lower hemoglobin than males of the same age range. A term infant has a normal hemoglobin level of 15 to 21 g/dl, followed by a physiologic nadir of 9.5 to 10 g/dl around 2 months of age. This is exaggerated in premature infants.

1. History should include iron sources in the diet. Infants with excessive intake (>24 oz per day) of cow's milk or low-iron formula are at risk. Allergy to cow's milk may also cause occult gastrointestinal blood losses. Goat's milk is associated with folate deficiency, and vitamin B12 deficiency occurs in those on macrobiotic diets. Increased iron requirements occur as a result of increased menstrual blood losses, pregnancy, and in prematurity. Impaired absorption of iron may be associated with malabsorptive syndromes such as inflammatory bowel disease or celiac disease. Pica may suggest lead poisoning. A neonatal history of hyperbilirubinemia may indicate a congenital hemolytic anemia, especially if there is a family history of anemia, splenectomy, or cholecystectomy. Sickle cell anemia is more common in those of African descent. Medications may lead to hemolysis, as in glucose-6-phosphate dehydrogenase (G6PD) deficiency. Infections and chronic disease are also associated with anemia. Travel history may reveal infections such as malaria.

In general, anemia (unless acute) may be asymptomatic until the hemoglobin level is less than 7 to 8 g/dl. Clinical features can include pallor, fatigue, irritability, and decreased exercise tolerance. A flow murmur may be present. Severe anemia may cause tachypnea, tachycardia, and ultimately heart failure. Chronic anemia may affect growth. Chronic hemolytic anemias may cause expansion of bone marrow with prominent cheek bones, frontal bossing, and dental malocclusion. Splenomegaly may be present. Lymphadenopathy and hepatosplenomegaly occur with infiltrative disease of the bone marrow. Examination may also reveal signs of systemic disease. A careful skin examination may reveal bruising or purpura.

2. Laboratory testing should include a CBC including red blood cell indices, a review of the peripheral blood smear, and a reticulocyte count. Anemias may be classified based on red blood cell size by using the mean corpuscular volume (MCV) to categorize anemias into microcytic, normocytic, and macrocytic.

Anemias may also be categorized based on reticulocyte counts, which are affected by the underlying cause. Low reticulocyte counts are seen with decreased production of red blood cells and increased reticulocyte counts with hemolysis or blood loss. In patients with moderate to severe anemia, this may appear elevated. It is therefore expressed as the corrected reticulocyte count (reticulocyte count × hemoglobin/normal hemoglobin for age). The reticulocyte count is expressed as a percent of the total number of RBCs.

Examination of the peripheral blood smear is also important and may reveal the diagnosis. Hypersegmentation of polymorphonuclear cells and macrocytosis indicate megaloblastic disease. Other findings may include spherocytes (spherocytic anemia, immune-mediated hemolytic anemia), sickle cells (sickle cell anemia), and Howell-Jolly bodies (asplenia). Blister or bite cells are seen in Glucose-6-phosphate dehydrogenase (G6PD) deficiency. Target cells may be seen in patients with iron deficiency, hemoglobinopathies, and thalassemia. Intraerythrocytic parasites may be seen on peripheral smear in patients with malaria. If necessary, bone marrow examination provides a definitive diagnosis in sideroblastic anemia, aplastic anemias, and malignancies.

3. The American Academy of Pediatrics recommends universal screening for anemia at age 1 year with determination of hemoglobin concentration. In addition, selective screening is recommended at any age for those with additional risk factors (e.g., prematurity or low birth weight, exclusive breast feeding beyond 4 months of age, early weaning to cow's milk).

Iron deficiency is the most common cause of anemia in children. If it is suggested by history and CBC (decreased hemoglobin, increased red blood cell distribution width and low MCV), a therapeutic trial of iron may be considered (3 to 6 mg/kg/day of elemental iron). Iron-deficiency anemia may be normocytic in the early stages. An increase in hemoglobin of 1 g/dl within 2 to 4 weeks confirms the diagnosis. Laboratory confirmation of iron-deficiency anemia by a low transferrin saturation (low serum iron, high total iron-binding capacity), and low ferritin may be considered in children who are at low risk and have unexplained iron deficiency.

4. Thalassemias are a group of genetic disorders of globin production. β-thalassemia trait is most common in children of Mediterranean or African descent. The red blood cell distribution width is normal, and hemoglobin A2 is increased. Children with β-thalassemia major (Cooley anemia) present during infancy with severe anemia, increased reticulocyte count, and features of bone marrow expansion. Children with β-thalassemia trait are asymptomatic. α-thalassemia may occur as an asymptomatic carrier state; as a trait with mild anemia and microcytosis; as hemoglobin H disease with a moderate hemolytic anemia, microcytosis, reticulocytosis, and splenomegaly; or as α-thalassemia major, which is generally incompatible with life. Hemoglobin H and α-thalassemia major disease usually occur in Asians. α-thalassemia is usually a diagnosis of exclusion because DNA sequencing is rarely done outside a laboratory setting.

5. Microcytic anemia is associated with lead poisoning (plumbism) as iron deficiency enhances the absorption of lead.

6. Anemia of chronic disease may be microcytic or normocytic, with increased erythrocyte sedimentation rate and decreased serum iron and total iron binding capacity (TIBC). The ferritin may be increased due to an inflammatory state. Because ferritin is an acute phase reactant and may be influenced by concurrent infection or inflammation, some experts recommend also obtaining a C-reactive protein (CRP) test. Anemia of chronic disease (ACD) is also known as "anemia of inflammation." It may be seen with systemic infections (e.g., HIV, osteomyelitis), autoimmune disorders (e.g., systemic lupus erythematosus, inflammatory bowel disease), and with malignancies.

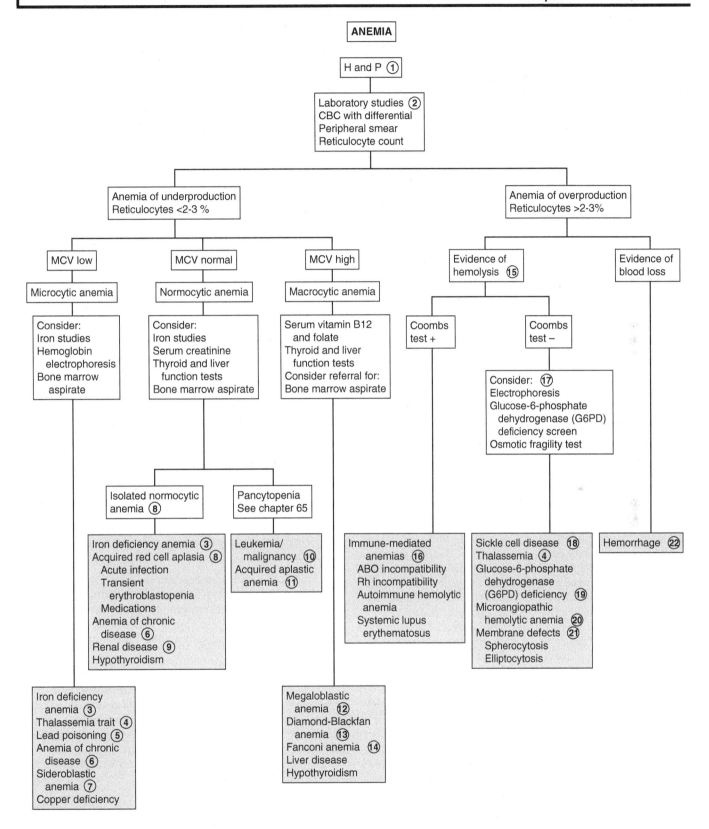

ANEMIA

H and P ①

Laboratory studies ②
CBC with differential
Peripheral smear
Reticulocyte count

Anemia of underproduction
Reticulocytes <2-3 %

Anemia of overproduction
Reticulocytes >2-3%

MCV low

MCV normal

MCV high

Evidence of
hemolysis ⑮

Evidence of
blood loss

Microcytic anemia

Normocytic anemia

Macrocytic anemia

Coombs
test +

Coombs
test −

Consider:
Iron studies
Hemoglobin
  electrophoresis
Bone marrow
  aspirate

Consider:
Iron studies
Serum creatinine
Thyroid and liver
  function tests
Bone marrow aspirate

Serum vitamin B12
  and folate
Thyroid and liver
  function tests
Consider referral for:
Bone marrow aspirate

Consider: ⑰
Electrophoresis
Glucose-6-phosphate
  dehydrogenase (G6PD)
  deficiency screen
Osmotic fragility test

Isolated normocytic
anemia ⑧

Pancytopenia
See chapter 65

Iron deficiency anemia ③
Acquired red cell aplasia ⑧
  Acute infection
  Transient
    erythroblastopenia
  Medications
Anemia of chronic
  disease ⑥
Renal disease ⑨
Hypothyroidism

Leukemia/
malignancy ⑩
Acquired aplastic
anemia ⑪

Immune-mediated
  anemias ⑯
ABO incompatibility
Rh incompatibility
Autoimmune hemolytic
  anemia
Systemic lupus
  erythematosus

Sickle cell disease ⑱
Thalassemia ④
Glucose-6-phosphate
  dehydrogenase
  (G6PD) deficiency ⑲
Microangiopathic
  hemolytic anemia ⑳
Membrane defects ㉑
  Spherocytosis
  Elliptocytosis

Hemorrhage ㉒

Iron deficiency
  anemia ③
Thalassemia trait ④
Lead poisoning ⑤
Anemia of chronic
  disease ⑥
Sideroblastic
  anemia ⑦
Copper deficiency

Megaloblastic
  anemia ⑫
Diamond-Blackfan
  anemia ⑬
Fanconi anemia ⑭
Liver disease
Hypothyroidism

Nelson Textbook of Pediatrics, 19e. Chapters 441-459
Nelsons Essentials, 6e. Chapter 150

7 Sideroblastic anemias are rare disorders of heme synthesis and may be acquired or hereditary. The peripheral smear shows hypochromic microcytic red blood cells mixed with normal cells, resulting in a very high red cell distribution width (RDW). Iron overload causes increased serum iron, ferritin, and iron saturation.

8 Acquired red cell aplasia may be due to acute infections, which may cause a transient mild anemia. A more severe form of transient red blood cell hypoplasia (aplastic crisis) may occur in patients with hemolytic anemias after infection with parvovirus B19, which causes erythema infectiosum (fifth disease). Transient erythroblastopenia of childhood is a temporary arrest of red blood cell production and occurs predominantly in children aged 6 months to 3 years. It often follows a viral illness. The temporary suppression of erythropoiesis results in reticulocytopenia and moderate to severe normocytic anemia. Hemoglobin levels are usually between 6 to 8 g/dL, neutropenia may be present and platelet counts are normal or elevated. Medications such as chloramphenicol may also cause red cell aplasia.

9 Chronic renal disease may cause anemia due to a deficiency of erythropoietin (EPO).

10 Leukemia and metastatic malignancy may cause bone marrow infiltration and normocytic anemia with thrombocytopenia and either leukocytosis or leukopenia. Blast cells may be seen on the peripheral smear.

11 Acquired aplastic anemia may be postinfectious (e.g., hepatitis, EBV, parvovirus B19), drug related (e.g., chloramphenicol, anticonvulsants, cytotoxic drugs, sulfonamides), toxin related (e.g., benzene), due to radiation exposure, or idiopathic. It is characterized by anemia, neutropenia, and thrombocytopenia. There is hypoplasia of the bone marrow.

12 Megaloblastic anemia (large RBCs with abnormal hypersegmented neutrophils due to vitamin B12 or folate deficiency is quite rare in children. Breast-fed infants of strictly vegetarian mothers may have vitamin B12 deficiency. Malabsorption of vitamin B12 may be due to a rare intrinsic factor deficiency (e.g., congenital pernicious anemia), resection of the ileum, or impaired absorption in inflammatory conditions (e.g., celiac disease).

Folate deficiency may be caused by decreased absorption due to resection or inflammatory disease of the small bowel or certain anticonvulsant drugs (e.g., phenytoin, primidone, phenobarbital). Folate deficiency may also be seen infants fed goat's milk, which is low in folate. Some medications (e.g., methotrexate, trimethoprim) can inhibit the action of folate. Increased folate requirements may occur in chronic hemolytic anemia (e.g., sickle cell).

13 Congenital hypoplastic anemia (Diamond-Blackfan anemia) occurs in the first year of life as severe, usually macrocytic anemia, and reticulocytopenia. Bone marrow examination shows a deficiency or absence of red blood cell precursors in an otherwise normally cellular bone marrow.

14 Fanconi anemia (FA) has a primarily autosomal recessive inheritance. The classic phenotype presents with pancytopenia and physical stigmata such as thumb and radial anomalies, growth failure, short stature and skin findings (e.g., hyperpigmentation, café-au-lait spots, vitiligo). Renal, cardiovascular and gastrointestinal malformations also occur. Approximately 10% of patients with FA are cognitively delayed. RBCs have

fetal characteristics (e.g., increased MCV, fetal hemoglobin). Thrombocytopenia usually appears first, with subsequent development of granulocytopenia and then macrocytic anemia. Ultimately, severe aplasia develops in most cases.

15 Hemolytic disorders are characterized by shortened RBC survival and reticulocytosis. There may be icterus, splenomegaly, gallstones, and significant family or neonatal history. Laboratory findings include abnormal cell morphology; increased red blood cell distribution width, indirect bilirubin, urine urobilinogen, and lactate dehydrogenase; decreased serum haptoglobin; and hemoglobinuria.

16 A positive antiglobulin (Coombs) test indicates an immune-mediated anemia. Isoimmune hemolytic anemia is the most common cause of neonatal anemia. Rh incompatibility is rare because of administration of Rh immune globulin to Rh-negative mothers. When it occurs it causes severe hemolysis and can occur as intrauterine hydrops fetalis or severe jaundice. The direct Coombs test is strongly positive. ABO incompatibility occurs when the mother is blood group O and the fetus is blood group A or B, and is usually less severe. Acquired autoimmune hemolytic anemia may occur with an underlying immunologic dysfunction (e.g., HIV, lymphoma) or after an acute infection, usually viral. It may be drug related (e.g., penicillins, cephalosporins), or idiopathic. The direct Coombs test result is positive, and spherocytes are seen on peripheral smear. Cold agglutinin disease occurs most commonly after infections from *Mycoplasma pneumonia* or viruses. It is characterized by increased cold agglutinin antibodies, which cause hemolysis after exposure to cold. Paroxysmal cold hemoglobinuria and, rarely, infectious mononucleosis also cause anemia with cold exposure.

17 In children with a negative Coombs test, other tests should be considered based on history, physical findings, and the CBC and smear. These may include hemoglobin electrophoresis, glucose-6-phosphate dehydrogenase screening, and osmotic fragility tests.

18 Sickle cell hemoglobinopathies are most common in children of Central African descent and less common in children of Mediterranean or Arabic descent. Sickle cell disease may occur combined with hemoglobin C or β-thalassemia, causing a less severe disorder. Diagnosis is by hemoglobin electrophoresis.

19 Glucose-6-phosphate dehydrogenase (G6PD) deficiency is an RBC enzyme defect. It is an X-linked disorder and occurs most often in patients of African or Mediterranean descent. Characteristic findings include "bite cells" and inclusion bodies called Heinz bodies. There is increased susceptibility of RBCs to oxidant injury due to infections, medications (e.g., sulfonamides, antimalarials, nitrofurantoin, nalidixic acid, chloramphenicol, methylene blue, vitamin K analogs), toxins (e.g., mothballs, large doses of vitamin C, benzene), and foods (e.g., fava beans).

20 Microangiopathic hemolytic anemia is a fragmentation hemolysis, which occurs due to mechanical injury of red blood cells. It may be seen along with thrombocytopenia in disseminated intravascular coagulation, hemolytic-uremic syndrome, Kasabach-Merritt syndrome (i.e., consumptive coagulopathy seen with large hemangiomas) and thrombotic thrombocytopenic purpura. The peripheral smear shows RBC fragments (e.g., helmet cells, schistocytes, spherocytes, burr cells).

21 Membrane defects include hereditary spherocytosis and elliptocytosis. Presenting features are anemia, jaundice, and splenomegaly. Diagnosis is confirmed by an osmotic fragility test.

22 A significant acute or subacute blood loss leads to anemia. The RBC morphology and size remain normal. It may require 3 to 5 days to produce an elevated reticulocyte count. Transfusion may be required to replace large blood losses when there are clinical manifestations such as fatigue, lightheadedness, tachycardia, dyspnea, or heart failure.

Bibliography

Baker RD, Greer FR: Diagnosis and prevention of iron deficiency and iron-deficiency anemia in infants and young children (0-3 years of age), *Pediatrics* 126(5):1040–1050, 2010.

Janus J, Moerschel SK: Evaluation of anemia in children, *Am Fam Physician* 81(12):1462–1471, 2010.

Chapter 62
BLEEDING

Bleeding disorders are caused by a disturbance in the normal hemostasis. Components of the hemostatic mechanism include platelets, anticoagulant proteins, procoagulant proteins, and components of the vessel walls. The first stage of hemostasis consists of formation of "platelet plug" followed by activation of coagulation pathways leading to formation of a fibrin clot.

(1) History should include age and acuity at onset of bleeding, triggers, whether bleeding was immediate or delayed, and whether it was prolonged or exaggerated. Severity of bleeding must be determined, such as nosebleeds requiring cautery or packing or surgeries requiring transfusions. It is very important to differentiate bruising due to child abuse. Perinatal history should include details regarding bruising or petechiae, bleeding with circumcision, cephalhematoma, CNS or gastrointestinal bleeding, unexplained anemia or jaundice, or bleeding after cord separation. A history of vitamin K administration and maternal drugs should be obtained. In adolescent girls a history of dysfunctional uterine bleeding would be important. A detailed family history should be obtained, including maternal obstetric history of bleeding. For X-linked disorders (e.g., hemophilias) a family history of male relatives on the maternal side should be solicited, and history of consanguinity for autosomal recessive conditions (Factor XIII deficiency). Medications such as aspirin, other nonsteroidal anti-inflammatory drugs (NSAIDs), anticoagulants, antibiotics, and anticonvulsants may be associated with bleeding. The bleeding site may indicate the etiology. Acute mucocutaneous bleeding may indicate idiopathic thrombocytopenic purpura. Generalized bleeding may be associated with disseminated intravascular coagulation (DIC), vitamin K deficiency, liver disease, or uremia. Mucosal bleeding, petechiae, and bruising may indicate disorders of platelets, blood vessels, or von Willebrand disease. Bleeding into soft tissues, muscles and joints, or excessive bleeding with surgery may be due to deficiency of coagulation factors (e.g., hemophilia). Various findings on physical examination may be helpful in determining the etiology. Heart murmurs may indicate endocarditis; arthropathy is suggestive of hemophilia; joint laxity is seen with Ehlers-Danlos syndrome; and thumb or radial anomalies are seen with Fanconi anemia or thrombocytopenia-absent radius (TAR) syndrome. Hepatosplenomegaly may indicate liver disease; lymphadenopathy may indicate a malignancy. Skin findings include hematomas, petechiae, ecchymoses, telangiectasia, purpura, poor wound healing, lax skin, and varicose veins.

(2) The critical evaluation for a bleeding disorder should begin with a few specific laboratory tests. A CBC including a platelet count may reveal thrombocytopenia or anemia. A peripheral smear can exclude pseudo-thrombocytopenia due to platelet clumping. Platelet morphology may indicate the diagnosis; platelets are small in Wiscott Aldrich syndrome and giant platelets are seen in Bernard Soulier syndrome. Prothrombin time (PT) and activated partial thromboplastin time (aPTT) are dependent on all coagulation factors except factor XIII. A clotting factor deficiency or the presence of an inhibitor can prolong

PT and aPTT. Testing for an inhibitor is done by mixing one part of patient plasma with one part pooled plasma; if the PT or aPTT corrects, there is a factor deficiency; if it does not correct, an inhibitor is present. Inhibitors include anticoagulants (e.g., heparin), autoantibodies against clotting factors, and lupus type anticoagulants. Fibrinogen function is measured by thrombin time or fibrinogen activity. In von Willebrand disease, the PTT may be prolonged, but testing should be considered if mucocutaneous bleeding disorder is suspected because screening laboratory results may be normal in von Willebrand disease. Testing may include a quantitative assay for von Willebrand factor (vWF) antigen, testing for vWF activity (ristocetin cofactor activity), testing for plasma factor VIII activity, determination of vWF structure (vWF multimers), and a platelet count. If the patient is taking medications that might interfere with hemostasis, all tests should be done or repeated after stopping the medication. Bleeding time indirectly measures platelet number, function and platelet-vessel wall interaction; it has low sensitivity. Platelet function studies may include PFA-100 as an initial screen for platelet function abnormalities but there are problems with sensitivity and specificity. If platelet function abnormality is seriously being considered, platelet aggregation studies are needed.

(3) Vitamin K deficiency is common in neonates, malnourished children, those receiving broad-spectrum antibiotics, and children with cholestatic liver disease. Hemorrhagic disease of the newborn is rarely seen anymore because of prophylactic administration on Vitamin K in the newborn nursery. Vitamin K deficiency may present as generalized bleeding into skin, gastrointestinal tract, and central nervous system. Dicumarol and rat poison (superwarfarin) also act by affecting vitamin K and, therefore, also vitamin K-dependent factors II, VII, IX, and X.

(4) Inhibitors may be directed against a specific coagulation factor or a reaction site in the coagulation pathway. Inhibitors against specific factors usually affect factors VIII, IX, or XI, causing prolonged PTT with normal PT. Lupus anticoagulant is directed against a reaction site and causes prolonged PT and PTT; it is more likely to cause thrombosis than bleeding.

(5) Deficiency of factor VIII is hemophilia A, and that of factor IX is hemophilia B or Christmas disease. These are transmitted as X-linked traits; therefore, family history of bleeding in males in the mother's family should be obtained. Hemophilia A or B usually occur as bleeding into muscles or joints and easy bruising. Because factor VIII does not cross the placenta, bleeding may occur during the neonatal period. Factor XI deficiency, or hemophilia C, has autosomal recessive transmission and milder symptoms than A and B. Factor XII or Hageman factor deficiency causes prolonged PTT but is usually asymptomatic.

(6) The most common cause of lifelong symptoms of mucocutaneous bleeding is von Willebrand disease due to deficiency of vWF, which is prevalent in approximately 1% of children. Inheritance is typically autosomal dominant. The vWF is a protein required for platelet plug formation; it is also a carrier for factor VIII. In severe deficiency of vWF there is also deficient factor VIII. PTT and bleeding time are often, but not always, abnormal, and so screening for vWF should always be considered when evaluating bleeding disorders. The PTT corrects with 1:1 mixing with pooled plasma. In addition, stress, medications, trauma, and difficult venipuncture may increase vWF levels. Levels of vWF are

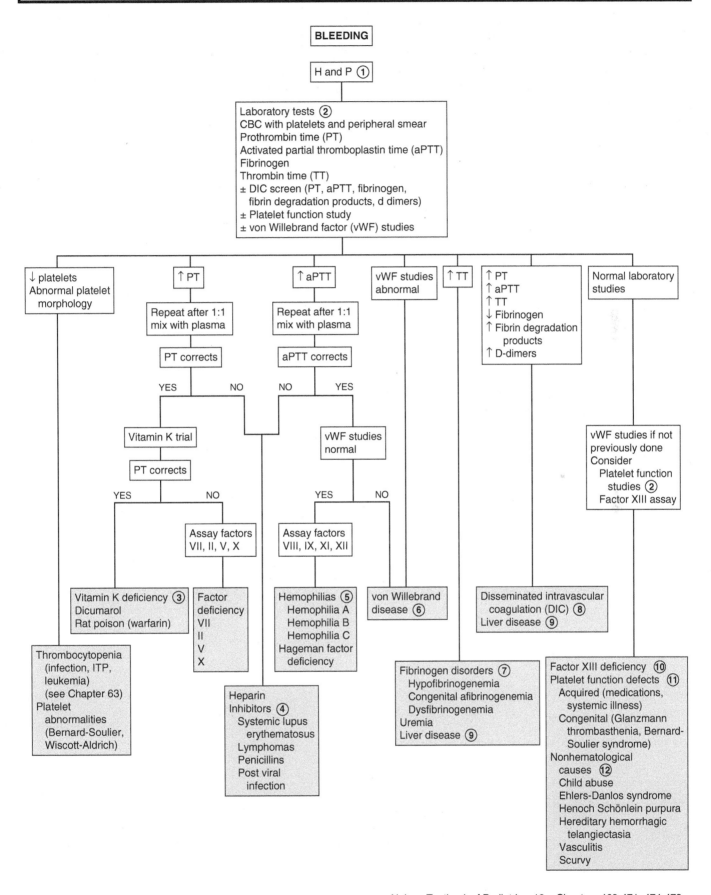

BLEEDING

H and P ①

Laboratory tests ②
CBC with platelets and peripheral smear
Prothrombin time (PT)
Activated partial thromboplastin time (aPTT)
Fibrinogen
Thrombin time (TT)
± DIC screen (PT, aPTT, fibrinogen,
    fibrin degradation products, d dimers)
± Platelet function study
± von Willebrand factor (vWF) studies

↓ platelets
Abnormal platelet
morphology

↑ PT

↑ aPTT

vWF studies
abnormal

↑ TT

↑ PT
↑ aPTT
↑ TT
↓ Fibrinogen
↑ Fibrin degradation
    products
↑ D-dimers

Normal laboratory
studies

Repeat after 1:1
mix with plasma

Repeat after 1:1
mix with plasma

PT corrects

aPTT corrects

YES   NO   NO   YES

Vitamin K trial

vWF studies
normal

PT corrects

YES   NO   YES   NO

vWF studies if not
previously done
Consider
    Platelet function
    studies ②
    Factor XIII assay

Assay factors
VII, II, V, X

Assay factors
VIII, IX, XI, XII

Vitamin K deficiency ③
Dicumarol
Rat poison (warfarin)

Factor
deficiency
VII
II
V
X

Hemophilias ⑤
Hemophilia A
Hemophilia B
Hemophilia C
Hageman factor
deficiency

von Willebrand
disease ⑥

Disseminated intravascular
coagulation (DIC) ⑧
Liver disease ⑨

Thrombocytopenia
(infection, ITP,
leukemia)
(see Chapter 63)
Platelet
abnormalities
(Bernard-Soulier,
Wiscott-Aldrich)

Heparin
Inhibitors ④
Systemic lupus
    erythematosus
Lymphomas
Penicillins
Post viral
    infection

Fibrinogen disorders ⑦
Hypofibrinogenemia
Congenital afibrinogenemia
Dysfibrinogenemia
Uremia
Liver disease ⑨

Factor XIII deficiency ⑩
Platelet function defects ⑪
Acquired (medications,
    systemic illness)
Congenital (Glanzmann
    thrombasthenia, Bernard-
    Soulier syndrome)
Nonhematological
    causes ⑫
Child abuse
Ehlers-Danlos syndrome
Henoch Schönlein purpura
Hereditary hemorrhagic
    telangiectasia
Vasculitis
Scurvy

Nelson Textbook of Pediatrics, 19e. Chapters 469-471, 474-478
Nelsons Essentials, 6e. Chapter 151

dependent on blood type and may be influenced by age. Interpretation of tests requires a qualified laboratory and often the assistance of a hematologist.

7 Thrombin time measures the last step in the clotting cascade, the conversion of fibrinogen to fibrin. Thrombin time is prolonged when fibrinogen levels are low (hypofibrinogenemia or afibrinogenemia), with dysfunctional fibrinogen (dysfibrinogenemia), or due to factors, which interfere with fibrin formation (e.g., heparin, fibrin split products). Congenital afibrinogenemia is a rare disorder. Although the blood is incoagulable, hemorrhage is rarely spontaneous and usually occurs with trauma or surgery.

8 DIC is a generalized consumption of clotting factors, anticoagulant proteins, and platelets. It is usually triggered by a severe illness, hypoxia, acidosis, tissue necrosis, and endothelial damage, and may be accompanied by shock. It may appear as a hemorrhagic or thrombotic disorder or both.

9 Liver failure affects all coagulation factors except factor VIII. In both DIC and liver failure there is prolonged PT, PTT, and thrombin time and decreased fibrinogen. Fibrin degradation products are elevated in DIC and are normal or elevated in liver failure. Platelets are decreased in DIC but may be normal or decreased with liver failure.

10 Factor XIII deficiency often presents in infancy as bleeding after separation of the umbilical stump and later as intracranial, gastrointestinal, and intra-articular bleeding. Results of routine coagulation studies are normal.

11 Platelet function defects may also be due to medications (e.g., aspirin, NSAIDs, alcohol, high doses of penicillin, valproate) as well as systemic illness (e.g., uremia, liver disease). Severe congenital platelet defects present shortly after birth; these include Glanzmann thrombasthenia (deficiency of a fibrinogen receptor) with normal platelet counts and Bernard-Soulier syndrome (deficiency of the von Willebrand receptor) with mild thrombocytopenia. If other tests are normal and examination does not suggest other nonhematological etiologies (see Footnote 12), platelet aggregation studies should be considered to evaluate for other less severe platelet function defects.

12 Many nonhematological conditions can mimic bleeding disorders. Significant bruising or bleeding with normal laboratory studies should prompt consideration of child abuse. Disorders of the vessel walls or their supporting tissues may have a similar presentation as a bleeding disorder but coagulation studies are usually normal. Petechiae and purpurae may be caused by an underlying vasculitis (Henoch-Schönlein purpura) or disorders affecting collagen structures (e.g., Ehlers-Danlos syndrome, scurvy). Hereditary hemorrhagic telangiectasia may present with epistaxis or gastrointestinal bleeding.

Bibliography

Journeycake JM, Buchanan GR: Coagulation disorders, *Pediatr Rev* 24(3): 83–91, 2003.

Sarnaik A, Kamat D, Kannikeswaran N: Diagnosis and management of bleeding disorder in a child, *Clin Pediatrics* 49(5):422–431, 2010.

Sharathkumar AA, Pipe SW: Bleeding disorders. *Pediatr Rev* 29(4): 121–130, 2008.

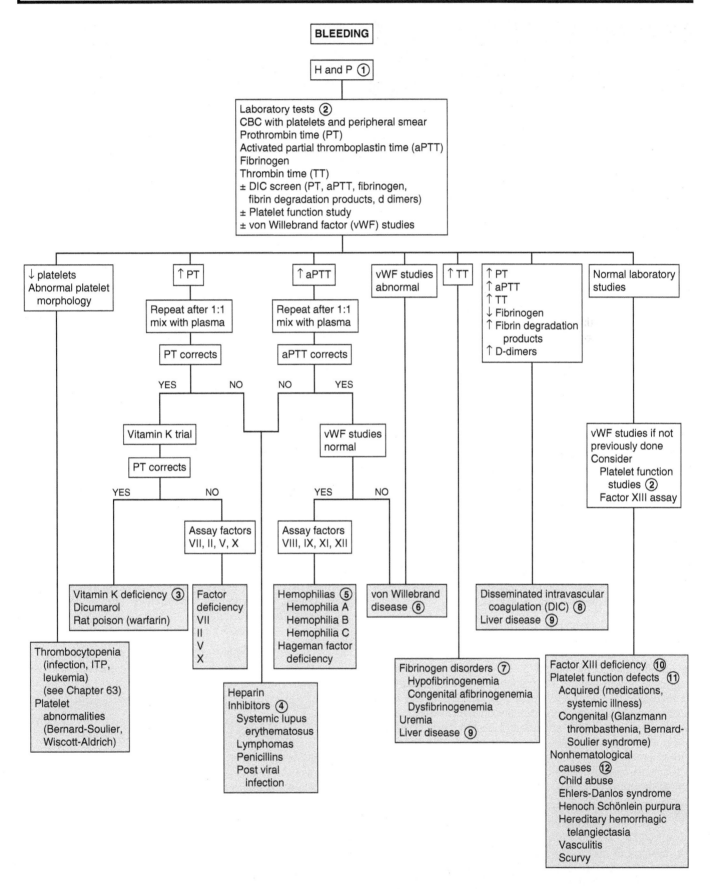

BLEEDING

H and P ①

Laboratory tests ②
CBC with platelets and peripheral smear
Prothrombin time (PT)
Activated partial thromboplastin time (aPTT)
Fibrinogen
Thrombin time (TT)
± DIC screen (PT, aPTT, fibrinogen,
  fibrin degradation products, d dimers)
± Platelet function study
± von Willebrand factor (vWF) studies

↓ platelets
Abnormal platelet
morphology

↑ PT

↑ aPTT

vWF studies
abnormal

↑ TT

↑ PT
↑ aPTT
↑ TT
↓ Fibrinogen
↑ Fibrin degradation
  products
↑ D-dimers

Normal laboratory
studies

Repeat after 1:1
mix with plasma

Repeat after 1:1
mix with plasma

PT corrects

aPTT corrects

YES   NO

NO   YES

Vitamin K trial

vWF studies
normal

vWF studies if not
previously done
Consider
  Platelet function
    studies ②
  Factor XIII assay

PT corrects

YES   NO

YES   NO

Assay factors
VII, II, V, X

Assay factors
VIII, IX, XI, XII

Vitamin K deficiency ③
Dicumarol
Rat poison (warfarin)

Factor
deficiency
VII
II
V
X

Hemophilias ⑤
  Hemophilia A
  Hemophilia B
  Hemophilia C
  Hageman factor
    deficiency

von Willebrand
disease ⑥

Disseminated intravascular
  coagulation (DIC) ⑧
Liver disease ⑨

Thrombocytopenia
(infection, ITP,
leukemia)
(see Chapter 63)
Platelet
abnormalities
(Bernard-Soulier,
Wiscott-Aldrich)

Heparin
Inhibitors ④
  Systemic lupus
    erythematosus
  Lymphomas
  Penicillins
  Post viral
    infection

Fibrinogen disorders ⑦
  Hypofibrinogenemia
  Congenital afibrinogenemia
  Dysfibrinogenemia
Uremia
Liver disease ⑨

Factor XIII deficiency ⑩
Platelet function defects ⑪
  Acquired (medications,
    systemic illness)
  Congenital (Glanzmann
    thrombasthenia, Bernard-
    Soulier syndrome)
Nonhematological
  causes ⑫
  Child abuse
  Ehlers-Danlos syndrome
  Henoch Schönlein purpura
  Hereditary hemorrhagic
    telangiectasia
  Vasculitis
  Scurvy

Nelson Textbook of Pediatrics, 19e. Chapters 469-471, 474-478
Nelsons Essentials, 6e. Chapter 151

Chapter 63
PETECHIAE/PURPURA

Petechiae are pinpoint, flat, red lesions caused by capillary bleeding into the skin. Purpura are red, purple, or brown lesions of the skin or mucosa may be raised and palpable. Petechiae are often caused by thrombocytopenia, but they may also be caused by platelet function defects or blood vessel defects. The presence of purpura in an ill child often implies disseminated intravascular coagulation (DIC). Thrombocytopenia is a decrease in platelet count by 2 standard deviations below the mean ($<150,000/mm^3$). Platelet counts $>50,000/mm^3$ are rarely associated with clinical bleeding in the absence of trauma. When the platelet count is $<20,000/mm^3$ there may be spontaneous bleeding.

1 History should include that of trauma. Localized petechiae may occur with trauma and predominantly on the face with prolonged crying or emesis; they may not require further evaluation. History of epistaxis, bleeding from the gums, menorrhagia, bleeding during surgery, and exposure to toxins, drugs, or radiation should be obtained, as well as noting the presence of infections or systemic illness. Viral illnesses and occasionally MMR vaccination may precede immune thrombocytopenia (ITP). Bloody diarrhea may be indicative of hemolytic uremic syndrome (HUS). Duration of symptoms and acuity of presentation may indicate if the cause is congenital or acquired. Congenital anomalies may be associated with platelet defects, as well as some familial conditions. Lymphadenopathy or hepatosplenomegaly may indicate infiltrative processes. Systemic symptoms (e.g., fever, weight loss) may indicate underlying malignancy or systemic disease. Examination for joint laxity (Ehlers-Danlos syndrome) and thumb and radial anomalies (Fanconi anemia or TAR [thrombocytopenia-absent radius] syndrome) should be done. In addition to petechiae and purpura, skin findings may include hematomas, ecchymoses, telangiectases, poor wound healing, and lax skin.

2 A CBC and review of peripheral smear is important. Clumping or aggregation of platelets due to interaction with anticoagulants in collection tubes or due to platelet cold agglutinins should be identified. Thrombocytopenia may be due to decreased production (hypoproductive), characterized by small platelets, destructive with large platelets, or due to sequestration. Hypoproductive conditions often involve the marrow and are associated with anemia and neutropenia. Peripheral smear may also show fragmented red blood cells consistent with microangiopathy (e.g., DIC, HUS). Leukocytosis suggests sepsis; blasts suggest leukemia, and leukocyte inclusions, congenital thrombocytopenias.

3 A common cause of immune-mediated thrombocytopenia in a well-appearing child is immune thrombocytopenic purpura (ITP). The platelet count is usually $<20,000/mm^3$, and the presence of megakaryocytes indicates a rapid turnover of platelets. History may reveal a preceding viral illness. Mucosal bleeding such as epistaxis and from the gastrointestinal tract may be present. Marrow examination should be considered in children with atypical presentation or with hepatosplenomegaly

or lymphadenopathy. (See Chapter 60.) In adolescents, particularly in girls, an antinuclear antibody (ANA) test may be considered to rule out systemic lupus erythematosus (SLE). HIV infection may also occur initially as thrombocytopenia, and the appropriate laboratory studies should be obtained if this is suggested. Drugs that may cause thrombocytopenia include quinidine, carbamazepine, phenytoin, sulfonamides, trimethoprim-sulfamethoxazole, and chloramphenicol.

4 Bernard-Soulier syndrome is severe congenital disorder of platelet function with autosomal recessive inheritance and characterized by thrombocytopenia with giant platelets. MYH9-related thrombocytopenia is a group of thrombocytopenia syndromes with autosomal dominant inheritance, characterized by large platelets and associated with anomalies such as sensorineural deafness and renal or eye disease.

5 Thrombocytopenia with small platelets (hypoproductive) may be associated with congenital syndromes. TAR syndrome is associated with severe thrombocytopenia, aplasia of the radii and thumbs, and renal and cardiac anomalies. It is a familial condition and may appear in the neonatal period. Similar features may be present in Fanconi pancytopenia, which usually presents in the third or fourth year of life. Wiskott-Aldrich syndrome, an X-linked recessive trait, includes eczema, thrombocytopenia, hemorrhage, and immunologic defects resulting in frequent infections. Congenital amegakaryocytic thrombocytopenia usually presents within the first week of life.

6 Fever and a petechial/purpuric rash should always alert the physician to the possibility of serious bacterial infection, in particular, infection with *Neisseria meningitidis*. Serious infections with other bacteria and rickettsial diseases can also produce this type of rash. (See Chapter 59.) Thrombocytopenia may or may not be present.

7 DIC is a generalized consumption of clotting factors, anticoagulant proteins, and platelets. It is usually triggered by a severe illness, hypoxia, acidosis, tissue necrosis, or endothelial damage and may be accompanied by shock. It may occur as a hemorrhagic or thrombotic disorder, or both. Fibrinogen is decreased. There is an increase in fibrin degradation products (FDPs) and D-dimers. PT and PTT are both prolonged.

8 HUS usually follows diarrheal infection (*Escherichia coli* O157:H7). Features include hemolytic anemia, thrombocytopenia, and acute renal insufficiency.

9 Thrombotic thrombocytopenic purpura is similar to HUS with thrombocytopenia and microangiopathic hemolytic anemia. It usually presents in adolescents and adults.

10 Kasabach-Merritt syndrome occurs in children with large cavernous hemangiomas of the trunk, extremities, or abdominal organs where platelets are trapped in the vascular bed. Peripheral smear shows thrombocytopenia and red blood cell fragments; bone marrow examination shows the normal number of megakaryocytes.

11 Thrombocytopenia occurs in patients with massive splenomegaly because the spleen sequesters platelets. Leukopenia and anemia may also be present. It is important to identify an etiology for the splenomegaly as part of the workup (See Chapter 28.)

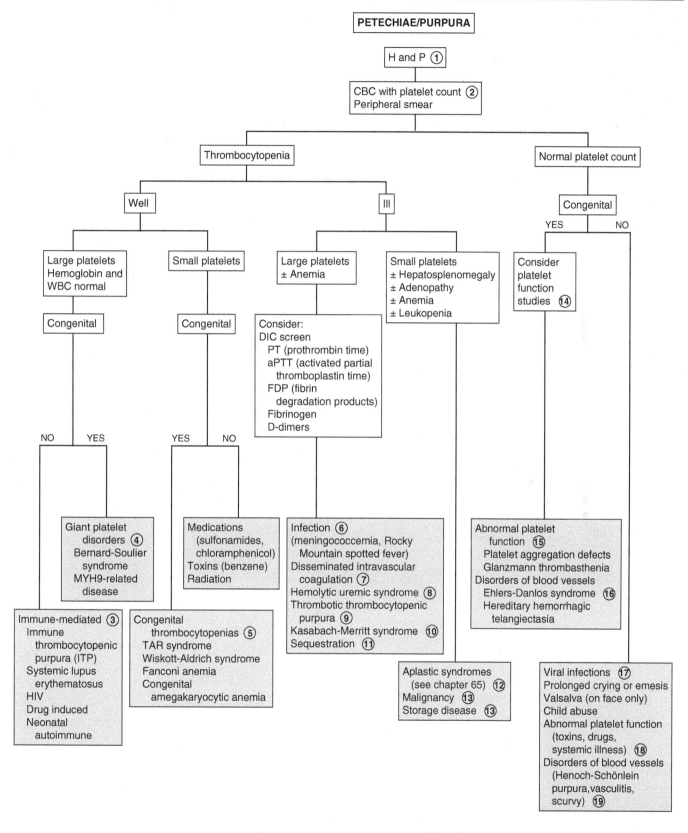

PETECHIAE/PURPURA

H and P ①

CBC with platelet count ②
Peripheral smear

Thrombocytopenia — **Normal platelet count**

Well — **Ill** — **Congenital** (YES / NO)

Large platelets
Hemoglobin and
WBC normal

Small platelets

Large platelets
± Anemia

Small platelets
± Hepatosplenomegaly
± Adenopathy
± Anemia
± Leukopenia

Consider
platelet
function
studies ⑭

Congenital (NO / YES)

Congenital (YES / NO)

Consider:
DIC screen
　PT (prothrombin time)
　aPTT (activated partial
　　thromboplastin time)
　FDP (fibrin
　　degradation products)
　Fibrinogen
　D-dimers

Giant platelet
　disorders ④
Bernard-Soulier
　syndrome
MYH9-related
　disease

Medications
　(sulfonamides,
　chloramphenicol)
Toxins (benzene)
Radiation

Infection ⑥
(meningococcemia, Rocky
　Mountain spotted fever)
Disseminated intravascular
　coagulation ⑦
Hemolytic uremic syndrome ⑧
Thrombotic thrombocytopenic
　purpura ⑨
Kasabach-Merritt syndrome ⑩
Sequestration ⑪

Abnormal platelet
　function ⑮
Platelet aggregation defects
Glanzmann thrombasthenia
Disorders of blood vessels
　Ehlers-Danlos syndrome ⑯
　Hereditary hemorrhagic
　　telangiectasia

Immune-mediated ③
Immune
　thrombocytopenic
　purpura (ITP)
Systemic lupus
　erythematosus
HIV
Drug induced
Neonatal
　autoimmune

Congenital
　thrombocytopenias ⑤
TAR syndrome
Wiskott-Aldrich syndrome
Fanconi anemia
Congenital
　amegakaryocytic anemia

Aplastic syndromes
　(see chapter 65) ⑫
Malignancy ⑬
Storage disease ⑬

Viral infections ⑰
Prolonged crying or emesis
Valsalva (on face only)
Child abuse
Abnormal platelet function
　(toxins, drugs,
　systemic illness) ⑱
Disorders of blood vessels
　(Henoch-Schönlein
　purpura, vasculitis,
　scurvy) ⑲

Nelson Textbook of Pediatrics, 19e. Chapters 477, 478
Nelson Essentials, 6e. Chapter 151

(12) With aplastic syndromes (congenital and acquired aplastic anemias) there is thrombocytopenia with small platelets, leukopenia, and anemia. (See Chapter 65.)

(13) Infiltration of the marrow by malignant cells or due to storage disorders interferes with platelet production. Malignancies may include acute lymphoblastic leukemia, lymphomas, histiocytosis X, as well as metastatic tumors (e.g., neuroblastoma). Other findings may include adenopathy, hepatosplenomegaly, masses, as well as other abnormalities of the peripheral smear. A bone marrow is diagnostic.

(14) Platelet function studies may include PFA-100 as an initial screen for platelet function abnormalities, but there are problems with sensitivity and specificity. If platelet function abnormality is seriously being considered, platelet aggregation studies are needed. Bleeding time indirectly measures platelet number and function and platelet-vessel wall interaction, and has low sensitivity.

(15) Congenital platelet function defects include Glanzmann thrombasthenia (deficiency of a fibrinogen receptor). Less severe platelet function defects may have more subtle presentation and may require platelet aggregation studies.

(16) In Ehlers-Danlos syndrome, features include joint laxity, hyperelastic skin and poor wound healing, often ecchymoses is present and occasionally petechiae.

(17) A number of viral infections also occur as petechial rashes. Most common of these is enterovirus infection, but rubella, measles, varicella, Ebstein-Barr virus (EBV), cytomegalovirus (CMV), herpes (HSV), and HIV may also be involved.

(18) Acquired platelet function defects may be acquired secondary to medications (aspirin, nonsteroidal antiinflammatory drugs, alcohol, high doses of penicillin, valproate, and others) as well as systemic illness (e.g., uremia, liver disease).

(19) Vasculitic disorders occur as hemorrhagic lesions of skin and mucous membranes and symptoms relating to involved organ systems. Coagulation studies are usually normal. Henoch-Schönlein purpura (HSP) presents as petechiae, palpable purpura over the buttocks and lower extremities, as well as arthritis, abdominal pain, and glomerulonephritis.

Bibliography

Consolini DM: Thrombocytopenia in infants and children. *Pediatr Rev* 32(4):135–151, 2011.

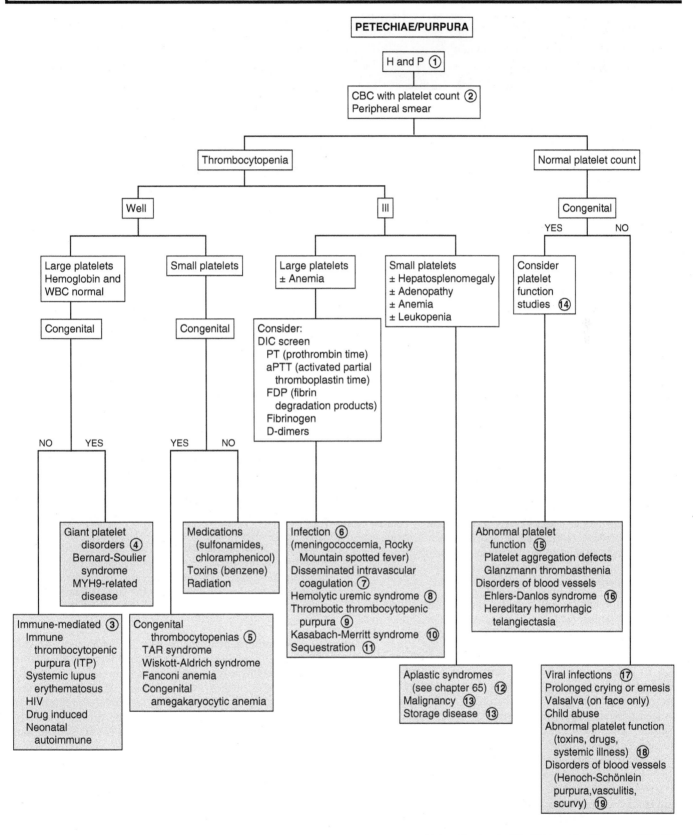

Nelson Textbook of Pediatrics, 19e. Chapters 477, 478
Nelson Essentials, 6e. Chapter 151

Chapter **64**
NEUTROPENIA

Neutropenia is an absolute decrease in the number of circulating neutrophils in the blood. It varies with age and race. In whites, the lower limit for normal absolute neutrophil counts (ANC = neutrophils + bands) is 1000 cells/µl in infants between 2 weeks and 1 year of age, and 1500 cells/µl in children older than 1 year. In blacks, the lower limits may be 200 to 600 cells/µl less than whites. The severity of neutropenia is helpful in predicting an increased likelihood of pyogenic infection. Mild neutropenia ranges from 1000 to 1500 cells/µl; moderate neutropenia ranges from 500 to 1000 cells/µl and severe neutropenia is <500 cells/µl.

1. History of any recent or recurrent infections, mouth ulcers and drug exposure should be obtained. This history should include fever, which may be a sign of infection. Infections may be both a cause and a consequence of neutropenia. The duration and severity of the neutropenia is important in determining infection risk. Severe neutropenia with counts <500 cells/µl is associated with the greatest risk of pyogenic infections, including cellulitis, abscesses (including perirectal), furuncles, pneumonia, septicemia, as well as oral infections such as stomatitis, gingivitis, and periodontitis. A detailed family history should include familial neutropenia and recurrent infections. A family history of short stature, dwarfism, skeletal abnormalities, and albinism may suggest congenital conditions associated with neutropenia. A careful physical examination is important in locating any sites of occult infection. The usual signs of infection (e.g., erythema, warmth) may not be present because of the neutropenia. Examination should also include evaluation for pallor indicating anemia, petechiae suggesting thrombocytopenia, lymphadenopathy, hepatosplenomegaly, and any other signs of underlying disease.

2. Although any severe infection may result in neutropenia, cyclic neutropenia and chronic neutropenia need to be excluded with twice weekly WBC counts for 6 to 8 weeks. Reticulocyte, platelet, and other leukocyte counts may also cycle.

3. In patients with fever and neutropenia, particularly if the child is ill appearing, cultures of blood, urine, and any suspected sites of infection should be done. Antibody responses, antigen detection tests, and polymerase chain reaction (PCR) methods may also be useful. In patients undergoing chemotherapy, cultures should also be obtained from central venous lines. These should include aerobic and anaerobic bacteria as well as fungi. In chronically infected sites, mycobacterial and anaerobic cultures are recommended. If diarrhea is present, obtain stool cultures for bacteria, viruses, and parasites. *Clostridium difficile* toxin should be sought. Tests for certain viruses may be considered in specific instances; for example, herpes cell culture and PCR testing from vesicular skin lesions or PCR testing for respiratory viruses in children with respiratory symptoms. It is important to note that mild neutropenia in a child with a febrile viral-appearing illness and without a history of recurrent significant infections may not need further evaluation.

4. There are many drugs that cause neutropenia, including chemotherapeutic drugs. A partial list is presented in the algorithm. An idiosyncratic reaction generally affects only neutrophils; other cell lines are usually unaffected.

5. The most common cause of transient neutropenia in children is viral infection. Viruses commonly causing neutropenia include hepatitis A and B, respiratory syncytial virus, influenza virus types A and B, measles, rubella, and varicella. It may also occur in early stages of infectious mononucleosis. Leukopenia may be seen in patients with HIV infection. This may be due to the virus or due to antiviral drugs.

6. There may be neutropenia associated with typhoid, paratyphoid, tuberculosis, brucellosis, tularemia, and rickettsial infections. In patients with an immunodeficiency, commonly cultured organisms include *Staphylococcus aureus*, coagulase-negative staphylococci, and gram-negative organisms, including *E. coli* and *Klebsiella pneumoniae*. *Candida* may also be cultured.

7. Severe malnutrition seen in anorexia nervosa and marasmus may also cause neutropenia.

8. Cyclic neutropenia is a congenital condition with regular fluctuation in neutrophil counts. The nadir occurs approximately every 21 days, often to an absolute neutrophil count of <200 cells/µl. During the neutropenic period there may be fever, oral ulcers, gingivitis, periodontitis, and pharyngitis with lymphadenopathy. More serious infections such as mastoiditis or pneumonia may also occur.

9. Congenital neutropenias include those associated with phenotypic abnormalities. Chédiak-Higashi syndrome is characterized by oculocutaneous albinism. There is an increased susceptibility to infection due to neutropenia, as well as defective function of the remaining neutrophils. Dyskeratosis congenita is associated with nail dystrophy, leukoplakia, and reticulated hyperpigmentation of the skin. Shwachman syndrome is characterized by dwarfism, growth failure, skeletal abnormalities, and exocrine pancreatic insufficiency, causing diarrhea, weight loss, and failure to thrive. Cartilage-hair hypoplasia features neutropenia with short-limbed dwarfism and fine hair.

10. Autoimmune neutropenia may be associated with other autoimmune diseases (e.g., systemic lupus erythematosus, autoimmune hemolytic anemia, and thrombocytopenia). It may also be associated with infection (e.g., infectious mononucleosis, HIV), malignancy (e.g., leukemia, lymphoma), and drugs. Antineutrophil antibodies may be present on testing; Coombs testing may identify associated hemolytic conditions.

11. Autoimmune neutropenia of infancy usually presents between ages 5 to 15 months. Patients usually have severe neutropenia with an ANC <500/µL, however the total WBC count is usually normal. Diagnosis is usually by the presence of antineutrophil antibodies, but multiple screenings may be needed to detect these, and avoid the need for bone marrow studies.

12. Immune neonatal neutropenia is similar to Rh-hemolytic anemia. It occurs due to maternal sensitization caused by fetal neutrophil antigens. The neutropenia may last for weeks and as long as 6 months. Antineutrophil antibodies are found in

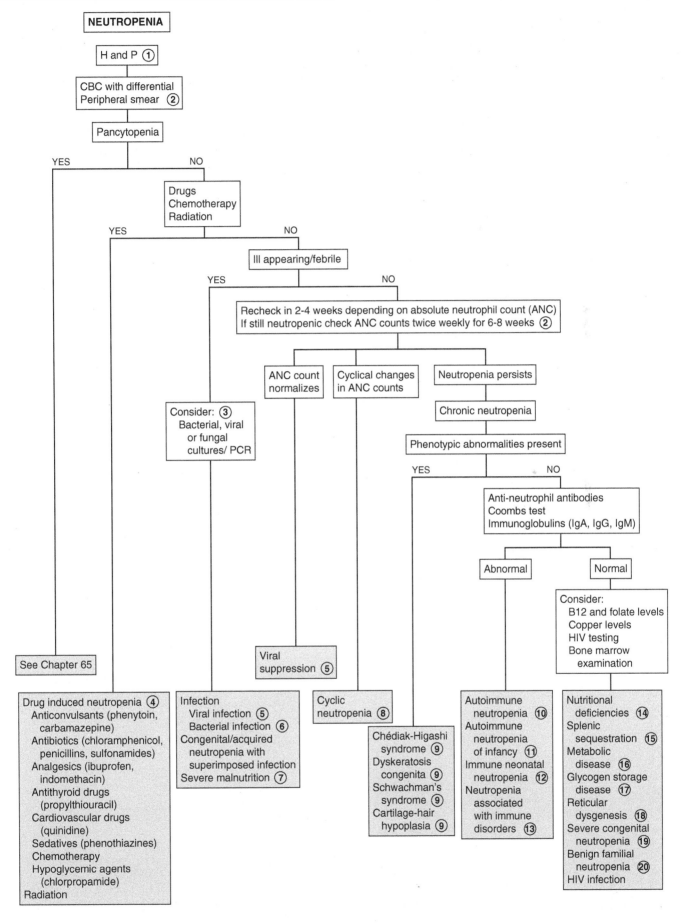

NEUTROPENIA

H and P ①

CBC with differential
Peripheral smear ②

Pancytopenia

YES — See Chapter 65

NO

Drugs
Chemotherapy
Radiation

YES

NO

Ill appearing/febrile

YES

Consider: ③
Bacterial, viral
or fungal
cultures/ PCR

NO

Recheck in 2-4 weeks depending on absolute neutrophil count (ANC)
If still neutropenic check ANC counts twice weekly for 6-8 weeks ②

ANC count
normalizes

Cyclical changes
in ANC counts

Neutropenia persists

Chronic neutropenia

Phenotypic abnormalities present

YES

NO

Anti-neutrophil antibodies
Coombs test
Immunoglobulins (IgA, IgG, IgM)

Abnormal

Normal

Consider:
B12 and folate levels
Copper levels
HIV testing
Bone marrow
examination

Viral
suppression ⑤

Drug induced neutropenia ④
  Anticonvulsants (phenytoin,
    carbamazepine)
  Antibiotics (chloramphenicol,
    penicillins, sulfonamides)
  Analgesics (ibuprofen,
    indomethacin)
  Antithyroid drugs
    (propylthiouracil)
  Cardiovascular drugs
    (quinidine)
  Sedatives (phenothiazines)
  Chemotherapy
  Hypoglycemic agents
    (chlorpropamide)
Radiation

Infection
  Viral infection ⑤
  Bacterial infection ⑥
Congenital/acquired
  neutropenia with
  superimposed infection
Severe malnutrition ⑦

Cyclic
neutropenia ⑧

Chédiak-Higashi
  syndrome ⑨
Dyskeratosis
  congenita ⑨
Schwachman's
  syndrome ⑨
Cartilage-hair
  hypoplasia ⑨

Autoimmune
  neutropenia ⑩
Autoimmune
  neutropenia
  of infancy ⑪
Immune neonatal
  neutropenia ⑫
Neutropenia
  associated
  with immune
  disorders ⑬

Nutritional
  deficiencies ⑭
Splenic
  sequestration ⑮
Metabolic
  disease ⑯
Glycogen storage
  disease ⑰
Reticular
  dysgenesis ⑱
Severe congenital
  neutropenia ⑲
Benign familial
  neutropenia ⑳
HIV infection

Nelson Textbook of Pediatrics, 19e. Chapters 81, 118, 125
Nelson Essentials, 6e. Chapter 74

maternal and infant serum. It can also occur in infants whose mothers have autoimmune neutropenia.

13 Neutropenia may be associated with disorders of immune dysfunction; these conditions include X-linked agammaglobulinemia, hyper-IgM syndrome, cartilage-hair hypoplasia, and HIV infection.

14 Nutritional deficiencies including those of vitamin B12, folate, and copper may be associated with neutropenia.

15 Reticuloendothelial sequestration secondary to splenic enlargement can lead to neutropenia; causes include portal hypertension, splenic disease, and splenic hyperplasia.

16 Many metabolic diseases are associated with neutropenia, such as hyperglycinemia, isovalericacidemia, propionicacidemia, methylmalonicacidemia, and tyrosinemia.

17 Neutropenia may also be noted in some glycogen storage disorder type 1b. Patients may present with hepatomegaly, hypoglycemia, elevated lactate, cholesterol, triglyceride, and uric acid levels as well as associated neutropenia.

18 Another congenital cause of neutropenia includes reticular dysgenesis, which is characterized by neutropenia and lymphopenia. Lymphoid tissue (e.g., tonsils, lymph nodes, Peyer patches, and lymphoid follicles) is absent.

19 In severe congenital neutropenia the ANC $<200/\mu L$. It presents in young infants with severe pyogenic infections of skin, mouth, and rectum. It has an autosomal dominant form and a recessive form (Kostmann disease).

20 Familial benign neutropenia is mild with no increased tendency for infection.

Bibliography

Segel GB, Halterman JS: Neutropenia in pediatric practice, *Pediatr Rev* 29: 12–24, 2008.

Walkovich K, Boxer LA: How to approach neutropenia in childhood, *Pediatr Rev* 34:173–184, 2013.

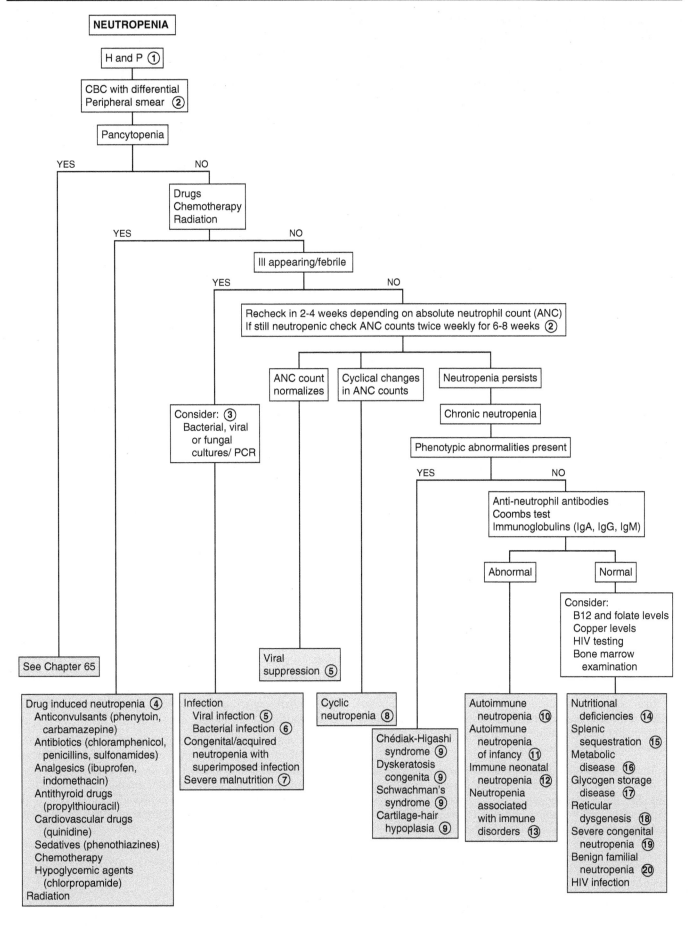

Nelson Textbook of Pediatrics, 19e. Chapters 81, 118, 125
Nelson Essentials, 6e. Chapter 74

Chapter 65
PANCYTOPENIA

Pancytopenia is caused by a decrease in production of erythrocytes, leukocytes, and platelets by the bone marrow. Clinically, this results in anemia, hemorrhage, and decreased resistance to infection. Severe aplastic anemia is diagnosed when at least two of the following are present: absolute neutrophil count (ANC) <500/µl, platelet count <20,000 µl, and corrected reticulocyte count <1%; the bone marrow contains <25% of the normal cellularity. Mild or moderate aplastic anemia (i.e., hypoplastic anemia) has a mild or moderate decrease in granulocytes, platelets, and erythrocytes, and there may be normal or increased bone marrow cellularity.

(1) History should include exposure to agents that are potentially myelosuppressive. These include radiation and chemotherapy (e.g., 6-mercaptopurine, methotrexate, nitrogen mustard). Other drugs include chloramphenicol, sulfonamides, phenylbutazone, and anticonvulsants. Chemicals and toxins include benzene and other aromatic hydrocarbons present in insecticides and herbicides. A history and physical examination compatible with certain viral infections should be sought. An increased susceptibility to infection may suggest an immunodeficiency syndrome. A family history of congenital anomalies, aplastic syndromes, and leukemias may indicate syndromes associated with constitutional aplastic pancytopenias. Physical examination may reveal the effects of the cytopenias, including anemia, which results in tachycardia and pallor; thrombocytopenia, which may cause bleeding, bruising, epistaxis, petechiae, or ecchymoses; and neutropenia, which may be associated with oral ulcerations and fevers. Examination should include identification of congenital anomalies associated with Fanconi and other syndromes (e.g., Down syndrome).

(2) When blasts are seen on peripheral smear, it indicates leukemia requiring referral for bone marrow examination. Leukoerythroblastosis (myelophthisic anemia) is usually due to invasion of the bone marrow and resulting release of immature cells including erythroblasts (nucleated erythrocytes), immature neutrophils and giant platelets.

(3) Laboratory findings suggesting hemolysis include abnormal cell morphology, increased reticulocyte count, increased red blood cell distribution width, indirect bilirubin, urine urobilinogen, and lactate dehydrogenase, decreased serum haptoglobin, and hemoglobinuria.

(4) The most common cause of mild or moderate pancytopenias in healthy patients is suppression due to infectious agents. Specific viruses include human parvovirus B19, hepatitis viruses (B, C, non-A non-B and non-C), dengue virus, cytomegalovirus, human herpes virus 6, and Epstein-Barr virus.

Patients with HIV may have pancytopenia for a number of reasons, including opportunistic infections, drugs used in treatment, and neoplasms associated with the disease. Other viruses that may cause cytopenias include measles, mumps, rubella, varicella, and influenza A. If a viral etiology is suggested, it is reasonable to recheck the CBC in a few weeks. If the pancytopenia persists or becomes more severe, referral to a hematologist for further evaluation is recommended.

(5) Patients with hemolytic anemia who have shortened red blood cell survival time are at risk of transient aplastic crisis. This is most commonly associated with parvovirus and may occur in children with sickle cell disease, thalassemia, hereditary spherocytosis, and other types of erythroid stress.

(6) Fanconi anemia is an autosomal recessive condition. Two thirds of affected children have congenital anomalies. These include microcephaly, microphthalmia, absent radii and thumbs, as well as heart and kidney abnormalities. There may be hypopigmentation of the skin and short stature.

(7) Dyskeratosis congenita is a rare form of ectodermal dysplasia associated with pancytopenia. Dermatologic manifestations include hyperpigmented skin, dystrophic nails, and mucous membrane leukoplakia.

(8) Schwachman-Diamond syndrome is characterized by neutropenia with exocrine pancreatic insufficiency (e.g., malabsorption, steatorrhea, failure to thrive). About 50% develop aplastic anemia.

(9) Pregnancy may be associated with aplastic anemia; estrogens may play a role.

(10) Paroxysmal nocturnal hemoglobinuria is characterized by intravascular hemolysis and hemoglobinuria as well as venous thrombosis. There is a strong association with aplastic anemia.

(11) Systemic diseases may be associated with pancytopenias. These may include systemic lupus erythematosus, metabolic diseases, brucellosis, sarcoidosis, and tuberculosis.

(12) Replacement of the marrow by malignant or nonhematopoietic cells may cause pancytopenias. Conditions include leukemia, lymphomas, and neuroblastoma metastases to the bone marrow. Osteopetrosis may cause obliteration of the marrow. Myelofibrosis may also be a cause. Myelodysplastic syndrome is rare in children; there is an increased risk of development with Down syndrome, Kostmann syndrome, Noonan syndrome, Fanconi anemia, trisomy 8 mosaicism, neurofibromatosis, and Schwachman syndrome.

(13) In autoimmune pancytopenia the Coombs (direct antiglobulin) test is usually positive. There is evidence of hemolysis with autoimmune hemolytic anemia. It is known as Evans syndrome when the patient has autoimmune hemolytic anemia and immune thrombocytopenic purpura (ITP). There may also be an associated autoimmune neutropenia. It may be associated with disorders such as systemic lupus erythematosus (SLE).

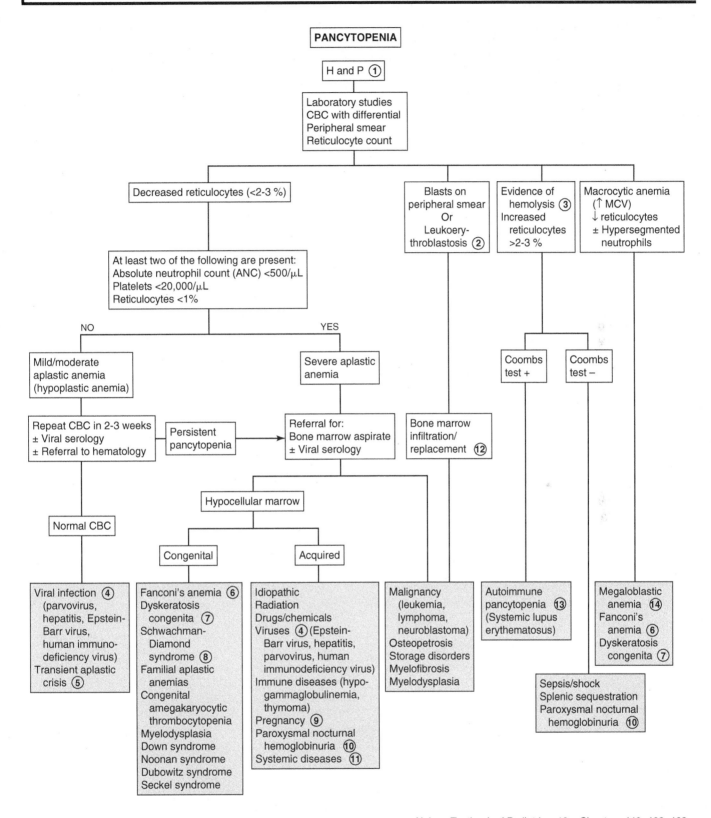

PANCYTOPENIA

H and P ①

Laboratory studies
CBC with differential
Peripheral smear
Reticulocyte count

Decreased reticulocytes (<2-3 %)

Blasts on peripheral smear Or Leukoery-throblastosis ②

Evidence of hemolysis ③ Increased reticulocytes >2-3 %

Macrocytic anemia (↑ MCV) ↓ reticulocytes ± Hypersegmented neutrophils

At least two of the following are present:
Absolute neutrophil count (ANC) <500/μL
Platelets <20,000/μL
Reticulocytes <1%

NO

YES

Mild/moderate aplastic anemia (hypoplastic anemia)

Severe aplastic anemia

Coombs test +

Coombs test –

Repeat CBC in 2-3 weeks ± Viral serology ± Referral to hematology

Persistent pancytopenia

Referral for: Bone marrow aspirate ± Viral serology

Bone marrow infiltration/ replacement ⑫

Hypocellular marrow

Normal CBC

Congenital

Acquired

Viral infection ④ (parvovirus, hepatitis, Epstein-Barr virus, human immuno-deficiency virus)
Transient aplastic crisis ⑤

Fanconi's anemia ⑥
Dyskeratosis congenita ⑦
Schwachman-Diamond syndrome ⑧
Familial aplastic anemias
Congenital amegakaryocytic thrombocytopenia
Myelodysplasia
Down syndrome
Noonan syndrome
Dubowitz syndrome
Seckel syndrome

Idiopathic
Radiation
Drugs/chemicals
Viruses ④ (Epstein-Barr virus, hepatitis, parvovirus, human immunodeficiency virus)
Immune diseases (hypo-gammaglobulinemia, thymoma)
Pregnancy ⑨
Paroxysmal nocturnal hemoglobinuria ⑩
Systemic diseases ⑪

Malignancy (leukemia, lymphoma, neuroblastoma)
Osteopetrosis
Storage disorders
Myelofibrosis
Myelodysplasia

Autoimmune pancytopenia ⑬ (Systemic lupus erythematosus)

Megaloblastic anemia ⑭
Fanconi's anemia ⑥
Dyskeratosis congenita ⑦

Sepsis/shock
Splenic sequestration
Paroxysmal nocturnal hemoglobinuria ⑩

Nelson Textbook of Pediatrics, 19e. Chapters 448, 462, 463
Nelson Essentials, 6e. Chapter 150

14 Megaloblastic anemia (large RBCs with abnormal hyper-segmented neutrophils due to vitamin B12 or folate deficiency is rare in children. Neutropenia and thrombocytopenia may be present, particularly in patients with long-standing and severe deficiencies.

Vitamin B12 deficiency may be seen in breast-fed infants of vegan mothers or with malabsorption due to a rare intrinsic factor deficiency (e.g., congenital pernicious anemia), resection of the ileum, or impaired absorption in inflammatory conditions (e.g., celiac disease).

Folate deficiency may be caused by decreased absorption due to resection or inflammatory disease of the small bowel or certain anticonvulsant drugs (e.g., phenytoin, primidone, phenobarbital). Folate deficiency may occur in infants fed goat's milk, which is low in folate). Some medications (e.g., methotrexate, trimethoprim) can inhibit the action of folate. Increased folate requirements may occur in chronic hemolytic anemia (e.g., sickle cell).

Bibliography
Sills RH, Deters A: Pancytopenia. In Sills RH, editor: *Practical Algorithms in Pediatric Hematology and Oncology*, Basel, Switzerland, 2003, Karger, pp 12–13.

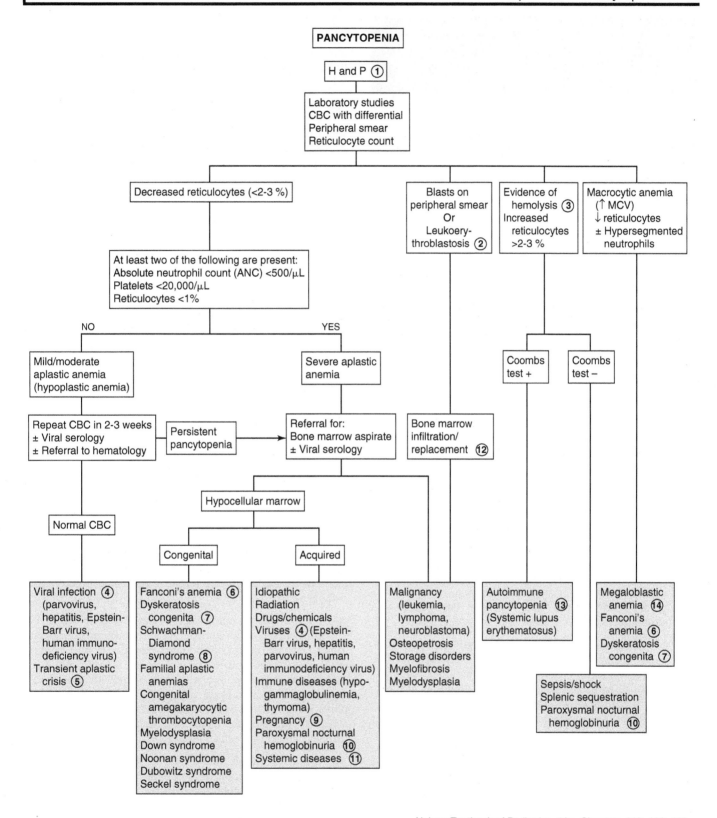

PANCYTOPENIA

H and P ①

Laboratory studies
CBC with differential
Peripheral smear
Reticulocyte count

Decreased reticulocytes (<2-3 %)

Blasts on peripheral smear Or Leukoery-throblastosis ②

Evidence of hemolysis ③ Increased reticulocytes >2-3 %

Macrocytic anemia (↑ MCV) ↓ reticulocytes ± Hypersegmented neutrophils

At least two of the following are present:
Absolute neutrophil count (ANC) <500/μL
Platelets <20,000/μL
Reticulocytes <1%

NO

Mild/moderate aplastic anemia (hypoplastic anemia)

YES

Severe aplastic anemia

Coombs test +

Coombs test −

Repeat CBC in 2-3 weeks
± Viral serology
± Referral to hematology

Persistent pancytopenia

Referral for:
Bone marrow aspirate
± Viral serology

Bone marrow infiltration/ replacement ⑫

Normal CBC

Hypocellular marrow

Congenital

Acquired

Viral infection ④
(parvovirus, hepatitis, Epstein-Barr virus, human immuno-deficiency virus)
Transient aplastic crisis ⑤

Fanconi's anemia ⑥
Dyskeratosis congenita ⑦
Schwachman-Diamond syndrome ⑧
Familial aplastic anemias
Congenital amegakaryocytic thrombocytopenia
Myelodysplasia
Down syndrome
Noonan syndrome
Dubowitz syndrome
Seckel syndrome

Idiopathic
Radiation
Drugs/chemicals
Viruses ④ (Epstein-Barr virus, hepatitis, parvovirus, human immunodeficiency virus)
Immune diseases (hypo-gammaglobulinemia, thymoma)
Pregnancy ⑨
Paroxysmal nocturnal hemoglobinuria ⑩
Systemic diseases ⑪

Malignancy
(leukemia, lymphoma, neuroblastoma)
Osteopetrosis
Storage disorders
Myelofibrosis
Myelodysplasia

Autoimmune pancytopenia ⑬
(Systemic lupus erythematosus)

Megaloblastic anemia ⑭
Fanconi's anemia ⑥
Dyskeratosis congenita ⑦

Sepsis/shock
Splenic sequestration
Paroxysmal nocturnal hemoglobinuria ⑩

Nelson Textbook of Pediatrics, 19e. Chapters 448, 462, 463
Nelson Essentials, 6e. Chapter 150

Chapter 66
EOSINOPHILIA

Eosinophilia is most commonly associated with exposure to an antigen, but the etiology may often be unclear. Normal absolute eosinophil counts are usually <450 cells/μL. Eosinophilia may be mild (500 to 1500 cells/μL), moderate (1500 to 5000 cells/μL), or severe (>5000 cells/μL).

1. History should include exposure to drugs that may cause hypersensitivity. Many rashes are associated with eosinophilia. These may be infectious or allergic. Travel history, particularly to tropical countries, is helpful in the diagnosis of parasitic infections. Exposure to cats and dogs may also be associated with parasites. Respiratory signs and symptoms (e.g., wheezing, cough, rales, and rhonchi) may indicate the presence of asthma or allergic rhinitis. If atopic disease is not suggested, a careful search for other causes is indicated. Gastrointestinal signs and symptoms such as weight loss, diarrhea, and failure to thrive may suggest either parasite infestation or chronic gastrointestinal disease associated with eosinophilia. A detailed history of medications and nutritional supplements should be obtained from patients with eosinophilia. Hematologic and oncologic conditions may also be associated with eosinophilia, as well as many chronic diseases. A family history of atopic disease (e.g., asthma, allergic rhinitis, and atopic dermatitis) should be obtained. Eosinophilia may be a familial condition. Because eosinophilia is associated with so many conditions, the algorithm focuses on more common pediatric causes.

2. If respiratory symptoms are present and asthma is not suggested, a chest x-ray should be obtained looking for eosinophilia associated lung diseases. Serologic tests for *Toxocara* may be done in children with exposure to pets, specifically cats or dogs. Stool studies for cysts and ova may reveal parasite infestation. Serologic and skin tests for aspergillosis and coccidioidomycosis may be considered in specific cases.

3. Löeffler syndrome is a transient allergic response to antigens, usually parasites or drugs. It is characterized by pulmonary infiltrates, which may resemble miliary tuberculosis, as well as by paroxysmal episodes of coughing, dyspnea, and pleurisy, usually without fever. Eosinophilia may be as high as 70%. The most common parasites causing Löeffler syndrome are *Toxocara* (*T. canis* and *T. cati*), *Ascaris lumbricoides*, *Strongyloides stercoralis*, and hookworm. *Echinococcus granulosus* may produce dyspnea, cough, and hemoptysis due to hydatid cysts in the lungs. Drugs that may cause Löeffler syndrome include aspirin, penicillin, sulfonamides, and imipramine.

4. Allergic bronchopulmonary aspergillosis (ABPA) is a hypersensitivity reaction characterized by recurrent bronchospasm, transient pulmonary infiltrates, and bronchiectasis. It occurs in children with chronic pulmonary disease (e.g., asthma, cystic fibrosis). Skin testing as well as testing for antibodies to *Aspergillus* antigen may aid in the diagnosis.

5. Sarcoidosis is a chronic granulomatous disease affecting primarily the lungs; however, it may affect any organ system. Pulmonary involvement includes parenchymal infiltrates, military nodules, and hilar and paratracheal lymphadenopathy. Pulmonary function test findings show a restrictive pattern.

6. Coccidioidomycosis is caused by *Coccidioides immitis*; it is endemic in California (San Joaquin valley), central and southern Arizona, and southwestern Texas. It may occur as a primary infection. Symptoms may include fever, rash, cough, chest pain, anorexia, malaise, and, occasionally, hemoptysis. A majority of cases are asymptomatic. Results of a chest examination are usually normal; however, chest x-ray findings may be significant for consolidation or pleural effusion. A residual cavity may develop in an area of consolidation. Diagnosis of coccidioidomycosis may be done using skin tests or serology. Negative skin test results do not exclude coccidioidal infection. Skin tests cannot distinguish recent from old infections.

7. Tropical pulmonary eosinophilia is caused by filarial infection of the lymph nodes and lungs. Signs and symptoms include cough, dyspnea, fever, weight loss, and fatigue; there may be rales and rhonchi on chest examination. Chest x-ray shows increased bronchovascular markings, discrete opacities, or diffuse miliary lesions. Hepatosplenomegaly and generalized lymphadenopathy may be present. Laboratory findings include eosinophilia (>2000/mm3), increased IgE levels, and high titers of antifilarial antibodies.

8. Eosinophilia is seen with many immunodeficiency syndromes. Wiskott-Aldrich syndrome is an X-linked recessive syndrome presenting as eczema, thrombocytopenia, and susceptibility to infections. Hyperimmunoglobulinemia E (hyper-IgE) syndrome is characterized by recurrent staphylococcal abscesses involving the skin, lungs, and joints.

9. Hypereosinophilic syndrome is a rare disorder characterized by sustained overproduction of eosinophils and signs and symptoms of organ involvement, including the heart, skin, liver, spleen, gastrointestinal tract, brain, and lungs. Although many cases are idiopathic, recent advances have determined pathogenesis.

10. Medications are often associated with eosinophilia; sometimes this is asymptomatic but it may also involve specific organs. Asymptomatic eosinophilia may occur with quinine, penicillins, cephalosporins, or quinolones. NSAIDs and nitrofurantoin may cause pulmonary involvement with eosinophilia. Cephalosporins may cause interstitial nephritis and eosinophilia. Drug reaction with eosinophilia and systemic symptoms (DRESS syndrome) can occur with multiple medications (e.g., carbamazepine, hydrochlorothiazide, cyclosporine)

11. Familial eosinophilia is usually benign, with no associated symptoms. Episodic angioedema is a familial syndrome associated with eosinophilia. Features include recurrent episodes of fever, urticaria, and angioedema.

Bibliography

Nutman TB: Evaluation and differential diagnosis of marked, persistent eosinophilia, *Immunol Allergy Clin North Am* 27(3):529–549, 2007.

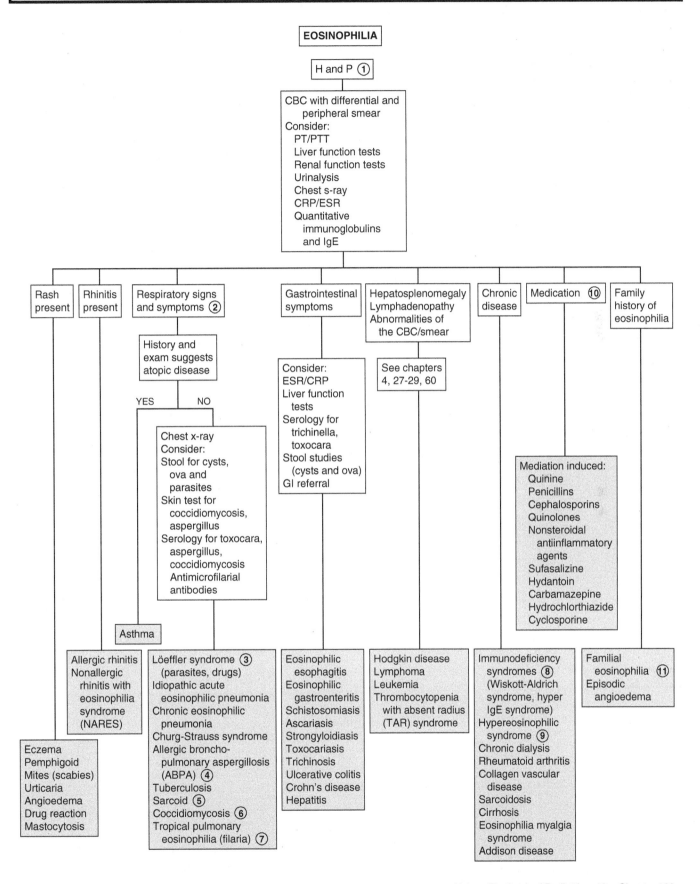

EOSINOPHILIA

H and P ①

CBC with differential and
peripheral smear
Consider:
 PT/PTT
 Liver function tests
 Renal function tests
 Urinalysis
 Chest s-ray
 CRP/ESR
 Quantitative
  immunoglobulins
  and IgE

Rash
present

Rhinitis
present

Respiratory signs
and symptoms ②

Gastrointestinal
symptoms

Hepatosplenomegaly
Lymphadenopathy
Abnormalities of
the CBC/smear

Chronic
disease

Medication ⑩

Family
history of
eosinophilia

History and
exam suggests
atopic disease

YES   NO

Chest x-ray
Consider:
Stool for cysts,
 ova and
 parasites
Skin test for
 coccidiomycosis,
 aspergillus
Serology for toxocara,
 aspergillus,
 coccidiomycosis
Antimicrofilarial
 antibodies

Consider:
ESR/CRP
Liver function
 tests
Serology for
 trichinella,
 toxocara
Stool studies
 (cysts and ova)
GI referral

See chapters
4, 27-29, 60

Mediation induced:
 Quinine
 Penicillins
 Cephalosporins
 Quinolones
 Nonsteroidal
  antiinflammatory
  agents
 Sufasalizine
 Hydantoin
 Carbamazepine
 Hydrochlorthiazide
 Cyclosporine

Asthma

Allergic rhinitis
Nonallergic
 rhinitis with
 eosinophilia
 syndrome
 (NARES)

Löeffler syndrome ③
 (parasites, drugs)
Idiopathic acute
 eosinophilic pneumonia
Chronic eosinophilic
 pneumonia
Churg-Strauss syndrome
Allergic broncho-
 pulmonary aspergillosis
 (ABPA) ④
Tuberculosis
Sarcoid ⑤
Coccidiomycosis ⑥
Tropical pulmonary
 eosinophilia (filaria) ⑦

Eosinophilic
 esophagitis
Eosinophilic
 gastroenteritis
Schistosomiasis
Ascariasis
Strongyloidiasis
Toxocariasis
Trichinosis
Ulcerative colitis
Crohn's disease
Hepatitis

Hodgkin disease
Lymphoma
Leukemia
Thrombocytopenia
 with absent radius
 (TAR) syndrome

Immunodeficiency
 syndromes ⑧
 (Wiskott-Aldrich
 syndrome, hyper
 IgE syndrome)
Hypereosinophilic
 syndrome ⑨
Chronic dialysis
Rheumatoid arthritis
Collagen vascular
 disease
Sarcoidosis
Cirrhosis
Eosinophilia myalgia
 syndrome
Addison disease

Familial
 eosinophilia ⑪
Episodic
 angioedema

Eczema
Pemphigoid
Mites (scabies)
Urticaria
Angioedema
Drug reaction
Mastocytosis

Nelson Textbook of Pediatrics, 19e. Chapter 123
Nelsons Essentials, 6e. Chapter 77, 93

Endocrine System

Chapter 67
SHORT STATURE

Short stature is defined as height less than 2 to 2.5 standard deviations (SD) below the mean for age. However, decreasing growth velocity is very important regardless of absolute height. It is important to distinguish normal (constitutional or familial) short stature from that due to a medical problem. Short stature must also be distinguished from failure to thrive (FTT), with associated poor weight gain. Because of the importance our culture places on height for males, boys are more likely to be brought to medical attention for this complaint. Many factors such as parental height and growth patterns, pubertal status, ethnicity, nutritional status, chronic illnesses, and emotional and psychological effects may influence stature. Infants of very low birth weight and small for gestational age (SGA) for various reasons (chromosomal disorders or syndromes, infections, or maternal alcohol use) are more likely to be of shorter stature.

1. History and physical examination should rule out any obvious dysmorphisms, syndromes, or diseases that may be associated with short stature. Birth history should include height and weight, prenatal exposures and illnesses, as well as perinatal problems. Prolonged jaundice, hypoglycemia, and small phallus suggest growth hormone (GH) deficiency; puffy extremities suggest Turner syndrome.

A careful analysis of the growth curve is essential. Growth velocity and growth patterns must be plotted. Weight-for-height ratio is also helpful in determining the cause of short stature. The target (mid-parental) should be determined. For boys: mid–parental height = [(maternal height + 13 cm) + paternal height]/2. For girls: mid–parental height = [(paternal height − 13 cm) + maternal height]/2. A height range can then be calculated; 8.5 cm below and above the mid–parental height represent the 3rd to 97th percentile for the child. The ratio of upper to lower body segment (U/L) ratio can differentiate whether short stature is proportionate (involving both trunk and lower extremities) or disproportionate. The U/L ratio is decreased in skeletal dysplasias involving the spine. It is increased in dysplasias involving long bones and also in precocious puberty.

A short child who remains along his or her growth percentile may have familial or constitutional delay. Progressive deviation below the curve suggests a congenital disorder (Turner syndrome, GH deficiency). Developmental delay is associated with syndromes such as Prader-Willi syndrome. Weight for age that is less than height for age suggests malnutrition or chronic illness. A history of cranial irradiation for CNS malignancies suggests GH deficiency. Midline defects may be associated with hypopituitarism.

2. A child with a family history of short stature or pubertal delay who is staying along his or her growth curve may be followed clinically.

3. A child with familial short stature has normal growth velocity with growth curves below but parallel to the normal growth curve and has normal pubertal development. These children have no endocrine disorder or systemic illness and have a family history of short stature. Bone age may be considered and

is normal. The final adult height is short but within targeted range based on parental height. If there is deviation from the growth curve, further evaluation is needed.

4. Constitutional delay of growth and adolescence is a normal variation, recognized more commonly in boys. There is pubertal delay, delayed bone age, and delayed growth spurt, with subsequent attainment of normal adult height. Bone age usually correlates with height age. There is often also a family history of delayed puberty (usually the father). Laboratory test results are normal. It may be difficult to distinguish these children from those with mild GH defects, chronic disease, or central hypogonadism.

5. If the child has decelerating growth patterns or is significantly short (≤2 SD), further evaluation should be guided by the clinical findings. Bone age radiography (BA) is used to assess skeletal maturity. A chronic illness may be suggested by the results of a CBC, ESR, chemistry profile, and UA. Hypothyroidism can be detected by obtaining free T_4 and TSH levels. Suspicion of Turner syndrome in girls with unexplained short stature requires a karyotype. GH deficiency may be screened for by obtaining an insulin-like growth factor (IGF)-1 and IGF binding protein 3 (IGFBP3); however, the definitive test involves GH levels in response to pharmacologic stimulation. Further evaluation by an endocrinologist is required.

6. We suggest using a weight/height ratio to organize a differential diagnosis for a child with short stature. This is an inexact method, and it is not a formal means of classification. The specific laboratory tests ordered should be based on the findings of the H and P. In general, however, weight for age less than height for age may indicate chronic illness or malnutrition, and weight for age greater than height for age may indicate endocrine disorders or genetic disorders and syndromes.

7. Children with weight disproportionately lower than height may be malnourished, malabsorbing, or have specific nutritional deficiencies (e.g., rickets). Chronic illness may be a cause. Screening laboratory tests (e.g., ESR, CBC, UA, and chemistry profile) may indicate the diagnosis. RTA may result in FTT and short stature. A low serum bicarbonate on the chemistry profile may be the clue. Further evaluation reveals a normal anion gap metabolic acidosis. (See Chapter 82.) If the reason is not evident, the evaluation should also include tests to exclude celiac disease (tissue transglutaminase, antigliadin antibodies, immunoglobulin [Ig]A), and testing for HIV should be considered when appropriate. Cystic fibrosis testing should be considered when newborn screen results are not available.

8. Emotional deprivation may retard growth and mimic hypopituitarism. The condition is known as psychosocial dwarfism. The mechanism is poorly understood, but the child may have functional hypopituitarism with low levels of IGF-1. Growth velocity is slow, and bone age is less than the chronological age. The child has short stature, and weight may be proportional to height or decreased compared to height. Puberty may be normal or premature. Close observation may reveal disturbed mother-child or family interactions. These children grow normally once they are removed from the poor environment.

9. Genetic syndromes or chromosomal abnormalities may be associated with short stature. If features of a particular syndrome are present, karyotype should be obtained; a comprehensive lab evaluation may not be necessary, and genetics

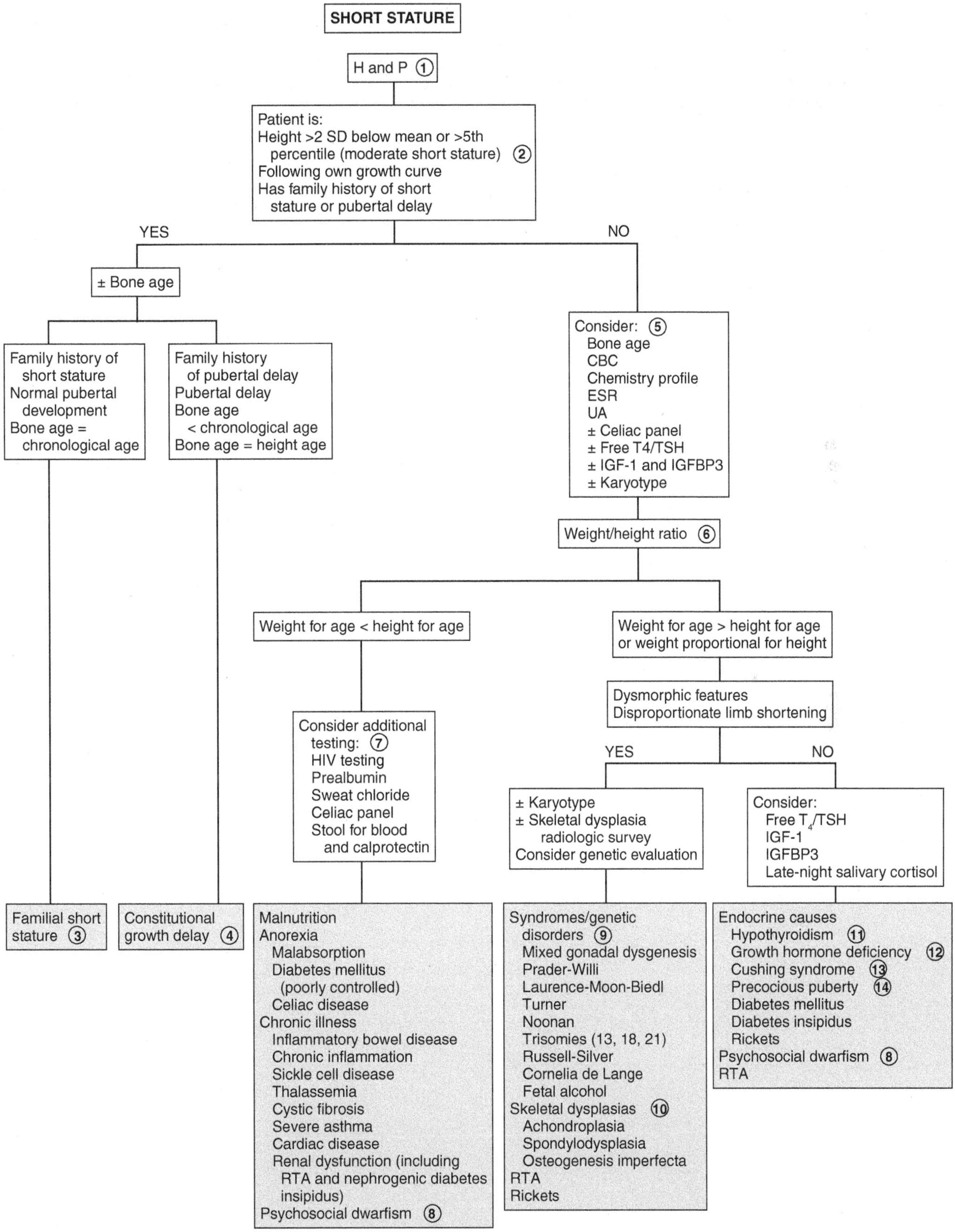

SHORT STATURE

H and P ①

Patient is:
Height >2 SD below mean or >5th
  percentile (moderate short stature) ②
Following own growth curve
Has family history of short
  stature or pubertal delay

YES

NO

± Bone age

Family history of
  short stature
Normal pubertal
  development
Bone age =
  chronological age

Family history
  of pubertal delay
Pubertal delay
Bone age
  < chronological age
Bone age = height age

Consider: ⑤
  Bone age
  CBC
  Chemistry profile
  ESR
  UA
  ± Celiac panel
  ± Free T4/TSH
  ± IGF-1 and IGFBP3
  ± Karyotype

Weight/height ratio ⑥

Weight for age < height for age

Weight for age > height for age
or weight proportional for height

Dysmorphic features
Disproportionate limb shortening

YES

NO

Consider additional
  testing: ⑦
  HIV testing
  Prealbumin
  Sweat chloride
  Celiac panel
  Stool for blood
    and calprotectin

± Karyotype
± Skeletal dysplasia
    radiologic survey
Consider genetic evaluation

Consider:
  Free T$_4$/TSH
  IGF-1
  IGFBP3
  Late-night salivary cortisol

Familial short
stature ③

Constitutional
growth delay ④

Malnutrition
Anorexia
  Malabsorption
  Diabetes mellitus
    (poorly controlled)
  Celiac disease
Chronic illness
  Inflammatory bowel disease
  Chronic inflammation
  Sickle cell disease
  Thalassemia
  Cystic fibrosis
  Severe asthma
  Cardiac disease
  Renal dysfunction (including
    RTA and nephrogenic diabetes
    insipidus)
Psychosocial dwarfism ⑧

Syndromes/genetic
  disorders ⑨
  Mixed gonadal dysgenesis
  Prader-Willi
  Laurence-Moon-Biedl
  Turner
  Noonan
  Trisomies (13, 18, 21)
  Russell-Silver
  Cornelia de Lange
  Fetal alcohol
Skeletal dysplasias ⑩
  Achondroplasia
  Spondylodysplasia
  Osteogenesis imperfecta
RTA
Rickets

Endocrine causes
  Hypothyroidism ⑪
  Growth hormone deficiency ⑫
  Cushing syndrome ⑬
  Precocious puberty ⑭
  Diabetes mellitus
  Diabetes insipidus
  Rickets
Psychosocial dwarfism ⑧
RTA

Nelson Textbook of Pediatrics, 19e. Chapters 13, 48, 76, 330, 529, 551, 556, 559, 580, 685
Nelson Essentials, 6e. Chapter 173

may be consulted for specific tests. The more common syndromes include Turner syndrome, 45,X/46,XY mixed gonadal dysgenesis, Down syndrome, and other trisomies. Turner syndrome should always be considered in short girls, because sometimes short stature may be the only feature. In mixed gonadal dysgenesis, puberty is delayed or absent and bone age is slightly delayed compared to chronological age. Syndromes such as Prader-Willi and Laurence-Moon-Biedl syndromes may present as hypogonadism, obesity, and mental retardation.

10 Bone dysplasias include skeletal dysplasias and osteochondrodysplasias. They usually present with short stature and abnormal body proportions (predominantly with short limbs or short trunks). Genetic consultation may be helpful.

11 Hypothyroidism may be congenital or acquired. Growth velocity is slow and bone age is delayed compared to chronological age. Children with Turner syndrome, Down syndrome, Klinefelter syndrome, or diabetes mellitus are also at risk for autoimmune hypothyroidism. Free T_4 is decreased and TSH is increased with acquired hypothyroidism. Low TSH and free T_4 suggest a hypothalamic/pituitary defect.

12 GH deficiency can be congenital or acquired. There may be isolated GH deficiency or panhypopituitarism. Congenital deficiencies are idiopathic, associated with midline defects (e.g., septooptic dysplasia, cleft palate, single central incisor), or inherited. The infants tend to be slightly smaller at birth (most are appropriate for gestational age); have hypoglycemia, jaundice, and micropenis; and show poor postnatal linear growth. Acquired GH deficiency may be due to CNS injury, infection, irradiation, or tumor. Bone age is delayed, and IGF-1 and IGFBP3 levels are often low. Levels are influenced by age, puberty, and nutrition. Further evaluation often requires referral to an endocrinologist for GH testing and testing for other pituitary hormone deficiencies (TSH, corticotropin, prolactin, gonadotropin deficiencies, or diabetes insipidus). Laron dwarfism features end-organ resistance to GH, with elevated GH levels and low levels of IGF-1 and IGFBP3.

13 Cushing syndrome is due to excessive levels of glucocorticoids, which may be exogenous (i.e., high doses of oral/topical corticosteroids) or endogenous due to excess corticotropin from pituitary tumors or ectopic production. Examination reveals an obese child who often has plethora, moon facies, buffalo hump, striae, acne, and hypertension. Hyperpigmentation occurs when excess corticotropin is present. Significant virilization may indicate an adrenal tumor. Growth velocity is slow, and bone age is delayed relative to chronological age.

14 Precocious puberty is characterized by early acceleration of growth, with advanced bone age. This is followed by early closure of epiphyses, which stops growth, leading to short stature. (See Chapters 69 and 70.)

Bibliography

Rose SR, Vogiatzi MG, Copeland KC: A general pediatric approach to evaluating a short child, *Pediatr Rev* 26:410–420, 2005.

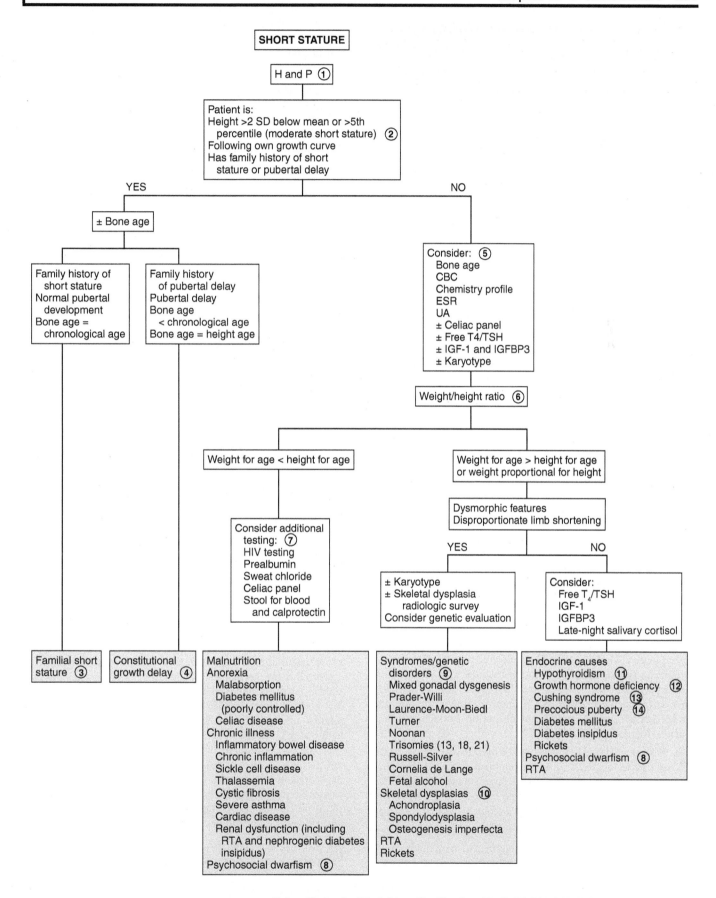

SHORT STATURE

H and P ①

Patient is:
Height >2 SD below mean or >5th
  percentile (moderate short stature) ②
Following own growth curve
Has family history of short
  stature or pubertal delay

YES / NO

YES:

± Bone age

Family history of
short stature
Normal pubertal
  development
Bone age =
  chronological age

Family history
  of pubertal delay
Pubertal delay
Bone age
  < chronological age
Bone age = height age

Familial short
stature ③

Constitutional
growth delay ④

NO:

Consider: ⑤
  Bone age
  CBC
  Chemistry profile
  ESR
  UA
  ± Celiac panel
  ± Free T4/TSH
  ± IGF-1 and IGFBP3
  ± Karyotype

Weight/height ratio ⑥

Weight for age < height for age

Weight for age > height for age
or weight proportional for height

Consider additional
  testing: ⑦
  HIV testing
  Prealbumin
  Sweat chloride
  Celiac panel
  Stool for blood
    and calprotectin

Dysmorphic features
Disproportionate limb shortening

YES / NO

YES:
± Karyotype
± Skeletal dysplasia
  radiologic survey
Consider genetic evaluation

NO:
Consider:
  Free T4/TSH
  IGF-1
  IGFBP3
  Late-night salivary cortisol

Malnutrition
Anorexia
  Malabsorption
  Diabetes mellitus
    (poorly controlled)
  Celiac disease
Chronic illness
  Inflammatory bowel disease
  Chronic inflammation
  Sickle cell disease
  Thalassemia
  Cystic fibrosis
  Severe asthma
  Cardiac disease
  Renal dysfunction (including
    RTA and nephrogenic diabetes
    insipidus)
Psychosocial dwarfism ⑧

Syndromes/genetic
  disorders ⑨
  Mixed gonadal dysgenesis
  Prader-Willi
  Laurence-Moon-Biedl
  Turner
  Noonan
  Trisomies (13, 18, 21)
  Russell-Silver
  Cornelia de Lange
  Fetal alcohol
Skeletal dysplasias ⑩
  Achondroplasia
  Spondylodysplasia
  Osteogenesis imperfecta
RTA
Rickets

Endocrine causes
  Hypothyroidism ⑪
  Growth hormone deficiency ⑫
  Cushing syndrome ⑬
  Precocious puberty ⑭
  Diabetes mellitus
  Diabetes insipidus
  Rickets
Psychosocial dwarfism ⑧
RTA

Nelson Textbook of Pediatrics, 19e. Chapters 13, 48, 76, 330, 529, 551, 556, 559, 580, 685
Nelson Essentials, 6e. Chapter 173

Chapter 68
PUBERTAL DELAY

Pubertal delay is defined as absence of development of secondary sexual characteristics (breast budding in girls, testicular enlargement in boys) by age 13 in girls and by age 14 in boys. It is related to abnormality of the hypothalamic-pituitary-gonadal axis. Pubic and axillary hair development are due to adrenal androgens and may be present in children with pubertal delay. For discussion of girls with some sexual maturation but with primary amenorrhea, please see Chapter 39.

1 History must include infections, chronic illness, endocrinopathies, trauma, chemotherapy, irradiation, CNS disorders, and syndromes. Growth patterns and growth velocity should be evaluated. Severe growth retardation may indicate growth hormone (GH) deficiency (see Chapter 67, Short Stature). History of heights of family members should be obtained. Also history of pubertal onset, menarche, and fertility of female relatives may indicate familial disorders such as pubertal delay, androgen insensitivity, and congenital adrenal hyperplasia. It is also important to obtain a history of gonadal tumors, autoimmune endocrine disorders, inborn errors of metabolism, and fragile X syndrome.

Examination includes careful measurements of height, weight, arm span, and body mass index (BMI). Patterns of growth (velocity) and sexual maturity rating (Tanner stage) should be assessed. Body proportions may be helpful; with GH deficiency, height age is less than weight age. Eunuchoidal proportions (arm span > height, long legs) are noted with hypogonadism. Androgen effects include phallic growth, increased testicular size, sexual hair, voice change, increased stature and muscle mass, hairline recession, and body odor. In girls, excessive androgens may lead to acne, hirsutism, or clitoromegaly. Estrogen effects include vaginal cornification/discharge, breast development, uterine size, and onset of menarche 2 to 2.5 years after breast budding. A careful CNS examination should include identification of midline facial defects and tests for olfaction (i.e., anosmia/hyposmia in Kallmann syndrome) as well as visual acuity. The presence of gynecomastia and galactorrhea should be noted. Skin examination includes café au lait spots (neurofibromatosis), tanning (adrenal insufficiency), and ichthyosis (congenital ichthyosis, Kallmann syndrome). Stigmata of specific syndromes may be identified on initial exam (e.g., Turner, fragile X, Prader-Willi, etc.).

2 Plasma FSH and LH levels can be used to classify the causes of pubertal delay into hypogonadotropic (↓FSH/LH) or hypergonadotropic (↑FSH/LH) hypogonadism. Bone age assessment, estradiol or testosterone levels, and prolactin and thyroid studies may be considered.

3 Stigmata of gonadal dysgenesis syndromes (e.g., Turner syndrome) include short stature, pigmented nevi, high-arched palate, low hairline, shield chest, ptosis, cutis laxa, pterygium coli (webbed neck), shortened fourth metacarpals, cubitus valgus, heart murmurs, nail changes, and deformed ears. There may be a history of congenital lymphedema. The 45,X karyotype is most common, but girls who are not diagnosed until their teens may have fewer examination findings and mosaicism (45,X/46,XX) may be present.

4 Mixed gonadal dysgenesis is a common cause of ambiguous genitalia in newborns. The karyotype usually shows mosaicism (45,X/46,XY). Patients often have a female phenotype and features of Turner syndrome. Some patients have no signs of masculinization, whereas in others there may be prepubertal clitoromegaly, with further virilization occurring at puberty.

5 Klinefelter syndrome is the most common cause of testicular failure; the karyotype is usually 47,XXY; mosaics are seen in 20%. The patients are usually tall and thin, testes are small, there is mild mental retardation, and gynecomastia may be present.

6 In pure gonadal dysgenesis, variants include XX or XY karyotype, with normal stature and streak gonads. In XY gonadal dysgenesis (Swyer syndrome), children have a female phenotype, but at pubertal age, breast development and menarche fail to occur.

7 Noonan syndrome has similar features to Turner syndrome but a normal karyotype.

8 The genetic male with androgen insensitivity (i.e., 46,XY disorder of sex development, testicular feminization) appears phenotypically female, with primary amenorrhea, breast development, and absence of pubic hair. There is wide variation in the degree of androgen resistance. Levels of LH are usually elevated, but FSH levels may be normal because estrogen from the testes may suppress it.

9 A cause of primary ovarian failure may be autoimmune oophoritis, which is associated with autoimmune endocrinopathies (thyroiditis, Addison disease, diabetes) and may be screened for with antiovarian antibodies. Resistant ovary syndrome is due to defects in the FSH or LH receptors. Premature gonadal failure may be associated with galactosemia, myotonic dystrophy, and fragile X–associated disorders. Anorchia is the absence of testes and must be distinguished from bilateral cryptorchidism. If testes cannot be palpated in boys with normal external genitalia, they have cryptorchidism. The testes are usually undescended or retractile, but rarely no testes are found even after investigation. This syndrome is known as "vanishing testes," congenital anorchia, or testicular regression syndrome. In cryptorchidism, owing to compromised Leydig cell function, normal testosterone levels may only be achieved with elevated FSH and LH levels. Irradiation or chemotherapy may also cause gonadal injury. Enzyme defects include 17-hydroxylase deficiency and 17-ketosteroid reductase deficiency, which result in hypertension, adrenal insufficiency, and deficiency of androgens and estrogens. The environmental influences that have been implicated in testicular dysgenesis syndrome include environmental chemicals that may act as endocrine disruptors (bisphenol A, phthalates), pesticides, phytoestrogens, and other chemicals. However, the evidence is only suggestive, not conclusive.

10 Constitutional delay is the most common cause of delayed puberty and is brought to medical attention more often in boys. There is a family history of delayed puberty, a consistent growth velocity, and a normal examination. Usually the bone age equals height age, which is less than the chronological age.

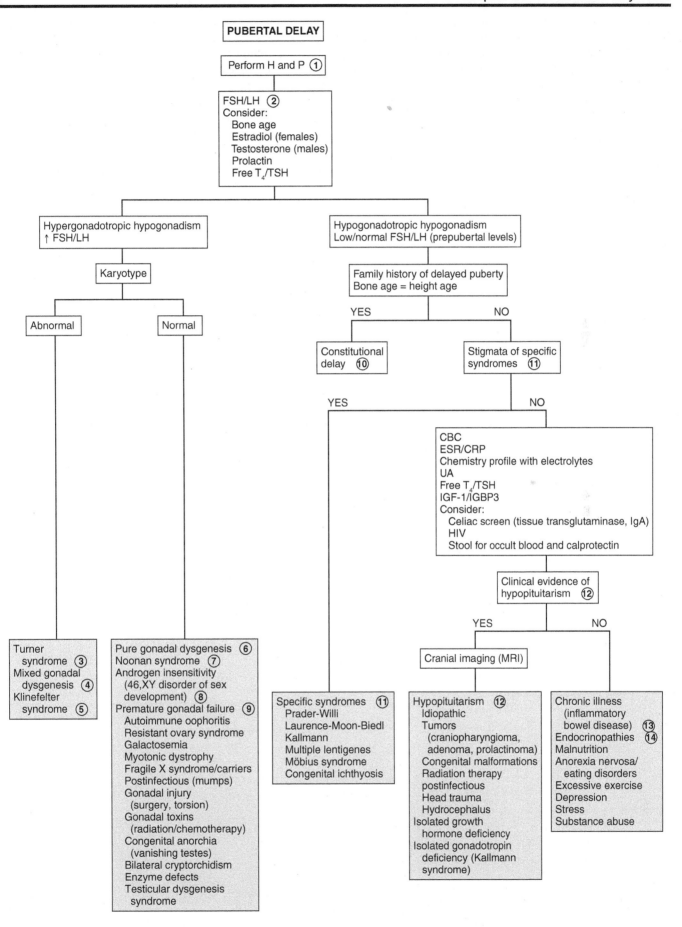

PUBERTAL DELAY

Perform H and P ①

FSH/LH ②
Consider:
  Bone age
  Estradiol (females)
  Testosterone (males)
  Prolactin
  Free T₄/TSH

Hypergonadotropic hypogonadism
↑ FSH/LH

Karyotype

Abnormal   Normal

Hypogonadotropic hypogonadism
Low/normal FSH/LH (prepubertal levels)

Family history of delayed puberty
Bone age = height age

YES   NO

Constitutional delay ⑩

Stigmata of specific syndromes ⑪

YES   NO

CBC
ESR/CRP
Chemistry profile with electrolytes
UA
Free T₄/TSH
IGF-1/IGBP3
Consider:
  Celiac screen (tissue transglutaminase, IgA)
  HIV
  Stool for occult blood and calprotectin

Clinical evidence of hypopituitarism ⑫

YES   NO

Cranial imaging (MRI)

Turner
syndrome ③
Mixed gonadal
dysgenesis ④
Klinefelter
syndrome ⑤

Pure gonadal dysgenesis ⑥
Noonan syndrome ⑦
Androgen insensitivity
  (46,XY disorder of sex
  development) ⑧
Premature gonadal failure ⑨
  Autoimmune oophoritis
  Resistant ovary syndrome
  Galactosemia
  Myotonic dystrophy
  Fragile X syndrome/carriers
  Postinfectious (mumps)
  Gonadal injury
    (surgery, torsion)
  Gonadal toxins
    (radiation/chemotherapy)
  Congenital anorchia
    (vanishing testes)
  Bilateral cryptorchidism
  Enzyme defects
  Testicular dysgenesis
    syndrome

Specific syndromes ⑪
  Prader-Willi
  Laurence-Moon-Biedl
  Kallmann
  Multiple lentigenes
  Möbius syndrome
  Congenital ichthyosis

Hypopituitarism ⑫
  Idiopathic
  Tumors
    (craniopharyngioma,
    adenoma, prolactinoma)
  Congenital malformations
  Radiation therapy
    postinfectious
  Head trauma
  Hydrocephalus
Isolated growth
  hormone deficiency
Isolated gonadotropin
  deficiency (Kallmann
  syndrome)

Chronic illness
  (inflammatory
  bowel disease) ⑬
Endocrinopathies
  ⑭
Malnutrition
Anorexia nervosa/
  eating disorders
Excessive exercise
Depression
Stress
Substance abuse

Nelson Textbook of Pediatrics, 19e. Chapters 76, 551, 577, 580, 582
Nelson Essentials, 6e. Chapter 174

11 Specific stigmata may be indicative of certain syndromes. In Prader-Willi syndrome, there is obesity, hyperphagia, short stature, and mild mental retardation. The hypogonadism is hypothalamic. Laurence-Moon-Biedl syndrome is associated with mild mental retardation, retinitis pigmentosa, syndactyly, polydactyly, and obesity. Pubertal delay is due to deficient gonadotropin-releasing hormone (GnRH), resulting in decreased FSH and LH. Kallmann syndrome (GnRH deficiency) is associated with midline defects (cleft lip/palate), congenital deafness, deficient sense of smell, and sometimes ichthyosis. Multiple lentigines syndrome includes cardiac defects, urologic abnormalities, short stature, and deafness. Other syndromes with hypogonadism include Möbius syndrome and congenital ichthyosis.

12 Clinical evidence that may suggest hypopituitarism include symptoms like growth failure, anosmia, midline facial defects, visual disturbances, and galactorrhea/hyperprolactinemia. Hypopituitarism with multiple tropic hormone deficiencies is usually idiopathic. However, it may be due to a tumor, trauma, congenital malformation (septooptic dysplasia), infiltrative diseases (tuberculosis, sarcoidosis, histiocytosis X), and cranial irradiation. Neuroimaging (MRI) should be considered to exclude these conditions. Patients with isolated GH deficiency usually have pubertal delay. Isolated gonadotropin deficiency is associated with a number of genetic disorders, including a subset with anosmia/hyposmia (Kallmann syndrome).

13 Systemic illness may affect both growth and pubertal development by GnRH suppression. Malnutrition, chronic illness such as renal failure, inflammatory bowel disease, celiac disease, recurrent infections, sickle cell disease, and malignancies may be causes.

14 Endocrinopathies include hypothyroidism, diabetes insipidus, Cushing disease, Addison's disease, and diabetes mellitus. In prolonged hypothyroidism, FSH and LH may be paradoxically increased. Hyperprolactinemia is more common in girls; it may be primary (idiopathic, pituitary adenoma) or secondary to disruption of the pituitary stalk or to hypothyroidism. Galactorrhea is present in 50%.

Bibliography

Emans SJ: Delayed puberty. In Emans SJ, Laufer MR, editors: *Pediatric and adolescent gynecology*, ed 6, Philadelphia, 2012, Lippincott Williams & Wilkins, Chapter 8.

Kaplowitz PB: Delayed puberty, *Pediatr Rev* 31:189–195, 2010.

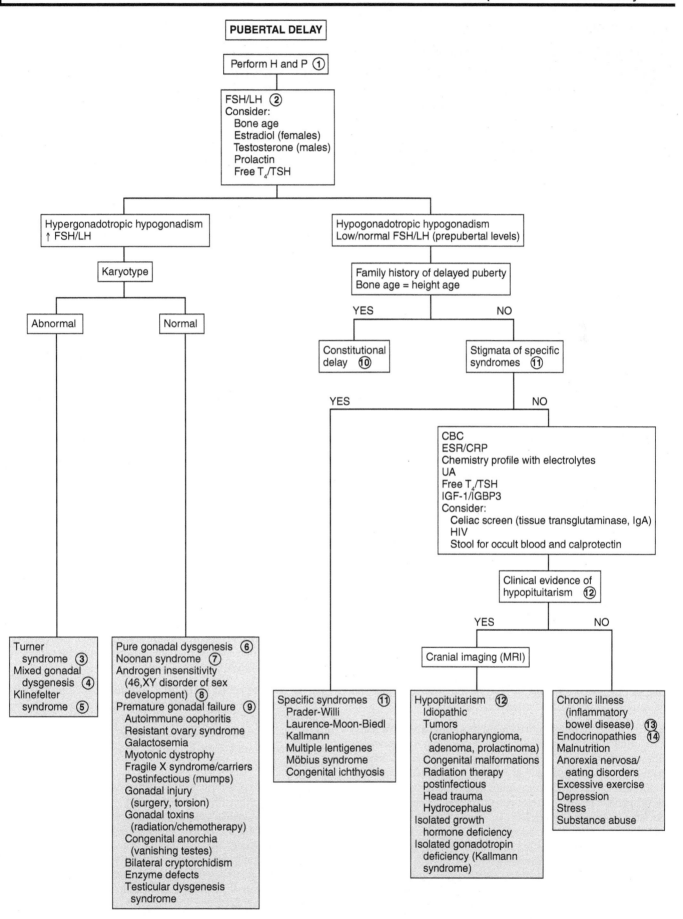

PUBERTAL DELAY

Perform H and P ①

FSH/LH ②
Consider:
  Bone age
  Estradiol (females)
  Testosterone (males)
  Prolactin
  Free T₄/TSH

Hypergonadotropic hypogonadism
↑ FSH/LH

Hypogonadotropic hypogonadism
Low/normal FSH/LH (prepubertal levels)

Karyotype

Family history of delayed puberty
Bone age = height age

Abnormal

Normal

YES

NO

Constitutional delay ⑩

Stigmata of specific syndromes ⑪

YES

NO

CBC
ESR/CRP
Chemistry profile with electrolytes
UA
Free T₄/TSH
IGF-1/IGBP3
Consider:
  Celiac screen (tissue transglutaminase, IgA)
  HIV
  Stool for occult blood and calprotectin

Clinical evidence of hypopituitarism ⑫

YES

NO

Cranial imaging (MRI)

Turner
  syndrome ③
Mixed gonadal
  dysgenesis ④
Klinefelter
  syndrome ⑤

Pure gonadal dysgenesis ⑥
Noonan syndrome ⑦
Androgen insensitivity
  (46,XY disorder of sex
  development) ⑧
Premature gonadal failure ⑨
  Autoimmune oophoritis
  Resistant ovary syndrome
  Galactosemia
  Myotonic dystrophy
  Fragile X syndrome/carriers
  Postinfectious (mumps)
  Gonadal injury
    (surgery, torsion)
  Gonadal toxins
    (radiation/chemotherapy)
  Congenital anorchia
    (vanishing testes)
  Bilateral cryptorchidism
  Enzyme defects
  Testicular dysgenesis
    syndrome

Specific syndromes ⑪
  Prader-Willi
  Laurence-Moon-Biedl
  Kallmann
  Multiple lentigenes
  Möbius syndrome
  Congenital ichthyosis

Hypopituitarism ⑫
  Idiopathic
  Tumors
    (craniopharyngioma,
    adenoma, prolactinoma)
  Congenital malformations
  Radiation therapy
    postinfectious
  Head trauma
  Hydrocephalus
Isolated growth
  hormone deficiency
Isolated gonadotropin
  deficiency (Kallmann
  syndrome)

Chronic illness
  (inflammatory
  bowel disease) ⑬
Endocrinopathies ⑭
Malnutrition
Anorexia nervosa/
  eating disorders
Excessive exercise
Depression
Stress
Substance abuse

Nelson Textbook of Pediatrics, 19e. Chapters 76, 551, 577, 580, 582
Nelson Essentials, 6e. Chapter 174

Chapter 69
PRECOCIOUS PUBERTY IN THE MALE

Precocious puberty in the male is defined as the beginning of secondary sexual characteristics before the age of 9 years. Isosexual puberty, with characteristic male sexual features, occurs as a result of normal male sex steroids. Heterosexual development with female characteristics (i.e., gynecomastia) is due to female sex steroids. Early pubarche is the isolated development of pubic or axillary hair.

1 History of growth patterns, chronological development of secondary sex characteristics, exposure to exogenous sex steroids (e.g., creams, lotions, meats, anabolic steroids), and family history of ambiguous genitalia or early pubertal development may be helpful. History of CNS disease, head injury, or irradiation may indicate a central cause. Symptoms including behavioral or emotional changes, headache, and vision problems require further assessment. Skin changes such as café au lait spots may indicate neurofibromatosis or McCune-Albright syndrome.

In boys, testicular enlargement is the earliest sign of puberty. Genital examination includes penile length and diameter and testicular volume, which is measured by orchidometer. Pubertal testes are more than 8 mL in volume or greater than 2.5 cm in longest diameter. Sexual Maturity Rating (SMR) or Tanner staging of pubic hair, and breasts in the case of gynecomastia, should be also be evaluated.

2 Central or gonadotropin-dependent precocious puberty is due to early activation of the hypothalamic-pituitary-gonadal axis. There is increased FSH and LH, acceleration of growth, testicular enlargement, and pubertal levels of testosterone. The bone age is advanced beyond the height age and chronological age.

3 Precocious puberty in males may be idiopathic, but up to 75% have an underlying CNS abnormality; therefore, imaging of the head, preferably by MRI, is imperative, in addition to a careful neurologic and visual examination.

4 Hypothalamic hamartomas are the most common brain lesion causing central precocious puberty and may be associated with seizures. Other CNS lesions causing central gonadotropin-dependent precocity usually involve the hypothalamus. These include postencephalitic scars, tuberculous meningitis, tuberous sclerosis, severe head trauma, and hydrocephalus (with or without associated myelomeningocele).

Neoplasms causing precocious puberty include astrocytomas, ependymomas, and optic tract tumors, including optic gliomas in children with neurofibromatosis type 1 (NF-1). Pineal or hypothalamic germinomas can cause central precocious puberty by secreting human chorionic gonadotropin (hCG), which stimulates the LH receptors in the Leydig cells of the testes.

5 McCune-Albright syndrome (MAS) is a rare disorder presenting with peripheral precocious puberty, café au lait skin pigmentation, and fibrous dysplasia of bone. It is more common in girls. When it presents in boys there may be overproduction of androgens, resulting in accelerated growth and skeletal maturation. Prolonged exposure to elevated levels of sex steroids may cause accelerated growth and skeletal maturation.

Although the precocious puberty is typically peripheral (gonadotropin independent), a secondary central (gonadotropin dependent) component may develop, also because of prolonged exposure to sex steroids. This secondary central precocious puberty may also be seen in late treatment of congenital adrenal hyperplasia (CAH).

6 If the FSH and LH levels are prepubertal and testosterone levels are elevated to pubertal levels, β-hCG levels should be checked. This hormone acts like LH, stimulating the testes to produce testosterone. Tumors producing β-hCG may be hepatomas, hepatoblastomas, teratomas, and chorioepitheliomas.

7 Prolonged untreated hypothyroidism may cause precocious puberty, in which case the bone age is delayed. TSH levels are elevated, and prolactin levels are mildly elevated. Although serum FSH is low and LH is undetectable, the elevated TSH appears to stimulate the FSH receptor (with no corresponding LH effects). Unlike in central precocious puberty, testicular enlargement occurs without increase in testosterone. Thus, the precocious puberty associated with hypothyroidism behaves as an incomplete form of central precocious puberty.

8 In autosomal dominant familial male-limited precocious puberty (testotoxicosis), β-hCG levels are normal and testosterone is elevated. There is autonomous production of testosterone from premature Leydig cell maturation; signs of puberty appear by age 2 to 3, and there is enlargement of the testes.

9 Elevated testosterone levels, particularly with asymmetric enlargement of one testis, may indicate a Leydig cell adenoma.

10 Another source of androgens is an adrenal tumor. Elevation of dehydroepiandrosterone sulfate (DHEAS) above 700 μg/dL or testosterone above 200 ng/dL warrants imaging for adrenal tumors. Adrenal tumors are also associated with increased dehydroepiandrosterone (DHEA) and androstenedione. Testosterone may be increased owing to production by the tumor or by peripheral conversion.

11 CAH is screened for by an early-morning 17-hydroxyprogesterone level. Levels below 200 ng/dL are normal; levels above 800 ng/dL are diagnostic of 21-hydroxylase deficiency, which is the most common form of CAH. Deficiency of 3β-hydroxysteroid dehydrogenase may result in precocious pubarche.

12 Premature pubarche is most commonly due to premature adrenarche, when there is an early increase in adrenal androgens. Testosterone and gonadotropin levels are prepubertal, and DHEAS may be moderately elevated but appropriate for stage 2 pubic hair. A 17-hydroxyprogesterone level may be considered to rule out late-onset CAH. Significantly elevated DHEAS or testosterone levels may require imaging studies to exclude a testicular or adrenal tumor. Clinical followup of premature adrenarche at 3-month intervals is usually adequate. Bone age is usually consistent with chronological age. If it is advanced, additional laboratory tests may be indicated. Idiopathic premature pubarche may be due to hypersensitivity of sexual hair follicles to androgen, and androgen levels are normal.

Bibliography

Muir A: Precocious puberty, *Pediatr Rev* 27:373–382, 2006.
Root AW: Precocious puberty, *Pediatr Rev* 21:10–19, 2000.

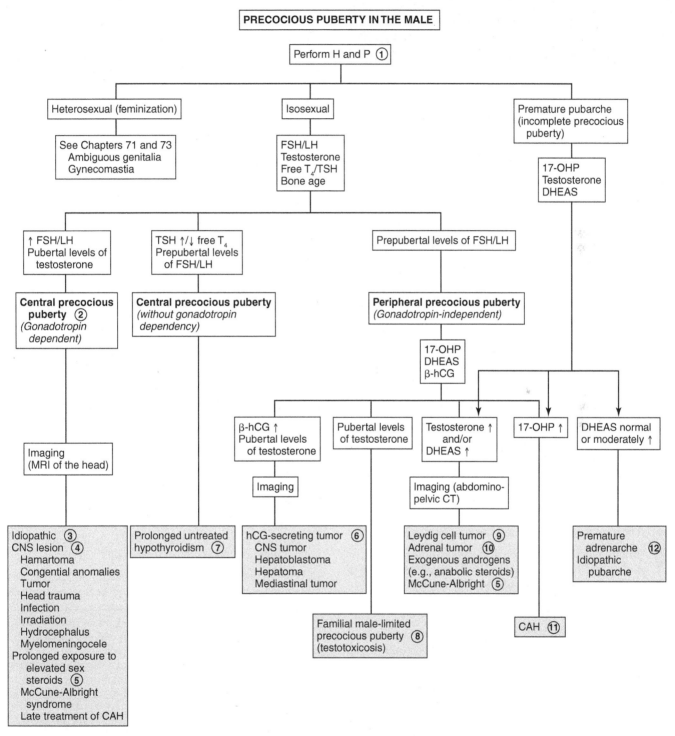

PRECOCIOUS PUBERTY IN THE MALE

Perform H and P ①

- **Heterosexual (feminization)**
  - See Chapters 71 and 73
  - Ambiguous genitalia
  - Gynecomastia

- **Isosexual**
  - FSH/LH
  - Testosterone
  - Free T₄/TSH
  - Bone age

  - ↑ FSH/LH
  - Pubertal levels of testosterone
    - **Central precocious puberty ②** *(Gonadotropin dependent)*
      - Imaging (MRI of the head)
        - Idiopathic ③
        - CNS lesion ④
          - Hamartoma
          - Congenital anomalies
          - Tumor
          - Head trauma
          - Infection
          - Irradiation
          - Hydrocephalus
          - Myelomeningocele
          - Prolonged exposure to elevated sex steroids ⑤
          - McCune-Albright syndrome
          - Late treatment of CAH

  - TSH ↑/↓ free T₄
  - Prepubertal levels of FSH/LH
    - **Central precocious puberty** *(without gonadotropin dependency)*
      - Prolonged untreated hypothyroidism ⑦

  - Prepubertal levels of FSH/LH
    - **Peripheral precocious puberty** *(Gonadotropin-independent)*
      - 17-OHP
      - DHEAS
      - β-hCG

      - β-hCG ↑
      - Pubertal levels of testosterone
        - Imaging
          - hCG-secreting tumor ⑥
            - CNS tumor
            - Hepatoblastoma
            - Hepatoma
            - Mediastinal tumor
          - Familial male-limited precocious puberty ⑧ (testotoxicosis)

      - Pubertal levels of testosterone

      - Testosterone ↑ and/or DHEAS ↑
        - Imaging (abdomino-pelvic CT)
          - Leydig cell tumor ⑨
          - Adrenal tumor ⑩
          - Exogenous androgens (e.g., anabolic steroids)
          - McCune-Albright ⑤

      - 17-OHP ↑
        - CAH ⑪

- **Premature pubarche (incomplete precocious puberty)**
  - 17-OHP
  - Testosterone
  - DHEAS

  - DHEAS normal or moderately ↑
    - Premature adrenarche ⑫
    - Idiopathic pubarche

β-hCG = β-human chorionic gonadotropin
DHEAS = dehydroepiandrosterone sulfate
17-OHP = 17-hydroxyprogesterone
CAH = congenital adrenal hyperplasia

Nelson Textbook of Pediatrics, 19e. Chapters 556, 578
Nelson Essentials, 6e. Chapter 174

Chapter 70
PRECOCIOUS PUBERTY IN THE FEMALE

Precocious puberty is defined by the onset of secondary sexual characteristics before the age of 8 years in girls. The lower limit of normal puberty may be age 6 for blacks and age 7 for whites. Isosexual puberty occurs because of normal female sex steroids. Heterosexual development is due to male sex steroids. Early pubarche is the isolated development of pubic or axillary hair. Premature thelarche is the isolated development of the breasts, with no other secondary sexual development.

1 History of growth patterns, chronological development of secondary sex characteristics, exposure to exogenous sex steroids (e.g., creams, lotions, meats, anabolic steroids), possible ambiguous genitalia, and family history of early pubertal development may be helpful. Evidence of CNS disease, such as behavioral or emotional changes, head trauma, hydrocephalus, headache, and vision problems, should be assessed. Skin changes such as café au lait spots may indicate McCune-Albright syndrome. Vaginal mucosal changes, enlargement of labia minora, and Tanner staging of pubic hair and breasts should be assessed. Rectoabdominal examination may indicate ovarian or abdominal masses. Virilization is indicated by excessive hirsutism, clitoromegaly, deepening voice, acne, and muscle development.

2 Central or gonadotropin-dependent precocious puberty is due to early activation of the normal physiologic pubertal development. There is increased FSH and LH, acceleration of growth, breast development, enlargement of the labia minora, vaginal mucosal change with enlargement of the ovaries and uterus, and pubertal levels of estradiol. The bone age is advanced beyond the height age and chronological age.

3 Childhood obesity has been associated with early puberty in girls and has been noted in children adopted from a developing country. Precocious puberty in females is often idiopathic, but a CNS lesion should be considered. Imaging of the head, preferably using MRI, is imperative, in addition to a careful neurologic and visual examination.

4 Hypothalamic hamartomas are the most common brain lesion causing central precocious puberty and may be associated with seizures. Other CNS lesions causing central gonadotropin-dependent precocity usually involve the hypothalamus. These include postencephalitic scars, tuberculous meningitis, tuberous sclerosis, severe head trauma, and hydrocephalus (with or without associated myelomeningocele).

Neoplasms causing precocious puberty include astrocytomas, ependymomas, and optic tract tumors, including optic gliomas in children with neurofibromatosis type 1 (NF-1).

5 McCune-Albright syndrome is a rare condition and is more common in girls than in boys; affected girls tend to have increased estrogen levels. It presents with a triad of peripheral precocious puberty, café au lait skin pigmentation, and fibrous dysplasia of bone. Vaginal bleeding often precedes significant breast development. A skeletal survey or technetium bone scan may identify polyostotic fibrous dysplasia. Prolonged exposure to elevated levels of sex steroids may cause accelerated growth and skeletal maturation.

Although the precocious puberty is typically peripheral (gonadotropin independent), a secondary central (gonadotropin dependent) component may develop, also because of prolonged exposure to sex steroids. This secondary central precocious puberty may also be seen in late treatment of congenital adrenal hyperplasia (CAH).

6 Prolonged untreated hypothyroidism may cause precocious puberty, in which case the bone age is delayed. TSH levels are elevated, and prolactin levels are mildly elevated. Although serum FSH is low and LH is usually undetectable, the elevated TSH appears to stimulate the FSH receptor (with no corresponding LH effects). Girls may have early breast development, galactorrhea, and recurrent menstrual bleeding. Precocious puberty associated with hypothyroidism behaves as an incomplete form of central precocious puberty.

7 If the FSH and LH levels are prepubertal and estradiol levels are elevated to pubertal levels, abdominopelvic imaging should be considered to exclude estrogen-secreting ovarian or adrenocortical tumors. The most common ovarian tumor causing precocious puberty is the granulosa cell tumor.

8 Autonomous ovarian follicular cysts are the most common estrogen-secreting masses. Plasma estradiol levels fluctuate with the size of the cyst. These may also result in premature thelarche.

9 Exogenous sources of estrogens include oral contraceptive pills and estrogen-containing tonics, lotions, and creams. Contamination of meat has been reported.

10 Benign premature thelarche is unilateral or bilateral breast enlargement, usually before age 2 years and resolving within 6 months to 6 years. No other signs of estrogenization are present. Plasma estrogen levels may be normal to slightly elevated. Laboratory studies are usually not indicated for premature thelarche. Clinical followup is adequate to detect progression to precocious puberty or onset of virilization. Regression followed by recurrence may indicate autonomous ovarian follicular cysts. Occurrence in children 3 years and older should prompt further evaluation.

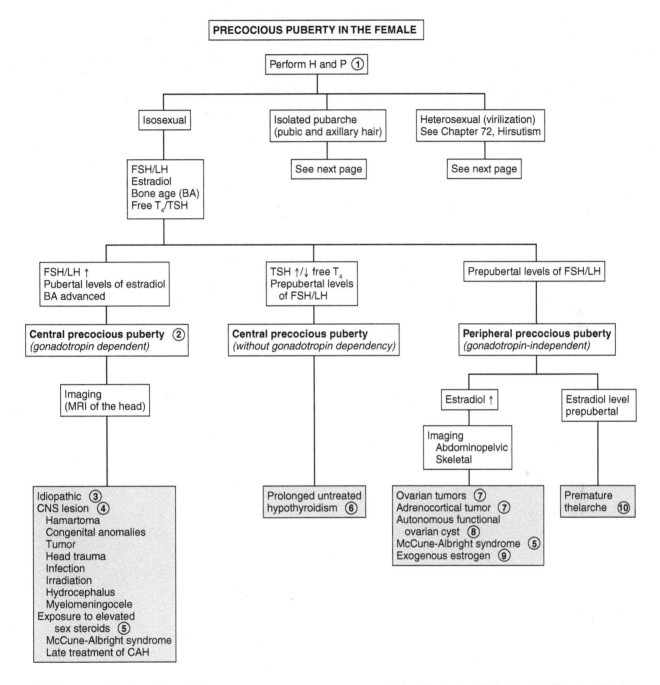

PRECOCIOUS PUBERTY IN THE FEMALE

Perform H and P ①

- Isosexual
- Isolated pubarche (pubic and axillary hair)
  - See next page
- Heterosexual (virilization) See Chapter 72, Hirsutism
  - See next page

FSH/LH
Estradiol
Bone age (BA)
Free T₄/TSH

FSH/LH ↑
Pubertal levels of estradiol
BA advanced

Central precocious puberty ②
(gonadotropin dependent)

Imaging
(MRI of the head)

Idiopathic ③
CNS lesion ④
  Hamartoma
  Congenital anomalies
  Tumor
  Head trauma
  Infection
  Irradiation
  Hydrocephalus
  Myelomeningocele
Exposure to elevated
  sex steroids ⑤
  McCune-Albright syndrome
  Late treatment of CAH

TSH ↑/↓ free T₄
Prepubertal levels
of FSH/LH

Central precocious puberty
(without gonadotropin dependency)

Prolonged untreated
hypothyroidism ⑥

Prepubertal levels of FSH/LH

Peripheral precocious puberty
(gonadotropin-independent)

- Estradiol ↑
  - Imaging
    Abdominopelvic
    Skeletal
  - Ovarian tumors ⑦
    Adrenocortical tumor ⑦
    Autonomous functional
      ovarian cyst ⑧
    McCune-Albright syndrome ⑤
    Exogenous estrogen ⑨
- Estradiol level
  prepubertal
  - Premature
    thelarche ⑩

CAH = congenital adrenal hyperplasia
DHEAS = dehydroepiandrosterone sulfate
17-OHP = 17 hydroxyprogesterone

Nelson Textbook of Pediatrics, 19e. Chapters 556, 581
Nelson Essentials, 6e. Chapter 174

(11) Premature adrenarche is the most common form of isolated precocious puberty, with an early increase in adrenal androgens. In addition to bone age, it is reasonable to obtain a 17-hydroxyprogesterone level to detect mild CAH due to 21-hydroxylase deficiency. Bone age is usually consistent with chronological age in premature adrenarche. Estradiol and gonadotropin levels are prepubertal, and dehydroepiandrosterone sulfate (DHEAS) may be moderately elevated (appropriate for stage 2 pubic hair). Girls with premature adrenarche are at increased risk for hyperandrogenism and polycystic ovary syndrome. Idiopathic premature pubarche may be due to hypersensitivity of sexual hair follicles to androgen.

If bone age is advanced or signs of virilization are present, further testing is needed.

(12) Virilization requires evaluation for androgen-producing adrenal or ovarian tumors, CAH, or exogenous androgen exposure, particularly in female athletes. CAH is screened for by an early-morning 17-hydroxyprogesterone level. Levels below 200 ng/dL are normal; levels above 800 ng/dL are diagnostic of 21-hydroxylase deficiency, which is the most common form of CAH. Bone age is greater than the chronological age. Deficiency of 3β-hydroxysteroid dehydrogenase may also result in precocious pubarche.

(13) Elevation of DHEAS above 700 µg/dL or testosterone above 200 ng/dL warrants imaging for adrenal or ovarian tumors. Bone age is usually greater than chronological age.

Bibliography

Muir A: Precocious puberty, *Pediatr Rev* 27:373–382, 2006.
Root AW: Precocious puberty, *Pediatr Rev* 21:10–19, 2000.

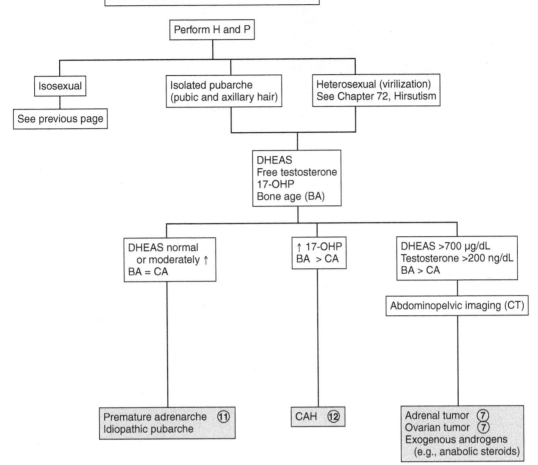

Chapter 71
ATYPICAL OR AMBIGUOUS GENITALIA

Evaluation of ambiguous genitalia in an infant requires a great deal of sensitivity. A geneticist, endocrinologist, and urologist should all be included. Bilateral cryptorchidism, unilateral cryptorchidism with incomplete scrotal fusion, subcoronal hypospadias, labial fusion, or clitoromegaly should prompt evaluation for ambiguous genitalia. Also consider evaluation in children with discordance between prenatal karyotype and appearance of the genitals or those with a family history of congenital adrenal hyperplasia (CAH).

A recent consensus statement proposed the term *disorders of sexual development* (DSD) to include "congenital conditions in which the chromosomal, gonadal, or anatomic sex is atypical." Some of these children present with ambiguous or atypical genitalia.

1. A careful history includes family history of male infants with increased scrotal pigmentation or rugae, infant deaths due to vomiting and dehydration (CAH), female relatives with amenorrhea or infertility (i.e., 46,XY DSD), and any variant sexual development. History of maternal drug exposure (hormones, spironolactone, and environmental chemical disruptors), virilization, or CAH should be obtained. Vomiting, dehydration, or failure to thrive may also suggest CAH.

Physical examination includes identification of stigmata of congenital malformation syndromes that may suggest the diagnosis. Hypertension, hyperpigmentation of the areolae and labioscrotal folds, dehydration, and poor weight gain may suggest CAH. A careful examination of genitalia is important, including measurement of clitoris/penis (a stretched penile length < 2.5 cm, or a clitoris > 1 cm, are abnormal at term). The urethral site, whether perineal or penile, should be determined. The presence of labioscrotal fusion and whether the gonad (almost always a testis) is palpable in the scrotum or inguinal rings should be assessed. A rectal examination is done to assess for the presence of a uterus. Often the cervix can be felt. Stigmata of other syndromes should be noted.

2. Initial evaluation for children with ambiguous genitalia should include 17-hydroxyprogesterone (17-OHP), electrolytes, imaging, and karyotype determination. In addition to US (pelvic, renal, adrenal) other imaging may include voiding cystourethrography and retrograde genitography. Pelvic CT or MRI may be needed for further evaluation. Endoscopy, laparotomy, and gonadal biopsy may be required for complete examination of genitalia with ovotesticular DSD.

CAH due to 21-hydroxylase deficiency is the most common cause of genital ambiguity in females. Currently, all U.S. states and many other countries include testing for 17-OHP levels as part of newborn screening programs. Infants with positive screening tests should be brought in for further testing (electrolytes and repeat 17-OHP).

3. 45,X/46,XY gonadal dysgenesis (mixed gonadal dysgenesis) is the second most common cause of ambiguous genitalia. There is wide phenotypic variation. Most children are short, and stigmata of Turner syndrome are present in one third of patients. There is mosaicism involving the Y chromosome, usually a streak gonad on one side and a dysgenetic or normal-appearing testis on the other. Müllerian and wolffian duct development correspond to the ipsilateral gonad.

4. Ovotesticular DSD (true hermaphroditism) is rare. Gonads contain both ovarian and testicular tissue. Both tissue types may be present in one gonad (ovotestis), or there may be a testis on one side and ovary on the other. About 70% have a 46,XX karyotype, 20% have 46,XX/46,XY mosaicism, and less than 10% of persons with ovotesticular DSD are 46,XY.

5. In partial gonadal dysgenesis the karyotype is 46,XY. It is a form of mixed gonadal dysgenesis.

6. 46,XY DSD may be due to defects in testicular differentiation. Patients have female external and internal genitalia; some have ambiguous genitals.

Defects in testicular differentiation include the following syndromes. Denys-Drash syndrome consists of nephropathy with ambiguous genitalia and bilateral Wilms tumor. Müllerian ducts are often present. WAGR syndrome includes *W*ilms tumor, *a*niridia, *G*U malformations, and mental *r*etardation. There is a deletion of 1 copy of chromosome 11p13. Males with this syndrome have atypical genitalia. Camptomelic syndrome is a form of short-limbed dysplasia. The gonads may contain elements of both ovaries and testes. In XY pure gonadal dysgenesis (Swyer syndrome), patients have normal stature, a female phenotype (including internal genitalia [uterus, fallopian tubes, vagina]), and streak gonads. They present with delayed puberty and hypergonadotropic primary amenorrhea (see chapters on Pubertal Delay and Amenorrhea).

7. Other causes of 46,XY DSD include defects in androgen action. In androgen resistance syndromes (testicular feminization) there is a defect in androgen receptors. Although testes are present but are often intraabdominal and testosterone and LH levels are high, external genitalia are female, the vagina is a blind pouch, the uterus is absent, but fallopian tube remnants may be present in approximately one third of patients. Diagnosis is usually at the time of puberty, when the phenotypic female presents with amenorrhea.

8. Defects in testicular hormones produce 46,XY males with inadequate masculinization. This was previously known as male pseudohermaphroditism. Boys with Leydig cell aplasia usually appear phenotypically female with mild virilization. Testes, epididymis, and vas deferens are present; the uterus and fallopian tubes are absent. Testosterone levels are low and LH is elevated.

CAH in 46,XY males may be due to the following enzyme deficiencies. Lipoid adrenal hyperplasia is a severe form of CAH, presenting in salt-wasting crisis (hyponatremia and hyperkalemia. Genetic males have no müllerian structures. Deficiency of 3β-hydroxysteroid dehydrogenase causes ambiguous genitalia in males and females and may also present with salt wasting. There is increased dehydroepiandrosterone (DHEA) and decreased androstenedione, testosterone, and estradiol. Deficiency of 17-hydroxylase/17,20-lyase causes ambiguous genitalia in

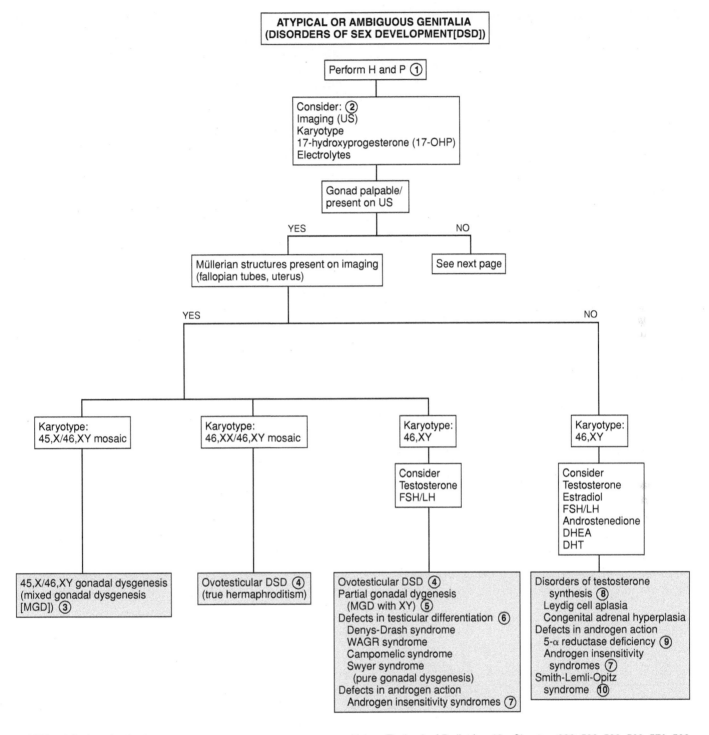

ATYPICAL OR AMBIGUOUS GENITALIA
(DISORDERS OF SEX DEVELOPMENT[DSD])

Perform H and P ①

Consider: ②
Imaging (US)
Karyotype
17-hydroxyprogesterone (17-OHP)
Electrolytes

Gonad palpable/
present on US

YES — Müllerian structures present on imaging
(fallopian tubes, uterus)

NO — See next page

YES

Karyotype:
45,X/46,XY mosaic

→ 45,X/46,XY gonadal dysgenesis
(mixed gonadal dysgenesis
[MGD]) ③

Karyotype:
46,XX/46,XY mosaic

→ Ovotesticular DSD ④
(true hermaphroditism)

Karyotype:
46,XY

Consider
Testosterone
FSH/LH

→ Ovotesticular DSD ④
Partial gonadal dygenesis
(MGD with XY) ⑤
Defects in testicular differentiation ⑥
Denys-Drash syndrome
WAGR syndrome
Campomelic syndrome
Swyer syndrome
(pure gonadal dysgenesis)
Defects in androgen action
Androgen insensitivity syndromes ⑦

NO

Karyotype:
46,XY

Consider
Testosterone
Estradiol
FSH/LH
Androstenedione
DHEA
DHT

→ Disorders of testosterone
synthesis ⑧
Leydig cell aplasia
Congenital adrenal hyperplasia
Defects in androgen action
5-α reductase deficiency ⑨
Androgen insensitivity
syndromes ⑦
Smith-Lemli-Opitz
syndrome ⑩

DHEA = dehydroepiandrosterone
DHT = dihydrotestosterone

Nelson Textbook of Pediatrics, 19e. Chapters 338, 538, 539, 569, 570, 582
Nelsons Essentials, 6e. Chapter 177

males, with hypertension, hypokalemia, and decreased serum androgens. In 17-ketosteroid reductase deficiency, müllerian ducts are absent and a shallow vagina is present.

9 In 5α-reductase deficiency, inadequate conversion of testosterone to dihydrotestosterone (DHT) occurs, which is necessary for fetal masculinization. Consequently, the newborn is characterized by a small phallus/ambiguous genitalia, hypospadias, bifid scrotum, and on occasion, scrotal/labial testes. A high testosterone-to-DHT ratio is diagnostic.

10 Smith-Lemli-Opitz syndrome (SLOS) is an autosomal recessive disorder characterized by growth retardation, microcephaly, ptosis, syndactyly, mental retardation, and genital ambiguity in males. Müllerian remnants are absent.

11 In XY gonadal agenesis syndrome (embryonic testicular regression syndrome) genitalia are female or atypical (ambiguous) in appearance. Müllerian structures are absent. It is presumed that testicles regress between the 8th and 12th weeks of gestation.

12 Anorchia (vanishing testes syndrome) is a form of testicular regression seen in 46,XY phenotypic boys who present with cryptorchidism. Presumably there was active fetal testicular function during the genital differentiation and with later regression (usually after 20th week). It may also be due to testicular torsion. Testosterone levels are low, and gonadotropin levels are elevated. If this occurs before 8 weeks of gestation, it results in Swyer syndrome, and female genitalia develop.

13 Elevated maternal androgens may be due to maternal ingestion of medications or hormones or to a virilizing adrenal or ovarian tumor in the mother, or may be idiopathic. The degree of virilization depends on the timing of fetal exposure.

14 Persistent müllerian duct syndrome may be seen in phenotypic males with cryptorchidism. Müllerian structures are often discovered during surgery for cryptorchidism.

15 CAH is the most common 46,XX DSD and is usually due to to 21-hydroxylase deficiency, with increased 17-OHP and adrenal androgens (e.g., dehydroepiandrosterone, androstenedione, and androstenediol). The severe form may occur as salt wasting (hyponatremia, hyperkalemia, acidosis), vomiting, dehydration, and circulatory collapse. Normal ovaries and müllerian structures are present. External genitalia changes depend on time of intrauterine exposure and can range from complete labioscrotal fusion to clitoral hypertrophy. In 11β-hydroxylase deficiency, 11-deoxycortisol and deoxycorticosterone levels are high, producing hypertension in infancy.

Bibliography

Lee PA, Houk CP, Ahmed SF, Hughes LA: International Consensus Conference on Intersex organized by the Lawson Wilkins Pediatric Endocrine Society and the European Society for Paediatric Endocrinology. Consensus Statement on Management of Intersex Disorders. International Consensus Conference on Intersex, *Pediatrics* 118:e488–500, 2006.

Emans SJH, Laufer MR: Ambiguous genitalia in the newborn and disorders of sex development. In Emans SJ, Laufer MR, editors: *Emans, Laufer, Goldstein's pediatric & adolescent gynecology,* ed 6, Philadelphia, 2012, Lippincott Williams & Wilkins.

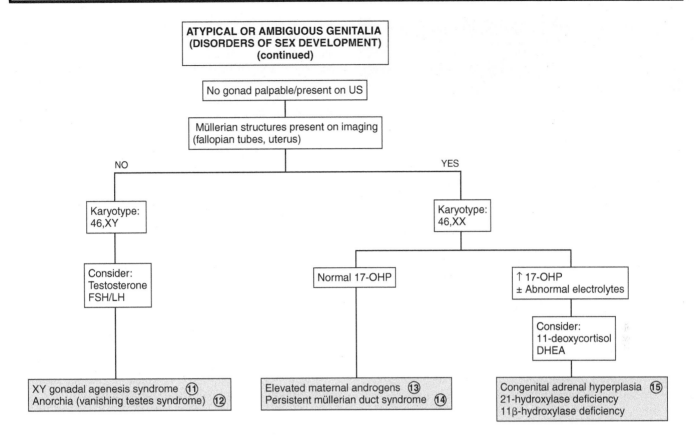

**ATYPICAL OR AMBIGUOUS GENITALIA
(DISORDERS OF SEX DEVELOPMENT)
(continued)**

No gonad palpable/present on US

Müllerian structures present on imaging
(fallopian tubes, uterus)

NO

YES

Karyotype:
46,XY

Karyotype:
46,XX

Consider:
Testosterone
FSH/LH

Normal 17-OHP

↑ 17-OHP
± Abnormal electrolytes

Consider:
11-deoxycortisol
DHEA

XY gonadal agenesis syndrome ⑪
Anorchia (vanishing testes syndrome) ⑫

Elevated maternal androgens ⑬
Persistent müllerian duct syndrome ⑭

Congenital adrenal hyperplasia ⑮
21-hydroxylase deficiency
11β-hydroxylase deficiency

Chapter 72
HIRSUTISM

Hirsutism implies an excessive growth of body hair in women and children in an adult male pattern. It is often due to androgen excess. Hirsutism is an increased density of terminal hair (coarse, adult type) and must be differentiated from hypertrichosis. Hypertrichosis is an increase in vellus hair (i.e., the downy hair seen in prepubertal years) and is often associated with drugs, malignancy, and anorexia. Hirsutism must also be distinguished from virilization (masculinization), which includes findings of increased muscle mass, voice changes, and clitoral enlargement in girls. Sexual hair grows in response to sex steroids. It grows on the face, lower abdomen, anterior thighs, chest, breasts, pubic area, and axilla. Androgens, especially testosterone, stimulate growth of sexual hair, whereas estrogens have an opposite effect. Other hormones (e.g., thyroxine, prolactin) also affect hair growth.

1. Increased androgen production usually causes hirsutism, acne, and increased oiliness of the skin. In extreme cases it causes virilization or masculinization, with male baldness patterns, clitoromegaly, deepening voice, increased muscle mass, and male body habitus. The age and rapidity of onset may indicate the etiology of the hirsutism. Rapid onset of virilization may indicate a tumor. Early onset of hirsutism is often seen with congenital adrenal hyperplasia (CAH). Amenorrhea or galactorrhea may indicate hyperprolactinemia. A history of CNS problems such as head trauma or encephalitis should be sought. Medications may at times be responsible and should be reviewed. A family history of hirsutism, polycystic ovary syndrome (PCOS), CAH, diabetes, hyperinsulinism, and infertility should be obtained. Careful examination should include the degree of virilization, and a search for thyromegaly, abdominal or pelvic masses, and skin changes (e.g., acanthosis nigricans or any chronic skin irritation such as from a cast). Features of PCOS include hirsutism, obesity, and oligomenorrhea. Presence of striae and a buffalo hump may indicate Cushing syndrome.

2. Idiopathic or familial hirsutism is seen in certain geographic areas, ethnic groups, or families. It is probably due to increased sensitivity of the skin's hair apparatus to normal levels of androgens, increased conversion of testosterone to dihydrotestosterone, or an excess of hair follicles. These women ovulate regularly and have normal menses and normal androgen levels.

3. Virilization during pregnancy may indicate a luteoma, which is an exaggerated response of ovarian stroma to chorionic gonadotropin; this regresses postpartum.

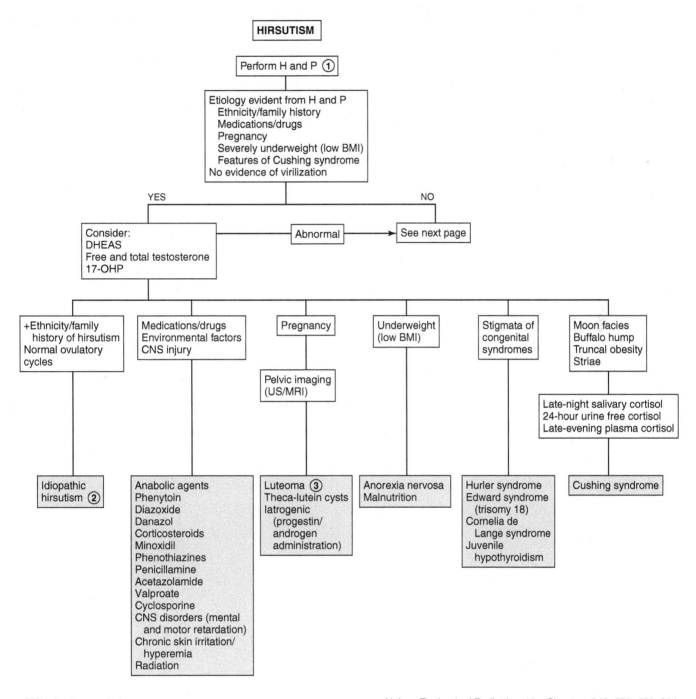

HIRSUTISM

Perform H and P ①

Etiology evident from H and P
   Ethnicity/family history
   Medications/drugs
   Pregnancy
   Severely underweight (low BMI)
   Features of Cushing syndrome
No evidence of virilization

YES   NO

Consider:
DHEAS
Free and total testosterone
17-OHP

Abnormal → See next page

+Ethnicity/family
  history of hirsutism
Normal ovulatory
cycles

Medications/drugs
Environmental factors
CNS injury

Pregnancy

Underweight
(low BMI)

Stigmata of
congenital
syndromes

Moon facies
Buffalo hump
Truncal obesity
Striae

Pelvic imaging
(US/MRI)

Late-night salivary cortisol
24-hour urine free cortisol
Late-evening plasma cortisol

Idiopathic
hirsutism ②

Anabolic agents
Phenytoin
Diazoxide
Danazol
Corticosteroids
Minoxidil
Phenothiazines
Penicillamine
Acetazolamide
Valproate
Cyclosporine
CNS disorders (mental
  and motor retardation)
Chronic skin irritation/
  hyperemia
Radiation

Luteoma ③
Theca-lutein cysts
Iatrogenic
  (progestin/
  androgen
  administration)

Anorexia nervosa
Malnutrition

Hurler syndrome
Edward syndrome
  (trisomy 18)
Cornelia de
  Lange syndrome
Juvenile
  hypothyroidism

Cushing syndrome

BMI = body mass index
DHEAS = dehydroepiandrosterone sulfate
HAIR-AN = hyperandrogenism, insulin resistance, acanthosis nigricans
17-OHP = 17-hydroxyprogesterone

Nelson Textbook of Pediatrics, 19e. Chapters 546, 570, 582, 654

(4) PCOS is the most common cause of hirsutism in adolescents. This is a spectrum of clinical disease that is ill defined, especially in adolescents. Features include persistent anovulation, irregular menstrual cycles, hirsutism, and obesity. On US evaluation the ovaries may appear normal or have a number of small cysts (25%). There is an increased sensitivity to gonadotropin-releasing hormones, resulting in an increase in LH levels and LH:FSH ratios. The elevated LH causes an increase in ovarian androgen production and a decrease in sex hormone–binding globulin (SHBG), resulting in an overall increase in free androgen, including testosterone and dehydroepiandrosterone sulfate (DHEAS). If anovulation or galactorrhea are present, consider a prolactin level and thyroid function tests to exclude hyperprolactinemia and hypothyroidism.

(5) Hyperandrogenism (HA) is often associated with insulin resistance (IR) and acanthosis nigricans (AN), otherwise known as the HAIR-AN syndrome. The mechanism of this syndrome is unknown; however, there is a defect in membrane insulin receptors. Testing for hyperinsulinism is therefore indicated in women with persistent anovulation, android obesity, and acanthosis nigricans.

(6) Elevation of DHEAS above 700 μg/dL (suggesting adrenal tumors), testosterone levels over 200 ng/dL (ovarian tumors), or history of rapid onset of virilizing symptoms warrants imaging for adrenal or ovarian tumors.

(7) Late-onset adrenal hyperplasia is screened for by an early-morning 17-hydroxyprogesterone level. Levels below 200 ng/dL are normal; levels above 800 ng/dL are diagnostic of 21-hydroxylase deficiency, which is the most common form of CAH. DHEAS and testosterone levels are also increased. Levels over 200 ng/dL require corticotropin testing for 3β-hydroxysteroid dehydrogenase and 11β-hydroxylase deficiency.

(8) If there is a history of ambiguous genitalia, consider karyotype testing to identify incomplete androgen insensitivity and mixed gonadal dysgenesis. Females with 45,X/46,XY mixed gonadal dysgenesis with Y-containing mosaics, or males with defects in androgen action (partial androgen insensitivity, 5a-reductase deficiency) who are phenotypically female, may develop signs of androgen stimulation at puberty. US may be needed to identify an intraabdominal gonad (testis or dysgenetic gonad). (See Chapter 71, Atypical or Ambiguous Genitalia.)

Bibliography

Emans SJH, Laufer MR: Androgen abnormalities in the adolescent girl. In Emans SJ, Laufer MR, editors: *Emans, Laufer, Goldstein's pediatric & adolescent gynecology,* ed 6, Philadelphia, 2012, Lippincott Williams & Wilkins.

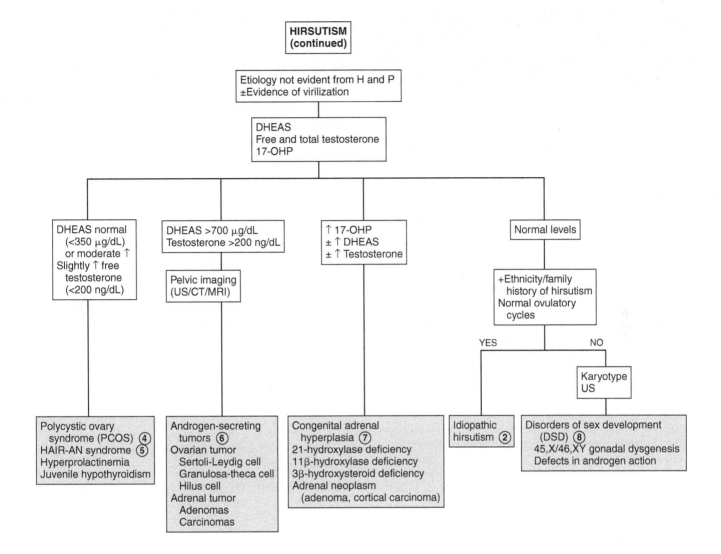

Chapter 73
GYNECOMASTIA

Gynecomastia is enlargement of the male breast tissue owing to a decrease in the ratio of androgens to estrogens. Testosterone weakly inhibits and estrogen strongly stimulates breast tissue development. In males, estrogen is usually produced by the aromatization of androgens in peripheral tissues. Macrogynecomastia is when the breast tissue is greater than 4 cm in diameter. It is similar to middle and late stages of female breast development and is less likely to resolve spontaneously. Asymmetry of breasts is common; however, any hardness of breast tissue or asymmetric placement of the nipple requires evaluation. Lipomastia, the fatty tissue in overweight boys, may cause pseudogynecomastia.

1 History should include a family history of permanent gynecomastia, as well as history of systemic or chronic illness, including endocrinopathies, renal failure, liver disease, and malnutrition. A careful history of drug or medication intake, including hormone-containing lotion, creams, foods, and other products, should be obtained. History of excessive alcohol intake as well as illicit drug intake (i.e., marijuana) should be sought. Gynecomastia that develops before the onset of other pubertal changes or before age 10 years or is associated with precocious or delayed puberty or macrogynecomastia requires further evaluation.

Physical examination should include a careful examination of the breast, including diameter and consistency of breast tissue and position of the nipple. Determination of pubertal staging and testicular size is also important.

2 Medications and drugs that can cause gynecomastia include hormones: estrogens in meat, milk, lotions, and oils; androgens, which are aromatized to estrogens; and human chorionic gonadotropin (hCG), which causes increased estradiol secretion from the testis.

3 Physiologic pubertal gynecomastia is common in adolescents. It occurs in up to 60% of boys aged 10 to 16 and usually resolves spontaneously (i.e., 75% within 2 years). The breast tissue is less than 4 cm in diameter and resembles breast budding in females. Signs of pubertal development usually precede gynecomastia by at least 6 months. Puberty is between Tanner stages II and IV. Obesity is commonly associated with gynecomastia and is usually due to increased aromatization of androgens to estrogen by adipose tissue. Gynecomastia may also persist longer in obese boys.

4 Lipomastia may also cause prominence of the breast tissue, known as pseudogynecomastia, and is usually seen in obese boys.

5 Familial gynecomastia may be X-linked or autosomal dominant; it may be due to increased aromatase activity.

6 Unilateral enlargement, especially with asymmetry and hard breast tissue, suggests local tumors. These are rare in adolescents. They may be caused by neurofibromas, dermoid cysts, lipoma, lymphangioma, metastatic neuroblastoma, leukemia, lymphoma, and rhabdomyosarcoma.

7 Gynecomastia may be seen in some chronic diseases such as cystic fibrosis, ulcerative colitis, cirrhosis, malnutrition followed by refeeding and acquired immunodeficiency syndrome (AIDS). It may be related to hepatic dysfunction. Uremia due to renal failure may cause testicular damage and decreased testosterone.

8 If there is no evident etiology for the gynecomastia, or there is evidence of hypogonadism, precocious puberty, or macrogynecomastia, obtain LH, FSH, estradiol, testosterone, dehydroepiandrosterone sulfate (DHEAS), free T_4, TSH, and hCG levels. If testes are smaller than 3 cm in diameter or 8 mL in volume or there is a history of ambiguous genitalia, a karyotype should also be obtained.

9 If DHEAS is increased, imaging for adrenal tumors is needed. Increased estradiol levels may require US of the liver, adrenals, and testes for hormone-producing tumors. Adrenal tumors usually cause feminization by conversion of androstenedione to estradiol. MRI imaging of the brain, chest, abdomen, and testes should be considered for evaluation for β-hCG–secreting tumors, which may also cause precocious puberty. Other hormone-producing tumors include LH-secreting pituitary tumors and prolactinomas, which cause galactorrhea but usually not gynecomastia. If galactorrhea is present, obtain a prolactin level. Karyotype may also be considered if there is a history of ambiguous genitalia at birth or if there is evidence of hypergonadotropic hypogonadism (testicular size <8 mL, ↑ FSH, ↑ LH).

10 In hypogonadism, gynecomastia develops during adrenarche owing to aromatization of adrenal androgens to estrogen. Klinefelter syndrome (47,XXY) usually presents as delayed puberty, gynecomastia, and small testes; patients with Klinefelter syndrome have decreased testosterone levels. In androgen insensitivity (XY), there is end-organ resistance to testosterone. In both conditions, Leydig cell action is retained, and there is secretion of estradiol in response to the increased LH. Testicular damage due to orchitis, injury, chemotherapy, or radiation, and congenital anorchia due to fetal testicular regression, may occur and present as gynecomastia at puberty. CNS injury (paraplegia) may be associated with decreased testicular function, leading to gynecomastia.

Enzyme defects of 17α-hydroxylase, 17/20-desmolase, and 17-ketosteroid reductase result in decreased synthesis of testosterone. Patients with these defects may also present with ambiguous genitalia at birth. Gynecomastia may also be seen in the gonadal dysgenesis.

11 Adrenal, testicular, and hepatocellular tumors may produce aromatase, causing increased estradiol. Familial gynecomastia is an autosomal dominant condition and may be due to increased aromatase activity.

12 Estrogen-secreting tumors are a rare cause of gynecomastia. Sex cord tumors with annular tubules (SCTAT) may occur in patients with Peutz-Jeghers syndrome. They are multifocal and may secrete estradiol.

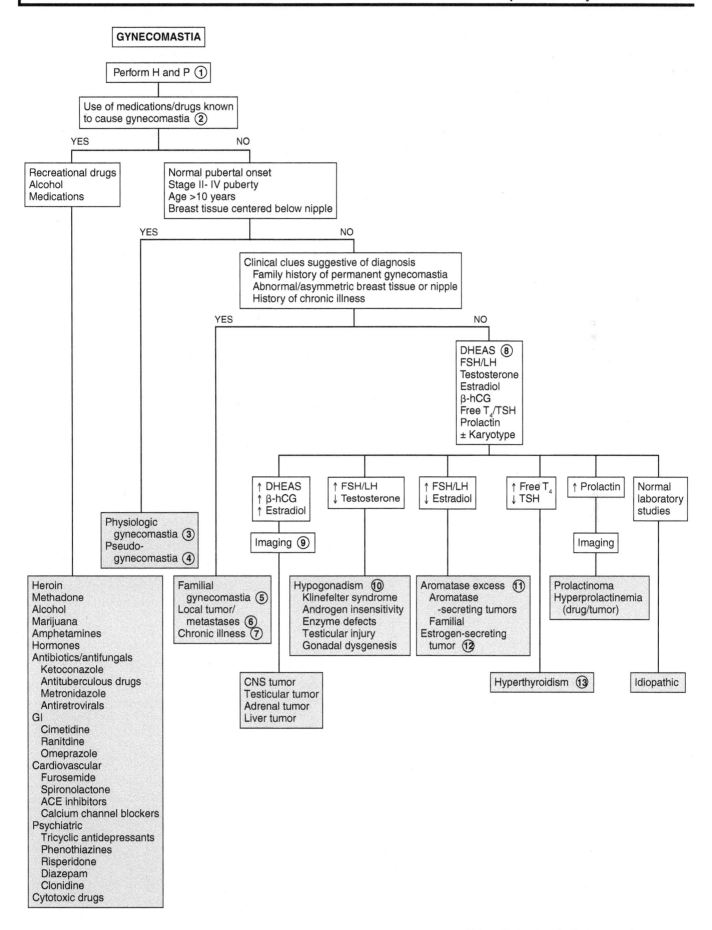

13 Gynecomastia is seen in a third of patients with thyrotoxicosis. It is primarily due to increased androstenedione, which is aromatized to estradiol. Hyperthyroidism also alters the androgen-to-estrogen ratio by increasing bound androgen and decreasing free testosterone.

Bibliography

Diamantopoulos SY: Gynecomastia and premature thelarche: A guide for practitioners, *Pediatr Rev* 28:57–68, 2007.

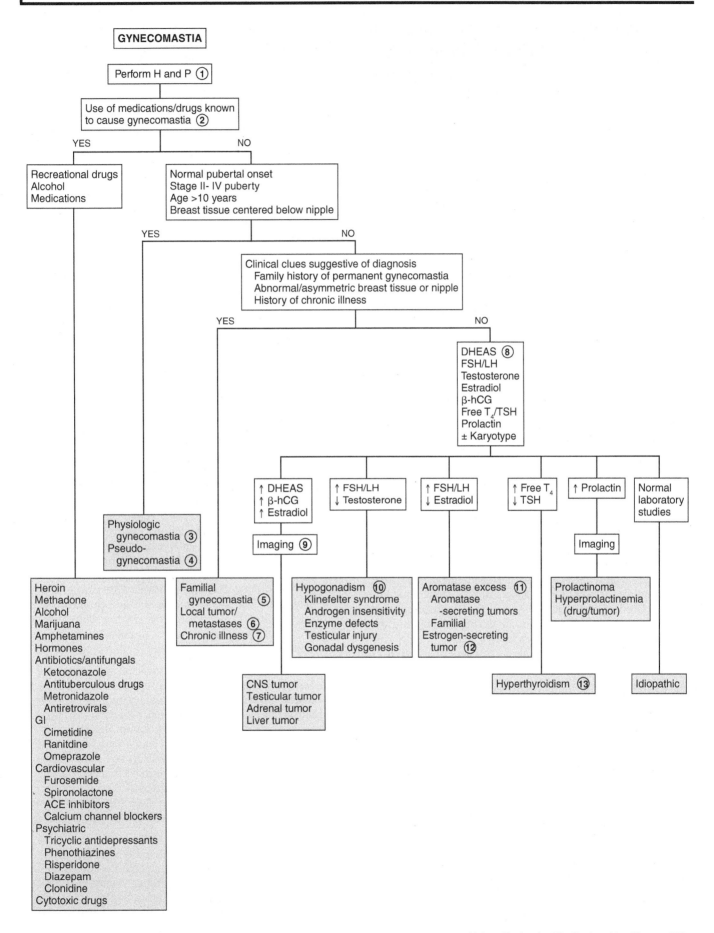

Chapter 74
OBESITY

Obesity among children is increasing. It is commonly defined by using the body mass index (BMI), which is a proxy for direct measurement of body fat. BMI = weight in kg / (height in meters)^2. Children older than 2 years with a BMI above the 95th percentile meet the criterion for obesity, and those with a BMI from the 85th to 95th percentiles are in the overweight range. Adults with a BMI of 30 or above meet the criterion for obesity, and those with a BMI of 25 to 30 fall in the overweight range. These children are at greater risk for obesity as an adult, which is associated with an increased risk of diabetes, hypertension, and atherosclerosis.

1. Children should be carefully evaluated for any disorder that may be associated with obesity. These disorders are rare and are usually associated with specific signs and symptoms. A drug history should be obtained because certain medications are associated with obesity. A history of headaches, visual changes, or CNS injuries or infections may indicate a hypothalamic cause. Short stature and delayed sexual development are often present. In girls, hirsutism, amenorrhea, or oligomenorrhea may suggest an underlying condition. Striae, buffalo hump, or truncal obesity, as well as acne and hypertrichosis, are present in Cushing syndrome. Dysmorphic features associated with syndromes should also be noted. Developmental delay is often a feature of these syndromes. Hyperinsulinemia should be considered in patients with hyperphagia who have an excessive increase in stature. Acanthosis nigricans is often present in obese children and has a strong association with insulin resistance. The presence of a goiter indicates thyroid disease. It is important to differentiate bigger or stockier children with larger skeletal frames from those who are obese.

2. Prader-Willi syndrome is associated with transient neonatal hypotonia, developmental delay, and intellectual disability. There is a hypogonadotropic hypogonadism and associated short stature. Feeding problems may occur during infancy, and extreme hyperphagia may occur in childhood and adolescence. The hands and feet are small. Strabismus is often present. FISH 15q11 microdeletion is present in 70% of cases.

3. Turner syndrome should be suspected in short females, particularly if there is a history of pubertal delay and amenorrhea. Features of this syndrome include webbed neck, low posterior hairline, small mandible, prominent ears, epicanthal folds, high-arched palate, broad chest with wide-spaced nipples, cubitus valgus, and hyperconvex fingernails. Diagnosis may be made by chromosome analysis.

4. Laurence-Moon-Biedl (Bardet-Biedl) syndrome is characterized by truncal obesity and retinal dystrophy/retinitis pigmentosa with progressive visual impairment. Other features include intellectual disability, digital anomalies (polydactyly, syndactyly), hypogenitalism, and nephropathy.

5. Alström-Hallgren syndrome is associated with nerve deafness, diabetes mellitus, and retinal degeneration with blindness, cataracts, and small testes in males.

6. Cohen syndrome is characterized by truncal obesity, hypotonia, muscle weakness, and mild intellectual disability. Characteristic craniofacial features include a high nasal bridge, maxillary hypoplasia, downslanting palpebral fissures, high-arched palate, short philtrum, strabismus, small jaw, open mouth, and prominent maxillary incisors. In addition, narrow hands and feet, short metacarpals and metatarsals, simian crease, hyperextensible joints, lumbar lordosis, and mild scoliosis are often present.

7. Carpenter syndrome is characterized by brachycephaly with craniosynostosis, lateral displacement of inner canthi and apparent exophthalmos, flat nasal bridge, low-set ears, retrognathism, and high-arched palate. The extremities may show brachydactyly, syndactyly, and polydactyly. Intellectual disability is present.

8. Albright hereditary osteodystrophy (i.e., pseudohypoparathyroidism type I) occurs as short stature, round face, short metacarpals and metatarsals, mental retardation, cataracts, coarse skin, brittle hair and nails, as well as hypocalcemia and hyperphosphatemia.

9. Biemond syndrome presents with cognitive impairment, coloboma of the iris, hypogonadism and polydactyly.

10. Gene disorders known to result in obesity including FTO (fat mass and obesity) and INSIG2 (insulin-induced gene 2) mutations, leptin or leptin receptor deficiency, and pro-opiomelanocortin deficiency.

11. Cushing syndrome is characterized by truncal obesity, with hypertension caused by high levels of cortisol arising from the adrenal cortex. Other features include "moon facies," plethora, hirsutism, buffalo hump, and striae. Prolonged exogenous administration of corticotropin or corticosteroids can cause similar features, referred to as "cushingoid" appearance. There may be signs of virilization, including hirsutism, acne, deepening of the voice, and clitoral enlargement in girls. Growth impairment occurs except when significant virilization is present, resulting in a period of normal or increased growth. Delayed puberty, amenorrhea, and oligomenorrhea in girls past menarche may occur. Laboratory findings include elevated evening cortisol levels (loss of normal diurnal rhythm with decreased evening cortisol levels) and increased urinary excretion of free cortisol and 17-hydroxycorticosteroids.

12. The classic polycystic ovaries syndrome is characterized by obesity, hirsutism, and secondary amenorrhea, with bilaterally enlarged polycystic ovaries. Laboratory findings are variable; total testosterone level is usually normal, but serum free testosterone level is often elevated and sex hormone–binding globulin level decreased. There is often an increased ratio of LH to FSH. Dehydroepiandrosterone sulfate (DHEAS) levels are normal or moderately elevated. Hyperandrogenism is often associated with insulin resistance and acanthosis nigricans. Testing for hyperinsulinism (i.e., fasting blood insulin and glucose) may be considered in women with persistent anovulation, android obesity, or acanthosis nigricans.

13. Hypoglycemic symptoms, particularly with rapid drop in glucose levels, may be due to activation of the autonomic nervous system and include perspiration, tachycardia, pallor, tremulousness, weakness, hunger, nausea, and vomiting. With a slower decrease in glucose level or prolonged hypoglycemia,

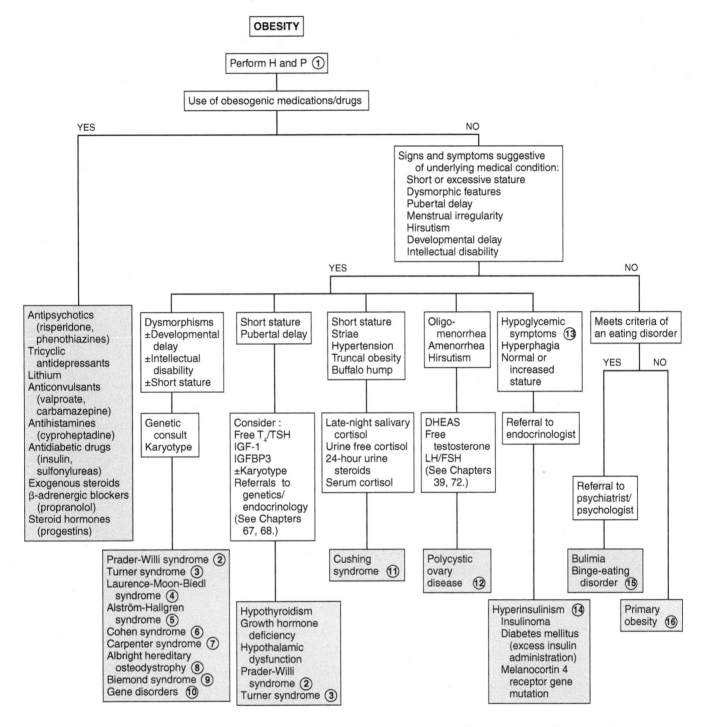

OBESITY

Perform H and P ①

Use of obesogenic medications/drugs

YES — NO

Signs and symptoms suggestive
of underlying medical condition:
Short or excessive stature
Dysmorphic features
Pubertal delay
Menstrual irregularity
Hirsutism
Developmental delay
Intellectual disability

YES — NO

Antipsychotics
(risperidone,
phenothiazines)
Tricyclic
antidepressants
Lithium
Anticonvulsants
(valproate,
carbamazepine)
Antihistamines
(cyproheptadine)
Antidiabetic drugs
(insulin,
sulfonylureas)
Exogenous steroids
β-adrenergic blockers
(propranolol)
Steroid hormones
(progestins)

Dysmorphisms
±Developmental
delay
±Intellectual
disability
±Short stature

Genetic
consult
Karyotype

Prader-Willi syndrome ②
Turner syndrome ③
Laurence-Moon-Biedl
syndrome ④
Alström-Hallgren
syndrome ⑤
Cohen syndrome ⑥
Carpenter syndrome ⑦
Albright hereditary
osteodystrophy ⑧
Biemond syndrome ⑨
Gene disorders ⑩

Short stature
Pubertal delay

Consider :
Free T₄/TSH
IGF-1
IGFBP3
±Karyotype
Referrals to
genetics/
endocrinology
(See Chapters
67, 68.)

Hypothyroidism
Growth hormone
deficiency
Hypothalamic
dysfunction
Prader-Willi
syndrome ②
Turner syndrome ③

Short stature
Striae
Hypertension
Truncal obesity
Buffalo hump

Late-night salivary
cortisol
Urine free cortisol
24-hour urine
steroids
Serum cortisol

Cushing
syndrome ⑪

Oligo-
menorrhea
Amenorrhea
Hirsutism

DHEAS
Free
testosterone
LH/FSH
(See Chapters
39, 72.)

Polycystic
ovary
disease ⑫

Hypoglycemic
symptoms ⑬
Hyperphagia
Normal or
increased
stature

Referral to
endocrinologist

Hyperinsulinism ⑭
Insulinoma
Diabetes mellitus
(excess insulin
administration)
Melanocortin 4
receptor gene
mutation

Meets criteria of
an eating disorder

YES — NO

Referral to
psychiatrist/
psychologist

Bulimia
Binge-eating
disorder ⑮

Primary
obesity ⑯

DHEAS = dehydroepiandrosterone sulfate

Nelson Textbook of Pediatrics, 19e. Chapter 44
Nelsons Essentials, 6e. Chapter 29

symptoms include headache, confusion, and visual disturbances. The symptoms of hypoglycemia in infants may be more subtle, such as cyanosis, apnea, hypothermia, hypotonia, poor feeding, lethargy, and seizures. In older children, hypoglycemia may cause behavior problems, inattention, ravenous appetite, or seizures.

14 Hyperinsulinemia may be due to an insulin-secreting pancreatic tumor, hypersecretion of the pancreatic beta cells, or a hypothalamic lesion. There is hyperinsulinemia with hyperphagia and increased linear growth. It may also be caused by excessive amounts of insulin in patients with diabetes mellitus. Melanocortin 4 receptor gene mutation is the most common known genetic cause for obesity that is severe and of early onset.

15 Eating disorders are more common in females and among whites. Most patients first develop symptoms during adolescence. Bulimia nervosa and binge-eating disorders are characterized by weight gain, in contrast to anorexia nervosa. In binge eating disorders, a "distorted" body image is often present.

Those affected may tend to eat alone and have feelings of guilt or disgust after binge eating. The hallmark of bulimia nervosa is binge eating followed by compensatory behavior such as purging, exercise, fasting, and laxative use.

16 In most cases, obesity is the result of a positive energy balance that is stored as adipose tissue. Factors associated with a positive balance include excessive intake of high-energy foods, inadequate exercise, sedentary lifestyle, low metabolic rate, and inadequate sleep. In primary obesity, screening for comorbidities is recommended. Screening tests may include fasting glucose and Hgb A_{1C} to screen for diabetes or prediabetes, serum ALT to screen for fatty liver, and a lipid panel for hyperlipidemias. Vitamin D levels may also be obtained; vitamin D deficiency is commonly associated with obesity.

Bibliography

American Academy of Pediatrics Committee on Adolescence: Identifying and treating eating disorders, *Pediatrics* 111:204–211, 2003.

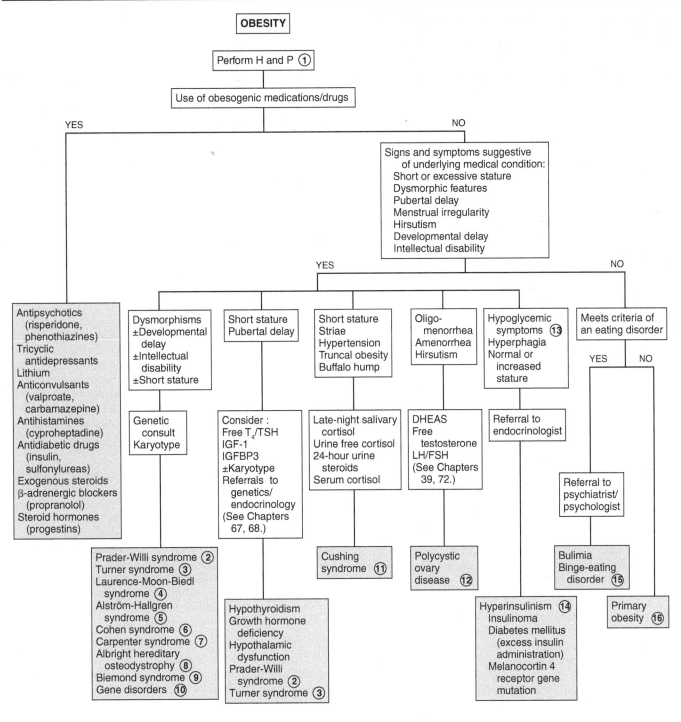

OBESITY

Perform H and P ①

Use of obesogenic medications/drugs

YES

NO

Signs and symptoms suggestive
of underlying medical condition:
Short or excessive stature
Dysmorphic features
Pubertal delay
Menstrual irregularity
Hirsutism
Developmental delay
Intellectual disability

YES

NO

Antipsychotics
(risperidone,
phenothiazines)
Tricyclic
antidepressants
Lithium
Anticonvulsants
(valproate,
carbamazepine)
Antihistamines
(cyproheptadine)
Antidiabetic drugs
(insulin,
sulfonylureas)
Exogenous steroids
β-adrenergic blockers
(propranolol)
Steroid hormones
(progestins)

Dysmorphisms
±Developmental
delay
±Intellectual
disability
±Short stature

Short stature
Pubertal delay

Short stature
Striae
Hypertension
Truncal obesity
Buffalo hump

Oligo-
menorrhea
Amenorrhea
Hirsutism

Hypoglycemic
symptoms ⑬
Hyperphagia
Normal or
increased
stature

Meets criteria of
an eating disorder

YES

NO

Genetic
consult
Karyotype

Consider :
Free T$_4$/TSH
IGF-1
IGFBP3
±Karyotype
Referrals to
genetics/
endocrinology
(See Chapters
67, 68.)

Late-night salivary
cortisol
Urine free cortisol
24-hour urine
steroids
Serum cortisol

DHEAS
Free
testosterone
LH/FSH
(See Chapters
39, 72.)

Referral to
endocrinologist

Referral to
psychiatrist/
psychologist

Prader-Willi syndrome ②
Turner syndrome ③
Laurence-Moon-Biedl
syndrome ④
Alström-Hallgren
syndrome ⑤
Cohen syndrome ⑥
Carpenter syndrome ⑦
Albright hereditary
osteodystrophy ⑧
Biemond syndrome ⑨
Gene disorders ⑩

Cushing
syndrome ⑪

Polycystic
ovary
disease ⑫

Bulimia
Binge-eating
disorder ⑮

Hypothyroidism
Growth hormone
deficiency
Hypothalamic
dysfunction
Prader-Willi
syndrome ②
Turner syndrome ③

Hyperinsulinism ⑭
Insulinoma
Diabetes mellitus
(excess insulin
administration)
Melanocortin 4
receptor gene
mutation

Primary
obesity ⑯

DHEAS = dehydroepiandrosterone sulfate

Nelson Textbook of Pediatrics, 19e. Chapter 44
Nelsons Essentials, 6e. Chapter 29

Chapter 75
POLYURIA

Polyuria is an excessive urine volume, usually over 2 L/m^2/day. It may be associated with increased thirst and drinking (polydipsia) and may be accompanied by nocturia or enuresis. Some conditions may appear as increased frequency of urination without increased volume (e.g., UTIs, urge syndrome). They may be difficult to distinguish from true polyuria by history alone and are therefore included in the algorithm.

1. History may include polyphagia, polydipsia, and weight loss, which may indicate diabetes mellitus (DM). Children may be prone to infections with *Candida* or pyogenic skin infections. Medications, heavy metals, and toxins may cause renal injury resulting in decreased reabsorption of glucose. Ingestion of substances that may produce osmotic diuresis, such as mannitol, glycerol, urea, and radiologic contrast materials, should be noted.

It is important to review fluid intake patterns. Children with psychogenic polydipsia often drink more during the day. Infants with polyuria due to diabetes insipidus (DI) often have failure to thrive and episodes of severe dehydration. There may be hyperthermia, irritability, vomiting, and constipation. They may be severely dehydrated with sunken fontanel, doughy skin turgor, and hypotension. Children with central DI do not perspire and may have anorexia. DI secondary to a CNS lesion may present with associated visual changes, sexual precocity, growth failure, and short stature. It is important to ask about a history of brain surgery or injury, because these may cause central DI. A weak urine stream may suggest obstructive uropathy.

2. UA revealing nitrite, leukocyte esterase, WBCs, and often bacteria suggests infection. (See Chapter 30.) The presence of glucose, with or without ketones, suggests DM; the presence of protein or blood may indicate renal disease. (See Chapters 32, 33.) A urine Sp gr above 1.020 makes DI unlikely. Urine and serum osmolality may be needed for complete evaluation.

3. DM is characterized by glucosuria and hyperglycemia, with a corresponding increase in serum and urine osmolality. The polyuria is due to an osmotic diuresis. Type 1, or insulin-dependent DM is more common in children. In early stages there may be vomiting, dehydration, and polyuria. In the later stages there may be Kussmaul respirations, severe abdominal pain, and CNS changes, leading ultimately to coma. In addition to glucosuria and hyperglycemia, there is ketonuria, ketonemia, and a metabolic acidosis. Type 2 or non–insulin-dependent DM is more common in adults, but it may be seen in older children and adolescents, particularly with obesity or family history. Ketosis is infrequent. An oral glucose tolerance test and Hgb A$_{1C}$ can confirm the diagnosis of type 2 DM. Secondary diabetes may be seen with cystic fibrosis or ingestion of drugs or poisons (e.g., the rat poison Vacor). Certain genetic syndromes may also be associated with DM, including Prader-Willi syndrome. Autoimmune diseases (e.g., Hashimoto thyroiditis, multiple endocrine deficiency syndrome) may also be associated with type 1 diabetes.

4. Renal glucosuria may be a congenital disorder or associated with Fanconi syndrome and other renal tubular disorders affecting renal absorption of glucose. Fanconi syndrome may be secondary to multiple myeloma, medications, and heavy metals. A transient glucosuria may also occur with stressful events, with or without mild hyperglycemia. This finding may indicate a decreased capacity for insulin secretion, and patients may need closer followup and glucose tolerance testing for DM.

5. The water deprivation test is usually performed after referral to a nephrologist. It is useful in differentiating DI from psychogenic DI.

6. DI is characterized by low urine Sp gr (usually , 1.005), low urine osmolality, and normal serum osmolality when hydration is adequate. With water restriction or deprivation, the serum sodium increases (as well as serum osmolality), whereas the patient remains unable to concentrate urine. The ratio of urine to plasma osmolality is less than 1.0. This test should be conducted in a controlled setting and discontinued if the body weight decreases by more than 3%.

7. Primary polydipsia is caused by an increase in water intake. It may be due to compulsive water drinking, which causes suppression of vasopressin secretion and results in a large volume of hypo-osmolar urine. The polyuria decreases at night as polydipsia stops during sleep. Polydipsia may also be seen in patients with psychiatric illnesses. Its etiology is unclear and may be associated with certain medications. Phenothiazines may cause a sensation of dry mouth, leading to increased fluid intake.

8. In nephrogenic DI, the kidney does not respond to antidiuretic hormone. It may be a primary condition (X-linked recessive), which usually appears in male infants as polyuria, polydipsia, and hypernatremic dehydration. Secondary DI may be seen in conditions causing a loss of medullary concentrating gradient, such as renal failure, tubular defects, and obstructive uropathy. Diseases such as sickle cell disease may cause renal damage and often may be associated with isosthenuria (urine Sp gr 5 1.010). Drugs (e.g., lithium) or metabolic diseases (e.g., hypokalemia, hypercalcemia) may decrease the effect of antidiuretic hormone on the tubule causing DI.

9. Any lesion affecting the neurohypophyseal unit may cause central DI. These include suprasellar and chiasmatic tumors (e.g., craniopharyngiomas, optic gliomas, germinomas). Infections (encephalitis) as well as infiltrative processes (leukemia, sarcoidosis, tuberculosis, histiocytosis, actinomycosis) may also be causes. Wolfram syndrome is associated with insulin-dependent DM, DI, optic atrophy, deafness, and neurogenic bladder. Imaging (CT/MRI) may be considered to exclude brain tumors, injuries, or infiltrative processes. In patients with accompanying growth failure or short stature, pituitary tests and thyroid function tests may be considered. A radioimmunoassay for vasopressin is available. Low levels indicate central DI.

Bibliography

Saborio P, Tipton GA, Chan JCM: Diabetes insipidus, *Pediatr Rev* 21:122–129, 2000.

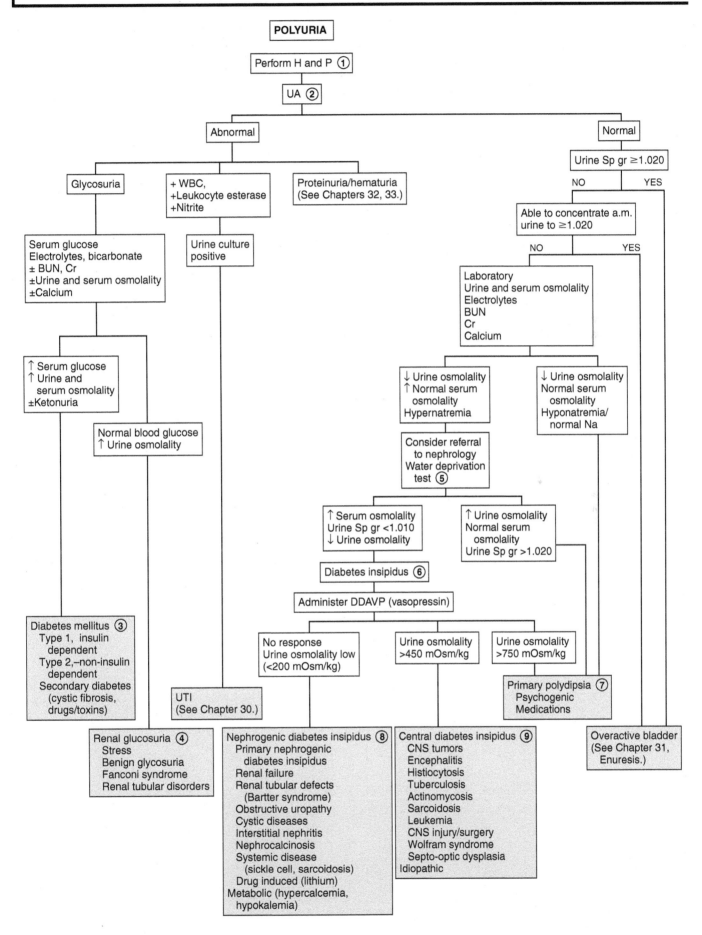

POLYURIA

Perform H and P ①

UA ②

Abnormal

Glycosuria

+ WBC,
+Leukocyte esterase
+Nitrite

Proteinuria/hematuria
(See Chapters 32, 33.)

Serum glucose
Electrolytes, bicarbonate
± BUN, Cr
±Urine and serum osmolality
±Calcium

Urine culture
positive

↑ Serum glucose
↑ Urine and
   serum osmolality
±Ketonuria

Normal blood glucose
↑ Urine osmolality

Diabetes mellitus ③
   Type 1, insulin
      dependent
   Type 2,–non-insulin
      dependent
   Secondary diabetes
      (cystic fibrosis,
      drugs/toxins)

UTI
(See Chapter 30.)

Renal glucosuria ④
   Stress
   Benign glycosuria
   Fanconi syndrome
   Renal tubular disorders

Normal

Urine Sp gr ≥1.020

NO   YES

Able to concentrate a.m.
urine to ≥1.020

NO   YES

Laboratory
Urine and serum osmolality
Electrolytes
BUN
Cr
Calcium

↓ Urine osmolality
↑ Normal serum
   osmolality
Hypernatremia

↓ Urine osmolality
Normal serum
   osmolality
Hyponatremia/
   normal Na

Consider referral
to nephrology
Water deprivation
test ⑤

↑ Serum osmolality
Urine Sp gr <1.010
↓ Urine osmolality

↑ Urine osmolality
Normal serum
   osmolality
Urine Sp gr >1.020

Diabetes insipidus ⑥

Administer DDAVP (vasopressin)

No response
Urine osmolality low
(<200 mOsm/kg)

Urine osmolality
>450 mOsm/kg

Urine osmolality
>750 mOsm/kg

Primary polydipsia ⑦
   Psychogenic
   Medications

Nephrogenic diabetes insipidus ⑧
   Primary nephrogenic
      diabetes insipidus
   Renal failure
   Renal tubular defects
      (Bartter syndrome)
   Obstructive uropathy
   Cystic diseases
   Interstitial nephritis
   Nephrocalcinosis
   Systemic disease
      (sickle cell, sarcoidosis)
   Drug induced (lithium)
   Metabolic (hypercalcemia,
      hypokalemia)

Central diabetes insipidus ⑨
   CNS tumors
   Encephalitis
   Histiocytosis
   Tuberculosis
   Actinomycosis
   Sarcoidosis
   Leukemia
   CNS injury/surgery
   Wolfram syndrome
   Septo-optic dysplasia
   Idiopathic

Overactive bladder
(See Chapter 31,
   Enuresis.)

Nelson Textbook of Pediatrics, 19e. Chapter 552
Nelsons Essentials, 6e. Chapters 35, 161

General

Chapter 76

FEVER WITHOUT A SOURCE

The most commonly used definition of fever is a rectal temperature of 38°C (100.4°F) or above. The terms *fever without a source* (FWS) and *fever without localizing signs* (FWLS) are used to describe fevers of a duration of less than 1 week that developed acutely in a previously well child in whom no likely cause for the fever is evident after a thorough H and P.

Prior to the development of the conjugated *Haemophilus influenza* type b (Hib) and pneumococcal vaccines, management guidelines (Boston, Rochester, Philadelphia) for fever in young children were aimed at identifying those at risk for bacteremia in order to reduce their risk of a subsequent serious bacterial infection (SBI) (meningitis, sepsis, osteomyelitis, septic arthritis, UTIs, pneumonias, bacterial enteritis). In the current era of widespread use of these conjugated vaccines, the risk of occult bacteremia in well-appearing children has been significantly reduced, diminishing the usefulness of such guidelines. Consensus remains strong, however, for the management of febrile infants younger than 3 months old, particularly those younger than 28 days old. A similar consensus exists regarding children who do not look well; any child who appears significantly ill or toxic should be hospitalized for further evaluation and treatment regardless of their age or immunization status.

(1) A rectal temperature is the best method of assessment of body core temperature and is recommended when evaluating infants younger than 3 months of age; axillary and tympanic membrane temperature measurements are not recommended. Infants with fever documented at home by a reliable caretaker should be treated the same as if the fever were documented by a healthcare worker. The role of bundling in the elevation of body temperature is controversial; bundling and a warm ambient temperature may contribute to an elevation in skin temperature more so than rectal temperature in young infants, but elevation into a febrile range is unlikely. Some studies suggest an infant with a normal temperature obtained 15 to 30 minutes after unbundling can be considered afebrile; others do not recommend attributing temperatures in the febrile range (especially temperatures >38.5°C) to bundling.

The birth history, including duration of ruptured membranes and history of maternal infections (group B strep, sexually transmitted infections) may be helpful, particularly in very young infants. A history of exposure to sick contacts and any use of medication (antibiotics, antipyretics) should also be elicited. A medical history of sickle cell disease, immunodeficiency, congenital heart disease, a central venous line, or malignancy is significant and will alter the approach to a febrile child. Individualized clinical judgment should be used when assessing fever in these high-risk children.

(2) If pleocytosis is present in the CSF or if there is a history of maternal herpes simplex (HSV) infection, consider adding acyclovir to the empirical treatment regimen.

(3) Urine should be obtained by either catheterization or suprapubic aspiration to avoid the risk of contamination. The addition of viral testing (culture, PCR) to CSF studies can aid in the identification of infants at low risk for SBIs; infants with an identified viral infection are at very low risk for bacterial infections. Stool should be examined for WBCs when diarrhea is present; culture should be sent if the microscopic analysis cannot be performed.

(4) Criteria established prior to the use of the current Hib and pneumococcal vaccines to identify infants as "low risk" for an SBI continue to be useful in the management of infants 29 to 90 days of age. A WBC of 15,000/mm^3 is generally considered the upper limit of values considered low risk for SBI (although <20, 000/mm^3 has also been proposed as a low-risk value, as has a WBC between 5000/mm^3 and 15,000/mm^3). A negative leukocyte esterase on urine dipstick and microscopic analysis showing fewer than 5 WBCs per high-power field and no bacteria on Gram stain suggest minimal risk for UTI.

(5) Some protocols may defer an LP and CSF studies if other labs indicate low risk for SBI; however, a strong consensus supports always obtaining CSF if empiric antibiotics are going to be administered. Definition of low risk CSF findings range between <5 to 10 WBC/mm^3 with negative Gram stains. The recommended empiric antibiotic therapy in young infants is ceftriaxone (50 mg/kg IM). In addition to fulfilling low-risk lab criteria, reliable follow-up in 24 hours should be ensured before planning outpatient treatment while culture results are pending. Parents should be instructed in the importance of urgent follow up whenever a child's clinical status seems to worsen.

(6) Well-appearing infants with an abnormal UA in the face of normal blood tests (normal absolute neutrophil count and band counts) can probably be safely treated with outpatient parental antibiotics for a presumed UTI. Children with a suspected UTI who appear severely ill or are vomiting should be hospitalized for IV antibiotic therapy. Beyond 2 months of age, oral therapy for suspected UTIs has been proven to be as efficacious as parenteral therapy.

FEVER WITHOUT A SOURCE (FWS)

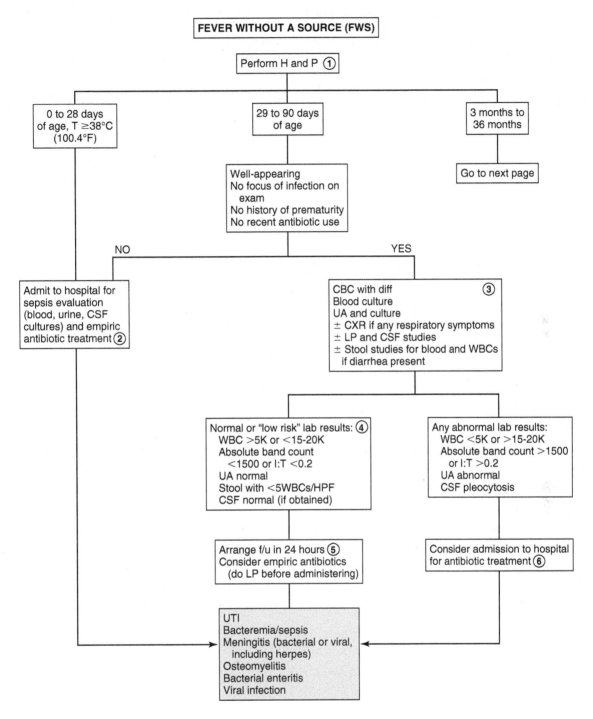

Nelson Textbook of Pediatrics, 19e. Chapters 169, 170
Nelsons Essentials, 6e. Chapter 96

7 A child who has received the primary series of 3 of a conjugated pneumococcal vaccine (PCV7 or PCV13) and a complete primary series of a conjugated *H. influenzae* vaccine (2 or 3 doses, depending on the product) is considered completely immunized. Because the primary series of pneumococcal vaccine cannot be completed until 6 months, all infants younger than 6 months are considered incompletely immunized.

8 Guidelines for evaluating fever in children who are incompletely immunized include using criteria for identifying risk of occult bacteremia, as well as clinical judgment. Reliability of parental followup should always be considered in management decisions for these children.

9 When blood cultures are positive for pathogens other than *Streptococcus pneumoniae*, the likelihood of a contaminant needs to be carefully considered. *Neisseria meningitidis*, *H. influenzae* type b, and *Staphylococcus aureus* are likely pathogens, and those children should be (if not already) admitted for a full sepsis evaluation and treatment. Other organisms may or may not be pathogens; if a contaminant is suspected and the child is well-appearing, continued outpatient observation may be appropriate.

10 Fever can rarely be caused by medications in children; although the onset can occur within days of administration of a drug, this etiology is usually not considered until the fever has been present for a more prolonged period. Anticonvulsants, allopurinol (and other chemotherapy agents), nitrofurantoin (and other antibiotics), and drugs with anticholinergic (atropine, antihistamines) and sympathomimetic (cocaine, amphetamines) effects are among the more common agents causing fever due to a variety of mechanisms (including, but not limited to, hypersensitivity). Other symptoms may or may not be associated.

11 Vaccine reactions may be a source of fever. Mild to moderate fever can occur after diphtheria and tetanus toxoids and acellular pertussis (DTaP) vaccines; extremely high fevers (>40.5°C) that were occasionally seen after administration of the previously used DTP whole-cell preparation are extremely rare following administration of the currently available acellular preparation. Fever occurs in approximately 5% to 15% of children within 5 to 12 days of receiving the measles, mumps, and rubella (MMR) vaccine; those receiving the combination MMR and varicella vaccine (MMRV) are more likely (22%) to develop fever.

12 A fever below 39°C in children 3 months of age or older is most likely to be a viral infection. It is reasonable in a well-appearing 3- to 36-month-old child to forego any lab evaluation and observe closely, assuming a reliable means of followup (phone, transportation) has been ensured. Careful instructions should be given to parents to return if the fever persists more than 2 to 3 days.

Many children with FWS are in the prodromal phase of an infectious illness and develop more specific signs or symptoms within several hours to days of the initial fever onset. In some diseases, such as Rocky Mountain spotted fever, leptospirosis, and measles, the fever may precede more specific signs by up to 3 days. In illnesses such as roseola, viral hepatitis, infectious mononucleosis, typhus, typhoid fever, and Kawasaki disease, a longer interval may occur between fever onset and more specific findings.

Bibliography

American Academy of Pediatrics: In Pickering LK, editor: *Red book: 2012 report of the Committee on Infectious Diseases*, ed 29, Elk Grove Village, Ill, 2012, AAP.

Baraff LJ, Bass JW, et al: Practice guidelines for the management of infants and children 0 to 36 months of age with fever without source, *Pediatrics* 92: 1, 1993.

Cheng TL, Partridge JC: Effect of bundling and high environmental temperature on neonatal body temperature, *Pediatrics* 92:238, 1993.

Grover G, Berkowitz CD, Thompson M, et al: The effects of bundling on infant temperature, *Pediatrics* 945:669, 1994.

Schnadower D, Kuppermann N, Macias CG, et al; American Academy of Pediatrics Pediatric Emergency Medicine Collaborative Research Committee: Febrile infants with urinary tract infections at very low risk for adverse events and bacteremia, *Pediatrics* 126:1074, 2010.

Subcommittee on Urinary Tract Infection, Steering Committee on Quality Improvement and Management: Urinary tract infection: Clinical practice guideline for the diagnosis and management of the initial UTI in febrile infants and children 2 to 24 months, *Pediatrics* 128:595, 2011.

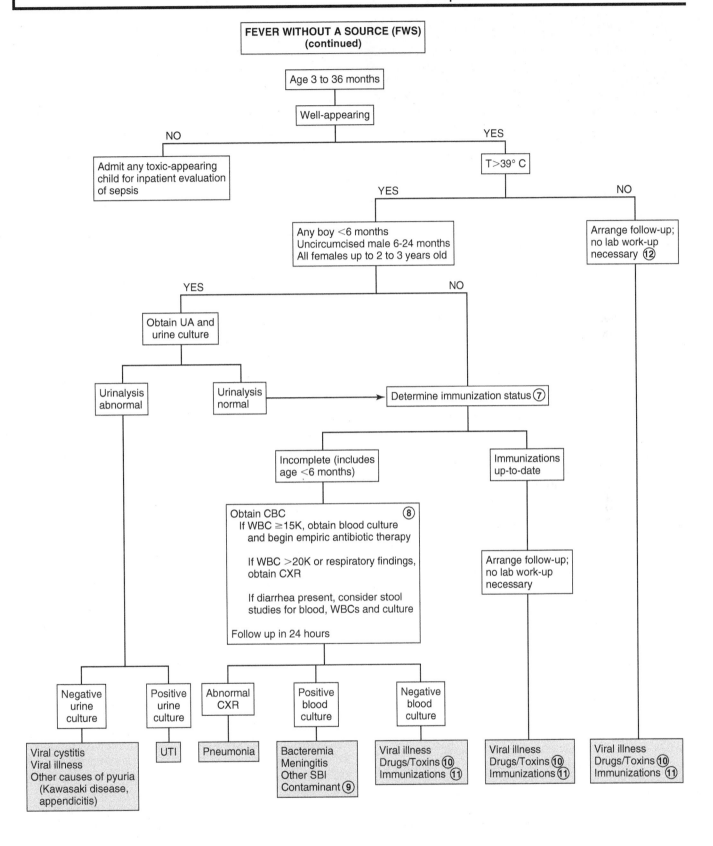

FEVER WITHOUT A SOURCE (FWS)
(continued)

Age 3 to 36 months

Well-appearing

NO / YES

Admit any toxic-appearing child for inpatient evaluation of sepsis

T>39° C

YES / NO

Any boy <6 months
Uncircumcised male 6-24 months
All females up to 2 to 3 years old

Arrange follow-up; no lab work-up necessary ⑫

YES / NO

Obtain UA and urine culture

Urinalysis abnormal

Urinalysis normal

Determine immunization status ⑦

Incomplete (includes age <6 months)

Immunizations up-to-date

Obtain CBC   ⑧
  If WBC ≥15K, obtain blood culture
  and begin empiric antibiotic therapy

  If WBC >20K or respiratory findings,
  obtain CXR

  If diarrhea present, consider stool
  studies for blood, WBCs and culture

Follow up in 24 hours

Arrange follow-up; no lab work-up necessary

Negative urine culture

Positive urine culture

Abnormal CXR

Positive blood culture

Negative blood culture

Viral cystitis
Viral illness
Other causes of pyuria
  (Kawasaki disease, appendicitis)

UTI

Pneumonia

Bacteremia
Meningitis
Other SBI
Contaminant ⑨

Viral illness
Drugs/Toxins ⑩
Immunizations ⑪

Viral illness
Drugs/Toxins ⑩
Immunizations ⑪

Viral illness
Drugs/Toxins ⑩
Immunizations ⑪

Chapter 77
FEVER OF UNKNOWN ORIGIN

The initial definition of fever of unknown origin (FUO) was proposed for adult patients in 1961 to provide a basis for data comparison across study populations; less consensus (from both a research and a practical standpoint) exists regarding a definition for children. One of the most commonly used definitions of FUO in pediatrics is a history of fever greater than 38.3°C (101°F) for 8 or more days in a child for whom an initial evaluation (inpatient or outpatient), including history and physical and preliminary lab evaluation, does not suggest a probable etiology of the fever. Extremely rare disorders can present with FUO in children, but the symptom is far more likely to be due to an uncommon presentation of a common illness. Infections are the leading cause of FUO in children, followed by connective tissue disorders, then neoplasm. The outcome of children with undiagnosed FUO is variable. Some without a diagnosis after a preliminary laboratory evaluation will eventually be diagnosed; no diagnosis, however, will be established for at least 10% to 20%. In general, the outcome for children with FUO is better than for adults with FUO.

1 The evaluation of FUO should be based on factors specific to each case, such as the age of a patient and their ability to report specific complaints, underlying medical conditions, and exposures. The history is by far the most essential component of an FUO evaluation. Requesting a family to keep a fever diary may be helpful. Fever patterns may be described as intermittent (when the temperature returns to normal at least once daily), remittent (temperature fluctuates but never normalizes), or sustained (minimal fluctuation); these categorizations, however, can be blurred by the use of antipyretics. A relapsing fever pattern (fever resolves for 1 or more days then recurs) can be characteristic of a few specific problems (malaria, Lyme disease); a pattern of recurrent fevers for more than 6 months is suggestive of metabolic defects, temperature dysregulation due to a CNS abnormality, or immunodeficiencies (particularly periodic disorders like cyclic neutropenia). The possibility of factitious fever should always be considered.

A surgical history (dental, abdominal, cardiac) may indicate a risk of endocarditis or abscesses. Ethnic background may be a clue to a very limited number of etiologies (nephrogenic diabetes insipidus, familial Mediterranean fever, familial dysautonomia). A complete review of systems is important; be sure to include GI, musculoskeletal (including joint complaints), and risk factors for HIV.

The social history should include exposures to ill contacts, animals (domestic, farm, wild), insect or tick bites, lake or well water, and travel. Inquire whether any travel prophylaxis was recommended and/or taken and about exposure to people who have traveled; artifacts, rocks, or soil that have been brought from distant areas could serve as vectors. Exposure to or ingestion of medications (including topicals, medications of household members, and illicit substances) and foods (game meat, raw meat, raw shellfish, unpasteurized milk) as well as dirt (or other pica) could be significant.

The PE should particularly note growth parameters, skin findings (rash, petechiae, sparse hair/eyebrows/eyelashes, bites or punctum), the ophthalmologic exam (conjunctivitis, abnormal corneal or pupillary reflexes, funduscopic abnormalities), ENT findings (nasal discharge, sinus tenderness, tooth abnormalities, smooth tongue, pharyngeal injection, gingival hypertrophy, dental abscesses), and a thorough musculoskeletal exam (arthritis, bone or muscle tenderness). Attempts should be made to examine a child while febrile to assess for the appearance of a rash with fever and the presence or absence of sweating. (Absence of sweating could indicate hereditary sensory and autonomic neuropathy or ectodermal dysplasia.) Sexually active females should always have a pelvic examination to assess for pelvic inflammatory disease (PID) and pelvic abscesses. A rectal exam should be performed to assess for an abscess or tumor, and stool should always be checked for occult blood.

2 Fever can be a reaction to several types of medication owing to a variety of mechanisms (not just allergy). Discontinuation of the drug followed by disappearance of the fever is suggestive of drug fever, although sometimes fever persists days to weeks as a result of slow excretion of the drug. Anticonvulsants, allopurinol (and other chemotherapy agents), nitrofurantoin (and other antibiotics), phenothiazines, drugs with anticholinergic effects (atropine, antihistamines) and sympathomimetic effects (cocaine, epinephrine, amphetamines) are among the more common causative agents.

3 The extent of urgency of the evaluation depends on the degree of illness in the child. Hospitalization is not usually necessary to evaluate FUO. It does offer the advantage, however, of close observation and following up on every lead. Blood cultures should be obtained aerobically unless anaerobic infection is suspected. Repeated cultures may be necessary to diagnose certain conditions such as endocarditis, osteomyelitis, or deep-seated abscesses causing bacteremia. Specific media need to be requested if particular infections are suspected (tularemia, leptospirosis, *Yersinia*); serology or PCR may be the preferred diagnostic method for some suspected pathogens. CXRs are commonly recommended in the initial testing for FUO; x-rays of sinuses, mastoids, and the GI tract should be performed selectively based on the clinical picture. Skin testing for tuberculosis (TB) with a PPD test is usually recommended. Both the CBC and inflammatory markers like ESR and CRP are often abnormal but nonspecific. Extreme WBC values (WBC >10K/mm^3, ANC <500/mm^3) are suggestive of bacterial infections; EBV infections are characterized by atypical lymphocytosis. An ESR greater than 100 mm/h warrants consideration of malignancy, autoimmune disease, Kawasaki disease, TB, and vasculitis. Lower values are nonspecific indicators of inflammation and may be more useful in monitoring disease course, whereas normal values should raise suspicion for factitious fever. CRP is similarly nonspecific; it normalizes more quickly than an ESR.

4 Malaria may be transmitted by a mosquito vector from an infected person (e.g., someone who has traveled in an endemic area) to another person. It can also be transmitted by contaminated syringe needles and blood. In persons who took appropriate antimalarial drugs while traveling, the disease may not manifest until several months later. The organism can be identified on blood smears. Trypanosomiasis and babesiosis are other parasites that can be identified on a blood smear. Splenomegaly is usually present; a relapsing fever pattern is characteristic.

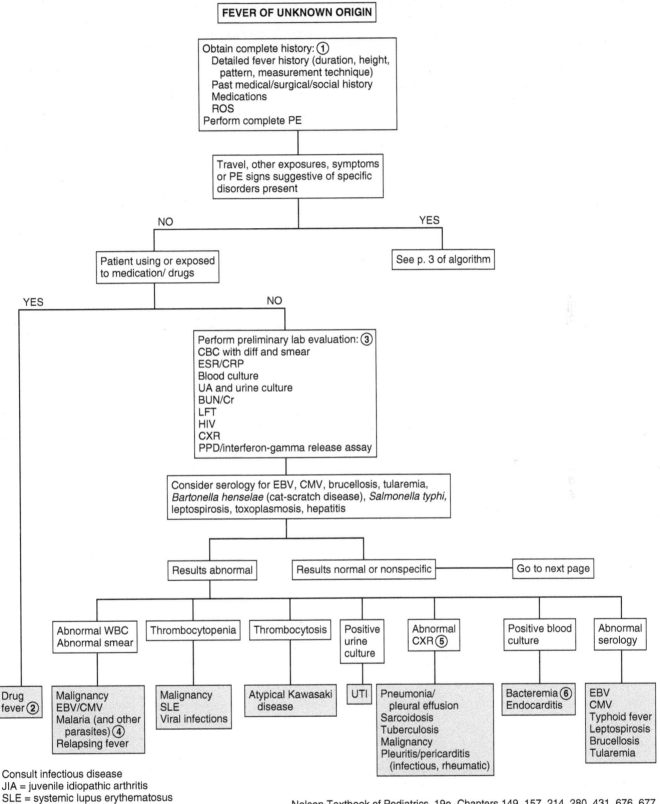

FEVER OF UNKNOWN ORIGIN

Obtain complete history: ①
  Detailed fever history (duration, height,
    pattern, measurement technique)
  Past medical/surgical/social history
  Medications
  ROS
Perform complete PE

Travel, other exposures, symptoms
or PE signs suggestive of specific
disorders present

NO — Patient using or exposed to medication/ drugs

YES — See p. 3 of algorithm

YES (from Patient using or exposed to medication/drugs)

NO — Perform preliminary lab evaluation: ③
CBC with diff and smear
ESR/CRP
Blood culture
UA and urine culture
BUN/Cr
LFT
HIV
CXR
PPD/interferon-gamma release assay

Consider serology for EBV, CMV, brucellosis, tularemia,
Bartonella henselae (cat-scratch disease), *Salmonella typhi*,
leptospirosis, toxoplasmosis, hepatitis

Results abnormal

Results normal or nonspecific — Go to next page

Abnormal WBC
Abnormal smear

Thrombocytopenia

Thrombocytosis

Positive urine culture

Abnormal CXR ⑤

Positive blood culture

Abnormal serology

Drug fever ②

Malignancy
EBV/CMV
Malaria (and other parasites) ④
Relapsing fever

Malignancy
SLE
Viral infections

Atypical Kawasaki disease

UTI

Pneumonia/
  pleural effusion
Sarcoidosis
Tuberculosis
Malignancy
Pleuritis/pericarditis
  (infectious, rheumatic)

Bacteremia ⑥
Endocarditis

EBV
CMV
Typhoid fever
Leptospirosis
Brucellosis
Tularemia

Consult infectious disease
JIA = juvenile idiopathic arthritis
SLE = systemic lupus erythematosus

Nelson Textbook of Pediatrics, 19e. Chapters 149, 157, 214, 280, 431, 676, 677
Nelsons Essentials, 6e. Chapters 96, 122

5 The finding of hilar adenopathy on CXR should raise suspicion for sarcoidosis, TB, or malignancy.

6 In cases of FUO, identification of bacteremia will usually indicate a more specific infection. For example, *Streptococcus viridans* is frequently associated with endocarditis, and *Staphylococcus aureus*, group A streptococci, pneumococcus, and *Kingella kingae* with bone and joint infections.

7 The possibility of factitious fever needs to be considered; it may be intentional (caregiver-fabricated illness, previously known as Munchausen syndrome by proxy) or unintentional (inappropriate heating of the thermometer or skin or mucosal surface before taking the temperature). Factitious fevers should be suspected when no recognizable circadian rhythm of the fevers can be identified; also be suspicious if vasoconstriction, sweating, tachypnea, and tachycardia are not associated with the fever.

8 Initial lab results, additional historical information or evolution of exam findings may help guide subsequent evaluation if the preliminary evaluation has not identified an etiology. An ANA level will be positive in systemic lupus erythematosus (SLE) but is not likely to be positive in systemic-onset juvenile idiopathic arthritis (JIA). Be aware that 30% of children without rheumatic disease will also have a positive ANA, so more specific immunologic testing (dsDNA or anti-Smith Abs) is recommended when a diagnosis of SLE is suspected. (It should definitely be obtained if there is a family history of lupus.) Elevated immunoglobulin levels may occur in systemic-onset JIA, certain immunodeficiencies, and HIV infection. Advanced imaging studies may identify tumors or abscesses, but cost, risk, and expected yield need to be considered; consultation with an infectious disease specialist should be considered prior to obtaining additional imaging or more specialized testing at this point in the evaluation in order to avoid a cycle of unfounded additional testing based on slightly abnormal but nonspecific results.

9 JIA is usually only diagnosed after an extended period of observation and evolution of more characteristic symptoms. The systemic form is most likely to present as an FUO with an intermittent fever pattern; arthritis is necessary for definitive diagnosis but may not develop for months. Serology may remain negative for an extended period. A characteristic salmon-colored rash frequently accompanies the fever. A slit lamp examination performed by an ophthalmologist may reveal uveitis.

10 Fever is more common in children than adults with inflammatory bowel disease. Evaluation should be considered in cases of prolonged FUO, even without specific GI symptoms (and especially if weight loss or impaired growth has occurred or if there is anemia, an elevated ESR, or occult blood in the stool).

11 Persons of Mediterranean descent (Armenians, Arabs, Sephardic Jews) may inherit familial Mediterranean fever, characterized by episodic fevers and abdominal pain. Ulster Scots may be at risk for nephrogenic diabetes insipidus, persons of Jewish descent may inherit familial dysautonomia, and Asians (particularly females) are at risk for Kikuchi-Fujimoto disease (a necrotizing lymphadenitis). Several other inherited (usually autosomal dominant) autoinflammatory disorders are recognized; they present with a spectrum of clinical manifestations in addition to fever.

```
┌─────────────────────────────┐
│  FEVER OF UNKNOWN ORIGIN    │
│       (continued)           │
└─────────────────────────────┘
```

```
┌──────────────────────────┐
│ Reconsider               │
│ factitious fever ⑦       │
│        OR                │
│ Resolution               │
└──────────────────────────┘
```

```
┌────────────────────────────────────────┐
│ Consider additional evaluation: ⑧      │
│ Serum ANA                              │
│ Serum immunoglobulins                  │
│ Serologies (if not already done)       │
│ Consult infectious disease             │
│ Other investigations:                  │
│    X-rays (sinus, mastoid, abdomen)    │
│    WBC scans (gallium, indium)         │
│    Immunoscintigraphy                  │
│    Bone scan                           │
│    Liver/spleen scan                   │
│    PET scan                            │
│    Bone marrow biopsy                  │
└────────────────────────────────────────┘
```

```
┌────────────────────────────────────────┐
│ JIA ⑨                                  │
│ SLE                                    │
│ Polyarteritis nodosa                   │
│ Osteomyelitis                          │
│ Abscess (intraabdominal, liver,        │
│    perinephric)                        │
│ Inflammatory bowel disease ⑩          │
│ Malignancy                             │
│ Hereditary periodic fever syndromes/   │
│    autoinflammatory disorders ⑪       │
│ Immunodeficiency                       │
└────────────────────────────────────────┘
```

12 The algorithm lists diagnoses suggested by particular elements of the history and physical. Repeating the history is important because parents and patients frequently remember historical elements that may be contributory. Physical findings often evolve.

13 Food outbreaks of salmonellosis have increased over the last few decades, likely because of processes related to mass food production and the use of antimicrobials in food animals. Salmonella is transmitted via food products and animals, including domestic animals (cats, dogs, reptiles, rodents, amphibians). Enteritis is the primary presentation of *Salmonella typhi*; nontyphoidal strains may cause GI as well as extraintestinal infections. Symptoms are frequently nonspecific, and repeated blood and stool cultures or serology should lead to a diagnosis.

Leptospirosis is one of the most common zoonoses in the world, and it frequently causes a biphasic illness. It is transmitted by contact with infected animals or soil or water contaminated with their urine; rats are the most common source of infection for humans, but many domestic and feral animals can be vectors. More cases are being recognized in urban and suburban areas, and occupational exposure is not always associated.

Brucellosis is uncommon in industrialized countries, but exposure to unpasteurized dairy products (especially goat's milk cheese) is a risk factor; symptoms are nonspecific, but the classic triad of fever, joint involvement, and hepatosplenomegaly generally occurs in most cases. Ingestion of squirrel or rabbit meat may be a risk factor for tularemia (*Francisella tularensis*); fever and lymph node involvement (including ulceration) are the most common of a variety of symptoms that can occur. Regional lymphadenitis is the most common symptom of catscratch disease (*Bartonella henselae*); scratches from kittens are more likely to transmit infection.

14 Lyme disease (due to *Borrelia burgdorferi*) is frequently diagnosed following the appearance of the characteristic erythema migrans rash (although the onset can also be more indolent, with nonspecific symptoms). A relapsing fever pattern is characteristic. Transmission is via bites from infected ticks that attach themselves to white-tailed deer; endemic U.S. areas are the Northeast and Midwest. A two-fold serologic testing process (enzyme-linked immunosorbent assay [ELISA] followed by confirmatory Western blot testing for positive or equivocal results) is recommended for diagnosis.

15 The onset of bacterial endocarditis may be fulminant or insidious; children with a preexisting cardiac lesion are at highest risk. A new or changing heart murmur, splenomegaly, and petechiae are common findings. Late findings in untreated cases may include Osler's nodes, Janeway lesions, and splinter hemorrhages of the nail beds. Repeated blood cultures (both aerobic and anaerobic should be obtained) may be negative; echocardiography may initially be negative.

16 In children, FUO is less likely due to pulmonary TB and more likely due to nonpulmonary TB (disseminated infection or infection of the liver, peritoneum, pericardium, or GU tract). A high index of suspicion based on a history of possible contacts should initiate further investigation of liver and bone marrow if CXR, skin testing, and lab testing are negative or inconclusive. Up to 50% of children with disseminated disease will demonstrate no response to their initial PPD. Results of interferon gamma release assays may also be negative in disseminated disease.

17 A CBC, CXR, and sinus CT or x-ray should be obtained when patients have complaints of prolonged upper or lower respiratory symptoms, regardless of the severity of the complaints. EBV and CMV can both cause mononucleosis-type syndromes with lymphadenopathy and pharyngitis; nontubercular mycobacteria may cause lymphadenitis.

18 Toxoplasmosis (due to the protozoan *Toxoplasma gondii*) is most often acquired by ingestion of undercooked meat that contains oocysts (or by ingestion of any matter contaminated with oocytes excreted by infected cats). Cervical and supraclavicular adenopathy is usually present.

19 A history of abdominal surgery is a risk factor for intraabdominal abscesses. Liver abscesses are occasionally found in the normal host, although they are more common in the immunocompromised patient. Blood cultures and LFTs are often normal, although hepatomegaly and right upper quadrant tenderness are usually evident on careful exam. Imaging may be necessary for diagnosis.

20 Osteomyelitis is often, but not always, clinically evident based on exam findings. Nonextremity infections (pelvis, vertebrae) are more likely to present as FUO, especially in younger children. Advanced imaging (bone scan, MRI) is most likely to aid in the diagnosis.

21 Fever repeatedly occurring in warm environments and the absence of sweating while febrile suggest ectodermal dysplasia (or factitious fever). Dental defects and sparse hair occur in the ectodermal dyplasias.

22 Severe brain damage may result in dysfunction of thermoregulation. Rarely, neurologically intact children have fevers due to central dysfunction.

23 Infantile cortical hyperostosis (Caffey disease) is suggested by swelling of soft tissues over the face and jaws, cortical thickening of long and flat bones, and tenderness over affected bony areas. The condition often becomes evident in the first year of life; persistent fevers are common.

24 Both hypothermia and extreme fevers occur in hereditary sensory and autonomic neuropathy (familial dysautonomia). Excessive sweating, insensitivity to pain, ataxia, and progressive scoliosis are also characteristic.

Bibliography

Lorin MI, Feigin RD: Fever without localizing signs and fever of unknown origin. In Cherry JD, Harrison G, Kaplan S, et al, editors: *Textbook of pediatric infectious diseases*, ed 6, Philadelphia, 2013, Elsevier Saunders, pp 837.

Long SS, Edwards KM: Prolonged, recurrent, and periodic fever syndromes. In Long SS, Pickering LK, Prober CG, editors: *Principles and practice of pediatric infectious diseases*, ed 4, Philadelphia, 2012, Elsevier Saunders, pp 117.

FEVER OF UNKNOWN ORIGIN
(continued)

Travel, other exposures, symptoms or PE signs suggestive of specific disorders present ⑫

Exposure to wild or domesticated animals

Zoonoses ⑬
  Cat scratch disease
  Tularemia
  Salmonellosis
  Brucellosis
  Leptospirosis
  Q fever
  Rat bite fever
  Psittacosis
  Toxoplasmosis
  Visceral larva migrans

Rash or petechiae

Lyme disease ⑭
JIA ⑨
Acute rheumatic fever
Endocarditis ⑮
Dermatomyositis
SLE
LE Kawasaki disease
Rocky Mountain spotted fever
Histiocytosis
Serum sickness
Tularemia
EBV

Travel
OR
Exposure to persons recently traveled

Coccidiomycosis
Histoplasmosis
Malaria
Blastomycosis
Lyme disease
Rocky Mountain spotted fever
Tuberculosis (TB) ⑯
Ehrlichiosis
Babesiosis
Typhoid fever
Other endemic diseases

ENT or respiratory symptoms ⑰

Sinusitis
Pulmonary disease (pneumonia, TB, abscess, sarcoid)
ANCA-associated vasculitis (Wegner's granulomatosis)
EBV
CMV
Mycobacteria
Mastoiditis
Malignancy
Thyroiditis

Ingestion of contaminated food or milk
OR
Pica

Visceral larva migrans
Toxoplasmosis ⑱
Salmonellosis
Brucellosis
Rat bite fever

Weight loss or impaired linear growth, nonspecific abdominal complaints, diarrhea

Hepatitis
Inflammatory bowel disease
Abscesses (intra abdominal, hepatic) ⑲
Malignancy
Enteritis (various pathogens)
Diabetes insipidus (central or nephrogenic)

Bone, joint, or muscle

Osteomyelitis ⑳
Malignancy
Trichinosis
Dermatomyositis
Polyarteritis nodosa
Arboviral infections
Hereditary periodic fever syndromes/ autoinflammatory disorders

Abnormal cardiac exam

Carditis (rheumatic fever)
Endocarditis ⑮
JIA ⑨
SLE
LE Viral pericarditis
Myocarditis

Recurrent fever (with periods of wellness in between)

Hereditary periodic fever syndromes/ autoinflammatory disorders ⑪

Other physical abnormalities (neurologic, cutaneous, dental, orthopedic)

Ectodermal dysplasia ㉑
CNS/hypothalamic disorders ㉒
Infantile cortical hyperostosis ㉓
Hereditary sensory and autonomic neuropathy (familial dysautonomia) ㉔
Hereditary periodic fever syndromes/ autoinflammatory disorders ⑪

Chapter 78
RECURRENT INFECTIONS

Recurrent infections are a frequent complaint, but only rarely are they caused by primary disorders of the immune system. More likely explanations for recurrent infections are frequent benign URIs, respiratory allergies, or a single prolonged infection in an otherwise normal child. Primary immunodeficiencies are rare; secondary immunodeficiencies due to infection, drugs, malnutrition, or protein loss are more common.

1 Data gathered from the H and P should help categorize a patient as probably well, probably allergic, chronically ill, or probably immunodeficient. Newborn screening results should be noted because an increasing number of states are screening for severe combined immunodeficiency (SCID).

Obtain a detailed history of the frequency and nature of the recurrent infections. High fevers and purulent secretions suggest bacterial infections; these cases are more likely to warrant consideration of an immune deficiency. Recurrent symptoms of a single site suggest allergy or local structural problems (anatomic obstruction, foreign bodies).

For young infants, an in-depth birth history should be obtained, including exposure to maternal infections (herpes simplex, HIV), a history of delayed umbilical cord separation (consistent with leukocyte adhesion deficiency) and risk factors for HIV. If the child was premature, inquire about associated complications (bronchopulmonary dysplasia, blood transfusions). Inquire about any chronic medical problems, conditions requiring indwelling equipment (catheters, shunts, prosthetic devices), and conditions disrupting the integrity of mucocutaneous barriers (dermal sinus tracks, burns, surgical wounds). Some autoimmune disorders (endocrine, rheumatic) can include primary immunodeficiencies as well.

The family history should inquire specifically about immunodeficiency disorders, as well as allergic disease, unexplained infant deaths, and risk factors for HIV in family members. The social history should inquire about risk factors for HIV in the patient plus exposure to environmental irritants (smoke, other fumes), animals, chemicals, and school or daycare attendance. Inquire about travel and any changes in the child's routine that may expose the child to new allergens or infectious contacts.

A complete physical exam is essential; signs of chronic disease (lung abnormalities, clubbing, impaired growth), cutaneous abnormalities, and findings suggestive of allergic disease (transverse nasal crease, allergic "shiners," posterior pharyngeal cobblestoning, swollen pale nasal mucosa) should all be carefully noted. Lymphadenopathy suggests chronic disease; absent lymph tissue (tonsils, lymph nodes, no thymus on CXR) suggest a congenital (lymphocyte) immune defect.

2 The majority of children with a complaint of recurrent infections are normal healthy children who are experiencing frequent URIs. Children who have a large family or attend daycare will experience 6 to 10 viral infections annually, mostly URIs and GI infections, until age 3 to 5 years. A minimal workup, if any, is usually all that is necessary.

3 Rarely, the CBC may reveal an unsuspected malignancy or a WBC abnormality (number, morphology). Further workup should be based on specific results.

4 Many children with recurrent respiratory symptoms have allergies; usually the diagnosis is made clinically. Although usually unnecessary, antigen-specific immunoglobulin panels (as-IgE) and skin testing are the most sensitive tests to identify allergens. Other labs are not recommended; both eosinophilia and total IgE levels are nonspecific (up to half of allergic patients have normal IgE levels).

5 A portion of children presenting with recurrent infections have an underlying chronic nonimmunologic problem. Structural or anatomic defects (cleft palate, congenital heart disease, pulmonary sequestration) are risk factors for recurrent local infections. Malnutrition, chronic illnesses, and protein-losing enteropathies alter immune function. Growth may or may not be normal, depending on the specific condition. Suggestive findings on physical examination include abnormal lung examination, digital clubbing, abdominal distention, hepatosplenomegaly, muscle wasting, and pallor. Secondary defects of the immune system, including the complement system, may develop owing to problems such as HIV infection, splenic dysfunction, malignancy, immunosuppression (due to chemotherapy or transplantation), and various causes of neutropenia.

6 Congenital asplenia may occur as part of a syndrome in association with congenital heart disease; functional asplenia occurs in children with sickle cell disease. Howell-Jolly bodies and pitted or pocked erythrocytes on the peripheral blood smear suggest asplenia. Asplenic children are at especially high risk for infection by pneumococci and *Haemophilus influenzae* as well as salmonellae, *Staphylococcus aureus*, gram-negative enteric bacilli, and meningococci. Children who have undergone surgical splenectomy are also at increased risk of serious bacterial infections, although their risk may be slightly lower because of the previous development of opsonizing antibodies.

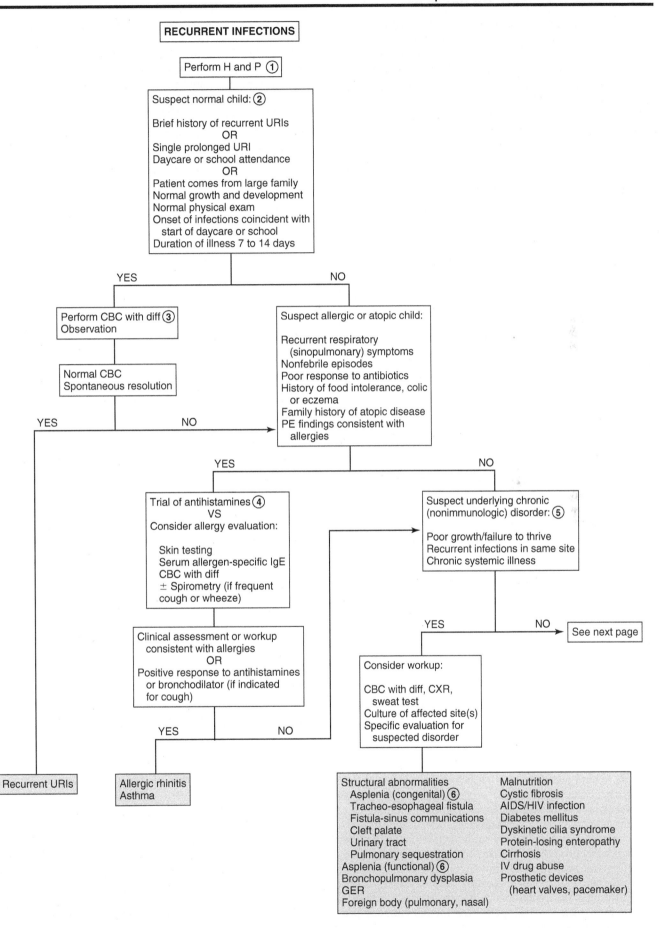

RECURRENT INFECTIONS

Perform H and P ①

Suspect normal child: ②

Brief history of recurrent URIs
OR
Single prolonged URI
Daycare or school attendance
OR
Patient comes from large family
Normal growth and development
Normal physical exam
Onset of infections coincident with start of daycare or school
Duration of illness 7 to 14 days

YES — Perform CBC with diff ③ / Observation

Normal CBC / Spontaneous resolution

YES — Recurrent URIs

NO — Suspect allergic or atopic child:

Recurrent respiratory (sinopulmonary) symptoms
Nonfebrile episodes
Poor response to antibiotics
History of food intolerance, colic or eczema
Family history of atopic disease
PE findings consistent with allergies

YES — Trial of antihistamines ④ / VS / Consider allergy evaluation:

Skin testing
Serum allergen-specific IgE
CBC with diff
± Spirometry (if frequent cough or wheeze)

NO — Suspect underlying chronic (nonimmunologic) disorder: ⑤

Poor growth/failure to thrive
Recurrent infections in same site
Chronic systemic illness

Clinical assessment or workup consistent with allergies
OR
Positive response to antihistamines or bronchodilator (if indicated for cough)

YES — Allergic rhinitis / Asthma

YES / NO — See next page

Consider workup:

CBC with diff, CXR, sweat test
Culture of affected site(s)
Specific evaluation for suspected disorder

Structural abnormalities
  Asplenia (congenital) ⑥
  Tracheo-esophageal fistula
  Fistula-sinus communications
  Cleft palate
  Urinary tract
  Pulmonary sequestration
Asplenia (functional) ⑥
Bronchopulmonary dysplasia
GER
Foreign body (pulmonary, nasal)

Malnutrition
Cystic fibrosis
AIDS/HIV infection
Diabetes mellitus
Dyskinetic cilia syndrome
Protein-losing enteropathy
Cirrhosis
IV drug abuse
Prosthetic devices
  (heart valves, pacemaker)

Nelson Textbook of Pediatrics, 19e. Chapters 119, 120, 124, 128
Nelsons Essentials, 6e. Chapters 72–75

7   A small percentage of children presenting with recurrent infections will have an underlying immunodeficiency; the true incidence is difficult to determine. Recurrent pneumonias are a common complaint, although children with immunodeficiencies usually experience infections of different sites and severity. In general, children with disorders of antibodies, the complement system, or phagocytic cells have recurrent infections with encapsulated bacteria; these children may exhibit normal growth and development. Failure to thrive, opportunistic infections, and serious infections from common viral pathogens early in life are more consistent with T-cell disorders in children.

8   An initial CBC with manual differential, CRP, and/or ESR and quantitative immunoglobulins constitute a practical initial evaluation for suspected immunodeficiencies; the results can be helpful in focusing the subsequent workup. Consideration of the age-appropriate CBC values is important. A normal ESR would make chronic bacterial or fungal infections less likely. Urgent consultation with immunology should be considered whenever the clinical picture and preliminary workup is suspicious of an immune disorder; providers need to be conscious of the possibility of lab artifact and the importance of not administering IVIG until blood for all appropriate lab tests has been drawn.

9   In B-cell or antibody production defects, the onset of frequent infections tends to occur after age 5 to 7 months when protective maternal antibody titers are waning. Infections tend to be caused by encapsulated organisms (*Streptococcus pneumoniae, H. influenzae* type b, group A streptococci); fungal and viral infections are less common, although severe enteroviral infections (encephalitis) do occur. Other clinical characteristics consistent with B-cell defects include reduced/absent tonsils and lymph nodes, which occur in X-linked agammaglobulinemia and X-linked hyper-IgM syndrome; in contrast, enlarged lymph nodes and spleen occur in common variable immunodeficiency (CVID) and autosomal recessive hyper-IgM syndrome. Cutaneous abnormalities (absent eyebrows, thin hair, severe eczema, refractory candidal infections after 4 months of age, petechiae, vitiligo, recurrent warts, severe molluscum) may also be clues to antibody production defects. Abnormal lung findings may suggest pneumonia or bronchiectasis (suggesting chronic pulmonary infections); digital clubbing may also occur.

10   The test for titers to vaccine antigens will assess response to protein (tetanus-diphtheria) and polysaccharide (pneumococcal) antigens. Repeat immunization and followup titers are generally recommended when titers are low. Response patterns need to be interpreted with consideration of patient age (children <age 2 years do not respond well to polysaccharide antigens). Global immune deficiencies are suggested by lack of response to both proteins and polysaccharides; a poor response to polysaccharide antigens only suggests less severe selective (IgG subclass) deficiencies. Isohemagglutinins (antibodies to RBC antigens) are natural antipolysaccharide antibodies; their absence also indicates a defect of antibody production, but they are not reliably present in the first 1 to 2 years of life (and they are not present at all in children with an AB blood type). One caveat to remember when evaluating antibody titers is that protein-losing states (enteropathy, nephrosis) and corticosteroid use may cause low IgG levels even though antibody production capacity is normal.

11   X-linked agammaglobulinemia (Bruton agammaglobulinemia) is an X-linked recessive disorder of severe hypogammaglobulinemia or agammaglobulinemia. Affected infants usually present with recurrent bacterial infections (OM, sinusitis, pneumonia, meningitis) around age 6 months. Occasionally a child may remain asymptomatic for a longer period (up to 2 years). These children have marked hypoplasia of lymphoid tissue on physical examination.

12   Common variable immunodeficiency is a group of disorders characterized by severe hypogammaglobulinemia. It is often associated with a sprue-like syndrome with diarrhea, protein-losing enteropathies, and failure to thrive. Chronic respiratory infections are the most common manifestation; *Giardia* infection is also common. These children have low circulating levels of IgG, IgM, and IgA but normal or increased numbers of B cells.

13   The hyper-IgM syndromes encompass a number of genetically and clinically heterogeneous disorders characterized by a defect that prevents B cells from switching from the production of IgM to other antibody classes (IgG, IgA, IgE). Most are characterized by absent or low IgG and IgA and normal or increased IgM.

14   IgA deficiency is the most common primary immunodeficiency. Affected children may be asymptomatic or have recurrent respiratory, GI, and urogenital tract infections; autoimmune disease (celiac disease, systemic lupus erythematosus) may also be associated. Four types of IgG subclass deficiencies are recognized, but the clinical significance of specific deficiencies is unclear, and subclass testing is not routinely recommended. The total IgG level is usually normal.

15   It is normal for infants to experience a variable physiologic hypogammaglobulinemia between 4 and 9 months of life. When prolonged or severe, recurrent viral and pyogenic infections may occur. The number of B cells and T cells is normal, and the infants respond appropriately to immunizations even though their immunoglobulin levels remain low until age 12 to 36 months.

16   Patients with hyper-IgE syndromes have characteristic facial features and suffer from recurrent "cold" (without inflammation) abscesses, pneumonias, and skin infections starting in infancy. IgE levels are extremely high, and T cells and phagocytic function are also affected.

17   Because B-cell function influences T-cell function, T-cell disorders will always be accompanied by some degree of B-cell dysfunction. Infections tend to be due to organisms that are typically considered opportunistic (viruses, fungi, protozoa) or less virulent and typically begin within the first several months of life. Other clinical features that should raise the suspicion for T-cell dysfunction include cutaneous abnormalities (absence of hair/nails/sweating, neonatal rashes, severe diaper rash, oral candidiasis, eczema, telangiectasias, petechiae), absence of lymphadenopathy with infections, and severe reactions (infections) in response to live virus vaccines. Tetany and abnormal facies may be present with DiGeorge syndrome.

18   HIV infection must be ruled out before primary disorders of T cells can be diagnosed.

19   SCID syndromes are a group of disorders of severe abnormalities in B- and T-cell function. Abnormal development of the thymus results in a small thymus, absent or low T cells,

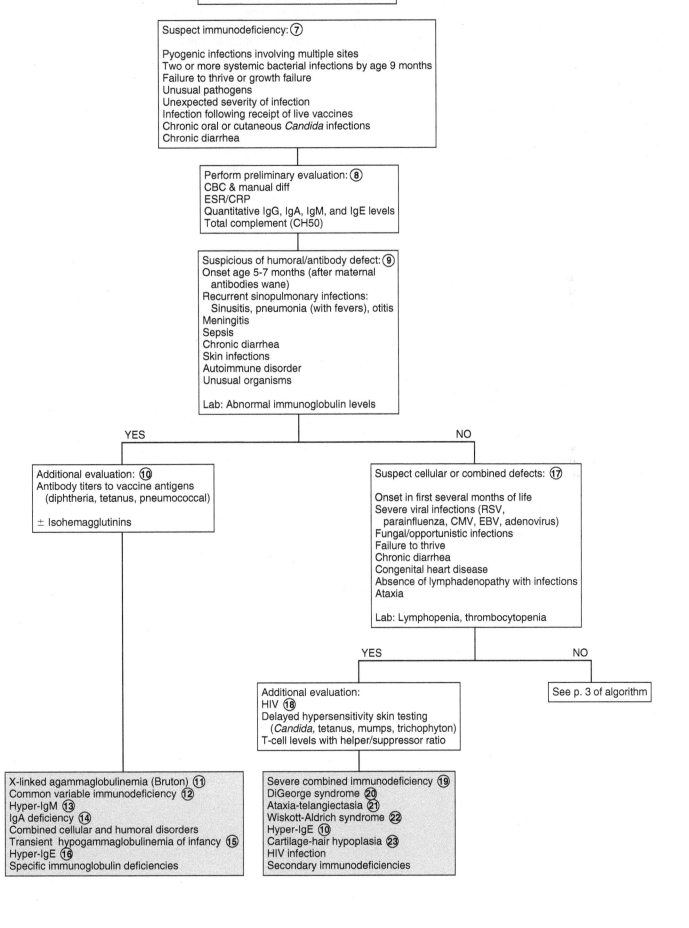

RECURRENT INFECTIONS (continued)

Suspect immunodeficiency: ⑦

Pyogenic infections involving multiple sites
Two or more systemic bacterial infections by age 9 months
Failure to thrive or growth failure
Unusual pathogens
Unexpected severity of infection
Infection following receipt of live vaccines
Chronic oral or cutaneous *Candida* infections
Chronic diarrhea

Perform preliminary evaluation: ⑧
CBC & manual diff
ESR/CRP
Quantitative IgG, IgA, IgM, and IgE levels
Total complement (CH50)

Suspicious of humoral/antibody defect: ⑨
Onset age 5-7 months (after maternal
    antibodies wane)
Recurrent sinopulmonary infections:
    Sinusitis, pneumonia (with fevers), otitis
Meningitis
Sepsis
Chronic diarrhea
Skin infections
Autoimmune disorder
Unusual organisms

Lab: Abnormal immunoglobulin levels

YES

NO

Additional evaluation: ⑩
Antibody titers to vaccine antigens
    (diphtheria, tetanus, pneumococcal)

± Isohemagglutinins

Suspect cellular or combined defects: ⑰

Onset in first several months of life
Severe viral infections (RSV,
    parainfluenza, CMV, EBV, adenovirus)
Fungal/opportunistic infections
Failure to thrive
Chronic diarrhea
Congenital heart disease
Absence of lymphadenopathy with infections
Ataxia

Lab: Lymphopenia, thrombocytopenia

YES

NO

Additional evaluation:
HIV ⑱
Delayed hypersensitivity skin testing
    (*Candida*, tetanus, mumps, trichophyton)
T-cell levels with helper/suppressor ratio

See p. 3 of algorithm

X-linked agammaglobulinemia (Bruton) ⑪
Common variable immunodeficiency ⑫
Hyper-IgM ⑬
IgA deficiency ⑭
Combined cellular and humoral disorders
Transient hypogammaglobulinemia of infancy ⑮
Hyper-IgE ⑯
Specific immunoglobulin deficiencies

Severe combined immunodeficiency ⑲
DiGeorge syndrome ⑳
Ataxia-telangiectasia ㉑
Wiskott-Aldrich syndrome ㉒
Hyper-IgE ⑩
Cartilage-hair hypoplasia ㉓
HIV infection
Secondary immunodeficiencies

and lymphopenia ($<2500/mm^3$ in children <5 years old) from birth. Growth is initially normal, but wasting typically occurs after symptom onset in the first few months of life; recurrent pneumonias, OM, failure to thrive, chronic diarrhea, and severe candidal (and other opportunistic) infections are common. Infections are characteristically *not* accompanied by lymphadenopathy. The addition of a test for SCID to newborn screening panels in an increasing number of states appears to be decreasing the morbidity and mortality for identified infants who receive early treatment.

20 Abnormal development of the branchial pouches (resulting in thymic hypoplasia) is the underlying defect in DiGeorge syndrome. The parathyroid glands, face, ears, aortic arch, and heart are also affected. Diagnosis is usually made early in life based on the congenital heart defects. The immunodeficiency is related to inadequate thymic function. The total lymphocyte count may range from very low to normal, but T-cell levels are usually depressed. Immunoglobulin levels may be normal, but antibody response to antigens is abnormal.

21 Ataxia-telangiectasia is an autosomal recessive disorder characterized by immunodeficiency, neurologic dysfunction, endocrine abnormalities, oculocutaneous telangiectasias, recurrent sinopulmonary infections, and a high rate of malignancy. The presenting symptom is usually ataxia beginning between 3 and 6 years of age. Varying degrees of both B-cell and T-cell dysfunction occur; absence of IgA is the most common immune abnormality, and IgE is also usually low.

22 Wiskott-Aldrich syndrome is an X-linked recessive disorder characterized by abnormal lymphocytes, platelets, and phagocytes. Patients experience severe eczema, bleeding (due to thrombocytopenia), and recurrent infections with encapsulated bacteria and opportunistic pathogens. Immunoglobulin levels vary. IgG is usually slightly low or normal, IgA and IgE are elevated, and IgM is decreased. Patients demonstrate abnormal responses to some antigens but no response to polysaccharide antigens (pneumococcal vaccine, *H. influenzae* type b vaccine). T-cell levels and the helper/suppressor ratio are normal, but their function is abnormal.

23 Cartilage-hair hypoplasia (short-limbed dwarfism) is an autosomal recessive immunodeficiency with skeletal abnormalities and sparse, unpigmented hair. Both B- and T-cell functions are affected; the immunodeficiency worsens with time.

24 The approach to neutropenia needs to consider production, destruction, and function of neutrophils. Specific testing can identify disorders of motility and chemotaxis, adhesion, microbicidal activity, and specific granule defects.

25 Leukocyte adhesion deficiency is characterized by neutrophilia but diminished inflammatory responses. These patients are susceptible to infections with *S. aureus*, enteric gram-negative pathogens and opportunistic pathogens. Impaired migration and phagocytic function result in infections without typical signs of inflammation (erythema, warmth, swelling). The newborn history will frequently reveal delayed separation of the umbilical cord.

26 Chronic granulomatous disease is a rare disorder of the microbicidal function of neutrophils. Catalase-positive microorganisms (*S. aureus*, *Serratia marcescens*) are ingested but not killed, owing to a defect in oxidative function. Recurrent pneumonias, skin infections, osteomyelitis, and lymphadenitis are the most common manifestations; focal infections are more common than sepsis. Granuloma development, occasionally with obstructive complications, can occur. Onset may occur early in infancy or as late as young adulthood.

27 Chédiak-Higashi syndrome is characterized by partial albinism, neutropenia, and abnormal giant cytoplasmic granules in multiple tissues. Recurrent infections of the skin, respiratory tract, and mucous membranes typically occur secondary to a defect in neutrophil degranulation. Bleeding time is usually prolonged. The presence of large melanosomes in melanocytes can confirm the diagnosis. Progressive neuropathies and a tendency to life-threatening histiocytosis can also occur. Chemotactic function is abnormal when assayed in control serum.

28 The complement system acts synergistically with the other components of the immune system to enhance the immune response to infectious agents. Any systemic infection with neisseria (*N. meningitides*, *N. gonorrhea*) should prompt an evaluation of the complement system. CH_{50} screens the classical pathway. Secondary complement disorders are common in autoimmune disorders.

29 Congenital deficiencies of all the components of the complement cascade have been described; a deficiency of C1 esterase inhibitor is associated with hereditary angioedema. Appropriate specimen handling is critical to obtaining accurate results in complement testing.

Bibliography

Ballow M: Approach to the patient with recurrent infections, *Clin Rev Allergy Immunol* 34:129–140, 2008.

Bonilla FA, Bernstein IL, Khan DA, et al: Practice parameter for the diagnosis and management of primary immunodeficiency, *Ann Allergy Asthma Immunol* 94:S1–S63, 2005.

Immune Deficiency Foundation: *Diagnostic and clinical care guidelines for primary immunodeficiency diseases,* ed 2, Towson, Md, 2009, IDF.

Slatter M, Cant AJ, Arkwright PD, et al: Clinical features that identify children with primary immunodeficiency diseases, *Pediatrics* 127:810, 2011.

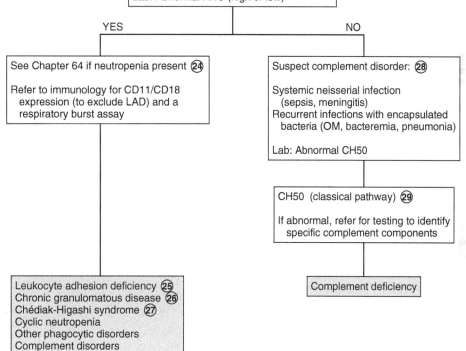

RECURRENT INFECTIONS (continued)

Suspect phagocytic cell disorder:

Skin infections (abscesses, cellulitis)
Lymphadenopathy/lymphadenitis
Deep-seated infections (osteomyelitis, hepatic or pulmonary abscesses)
Pulmonary aspergillosis
Recurrent pneumonia
Oral lesions (gingivitis, ulcers)
Abscesses due to unusual pathogens
History of delayed umbilical cord separation
Poor wound healing
Open sores with scant pus
Unexplained systemic symptoms (fever, malaise, fatigue)

Lab: Abnormal ANC (high or low)

YES

See Chapter 64 if neutropenia present 24

Refer to immunology for CD11/CD18 expression (to exclude LAD) and a respiratory burst assay

Leukocyte adhesion deficiency 25
Chronic granulomatous disease 26
Chédiak-Higashi syndrome 27
Cyclic neutropenia
Other phagocytic disorders
Complement disorders

NO

Suspect complement disorder: 28

Systemic neisserial infection (sepsis, meningitis)
Recurrent infections with encapsulated bacteria (OM, bacteremia, pneumonia)

Lab: Abnormal CH50

CH50 (classical pathway) 29

If abnormal, refer for testing to identify specific complement components

Complement deficiency

Chapter 79
IRRITABLE INFANT (Fussy or Excessively Crying Infant)

(Background: The semantics of traditional medical teachings were such that the term "irritable infant" implied an infant needed to be evaluated for a serious or life-threatening condition [e.g., meningitis]. Current literature uses terms such as "fussy" or "excessively crying" to describe less severe clinical presentations with less critical connotations.)

Parents are frequently concerned by what they consider to be excessive crying or fussiness in an infant without an obvious apparent reason. Most children presenting with this history will be normal or have a non-serious medical condition, but a very small proportion (5%) will have a serious medical disorder. The challenge to the practitioner is to identify those infants who are affected by a serious organic or life-threatening disorder. This algorithm includes common conditions that are frequently overlooked, but it should not be considered all inclusive. (Febrile infants or those presenting with respiratory distress or other significant symptoms will be evaluated and managed according to their clinical presentation.)

1 A thorough history and physical will yield a diagnosis in a majority of crying infants. The history should include the fever history, birth history (including newborn screen results), a past medical history, a thorough review of symptoms, plus a social, developmental, and feeding history. A thorough unclothed physical examination is essential; be particularly vigilant with the otolaryngologic, ophthalmologic, cutaneous, and musculoskeletal exams. (Include palpation of long bones and careful examination of digits in the musculoskeletal exam.) Growth parameters should be noted. Labs or imaging based on positive elements of the history and physical may be indicated; be aware that the yield of diagnostic tests *not* suggested by the history and physical is very low.

2 Judgment must be used in determining whether certain subtle or minor physical findings (abrasions, insect bites, stomatitis) are causative. In cases of severe or persistent irritability, follow-up and possibly additional evaluation may be necessary.

3 Tourniquet syndrome refers to a thin filamentous material (hair, thread) that has wrapped around an appendage and is causing vascular compromise. Careful examination of digits is essential; fingers, toes, penis, and even the uvula have been reported as affected sites. An area of well-demarcated discoloration or swelling on a distal appendage is suspicious; be aware that accompanying edema and duskiness can obscure the strangulating item, making diagnosis difficult. Rapid diagnosis is necessary to minimize morbidity. Surgical intervention is frequently needed, especially for cases of penile strangulation.

4 Intussusception typically presents with a sudden onset of paroxysmal colicky episodes of pain. Vomiting is common; affected infants and toddlers are initially normal between episodes and gradually become weaker and more lethargic. Most (≈60%) will pass stool with gross blood and mucous ("currant jelly"), but this may not occur for up to 1 or 2 days after symptom onset. Abdominal US followed by enema (air, saline, water-soluble contrast) is the preferred diagnostic and therapeutic approach.

5 Test stool for occult blood in fussy infants with nonspecific GI symptoms. Mild cases of protein-induced enterocolitis (non–IgE-mediated hypersensitivity or food allergy) may present with very nonspecific symptoms (spitting, slightly loose stools, fussy). Fecal occult blood is frequently positive. Consider a trial of a hypoallergenic formula if suspicious of the diagnosis. Consider allergy consultation for long-term recommendations.

6 Hand-foot syndrome (dactylitis) is often the first clinical manifestation of sickle cell disease. Infants present with irritability and painful, usually symmetric, swelling of the hands and feet.

7 If the initial history and physical examination do not suggest a diagnosis, consider the ability to console the infant during the evaluation. An infant who can be consoled during the initial period of observation and has normal results on physical examination is not likely to have a serious illness. Follow-up should be recommended within 24 hours for any infant being evaluated for excessive fussiness or crying, even if consolable or a diagnosis seems evident; sometimes an alternative or definitive diagnosis may become evident within 1 or 2 days of the initial presentation. In addition, parents should be counseled carefully about worrisome signs and symptoms and reasons to follow up sooner.

8 Appropriate age (most infants start teething around age 6 months), evidence of erupting teeth, increased salivation, and relief with chewing on a cold object suggest teething.

9 Normal crying may be reported as excessive by inexperienced or stressed parents. Normally, crying increases from birth until about 6 weeks of age, with an average maximum of 2.5 to 3 hours per day. The crying tends to be concentrated between 3 and 11 PM. A wide range of normal variation in crying time is recognized. An acute change in a child's crying pattern is more worrisome than the actual duration.

10 Mild fussiness is associated with several of the standard childhood vaccines; local soreness at the injection site is generally considered the cause. Significant irritability related to vaccines is unusual; other etiologies should be considered.

11 A common definition of colic is recurrent episodes of excessive crying or fussiness at predictable times of the day, usually the evening, lasting more than 3 hours, and occurring on more than 3 days per week in otherwise normal infants. Onset is usually around 3 weeks of age, and the condition typically resolves by 3 to 4 months of age. Parental education and reassurance are necessary and important.

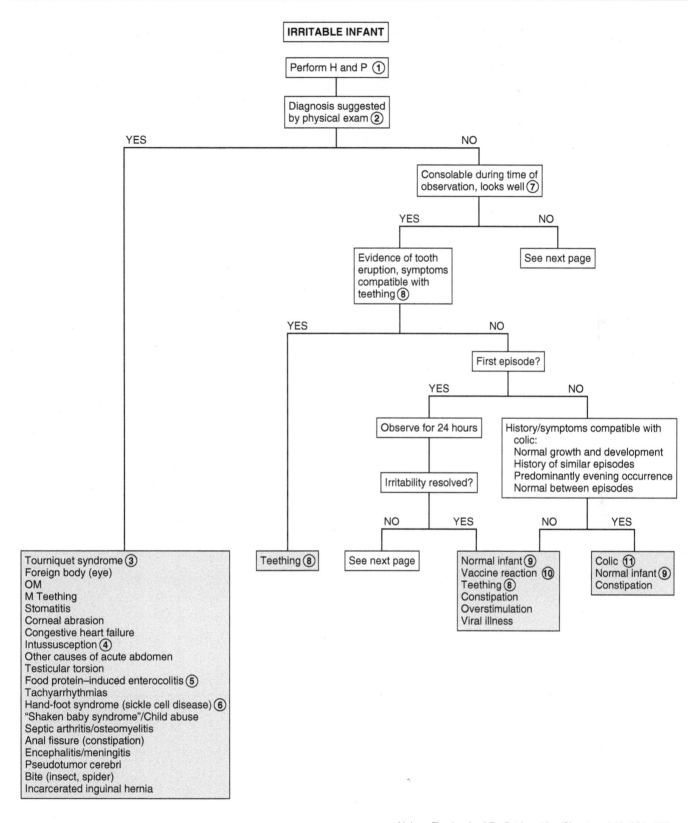

IRRITABLE INFANT

Perform H and P ①

Diagnosis suggested by physical exam ②

YES

NO

Consolable during time of observation, looks well ⑦

YES

NO

Evidence of tooth eruption, symptoms compatible with teething ⑧

See next page

YES

NO

First episode?

YES

NO

Observe for 24 hours

History/symptoms compatible with colic:
 Normal growth and development
 History of similar episodes
 Predominantly evening occurrence
 Normal between episodes

Irritability resolved?

NO

YES

NO

YES

Teething ⑧

See next page

Normal infant ⑨
Vaccine reaction ⑩
Teething ⑧
Constipation
Overstimulation
Viral illness

Colic ⑪
Normal infant ⑨
Constipation

Tourniquet syndrome ③
Foreign body (eye)
OM
M Teething
Stomatitis
Corneal abrasion
Congestive heart failure
Intussusception ④
Other causes of acute abdomen
Testicular torsion
Food protein–induced enterocolitis ⑤
Tachyarrhythmias
Hand-foot syndrome (sickle cell disease) ⑥
"Shaken baby syndrome"/Child abuse
Septic arthritis/osteomyelitis
Anal fissure (constipation)
Encephalitis/meningitis
Pseudotumor cerebri
Bite (insect, spider)
Incarcerated inguinal hernia

Nelson Textbook of Pediatrics, 19e. Chapters 145, 325, 456
Nelsons Essentials, 6e. Chapters 11, 84

12 A UA and culture are the most likely diagnostic tests to yield a positive result. Other testing has a very low yield unless the history and physical suggests an indication for it.

13 Abstinence syndromes may occur in infants born to substance-abusing mothers; withdrawal symptoms include irritability, vomiting, diarrhea, hypertonicity, poor feeding, and sleep problems. Withdrawal usually occurs in the first week of life but may be delayed up to 2 to 3 weeks if the mother was using methadone. Beyond the neonatal period, breastfeeding infants may experience fussiness and irritability due to transfer of maternal drugs (decongestants, caffeine, nicotine, cocaine). Environmental toxins (carbon monoxide) may rarely be a cause of nonspecific infant fussiness.

14 The risk/benefit ratio of performing additional testing must be weighed against the option of simply ensuring follow-up and reassessment in 24 hours. Very rarely will an infant with persistent or severe irritability of unclear cause warrant hospitalization for observation and additional evaluation.

15 A head CT will diagnose intracranial hemorrhage (suspicious of child abuse) or other causes of increased ICP.

Meningitis needs to be considered in cases of severe or inconsolable irritability; some infants will present afebrile. A head CT should be obtained before performing an LP in these infants to rule out increased ICP.

16 Acidosis, hypernatremia, hypocalcemia, and hypoglycemia are rare but serious causes of irritability in infants. Inborn errors of metabolism should be considered when there is associated vomiting, neurologic symptoms, failure to thrive, or a positive family history, including unexplained neonatal deaths.

Bibliography

Freedman SB, Al-Harthy N, Thull-Freedman J: The crying infant: Diagnostic testing and frequency of serious underlying disease, *Pediatrics* 123:841–848, 2009.

Herman M, Le A: The crying infant, *Emerg Med Clin North Am* 25:1137–1159, 2007.

Pawel BB, Henretig FM: Crying and colic in early infancy. In Fleisher G, Ludwig S, editors: *Textbook of pediatric emergency medicine*, ed 6, Philadelphia, 2010, Lippincott Williams & Wilkins, pp 203–205.

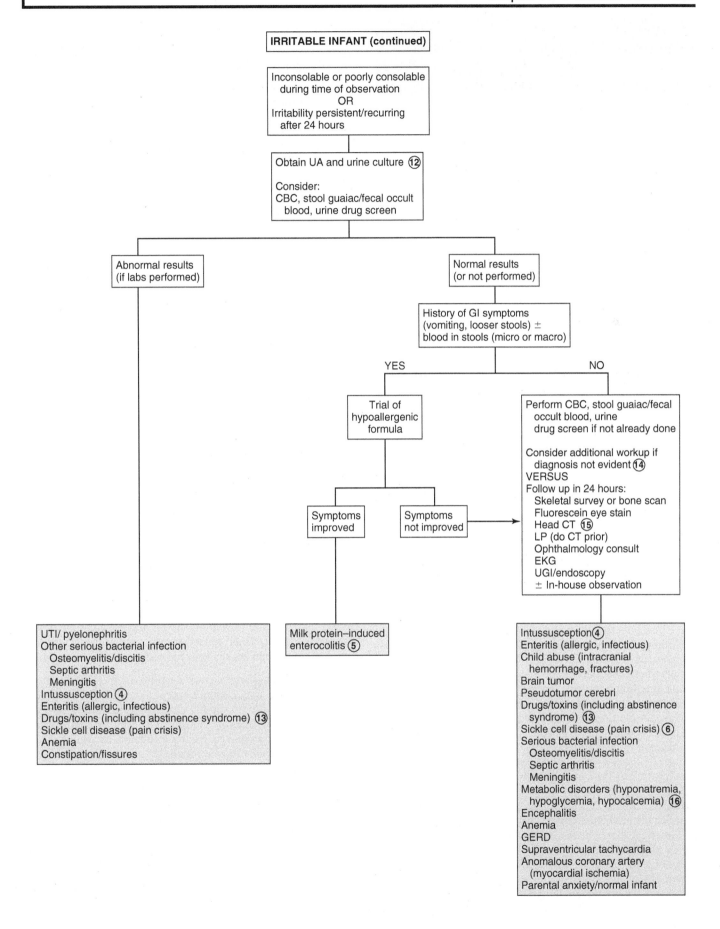

IRRITABLE INFANT (continued)

Inconsolable or poorly consolable during time of observation
OR
Irritability persistent/recurring after 24 hours

Obtain UA and urine culture ⑫

Consider:
CBC, stool guaiac/fecal occult blood, urine drug screen

Abnormal results (if labs performed)

Normal results (or not performed)

History of GI symptoms (vomiting, looser stools) ± blood in stools (micro or macro)

YES

NO

Trial of hypoallergenic formula

Perform CBC, stool guaiac/fecal occult blood, urine drug screen if not already done

Consider additional workup if diagnosis not evident ⑭
VERSUS
Follow up in 24 hours:
  Skeletal survey or bone scan
  Fluorescein eye stain
  Head CT ⑮
  LP (do CT prior)
  Ophthalmology consult
  EKG
  UGI/endoscopy
  ± In-house observation

Symptoms improved

Symptoms not improved

UTI/ pyelonephritis
Other serious bacterial infection
  Osteomyelitis/discitis
  Septic arthritis
  Meningitis
Intussusception ④
Enteritis (allergic, infectious)
Drugs/toxins (including abstinence syndrome) ⑬
Sickle cell disease (pain crisis)
Anemia
Constipation/fissures

Milk protein–induced enterocolitis ⑤

Intussusception④
Enteritis (allergic, infectious)
Child abuse (intracranial hemorrhage, fractures)
Brain tumor
Pseudotumor cerebri
Drugs/toxins (including abstinence syndrome) ⑬
Sickle cell disease (pain crisis) ⑥
Serious bacterial infection
  Osteomyelitis/discitis
  Septic arthritis
  Meningitis
Metabolic disorders (hyponatremia, hypoglycemia, hypocalcemia) ⑯
Encephalitis
Anemia
GERD
Supraventricular tachycardia
Anomalous coronary artery (myocardial ischemia)
Parental anxiety/normal infant

Chapter 80
FAILURE TO THRIVE

Failure to thrive (FTT) describes a condition of poor growth as a result of inadequate calories in infants and young children. A precise definition is lacking, as is a recommended uniform approach to the problem. The "organic" versus "nonorganic" etiology dichotomy has been replaced by the recognition that most cases of FTT are due to inadequate nutrition secondary to an often complex combination of biological and environmental factors. Rarely is an underlying serious organic disorder contributory. Broader consideration of the multifactorial aspect of FTT is occurring; simply ruling out an organic etiology is typically a costly (and misguided) approach to evaluation of FTT.

Definitions of FTT include failing to grow at a rate consistent with expected standards, the deceleration of growth velocity with subsequent crossing of at least 2 major percentile lines, a weight less than the 3rd percentile for age (which, by definition, includes 3% of the population), weight less than 80% of ideal weight for age, and a weight/height ratio of less than the 3rd to 5th percentile. Weight generally drops off before length or head circumference in malnutrition, but be aware that the weight/length ratio may normalize in prolonged cases of malnutrition (after linear growth is affected). The lack of a clear definition to help distinguish between normal variants of growth (constitutional growth delay, short stature due to extreme prematurity) and FTT challenges the clinician because the latter warrants intervention; its impact extends to developmental and behavioral outcomes, not just physical growth.

1. Careful, nonjudgmental observation of the parent-child interaction is important. Sensitive questions about how difficult the child is to take care of, the parents' impression of the problem, and the relationship and shared responsibilities between the parents should be asked. Postpartum depression can affect bonding and have a negative impact on feeding interactions and increase the risk of neglect. FTT due to inadequate intake may be related to financial limitations of the parents.

A complete history, including a thorough review of systems, and physical examination should be performed. Inquire specifically about risk factors for HIV infection and travel to or from a developing country. A family history of growth patterns (short stature, constitutional growth delay) may also be helpful.

Accurate plotting of serial measurements of height, weight, and head circumference is essential in the evaluation of FTT. The World Health Organization (WHO) growth charts for children younger than age 2 years are preferred over the Centers for Disease Control and Prevention growth charts; they identify a lower proportion of underweight children. Growth charts for premature infants are available; after 1 to 2 months of age (beyond the values on the premature growth chart), correction for gestational age for weight should be made until 24 months, for head circumference until 18 months, and for length/height until 40 months by accounting for gestation-adjusted age on the standard WHO growth charts. It is important to ensure standing height is not documented as recumbent length on growth charts ("we are all longer than we are tall"). The age of onset of growth failure

should be noted; poor growth since birth suggests a prenatal or congenital etiology (chromosomal disorder, congenital infection, teratogen), whereas problems starting after the initiation of solid foods could be a clue to oral-motor dysfunction or celiac disease.

2. Most causes of developmental delay can result in FTT. Even mild neurologic disabilities can significantly impact a child's ability to achieve adequate caloric intake. A small head that predates the FTT suggests a prenatal insult, such as hypoxic-ischemic encephalopathy or a congenital viral infection, including HIV. Dysmorphic features suggest chromosomal abnormalities. Prenatal exposures to anticonvulsants or alcohol are also risk factors for developmental delay and FTT. Other diagnoses to consider include neuromuscular disorders, congenital syndromes, and metabolic disorders. Special consideration is required regarding the expected growth and caloric needs of children with more severe disabilities. Subcutaneous fat (triceps skinfold measurement) may be a more appropriate growth assessment than growth chart parameters for some of these children.

3. Oral-motor dysfunction is common in children with developmental delay of any severity. The condition may be subtle and tends to manifest when a child begins taking more textured solid foods. Evaluation by a speech pathologist, including a video fluoroscopic swallow study (VFSS), may be necessary.

4. Although organic causes of FTT are more the exception than the rule, a careful history and physical will usually suggest an underlying medical problem if present. Any disease, depending on its severity and chronicity, may produce FTT.

5. An in-depth diet and feeding history should include dietary content (food types, volume, preparation) as well as inquiries about how easy the child is to feed—food aversion, parental anxiety, or misconceptions about feeding cues or appropriate nutrition can all contribute to inadequate caloric intake. Asking parents to provide a 24-hour dietary recall or a food diary for 2 to 3 days is often helpful. Quantify water, milk, and juice intake. Ask about formula preparation and substitution and the process of feeding and mealtimes in the household. For example, ask about whether everyone in the family eats their meals together and whether any distractions are present during meals. Nutritional intervention should begin at the time of the assessment. Nutritional education and counseling should be provided to parents, ideally with the assistance of a nutritionist.

6. Other psychosocial factors contributing to inadequate caloric intake include family mental health disorders, substance abuse, and other family chaos (homelessness, intimate partner violence, unemployment). Neglect can occur when parents perceive a child as having a difficult temperament or being poorly responsive when feeding.

7. There is no recognized ideal panel of screening tests for FTT. Ideally tests should be considered according to the suspected disorder; the algorithm lists a reasonable selection for when no clinical diagnosis is suspected. Review of the newborn screen should provide results of screening for cystic fibrosis and congenital hypothyroidism. Most newborn screening processes use a combination of immunoreactive trypsinogen levels and limited DNA testing to identify children with cystic fibrosis; confirmatory sweat analysis is recommended when results are abnormal. This approach is about 95% sensitive.

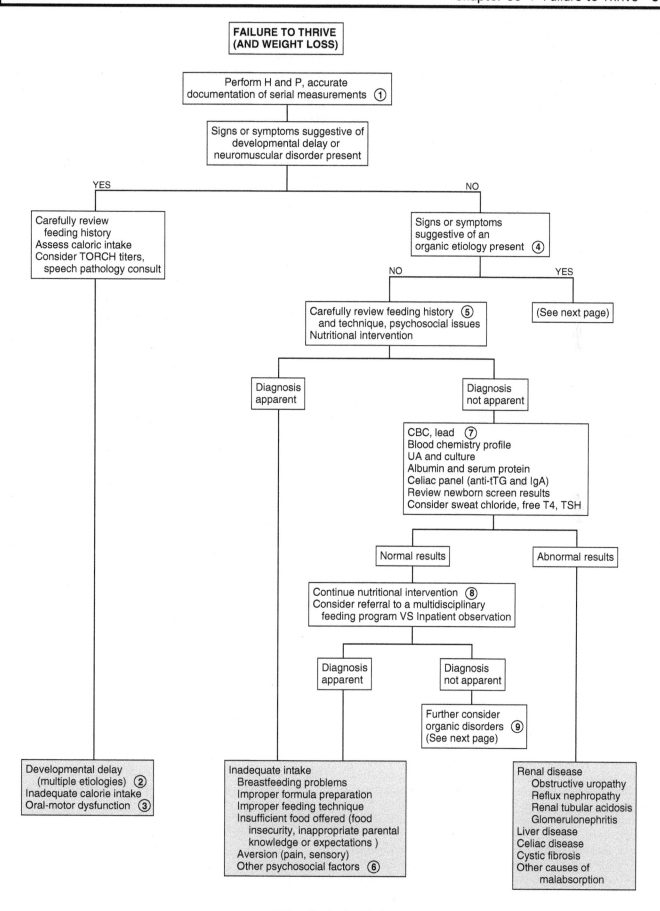

FAILURE TO THRIVE (AND WEIGHT LOSS)

Perform H and P, accurate documentation of serial measurements ①

Signs or symptoms suggestive of developmental delay or neuromuscular disorder present

YES → Carefully review feeding history / Assess caloric intake / Consider TORCH titers, speech pathology consult

NO → Signs or symptoms suggestive of an organic etiology present ④

NO → Carefully review feeding history ⑤ and technique, psychosocial issues / Nutritional intervention

YES → (See next page)

Diagnosis apparent

Diagnosis not apparent

CBC, lead ⑦
Blood chemistry profile
UA and culture
Albumin and serum protein
Celiac panel (anti-tTG and IgA)
Review newborn screen results
Consider sweat chloride, free T4, TSH

Normal results

Abnormal results

Continue nutritional intervention ⑧
Consider referral to a multidisciplinary feeding program VS Inpatient observation

Diagnosis apparent

Diagnosis not apparent

Further consider organic disorders ⑨ (See next page)

Developmental delay (multiple etiologies) ②
Inadequate calorie intake
Oral-motor dysfunction ③

Inadequate intake
Breastfeeding problems
Improper formula preparation
Improper feeding technique
Insufficient food offered (food insecurity, inappropriate parental knowledge or expectations)
Aversion (pain, sensory)
Other psychosocial factors ⑥

Renal disease
Obstructive uropathy
Reflux nephropathy
Renal tubular acidosis
Glomerulonephritis
Liver disease
Celiac disease
Cystic fibrosis
Other causes of malabsorption

Nelson Textbook of Pediatrics, 19e. Chapters 149, 157, 214, 280, 431, 676, 677
Nelsons Essentials, 6e. Chapters 96, 122

8 If a cause is not apparent after a thorough history and physical and preliminary laboratory evaluation, and no improvement has occurred with initial nutritional interventions, involvement with a more intensive multidisciplinary team is ideal (if available). Therapists, nutritionists, social workers, speech pathologists, and psychologists or developmental specialists can all make valuable contributions to the management of a child with FTT, regardless of the cause; the availability of such comprehensive teams is, however, limited in most places. Hospitalization is indicated in cases of suspected abuse or neglect for the purpose of ensuring patient safety, in extreme cases of malnutrition in which a child is at risk for refeeding syndrome, and when more intense surveillance is needed because outpatient evaluation and intervention has not resulted in any improvement. The benefits of hospitalization are limited by short stays (due to payer mandates) and the multiple variables an inpatient setting creates. Long-term outpatient and in-home therapies are preferred options.

9 When a period of multidisciplinary involvement and observation still fail to improve growth or suggest an etiology, further consideration should be given to organic disorders, especially those that may present with subtle symptoms. Assessing for malabsorption disorders is reasonable because they may occur without obvious diarrhea. Also remember that GER can be present without obvious spitting up or vomiting.

10 If GI causes are not identified in a child with a history of vomiting, neuroimaging should also be considered, since increased ICP due to a variety of etiologies (including abusive head trauma) may be the cause.

11 Food protein–induced syndromes (enterocolitis, proctocolitis, enteropathy) are non–immunoglobulin (Ig)E-mediated hypersensitivity reactions that can manifest as vomiting and/or diarrhea, with a wide range of clinical severity and usually begin in infancy.

12 Children with Hirschsprung disease may have a history of delayed passage of meconium, Down syndrome, or positive family history. Most cases will be diagnosed in the first days of life with abdominal distention, vomiting, and constipation. Occasionally, older children will present with FTT, abdominal distention, and constipation. A few will demonstrate intermittent diarrhea. Absent stool on rectal examination and immediate passage of stool and gas after the rectal examination are also suggestive. A rectal suction biopsy demonstrating absent ganglion cells is necessary for diagnosis.

13 Inborn errors of metabolism in the neonate are typically severe and life threatening. The infants are usually normal at birth and often rapidly deteriorate over the hours to days after their birth. Signs and symptoms are nonspecific and include vomiting, lethargy, poor feeding, convulsions, and coma. These infants are often presumed to have sepsis. The physical examination may be normal or may reveal signs related to the CNS, hepatomegaly, or occasionally, a characteristic odor that may aid in diagnosis.

A high index of suspicion is necessary and should be increased by a history of consanguinity and/or a family history of neonatal deaths. For a metabolic workup, blood and urine should be obtained during episodes of suggestive symptoms. Blood tests should include a CBC, electrolytes (calculate anion gap), ABG, glucose, ammonia, lactate, carnitine, acylcarnitine, and serum amino acids. Urine should be analyzed for ketones, reducing substances, organic acids, and carnitine. Consider amylase or lipase, particularly in older children who also complain of abdominal pain.

Mild variants of most inborn errors do occur and have an insidious presentation. Be suspicious when there is a history of unexplained mental retardation, seizures, an unusual odor (especially if manifest during an acute illness), or a family history of metabolic disorders or unexplained infant deaths. Some children will experience intermittent episodes of severe illness, including unexplained vomiting, acidosis, and mental deterioration or coma.

14 Celiac disease is the most common food protein–induced enteropathy. It typically presents as intestinal symptoms (diarrhea, bloating, FTT, irritability, poor appetite) in the first 2 years of life after the introduction of gluten-containing products (wheat, rye, barley, other grains) into the diet. Anti–tissue transglutaminase (anti-tTG) antibody is the preferred screening test in most institutions; an IgA endomysial (EMA) antibody titer is a reasonable alternative. Be aware that anti-tTG may be absent in 10% of children younger than age 2 with celiac disease. Checking total serum IgA is also recommended because IgA deficiency is common in celiac disease; if present, additional serology or intestinal biopsy may be necessary for diagnosis.

15 Cystic fibrosis may manifest at birth with meconium ileus or later with steatorrhea, FTT, and cough. Not all cases develop pancreatic insufficiency; of those that do, the malabsorption may not be evident until after the neonatal period. Shwachman syndrome is characterized by pancreatic insufficiency and chronic neutropenia.

16 Even the most exhaustive efforts and thorough evaluation may occasionally fail to determine the cause of a case of FTT. Maintaining involvement and recurrent evaluation over time may be the key to diagnosis.

17 Eating disorders should always be carefully considered in adolescents, regardless of associated complaints.

18 In children without other obvious associated disorders, iatrogenic causes of anorexia (drug therapy, unpalatable therapeutic diets) and depression should be considered.

19 It is important to inquire about risk factors for HIV because it may present only as FTT with lymphadenopathy and developmental delay. Associated infections are not always present.

20 Nearly any chronic disease can lead to FTT secondary either to altered intake, increased needs, or excessive irritability.

Bibliography

Gahagan S: Failure to thrive: A consequence of undernutrition, *Pediatr Rev* 27:e1, 2006.

Jaffe AC: Failure to thrive: Current clinical concepts, *Pediatr Rev* 32:100, 2011.

Schwartz D: Failure to thrive: An old nemesis in the new millennium, *Pediatr Rev* 21:257, 2000.

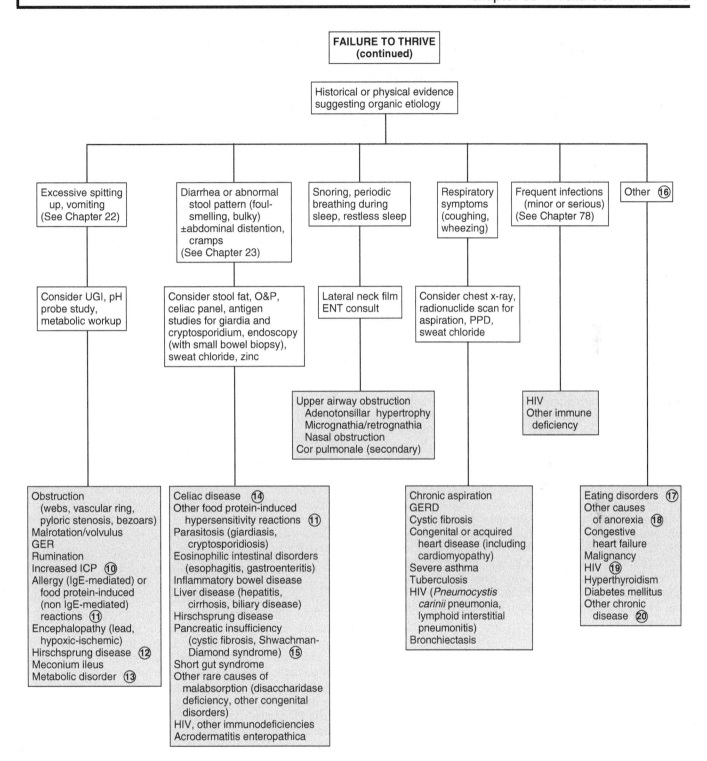

Chapter 81
SLEEP DISTURBANCES

Sleep problems or disturbances are a common concern of parents. They may be classified as dyssomnias (disturbance in amount or timing of sleep), parasomnias (abnormal sleep behaviors such as nightmares and night terrors), and disruptions due to other physical or mental conditions. It is important to understand the normal maturation of the sleep cycle of newborns, infants, and children. In the first year, infants often wake many times during the night, but they may not always cry. The average newborn sleeps about 16.5 hours a day, with relatively undifferentiated sleep cycles. Sleep/wake cycles become more clearly established by 3 to 4 months of age, with an increasing proportion of nighttime sleep. However, there is a great deal of individual variation. In evaluating sleep disorders, it is important to identify inappropriate parental expectations, excessive parental anxiety or stress, as well as parental behaviors that may reinforce the sleep problems.

1 History and physical examination should first of all identify any underlying organic etiology for the sleep disturbance. This may be easier to identify in cases of an acute change in sleep due to illness or injury. A drug and medication history should include caffeine-containing beverages and over-the-counter medications such as cold preparations. Maternal behaviors and attachment as well as psychosocial stress have an important role in sleep problems. Perinatal factors such as birth asphyxia and prematurity contribute to increased wakefulness. Children with developmental delay and autism commonly have sleep problems. The sleeping environment (e.g., temperature, noise, television in room) should also be assessed.

A screening tool (BEARS) is helpful in determining causes of sleep disturbances. It includes five sleep domains, each with trigger questions: **B**edtime problems, **E**xcessive daytime sleepiness, **A**wakenings during the night, **R**egularity and duration of sleep, and **S**noring.

Snoring may indicate obstructive sleep apnea; other symptoms may include choking and gasping. A history of repetitive kicking movements may suggest periodic leg movement disorders. An overnight sleep study may be indicated if history suggests obstructive sleep apnea, periodic leg movement disorders, or excessive daytime sleepiness.

2 If possible, parents should be asked to keep a sleep log. This should include the following information: the time the child awoke in the morning, the time and duration of daytime naps, the time the child is put to bed at night, the time the child fell asleep, the time(s) awakened at night, and what the parent did. It is also important to review sleep practices and influences. The term *sleep hygiene* is used to describe habits acquired for readying for, falling, and staying asleep. Bedtime settling practices create sleep associations and include rituals and routines used, such as bedtime stories or songs, rocking, or comforting. The child's temperament and ability to self-soothe (e.g., thumb sucking, transitional objects) are important in the ability to fall asleep and maintain sleep. Feeding practices play an important role. Breast-fed infants may be more likely to

wake up for feeding. Bed sharing is controversial. In countries where bed sharing is common, it does not seem to be associated with sleep problems; studies in the United States suggest an association. Bed sharing is unsafe for younger children and has been associated with sudden infant death syndrome (SIDS) and other sleep-related causes of infant deaths. One must also determine whether the bed sharing arrangement is due to the parents' beliefs or a response to a sleep problem.

3 Obstructive sleep apnea is due to recurring episodes of upper airway obstruction and is associated with hypoxemia and hypercapnia. There may be a history of snoring and mouth breathing, with episodes of apnea. It is often associated with airway obstruction due to hypertrophy of the tonsils and adenoids. Sleep apnea is associated with obesity and craniofacial abnormalities (micrognathia, Pierre-Robin syndrome). It may result in daytime hypersomnia and behavior problems. An overnight polysomnogram (sleep study) is helpful in making the diagnosis of obstructive sleep apnea.

4 Stimulant medications or caffeine-containing products are known to cause sleep problems. Additionally, corticosteroids may disrupt sleep. Some medications such as antihistamines and anticonvulsants may cause excessive sleepiness during the day.

5 Sleep problems may be due to acute illness, such as otitis media, URI, and UTI. Other possible causes include teething, food allergy, atopic disease, GER, and diaper dermatitis.

6 Injuries such as corneal abrasion, occult fracture, and those secondary to child abuse should be identified.

7 Children with neurodevelopmental disorders can have subclinical or nocturnal seizures, thereby causing sleep disruptions. Children with blindness, cognitive delay, autism spectrum disorders, and some chromosomal syndromes (fragile X) often have sleep disturbances.

8 Behavioral insomnia of childhood includes the sleep-onset association type and the limit-setting type. Sleep-onset association disorder describes a child who requires certain activities to fall asleep, such as rocking, singing, playing, or feeding and does not develop the ability to self-soothe. Some associations may be helpful in preparing the child for bed (reading); others may create problems (rocking) if the child tends to wake up and require the same behavior repeated to fall asleep. Trained night feeders are babies who have a prolonged need for nighttime feeding. Beyond 6 months of age, most night feeding may be considered a learned behavior. It is present in approximately 5% of children aged 6 months to 3 years. It may be considered a form of sleep-onset association disorder, because the child requires food or drink to return to sleep.

Bedtime struggles such as stalling and refusing to go to bed are more common in preschoolers and older children. They are often due to parental difficulties in setting limits such as consistent bedtimes and enforcing bedtime rules. The child's temperament plays an important role, with struggles for autonomy and attention-seeking behaviors further complicating the situation. Problems may begin after 6 to 9 months of age with the acquisition of developmental skills such as object permanence, with consequent separation anxiety and the ability to pull to stand, which the child may use to avoid going to bed. Difficulty settling to sleep may occur during an acute illness and may persist after recovery.

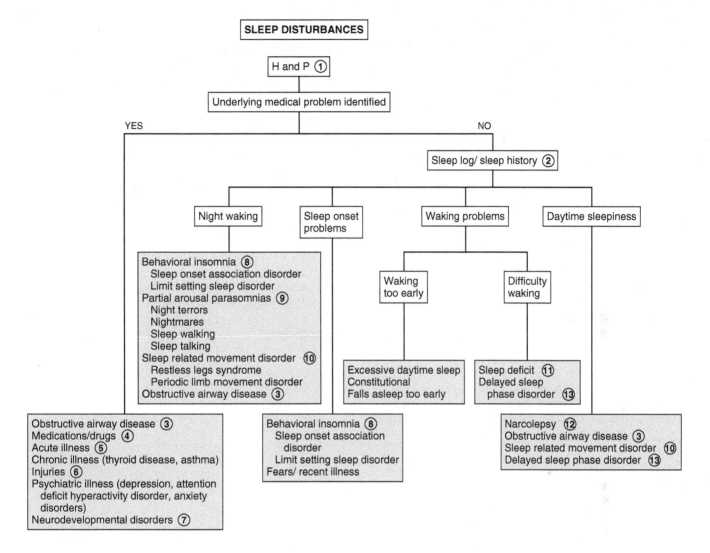

SLEEP DISTURBANCES

H and P ①

Underlying medical problem identified

YES

NO

Sleep log/ sleep history ②

Night waking

Sleep onset problems

Waking problems

Daytime sleepiness

Behavioral insomnia ⑧
  Sleep onset association disorder
  Limit setting sleep disorder
Partial arousal parasomnias ⑨
  Night terrors
  Nightmares
  Sleep walking
  Sleep talking
Sleep related movement disorder ⑩
  Restless legs syndrome
  Periodic limb movement disorder
Obstructive airway disease ③

Waking too early

Difficulty waking

Excessive daytime sleep
Constitutional
Falls asleep too early

Sleep deficit ⑪
Delayed sleep
  phase disorder ⑬

Obstructive airway disease ③
Medications/drugs ④
Acute illness ⑤
Chronic illness (thyroid disease, asthma)
Injuries ⑥
Psychiatric illness (depression, attention
  deficit hyperactivity disorder, anxiety
  disorders)
Neurodevelopmental disorders ⑦

Behavioral insomnia ⑧
  Sleep onset association
    disorder
  Limit setting sleep disorder
Fears/ recent illness

Narcolepsy ⑫
Obstructive airway disease ③
Sleep related movement disorder ⑩
Delayed sleep phase disorder ⑬

Nelson Textbook of Pediatrics, 19e. Chapter 17
Nelsons Essentials, 6e. Chapter 15

9 Parasomnias or disorders of arousal include night terrors and nightmares, as well as sleep walking and talking. Night terrors occur early in the night during partial arousal from deep non–rapid eye movement (non-REM) sleep. The child may cry or scream and show signs of agitation; the child may appear disoriented or confused and seems unaware of the parent's presence. He or she may be difficult to arouse and on awakening usually has no memory of the event. This occurs most commonly in children aged 2 to 6 years. Nightmares usually occur later during the night during REM sleep. The child usually remembers the dream vividly, seems upset on waking, but can be comforted by the parent. The peak age at onset of nightmares is 3 to 5 years, but they can occur at any age, presumably even in preverbal children. Sleep walking (somnambulism) occurs, like sleep terrors, during non-REM sleep. The most common age at onset is 4 to 8 years of age. Safety of the child is the primary concern with this disorder. Sleep talking (somniloquy) is not specific to any stage of sleep and has no clinical significance except that it may occur during nightmares or night terrors.

10 Restless legs syndrome (RLS) is a disorder characterized by uncomfortable sensations in the lower extremities, accompanied by a strong urge to move the legs. RLS is a clinical diagnosis, and the patient is aware of the symptoms. With periodic limb movement disorder (PLMD), there are periodic repetitive limb jerks occurring at frequent intervals. These movements usually occur during sleep and involve the leg, with extension of the big toe and dorsiflexion of the ankle. The patient is unaware of these movements. The diagnosis may be confirmed by overnight polysomnography. Both RLS and PLMD may be associated with low serum iron levels.

11 A child who has difficulty waking up in the morning often has a sleep deficit. This is most common in adolescents because of increased activities and demands on their time. There is often an increased physiologic need for sleep at this time as well.

12 Narcolepsy is a rare disorder with a characteristic irresistible daytime sleepiness. It may be associated with cataplexy (i.e., sudden loss of muscle tone with maintained consciousness) and rarely with hallucinations and sleep paralysis. It is rare in children; however, 25% of adults with narcolepsy report initial presentation during adolescence. Confirmation of the diagnosis requires referral to a sleep laboratory for polysomnography.

13 Delayed sleep phase disorder is due to a disorder of circadian rhythms and is common in adolescents. There is late sleep onset with subsequent delayed wakening time. This causes difficulty adjusting to normal school or work times.

Bibliography

AAP Task Force on Sudden Infant Death Syndrome: SIDS and other sleep-related infant deaths: Expansion of recommendations for a safe infant sleeping environment, *Pediatrics* 128:e1341–e1367, 2011.

Bhargave S: Diagnosis and management of common sleep problems in children, *Pediatr Rev* 32:91–99, 2011.

Owens JA, Dalzell J: Use of the 'BEARS' sleep screening tool in a pediatric residents' continuity clinic: A pilot study, *Sleep Med* 6:63–69, 2005.

Fluids and Electrolytes

Chapter 82
ACIDEMIA

Acidemia is a blood pH less than 7.35. Excessive acidity of body fluids (acidosis) may be acute or chronic, primarily metabolic (decreased plasma bicarbonate), or primarily respiratory (increased partial pressure of CO_2). It may occur as part of a mixed acid-base disorder.

1 In acute acidosis, inquire about diarrhea or other GI losses, medications, and possibility of ingestions. In young infants a history of poor feeding, failure to thrive, vomiting, lethargy, or seizures may indicate an inborn error of metabolism. Poor growth may be a clue to RTA in older children. Nonspecific symptoms of acidosis may include hyperventilation and Kussmaul breathing (i.e., deep, rapid respirations). Unusual breath odors may suggest diabetic ketoacidosis or ingestions.

2 The diagnosis is made by laboratory values. The pH reflecting extracellular free hydrogen ion $[H^+]$ concentration, partial pressure of CO_2 (PCO_2), and plasma bicarbonate level (HCO_3^-) are considered in clinical acid-base disorders. Their relationship is described by this modified version of the Henderson-Hasselbalch equation:

$$[H^+] = 24 \times PCO_2/HCO_3^-$$

When the HCO_3^- level is decreased, an increased respiratory rate occurs as a compensatory mechanism to try to maintain a normal pH. Renal compensation (i.e., secretion of excess H^+ and reabsorption of bicarbonate) is necessary to ultimately correct the acidosis, because the lungs cannot create an absolute loss or gain of H^+ ions.

In mixed acid-base disorders, a combination of simple disorders occurs, such as in the child with chronic lung disease who experiences a combined metabolic alkalosis and respiratory acidosis. Guidelines exist for expected renal and respiratory compensation of acidemia. Mixed disorders should be suspected when the compensatory response differs from the predicted response. Compensation never overcorrects the pH and rarely corrects the pH to normal values.

Urine pH and urine electrolytes should be included in the preliminary analysis if RTA is suspected. A serum osmolality value will aid in narrowing the diagnosis of a metabolic acidosis with an increased anion gap.

3 Neuromuscular disorders that can result in a respiratory acidosis include brainstem or spinal cord disorders, including tumors, Guillain-Barré syndrome, polio, myasthenia gravis, muscular dystrophy, botulism, encephalopathy, and drugs (e.g., depressants, sedatives).

4 The anion gap (AG) reflects unmeasured anions, which, in combination with bicarbonate (HCO_3^-) and chloride (Cl^-), counterbalance the positive charge of the sodium (Na^+) ions.

$$AG = Na^+ - (Cl^- + HCO_3^-)$$

The normal anion gap is 4 to 11 mEq/L, although variations exist among laboratories. Elevation occurs secondary to an excess accumulation of acids (endogenous or ingested) or inadequate excretion of acids. Hyperchloremia occurs in a metabolic acidosis with a normal anion gap. An anion gap lower than expected may occur in the presence of hyperkalemia, hypercalcemia, hypoalbuminemia, hypermagnesemia, bromide intoxication, or laboratory error.

5 Ingestions should be suspected in young children or depressed adolescents at risk for suicide with an acute onset of symptoms (usually multisystemic), a history of previous accidental ingestions, or an altered level of consciousness.

6 A difference of greater than 10 to 15 mOsm/L between the measured serum osmolality and calculated serum osmolality suggests unmeasured osmotic particles (e.g., methanol, ethylene glycol).

$$\text{Calculated serum osmolality} = 2\,[\text{serum } Na^+ + K^+]$$
$$+ \text{BUN}/2.8$$
$$+ \text{glucose}/18$$

7 Ethylene glycol (radiator antifreeze) ingestion causes neurologic symptoms, respiratory failure, cardiovascular collapse, and renal failure. The increased anion gap is due to the accumulation of the metabolite formic acid. Lactic acidosis also frequently occurs.

8 Methanol (wood alcohol) ingestion causes GI and neurologic symptoms. A severe blinding retinitis can also occur. The anion gap is due to the metabolites glyoxylic acid, formic acid, and oxalic acid. Lactic acidosis also occurs.

9 Salicylate ingestion in children is characterized by neurologic symptoms (e.g., coma, altered mental status, seizures) and hyperventilation. Fever may be prominent in infants. Younger children are more susceptible to metabolic acidosis. Respiratory alkalosis is the predominant acid-base abnormality in older patients.

10 Starvation, glycogen storage disease (type 1), and inborn errors of amino acid or organic acid metabolism are less common causes of ketoacidosis.

11 Lactic acidosis with blood lactate levels of 5 mEq/L or higher most commonly is due to hypotension, hypovolemia, or sepsis. Other causes include exercise, ethanol ingestion, and inborn errors of metabolism, particularly mitochondrial and disorders of carbohydrate metabolism.

12 An increased anion gap in renal failure occurs because impaired H^+ excretion prevents appropriate regeneration of HCO_3^-. Anions such as sulfate and phosphate also accumulate.

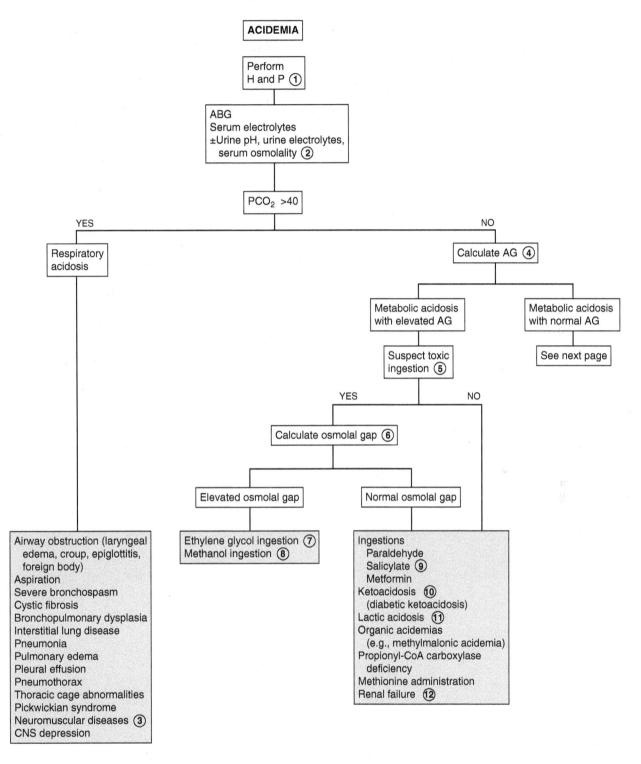

13 Hyperkalemia can develop without the effect of aldosterone. It may be due to primary aldosterone deficiency or result from acquired kidney disease, resulting in low renin levels.

14 Type IV RTA is characterized by a deficiency of or impaired distal tubular response to aldosterone.

15 In pseudohypoaldosteronism, both renin and aldosterone levels are elevated, but the response of the distal tubule to the aldosterone is impaired.

16 Certain medications (e.g., potassium-sparing diuretics, nonsteroidal antiinflammatory drugs, β-blocking agents, angiotensin-converting enzyme inhibitors, cyclosporine) can cause a functional hypoaldosteronism.

17 Urine pH should be measured on a fresh urine specimen. Serum electrolytes should be collected at the same time for the HCO_3^- level. The urine specimen can be taken at any time but should be obtained while the patient is still acidotic.

The urine pH reflects only free H^+ ($<1\%$ of the total H^+ excreted). It is often helpful to consider it in conjunction with a measure of net acid excretion, primarily urine ammonium concentration. Synthesis of ammonia (NH_3) and its subsequent excretion as ammonium (NH_4^+) are increased in most cases of systemic acidosis. The urinary anion gap is used to estimate the production of ammonium ion:

$$\text{Urine AG} = (\text{Urine } Na^+ + \text{Urine } K^+) - \text{Urine } Cl^-$$

The lower or more negative the gap, the greater the acid secretion in the form of NH_4^+.

18 RTA is characterized by an inability to adequately acidify the urine in the presence of a normal anion gap (hyperchloremic) acidosis. It may occur primarily or in association with multiple inherited disorders or acquired systemic disorders. In the distal and proximal subtypes, volume contraction results in an aldosterone-mediated hypokalemia.

In distal (type I or classic) RTA, a permanent deficiency of H^+ secretion by the distal tubules results in wasting of a portion of the filtered load of HCO_3^-. The HCO_3^- wasting persists even in the presence of severe systemic acidosis; urine pH is never more acidic than 5.8. The urine anion gap is a small or low negative value.

In proximal RTA (type II or HCO_3^- wasting) a defect in the proximal tubular reabsorption of HCO_3^- results in a higher load of HCO_3^- being presented to the distal tubule. In mild acidosis, this excess HCO_3^- is lost in the urine because its amount exceeds the capacity of the distal tubule for reabsorption in the normal distal tubule. In more severe acidosis a lower amount of HCO_3^- is filtered and is able to be reabsorbed in the normal distal tubule. Because distal acidification mechanisms are intact in proximal RTA, urine pH will become more acidic (pH <5.5) under these circumstances. The urine anion gap is a high negative value, regardless of the severity or duration of the acidosis. Accompanying hypokalemia can be severe.

19 Rapid volume expansion with non–HCO_3^--containing solutions can cause transient small HCO_3^- losses in the urine.

20 Premature infants and neonates with renal function that is normal for maturation may demonstrate a mild metabolic acidosis due to a transient reduced threshold for HCO_3^- reabsorption. This normally corrects by 4 to 6 weeks in the premature infant and by 3 weeks in the term infant.

21 Increased HCO_3^- losses in diarrhea can contribute to a metabolic acidosis.

Bibliography

Brewer ED: Disorders of acid-base balance, *Pediatr Clin North Am* 37: 429–447, 1990.
Hanna JD, Scheinman JI, Chan JC: The kidney in acid-base balance, *Pediatr Clin North Am* 42:1365–1395, 1995.

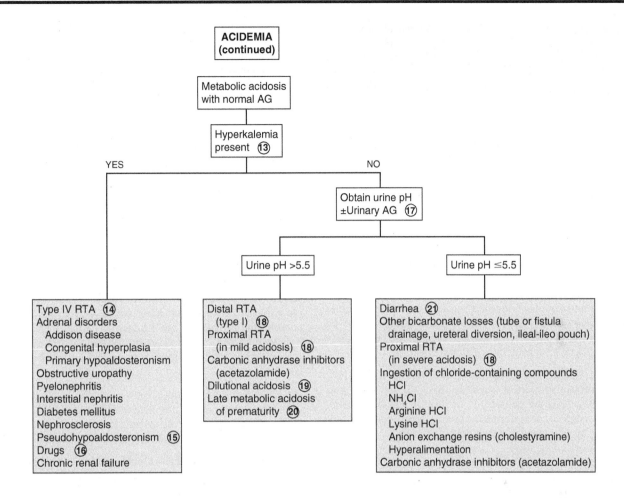

AG = Anion gap
RTA = Renal tubular acidosis
PCO$_2$ = Partial pressure of CO$_2$

Chapter 83

ALKALEMIA

Alkalemia is a serum pH above 7.45. The term *alkalosis* refers to the process resulting in excess total body bicarbonate (HCO_3^-) or deficit of total body hydrogen. The disorder may be acute or chronic, primarily metabolic, or primarily respiratory or occur as a part of a mixed acid-base disorder.

1. The history should inquire about underlying medical problems and medication use, as well as potential losses of GI fluid (e.g., vomiting, diarrhea, nasogastric drainage). The diet history should inquire about the possibility of ingestion of natural licorice, but most licorice in the United States is artificially flavored. A prenatal history of polyhydramnios and history of prematurity may suggest a primary renal hypokalemic syndrome (e.g., Bartter syndrome). Older children should be asked about use of chewing tobacco, because some brands may contain an acid with a mineralocorticoid effect.

2. The pH (reflecting extracellular free hydrogen ion [H^+] concentration), partial pressure of CO_2 (PCO_2), and plasma HCO_3^- level are considered in clinical acid-base disorders. Their relationship is described by this modified version of the Henderson-Hasselbalch equation:

$$[H^+] = 24 \times PCO_2 / HCO_3^-$$

In response to an increased pH, the body normally attempts to decrease total serum HCO_3^- (renal compensation) and increase PCO_2 (respiratory compensation).

3. Respiratory alkalosis occurs when a primary decrease in PCO_2 causes an increase in the pH to greater than 7.45. Hyperventilation of various causes is the most common etiology. Tachypnea is often obvious initially. In chronic respiratory alkalosis, the respiratory rate may approach normal, with the patient taking deeper breaths.

4. A metabolic alkalosis occurs when a primary increase in extracellular HCO_3^- causes a rise in the pH above 7.45. The etiology may be loss of H^+, gain of HCO_3^-, or loss of extracellular fluid, with chloride losses exceeding HCO_3^- losses. Factors that prevent renal excretion of HCO_3^- (e.g., renal failure, volume depletion, profound hypokalemia) must be present to maintain a metabolic alkalosis. Volume depletion results in aldosterone-mediated sodium retention in exchange for potassium and H^+ secretion, which maintains an alkalosis (i.e., contraction alkalosis) with a paradoxical aciduria. Hypokalemia is a stimulus for additional renal H^+ secretion.

5. If the etiology of a metabolic alkalosis is not clear from the H and P, a spot urine chloride test will aid in the diagnosis.

6. The loss of hydrochloric acid (HCl) due to vomiting or nasogastric fluid drainage leads to increased gastric HCl production, which is accompanied by systemic HCO_3^- production. The alkalosis is further maintained by volume depletion that results in aldosterone-mediated renal absorption of sodium in exchange for H^+ and potassium secretion.

7. High urinary chloride losses (e.g., sodium chloride) occur shortly after beginning diuretic therapy. Urinary chloride losses are minimized with prolonged therapy because of chloride depletion and subsequent volume contraction. The volume contraction results in aldosterone-mediated sodium and closely linked chloride reabsorption and H^+ secretion.

8. In congenital chloride-wasting diarrhea, a rare inherited disorder, a defect of the normal chloride-for-HCO_3^- exchange in the ileum and colon leads to increased GI losses of chloride and subsequent metabolic alkalosis.

9. Infants with cystic fibrosis require more sodium chloride than is contained in usual formulas or breast milk. High losses of sodium chloride in sweat that are not countered by dietary intake can cause volume contraction and mild metabolic alkalosis.

10. Rapid recovery from compensated chronic respiratory acidosis can cause posthypercapnia metabolic alkalosis. This scenario is most likely to occur in infants with bronchopulmonary dysplasia who have experienced sodium chloride losses and volume depletion from diuretic use. After correction of the hypercapnia and despite normalization of the pH, renal HCO_3^- reabsorption is favored until volume and chloride depletion is corrected.

11. Ingestion of exogenous sources of alkali (e.g., citrate, acetate, lactate, HCO_3^-) is occasionally sufficient to generate a metabolic alkalosis. Excessive transfusions with citrated blood or Plasmanate containing acetate are other possible causes.

12. High levels of urinary chloride indicate some impairment of urinary reabsorption of chloride. The presence or absence of hypertension can help clarify the diagnosis.

13. Mineralocorticoid excess typically results in volume expansion and hypertension. Congenital adrenal hyperplasia with deficiencies of the 11-hydroxylase or 17-hydroxylase enzymes results in levels of desoxycorticosterone (an aldosterone precursor) high enough to exert a significant mineralocorticoid effect. Natural licorice and some chewing tobaccos have glycyrrhizic acid that creates a mineralocorticoid effect.

14. Bartter syndrome is a rare renal tubular disorder characterized by hypokalemic metabolic alkalosis, urinary chloride wasting, increased plasma renin and aldosterone levels, and normal to low BP. Children exhibit failure to thrive, short stature, polyuria, polydipsia, and tendency to get dehydrated. Gitelman syndrome is a similar but more benign tubular disorder characterized by hypokalemia and urinary magnesium wasting. Children with this syndrome exhibit short stature and are prone to febrile seizures and hypomagnesemic-tetanic episodes. The two disorders can be distinguished by urinary calcium levels, which are high in Bartter syndrome and low in Gitelman syndrome.

Bibliography

Avner E: Clinical disorders of water metabolism, *Pediatr Ann* 24:23, 1995.

Brewer ED: Disorders of acid-base balance, *Pediatr Clin North Am* 37: 429–447, 1990.

Hanna JD, Scheinman JI, Chan JC: The kidney in acid-base balance, *Pediatr Clin North Am* 42:1365–1395, 1995.

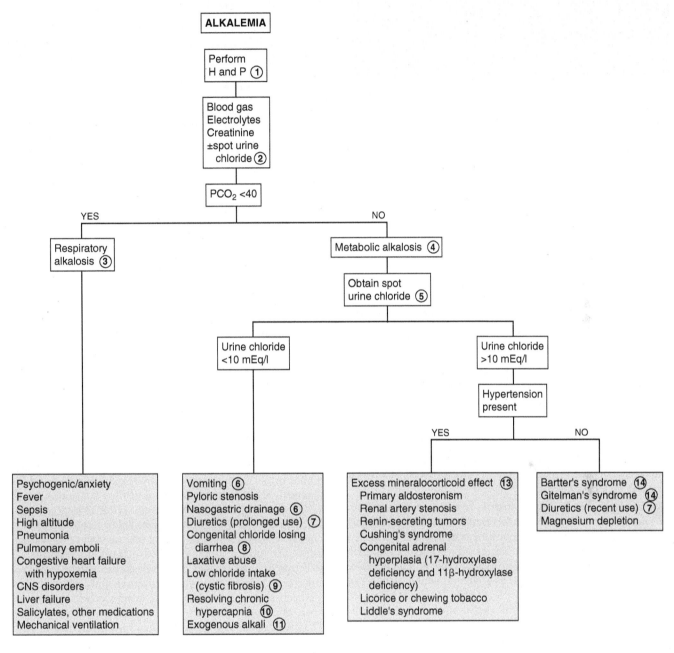

ALKALEMIA

Perform H and P ①

Blood gas
Electrolytes
Creatinine
±spot urine
 chloride ②

PCO₂ <40

YES

NO

Respiratory alkalosis ③

Metabolic alkalosis ④

Obtain spot urine chloride ⑤

Urine chloride <10 mEq/l

Urine chloride >10 mEq/l

Hypertension present

YES

NO

Psychogenic/anxiety
Fever
Sepsis
High altitude
Pneumonia
Pulmonary emboli
Congestive heart failure
  with hypoxemia
CNS disorders
Liver failure
Salicylates, other medications
Mechanical ventilation

Vomiting ⑥
Pyloric stenosis
Nasogastric drainage ⑥
Diuretics (prolonged use) ⑦
Congenital chloride losing
  diarrhea ⑧
Laxative abuse
Low chloride intake
  (cystic fibrosis) ⑨
Resolving chronic
  hypercapnia ⑩
Exogenous alkali ⑪

Excess mineralocorticoid effect ⑬
  Primary aldosteronism
  Renal artery stenosis
  Renin-secreting tumors
  Cushing's syndrome
  Congenital adrenal
    hyperplasia (17-hydroxylase
    deficiency and 11β-hydroxylase
    deficiency)
  Licorice or chewing tobacco
  Liddle's syndrome

Bartter's syndrome ⑭
Gitelman's syndrome ⑭
Diuretics (recent use) ⑦
Magnesium depletion

PCO_2 = Partial pressure of CO_2

Nelson Textbook of Pediatrics, 19e. Chapter 52

Chapter 84
HYPERNATREMIA

Sodium (Na^+) is the primary cation of the ECF compartment and is the major osmotically active solute in the ECF. Osmolality is the measurement of the number of solute particles in a unit of volume. It can be measured or estimated by the formula:

$$\text{Calculated serum osmolality} = 2\,[\text{serum } Na^+ + K^+] + BUN/2.8 + glucose/18$$

The body responds to changes in osmolality by increasing or suppressing thirst and antidiuretic hormone (ADH) release.

1 Signs and symptoms of hypernatremia are nonspecific. Thirst will be increased as long as the brain's thirst centers are intact. Excessive thirst to the point it disrupts sleep or play and enuresis may be a clue to diabetes. Neurologic symptoms (e.g., irritability, lethargy, confusion, seizures) may be present in severe cases.

Inquire about volume losses (diarrhea, vomiting), oral intake, and urine output. Specifically ask about formula preparation and the possibility of excessive salt intake (e.g., of table salt or sea water). Polyuria and polydipsia may suggest diabetes mellitus (DM) or insipidus (DI). Infants with fever, very low-birth-weight infants, and children with cystic fibrosis or heat stroke are at risk for hypernatremia because of excessive (hypotonic) sweat losses. The medical history should also inquire about renal disease and CNS disease or hemorrhage, which may be a risk factor for central DI.

2 The approach to hypernatremia is best initiated with an assessment of the patient's volume status. Hypovolemia manifests as lethargy, dry mucous membranes, and decreased skin turgor. Infants will exhibit decreased tearing and a sunken fontanel. Tachycardia, orthostatic hypotension, and oliguria are also common. Fever may occur as both a cause and an effect of hypernatremic dehydration. The signs of ECF volume losses are less pronounced in hypernatremic dehydration than in hyponatremic dehydration.

Patients appear to have a normal volume status (euvolemia) when total body water is decreased in the presence of normal or near-normal sodium content. This situation occurs secondary to inadequate water intake or solute-free water losses. These water losses may be extrarenal or renal (DI). Extrarenal losses will produce hypertonic urine. Urine sodium may be variable. Renal losses result in hypotonic urine.

Hypervolemia occurs when total body water is essentially normal in the presence of increased total body sodium. Manifestations of excess ECF volume include edema and congestive heart failure.

3 Diarrhea is most likely to lead to hyponatremic or isonatremic dehydration; hypernatremic dehydration is likely if fluid intake is low (vomiting, anorexia), fever is present (increased free water insensible losses), or hypertonic fluids are being given.

4 Insensible water losses from the respiratory tract occur secondary to hyperventilation or respiratory distress. Dermal losses are common in infants placed on a radiant warmer and in settings of increased ambient temperature.

5 Although adipsia is rare, it can occur as a primary entity or secondary to hypothalamic lesions, hydrocephalus, or head trauma.

6 Hypotonic urine and polyuria in the presence of hypernatremia suggest DI. DI, which presents with polyuria and polydipsia, represents an inability to concentrate urine because of either a lack of ADH production (central DI) or renal resistance to ADH (nephrogenic DI). DI is an inability to effectively conserve urinary water. Hypernatremia in DI most often occurs when access to water is restricted. Because young children do not usually have control over their fluid intake, most pediatric cases of DI occur as hypovolemia.

7 A water deprivation test should be carefully monitored in the hospital and should be done during daytime hours rather than overnight. During water deprivation, the body weight should not be allowed to decline by more than 3%.

8 The response to intramuscular aqueous vasopressin (0.1-0.2 units/kg) will help confirm the diagnosis of DI and distinguish between central and renal causes.

9 Central DI is probably the diagnosis if, after administration of vasopressin, the urine/serum ratio becomes greater than 1. Psychogenic polydipsia usually does not result in hypernatremia. If the administration of vasopressin produces a higher urinary concentration than dehydration does, DI is the diagnosis regardless of the level of urinary concentration. Psychogenic polydipsia usually does not result in hypernatremia.

Central DI may be primary (familial or nonfamilial) or secondary to head trauma or several disease states (suprasellar or intrasellar tumors, granulomatous disease, histiocytosis, CNS infection or hemorrhage). ADH release can also be inhibited by stress (e.g., pain from surgery or trauma) and certain drugs and medications (e.g., α-adrenergic agonists, alcohol, opiate antagonists, phenytoin, clonidine) and carbon monoxide poisoning. The disorder has also been associated with cleft lip and palate.

10 Nephrogenic DI may be congenital or secondary to multiple types of renal disease. Males with primary nephrogenic DI are likely to have a significant history of polyuria, polydipsia, and previous episodes of hypernatremic dehydration. Females with a primary defect have milder symptoms and tend to be diagnosed later in life. It can also be caused by drugs or medications (e.g., lithium, demeclocycline, methoxyflurane, amphotericin B, cyclophosphamide, propoxyphene, cisplatin, angiographic dyes, osmotic diuretics), hypokalemia, and hypercalcemia.

Bibliography

Avner E: Clinical disorders of water metabolism, *Pediatr Ann* 24:23, 1995.
Conley SB: Hypernatremia, *Pediatr Clin North Am* 37:365–372, 1990.

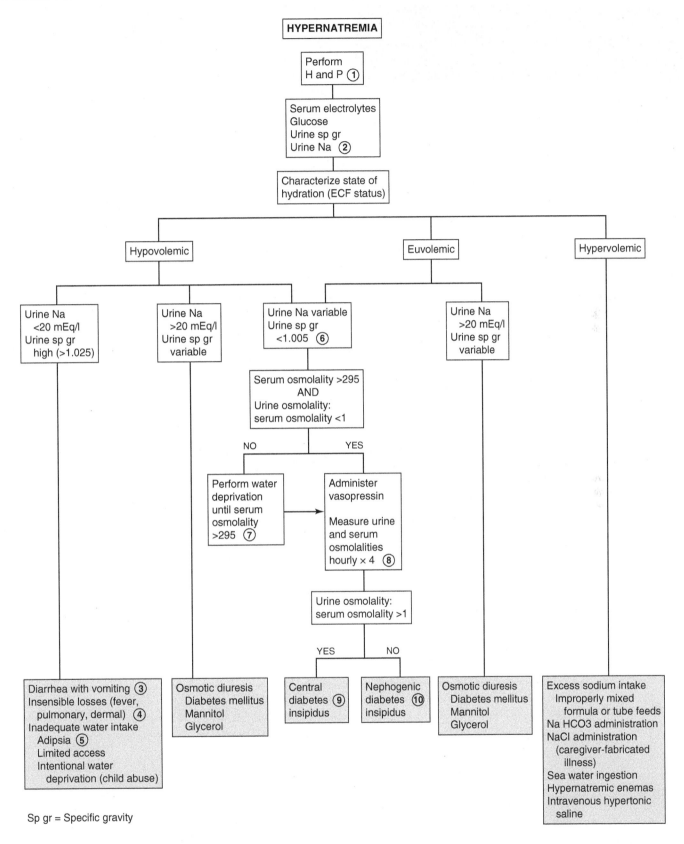

HYPERNATREMIA

Perform H and P ①

Serum electrolytes
Glucose
Urine sp gr
Urine Na ②

Characterize state of hydration (ECF status)

Hypovolemic

Euvolemic

Hypervolemic

Urine Na
<20 mEq/l
Urine sp gr
high (>1.025)

Urine Na
>20 mEq/l
Urine sp gr
variable

Urine Na variable
Urine sp gr
<1.005 ⑥

Urine Na
>20 mEq/l
Urine sp gr
variable

Serum osmolality >295
AND
Urine osmolality:
serum osmolality <1

NO   YES

Perform water
deprivation
until serum
osmolality
>295 ⑦

Administer
vasopressin

Measure urine
and serum
osmolalities
hourly × 4 ⑧

Urine osmolality:
serum osmolality >1

YES   NO

Diarrhea with vomiting ③
Insensible losses (fever,
    pulmonary, dermal) ④
Inadequate water intake
    Adipsia ⑤
    Limited access
    Intentional water
        deprivation (child abuse)

Osmotic diuresis
    Diabetes mellitus
    Mannitol
    Glycerol

Central
diabetes ⑨
insipidus

Nephogenic
diabetes ⑩
insipidus

Osmotic diuresis
    Diabetes mellitus
    Mannitol
    Glycerol

Excess sodium intake
Improperly mixed
    formula or tube feeds
Na HCO3 administration
NaCl administration
    (caregiver-fabricated
    illness)
Sea water ingestion
Hypernatremic enemas
Intravenous hypertonic
    saline

Sp gr = Specific gravity

Nelson Textbook of Pediatrics, 19e. Chapters 52 and 552

Chapter 85
HYPONATREMIA

Sodium (Na^+) is the primary cation of the ECF compartment and is the major osmotically active solute in the ECF. Osmolality is the measurement of the number of solute particles in a unit of volume. It can be measured or estimated by the formula:

$$\text{Calculated serum osmolality} = 2\,[\text{serum } Na^+ + K^+] + BUN/2.8 + \text{glucose}/18$$

The body responds to changes in osmolality by increasing or suppressing thirst and antidiuretic hormone (ADH) release.

1. The history should inquire about GI losses (e.g., vomiting, diarrhea). Ask about fluid intake, urine output, medications, and possibility of a toxic ingestion. For infants, inquire specifically about formula preparation and amount of free water ingested. Ingestions should be suspected in young children aged 1 to 5 years with an acute onset of symptoms, a history of previous accidental ingestions, neurologic symptoms, or an unusual breath odor. Signs of hyponatremia usually manifest when the sodium level falls rapidly below 120 mEq/L. Signs and symptoms may include apathy, anorexia, nausea, vomiting, altered mental status, and seizures. Musculoskeletal symptoms include cramps and weakness.

2. If the preliminary laboratory evaluation reveals a significantly elevated BUN and Cr value not believed to be caused by dehydration, a pediatric nephrologist should be consulted for further evaluation of presumed renal failure.

3. Hyponatremia most commonly occurs in conjunction with a hypotonic state. The presence of lipemic serum or clinical clues suggestive of diabetes mellitus (e.g., polyuria, polydipsia, weight loss, hyperglycemia) or a possible ingestion should prompt consideration of nonhypotonic states.

4. Older methods of electrolyte measurement determined sodium in mEq/L of plasma, as opposed to plasma water, which could yield an artificially low sodium value (pseudohyponatremia) in the presence of hyperlipidemia (nephrotic syndrome) or hyperproteinemia, which is rare in children. Newer methods use ion-selective electrodes to measure serum sodium activity directly in plasma water and do not produce this artifact.

5. Hyponatremia occurs in a hypertonic setting when an osmotically active solute has been added to the ECF. A difference of greater than 10 to 15 mOsm/L between the measured serum osmolality and the calculated serum osmolality is suggestive of a nonglucose solute in the ECF and may be the first clue to certain ingestions (e.g., of methanol, ethanol).

6. Assessment of the patient's overall volume status is essential in the evaluation of hyponatremia.

Hypovolemia (dehydration) manifests as lethargy, dry mucous membranes, and decreased skin turgor. Infants will exhibit decreased tearing and a sunken fontanel. Tachycardia, orthostatic hypotension, and oliguria are also common.

Patients appear to have a normal volume status (euvolemia) when total body sodium is normal or near normal in the presence of a slight excess of body water. Most patients presenting with euvolemic hyponatremia have a syndrome of inappropriate antidiuretic hormone secretion (SIADH). Although characterized as euvolemic, many of these patients will have a slightly increased but clinically unimportant ECF volume.

Hypervolemia occurs when total body water is increased to a greater degree than total body sodium in either edema-forming states or renal failure.

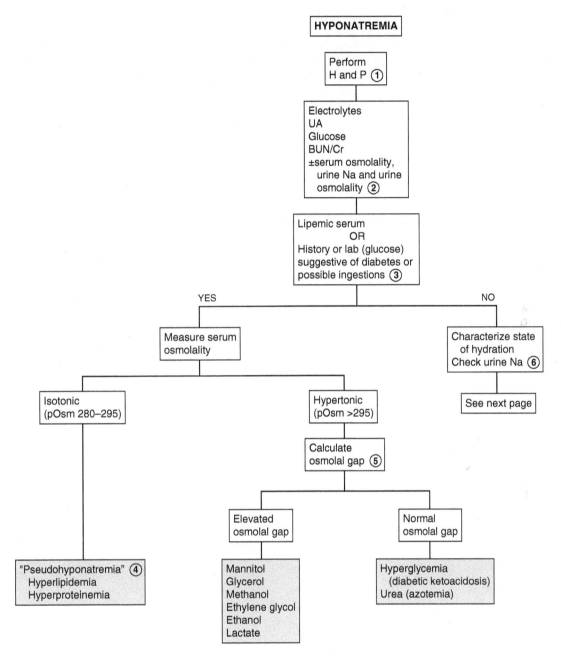

Nelson Textbook of Pediatrics, 19e. Chapters 553 and 52

7 Renal disorders causing sodium wasting include nephritis, medullary cystic disease, polycystic kidney disease, and obstructive uropathies. Premature infants may have limited reabsorption of sodium, leading to salt wasting.

In proximal renal RTA, reduced proximal tubular reabsorption of bicarbonate results in an obligatory loss of sodium. Type IV RTA is caused by either a lack of aldosterone or an insensitivity to it (i.e., pseudohypoaldosteronism), resulting in increased renal losses of sodium.

8 Conditions in which isotonic fluid translocates to a "third space" include burns, pancreatitis, muscle trauma, peritonitis, and ascites.

9 Water intoxication as a cause of hyponatremia occurs in children receiving IV fluids in the presence of some level of impaired water excretion. For instance, infants are less efficient at excreting water and therefore are at higher risk for water intoxication. Infants younger than 6 months of age fed excessive amounts of water may also develop hyponatremia and seizures. Rare causes include tap water enemas and swallowed swimming pool water. Psychogenic polydipsia is most likely to occur in mentally disturbed patients.

10 The syndrome of SIADH is characterized by a sustained or intermittent secretion of ADH that is inappropriate based on the volume status and serum osmolality. The urine osmolality is generally higher than the serum osmolality and higher than expected for the degree of hyponatremia. The urine sodium is usually higher than expected for the degree of hyponatremia in SIADH. The diagnosis is one of exclusion and should only be made in the presence of normal renal, adrenal, pituitary, and thyroid function, and in the absence of hypovolemia, dehydration, and edema. The condition can be due to numerous causes, including CNS disorders, pulmonary disorders, tumors, and medications. Postoperative pain and stress are also causes.

11 In glucocorticoid deficiency, ADH release is not maximally suppressed. The condition resembles SIADH, except that it will respond to exogenous glucocorticoid.

12 A reset osmostat is a variant of SIADH affecting chronically ill children. The plasma osmolality level at which ADH release occurs is reset downward, so that these patients have chronic hyponatremia. Water loading decreases ADH secretion, and sodium loading increases ADH secretion and concentrates the urine.

13 Hypervolemia occurs when total body water is increased to a greater degree than total body sodium. Patients usually have an impaired ability to excrete water and may have decreased intravascular volume. A manifestation of excess ECF volume is peripheral edema, as noted in cirrhosis and heart failure. All cases are further complicated by an increased secretion of ADH, which leads to further water retention.

Bibliography

Avner E: Clinical disorders of water metabolism, *Pediatr Ann* 24:23, 1995.
Berry PL, Belsha CW: Hyponatremia, *Pediatr Clin North Am* 37:351–363, 1990.
Trachtman H: Sodium and water homeostasis, *Pediatr Clin North Am* 42:1343–1363, 1995.

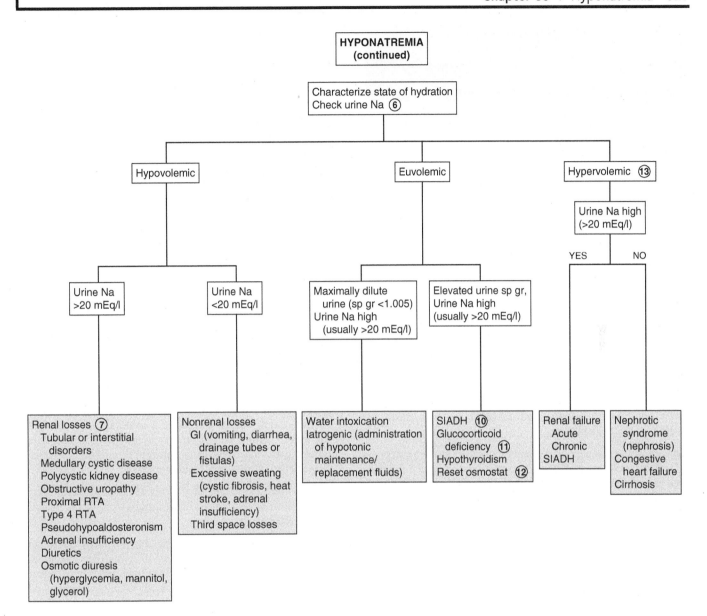

SIADH = Syndrome of inappropriate antidiuretic hormone secretion

Chapter 86
HYPOKALEMIA

Potassium is the main cation of the intracellular fluid (ICF) compartment. The ECF concentration is carefully regulated to maintain a value around 4 mEq/L. Potassium (K^+) plays a critical role in the excitability of nerve and muscle cells and contractility of muscles (smooth, skeletal, cardiac). Aldosterone normally regulates renal excretion of potassium. Aldosterone also causes sodium reabsorption and H^+ secretion in the distal tubule. Aldosterone similarly affects potassium excretion in the stool. Hypokalemia is defined as a serum potassium concentration < 3.5 mEq/L.

1. The history should inquire about medications, underlying medical problems, and diet, including pica and the use of salt substitutes. Muscle weakness, hyporeflexia, and intestinal ileus are manifestations of hypokalemia. Cardiac arrhythmias are the most serious complications. Flattened T waves, a short PR interval, and a prolonged QT interval are characteristic EKG abnormalities. A U wave may develop after the QRS complex. Patients may also be lethargic or confused and may have muscle cramping, rhabdomyolysis, and myoglobinuria in cases of severe potassium depletion.

2. Acid-base disorders and disturbances in chloride or magnesium levels may contribute to potassium imbalance and will need to be corrected before correcting the potassium problem.

3. GI losses of potassium are exacerbated by accompanying volume depletion and subsequent increased aldosterone effects.

4. If the etiology of hypokalemia is unclear from the history, a urine potassium level may aid in distinguishing between renal and nonrenal losses.

5. Transcellular shifts of potassium occur in an effort to maintain electrical neutrality in varying conditions. In metabolic acidosis, potassium shifts out of the cell in exchange for intracellular buffering of H^+. The opposite exchange occurs to a lesser degree in metabolic alkalosis. These shifts also occur in acid-base disturbances that are primarily respiratory, although to a lesser degree.

6. Insulin, catecholamines, and β-agonists (albuterol) acutely shift potassium intracellularly.

7. Potassium uptake by rapidly forming new RBCs and platelets in the treatment of megaloblastic anemia can result in hypokalemia. Similarly, transfusion of frozen washed RBCs (not stored in acid-citrate-dextran) may lower potassium levels because of increased cellular uptake.

8. Rarely, episodic weakness or paralysis can be due to transient changes in potassium levels. The familial forms result from mutations in genes that affect ion channels in muscle. In the hypokalemic version, triggers such as exercise, stress, β_2-agonists, or eating a heavy meal cause a sudden intracellular shift of potassium. Barium poisoning from foods (not radiologic barium) can cause a similar paralysis. In the hyperkalemic version, symptoms follow rest after exercise or ingestion of potassium. Both are autosomal dominant disorders.

9. Chronic clay ingestion contributes to hypokalemia by binding dietary potassium. Nutritional potassium deficiency is otherwise uncommon in patients with normal diets.

10. Gentamicin, amphotericin B, and chemotherapeutic agents can damage renal tubules, resulting in potassium wasting. Hypercalcemic states also induce renal damage.

11. Glycyrrhizic acid is a component of natural licorice, rarely used today, which can exert a mineralocorticoid effect. Some infants with Cushing syndrome may have tumors of the adrenal cortex that result in overproduction of aldosterone, as well as cortisol and other corticosteroids.

12. Increased excretion of cations (K^+, H^+) accompanies excretion of nonreabsorbable anions as a means of maintaining electrical neutrality.

13. Bartter syndrome is characterized by hypokalemia secondary to renal losses, normal BP, and vascular insensitivity to pressor agents. Renin and aldosterone levels are elevated. Clinical manifestations include growth failure, weakness, constipation, polyuria, and dehydration. Gitelman and Liddle syndromes are other rare primary hypokalemic tubulopathies.

Bibliography

Brem AS: Disorders of potassium homeostasis, *Pediatr Clin North Am* 37:419–427, 1990.
Watkins SL: Disorders of potassium balance, *Pediatr Ann* 24:31, 1995.

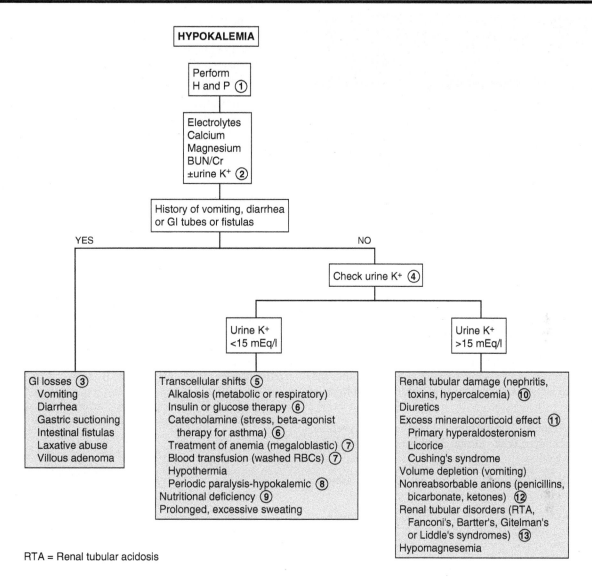

HYPOKALEMIA

Perform H and P ①

Electrolytes
Calcium
Magnesium
BUN/Cr
±urine K+ ②

History of vomiting, diarrhea or GI tubes or fistulas

YES

NO

Check urine K+ ④

Urine K+ <15 mEq/l

Urine K+ >15 mEq/l

GI losses ③
    Vomiting
    Diarrhea
    Gastric suctioning
    Intestinal fistulas
    Laxative abuse
    Villous adenoma

Transcellular shifts ⑤
    Alkalosis (metabolic or respiratory)
    Insulin or glucose therapy ⑥
    Catecholamine (stress, beta-agonist
        therapy for asthma) ⑥
    Treatment of anemia (megaloblastic) ⑦
    Blood transfusion (washed RBCs) ⑦
    Hypothermia
    Periodic paralysis-hypokalemic ⑧
Nutritional deficiency ⑨
Prolonged, excessive sweating

Renal tubular damage (nephritis,
    toxins, hypercalcemia) ⑩
Diuretics
Excess mineralocorticoid effect ⑪
    Primary hyperaldosteronism
    Licorice
    Cushing's syndrome
Volume depletion (vomiting)
Nonreabsorbable anions (penicillins,
    bicarbonate, ketones) ⑫
Renal tubular disorders (RTA,
    Fanconi's, Bartter's, Gitelman's
    or Liddle's syndromes) ⑬
Hypomagnesemia

RTA = Renal tubular acidosis

Nelson Textbook of Pediatrics, 19e. Chapter 52

Chapter 87
HYPERKALEMIA

Potassium is the main cation of the intracellular fluid (ICF) compartment. The ECF concentration is carefully regulated to maintain a value around 4 mEq/L. Potassium (K^+) plays a critical role in the excitability of nerve and muscle cells and contractility of muscles (smooth, skeletal, cardiac). Aldosterone normally regulates renal excretion of potassium. Aldosterone also causes sodium reabsorption and H^+ secretion in the distal tubule. Aldosterone similarly affects potassium excretion in the stool. Hyperkalemia is defined as a serum potassium concentration above 5.5 mEq/L.

1. The history should inquire about medications, underlying medical problems, and diets, including pica and the use of salt substitutes. Hyperkalemia may manifest with muscle weakness, as well as tingling, paresthesias, and paralysis. EKG changes include narrow peaked T waves and shortened QT interval initially. At higher serum potassium levels, delayed depolarization results in a widened QRS and P wave that may precede more serious arrhythmias (e.g., ventricular fibrillation, asystole).

2. Increased intake of potassium is a rare cause of hyperkalemia in children with normal renal function. Salt substitutes may be a cause.

3. Acute or chronic renal disorders may be responsible for impaired excretion of potassium.

4. Type IV renal tubular acidosis (RTA) is characterized by a deficiency of aldosterone or impaired aldosterone responsiveness. Pseudohypoaldosteronism is a subtype of type IV RTA that is characterized by high levels of aldosterone but an impaired distal tubular response to it.

5. Trauma, use of cytotoxic agents, massive hemolysis, rhabdomyolysis, and (to a lesser extent) intense exercise can release potassium as a result of tissue breakdown.

6. Transcellular shifts of potassium occur in an effort to maintain electrical neutrality in varying conditions. In metabolic acidosis, potassium shifts out of the cell in exchange for intracellular buffering of H^+. The opposite exchange occurs to a lesser degree in metabolic alkalosis. These shifts also occur in acid-base disturbances that are primarily respiratory, although to a lesser degree.

7. Potassium accompanies the osmotic shift of water from ICF to ECF in hypertonic states.

8. Rarely, episodic weakness or paralysis can be due to transient changes in potassium levels. The familial forms result from mutations in genes that affect ion channels in the muscle. In the hyperkalemic version, symptoms follow rest after exercise or ingestion of potassium. In the hypokalemic version, triggers such as exercise, stress, β_2-agonists, or a heavy meal cause a sudden intracellular shift of potassium. Barium poisoning from foods (not radiologic barium) can cause a similar paralysis. Both are autosomal dominant disorders.

Bibliography
Brem AS: Disorders of potassium homeostasis, *Pediatr Clin North Am* 37: 419–427, 1990.
Watkins SL: Disorders of potassium balance, *Pediatr Ann* 24:31, 1995.

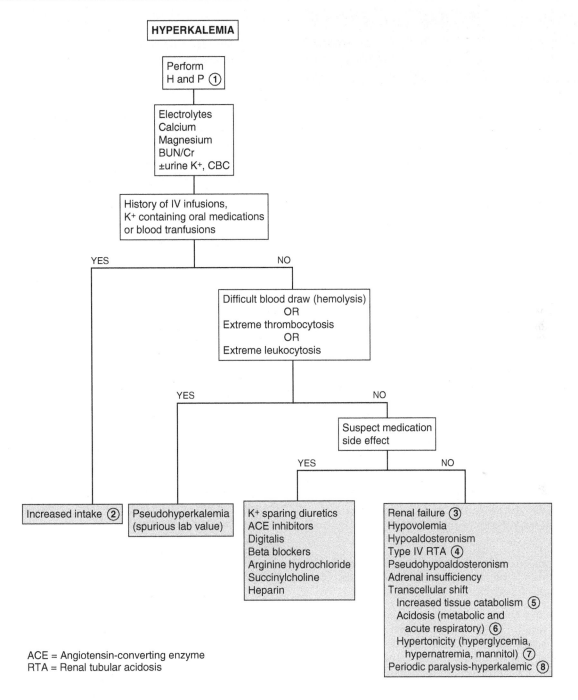

HYPERKALEMIA

Perform
H and P ①

Electrolytes
Calcium
Magnesium
BUN/Cr
±urine K⁺, CBC

History of IV infusions,
K⁺ containing oral medications
or blood tranfusions

YES   NO

Difficult blood draw (hemolysis)
OR
Extreme thrombocytosis
OR
Extreme leukocytosis

YES   NO

Suspect medication
side effect

YES   NO

Increased intake ②

Pseudohyperkalemia
(spurious lab value)

K⁺ sparing diuretics
ACE inhibitors
Digitalis
Beta blockers
Arginine hydrochloride
Succinylcholine
Heparin

Renal failure ③
Hypovolemia
Hypoaldosteronism
Type IV RTA ④
Pseudohypoaldosteronism
Adrenal insufficiency
Transcellular shift
    Increased tissue catabolism ⑤
    Acidosis (metabolic and
        acute respiratory) ⑥
    Hypertonicity (hyperglycemia,
        hypernatremia, mannitol) ⑦
Periodic paralysis-hyperkalemic ⑧

ACE = Angiotensin-converting enzyme
RTA = Renal tubular acidosis

Nelson Textbook of Pediatrics, 19e. Chapter 52

Chapter 88
HYPOCALCEMIA

Serum calcium concentration in the ECF is maintained by parathyroid hormone (PTH), which acts on the kidneys and bones, and by 1,25-dihydroxyvitamin D, which acts on the intestines and bones. About 50% of the calcium is in the biologically important ionized form, 40% is protein bound (i.e., mainly albumin), and 10% is complexed to anions (e.g., bicarbonate, citrate, sulfate, phosphate, and lactate). Mild hypocalcemia is usually asymptomatic. Symptoms and signs of more severe hypocalcemia include paresthesias of the extremities, Chvostek sign, Trousseau sign, muscle cramps or spasm, laryngospasm, tetany, and seizures. Cardiac manifestations include a prolonged QT interval, which may progress to heart block.

1. Calcium levels are affected by serum albumin levels and by pH. A low serum albumin will lower the total serum calcium, and acidic pH will decrease protein binding and increase ionized calcium levels. It is important to obtain an ionized calcium level. If this test is not available, in order to correct for hypoalbuminemia, 0.2 mmol/L (0.8 mg/dL) of calcium must be added to the total calcium level for each 1 g/dL decrease in serum albumin from the normal 4.0 g/dL. Similarly, for each 0.1 decrease in pH, ionized calcium rises by 0.05 mmol/L. However, these corrections are a poor substitute for ionized calcium level.

2. Hypoalbuminemic states result in a lower serum calcium level. The ionized calcium that is the biologically important level is usually normal, but it should be confirmed. Causes include liver disease, protein-losing enteropathy, and nephrotic syndrome.

3. Endotoxic shock is associated with hypocalcemia, although the mechanism is unknown. Hypocalcemia may also occur with rapid correction or overcorrection of acidosis.

4. Aplasia or hypoplasia of the parathyroid glands is often associated with DiGeorge/velocardiofacial syndrome. Many of the children have transient neonatal hypocalcemia; however, the hypocalcemia may recur later in life. Associated anomalies include conotruncal heart defects, velopharyngeal insufficiency, cleft palate, renal anomalies, and partial to complete aplasia of the thymus with varying severities of immunodeficiency.

5. Surgical hypoparathyroidism is a complication of thyroidectomy.

6. Autoimmune hypoparathyroidism is usually associated with other autoimmune disorders such as Addison disease and chronic mucocutaneous candidiasis. Other associations, including vitiligo, alopecia areata, pernicious anemia, and malabsorption may not appear until adulthood. Parathyroid antibodies are present.

7. Maternal hyperparathyroidism during pregnancy may cause a transient neonatal hypocalcemia. It may persist for weeks or months. Symptoms such as tetany may be delayed, especially in breast-fed infants.

8. Vitamin D deficiency occurs in dark-skinned breast-fed infants who live in areas with less sunlight. It may also occur in infants fed with unfortified cow's milk. Inadequate exposure to ultraviolet light, particularly in dark-skinned children, may also cause vitamin D deficiency. Inadequate absorption of vitamin D or calcium may be seen in diseases such as celiac disease, liver disease (including biliary cirrhosis), and cystic fibrosis. Phenobarbital and phenytoin interfere with metabolism of vitamin D. Renal failure also decreases vitamin D synthesis. Clinical manifestations of vitamin D deficiency include rickets, which occurs as a result of the body's attempt to maintain serum calcium levels. Vitamin D deficiency is best determined by obtaining a 25-OH vitamin D level; 1.25(OH)2 vitamin D can be normal with deficiency.

9. Vitamin D–dependent rickets (vitamin D–resistant rickets) type I usually presents between the ages of 3 and 6 months in children receiving adequate quantities of vitamin D. This is believed to be caused by decreased activity of the enzyme 25-hydroxy-1α-hydroxylase, resulting in decreased serum levels of 1,25-dihydroxyvitamin D. Alkaline phosphatase and PTH are increased, and serum phosphorus is low.

10. In pseudohypoparathyroidism (i.e., Albright hereditary osteodystrophy), the parathyroid glands are normal or even hyperplastic. PTH levels are normal or elevated; however, there is a peripheral resistance to PTH. This syndrome is associated with tetany and a distinctive phenotype with brachydactyly, skeletal abnormalities, short stature, and mild mental retardation.

11. Hyperphosphatemia may be associated with renal failure. It can occur secondary to rapid cell destruction due to chemotherapy (i.e., tumor lysis syndrome). Trauma leading to rhabdomyolysis causes release of cellular phosphorus. Hyperphosphatemia may also result from exogenous phosphate in the form of laxatives and enemas.

12. Pancreatitis causes release of pancreatic lipase, resulting in degradation of omental fat and binding of calcium in the peritoneum.

13. "Hungry bone" syndrome may occur during initial therapy to correct chronic hyperparathyroidism, leading to a sudden fall in phosphorus and calcium levels. Calcium and phosphorus are rapidly absorbed into severely demineralized bones.

14. Vitamin D–dependent rickets (type II) is a hereditary disorder due a receptor defect, resulting in hypocalcemia despite elevated levels of 1,25-dihydroxyvitamin D.

15. Hypocalcemia may also occur with alkalosis or rapid correction or overcorrection of acidosis.

16. Hypomagnesemia often coexists with hypocalcemia and may be due to decreased absorption (e.g., in malabsorption syndromes) or intake. Familial hypomagnesemia with secondary hypocalcemia usually appears between the second and sixth weeks of life. Aminoglycoside therapy may cause increased urinary losses of magnesium. PTH may be normal or decreased.

Bibliography

Bushinsky DA, Monk RD: Calcium, *Lancet* 352:306–311, 1998.
Fouser L: Disorders of calcium, phosphorus, and magnesium, *Pediatr Ann* 24:38–46, 1995.

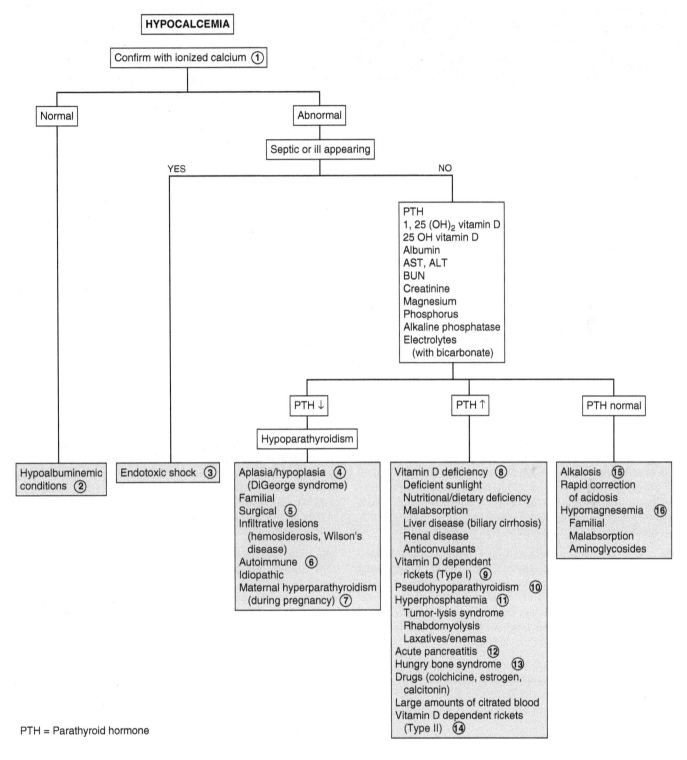

HYPOCALCEMIA

Confirm with ionized calcium ①

Normal

Abnormal

Septic or ill appearing

YES

NO

PTH
1, 25 $(OH)_2$ vitamin D
25 OH vitamin D
Albumin
AST, ALT
BUN
Creatinine
Magnesium
Phosphorus
Alkaline phosphatase
Electrolytes
  (with bicarbonate)

PTH ↓

Hypoparathyroidism

PTH ↑

PTH normal

Hypoalbuminemic conditions ②

Endotoxic shock ③

Aplasia/hypoplasia ④
  (DiGeorge syndrome)
Familial
Surgical ⑤
Infiltrative lesions
  (hemosiderosis, Wilson's
  disease)
Autoimmune ⑥
Idiopathic
Maternal hyperparathyroidism
  (during pregnancy) ⑦

Vitamin D deficiency ⑧
  Deficient sunlight
  Nutritional/dietary deficiency
  Malabsorption
  Liver disease (biliary cirrhosis)
  Renal disease
  Anticonvulsants
Vitamin D dependent
  rickets (Type I) ⑨
Pseudohypoparathyroidism ⑩
Hyperphosphatemia ⑪
  Tumor-lysis syndrome
  Rhabdomyolysis
  Laxatives/enemas
Acute pancreatitis ⑫
Hungry bone syndrome ⑬
Drugs (colchicine, estrogen,
  calcitonin)
Large amounts of citrated blood
Vitamin D dependent rickets
  (Type II) ⑭

Alkalosis ⑮
Rapid correction
  of acidosis
Hypomagnesemia ⑯
  Familial
  Malabsorption
  Aminoglycosides

PTH = Parathyroid hormone

Nelson Textbook of Pediatrics, 19e. Chapters 565 and 48

Chapter 89
HYPERCALCEMIA

Serum calcium concentration in the ECF is maintained by parathyroid hormone (PTH) and 1,25-dihydroxyvitamin D. PTH acts on the kidneys and bones and stimulates the production of 1,25-dihydroxyvitamin D, which acts on the intestines and bones. About 50% of the calcium is in the biologically important ionized form, 40% is protein bound (mainly albumin), and 10% is complexed to anions (bicarbonate, citrate, sulfate, phosphate, and lactate). Calcium levels are affected by serum albumin levels and pH. An elevated serum albumin concentration will appear to raise the total serum calcium concentration; an alkaline pH will increase protein binding and decrease ionized calcium levels. It is important to obtain an ionized calcium level.

Mild hypercalcemia is usually asymptomatic. With more severe hypercalcemia there may be neurologic features ranging from drowsiness to depression, stupor, and coma. GI manifestations such as constipation, nausea, vomiting, anorexia, and ulcers may occur. Hypercalciuria leads to nephrogenic diabetes insipidus, resulting in polyuria. Other renal effects of hypercalcemia include nephrolithiasis and nephrocalcinosis.

1 Primary hyperparathyroidism is caused by excessive production of PTH, owing to adenoma or hyperplasia. Incidence may be sporadic or may occur as part of the multiple endocrine neoplasia (MEN) syndromes, with involvement of the pancreas and the anterior pituitary. Hyperparathyroidism–jaw tumor syndrome is characterized by parathyroid adenomas and fibro-osseous jaw tumors. Patients may also have polycystic kidney disease, renal hamartomas, and Wilms tumor.

2 Secondary hyperparathyroidism is increased production of PTH in response to hypocalcemia, as in chronic renal failure. If this persists for a prolonged period, the glands begin to autonomously produce PTH even after the underlying reason for the hypocalcemia has been corrected, as after renal transplant. This is known as tertiary hyperparathyroidism and results in hypercalcemia.

3 Hypercalcemia may occur in association with malignancies (e.g., neuroblastoma, leukemia, renal tumors). This may be due to ectopic production of PTH; however, ectopic production of PTH-related peptide (PTHrP) is more common.

4 Hypercalcemia is present in 10% of children with Williams syndrome; the cause is unknown. Features of the syndrome include feeding difficulties, elfin facies, growth delay, gregarious personality, supravalvular aortic stenosis, renovascular disease, and developmental delay.

5 In familial hypocalciuric hypercalcemia (familial benign hypercalcemia), the patients are usually asymptomatic and PTH levels are inappropriately normal. The calcium-to-Cr clearance ratio is decreased in spite of the hypercalcemia.

6 Idiopathic hypercalcemia of infancy manifests during the first year of life with failure to thrive and hypercalcemia. There is increased absorption of calcium. Levels of 1,25-dihydroxyvitamin D may be normal or elevated. PTH and phosphorus levels are normal.

7 Ectopic production of vitamin D may occur with granulomatous disease, such as sarcoidosis (30%-50%) and tuberculosis. It may rarely occur with tumors. The excessive 1,25-dihydroxyvitamin D suppresses the production of PTH.

8 Hypervitaminosis A results in excessive bone resorption. Thiazide diuretics cause increased renal calcium reabsorption. Milk-alkali syndrome is caused by the consumption of large amounts of calcium-containing nonabsorbable antacids, leading to hypercalcemia, alkalemia, nephrocalcinosis, and renal insufficiency.

9 Malignancy may cause hypercalcemia. Most commonly it is secondary to production of PTH-related peptide but can also be caused by bone lysis, tumor production of 1,25-dihydroxyvitamin D, or ectopic PTH. In thyrotoxicosis, PTH is suppressed. Hypercalcemia is due to excessive bone resorption caused by the thyroid hormone. Patients undergoing dialysis may develop hypercalcemia, especially if they receive calcium supplements or are dialyzed against a high-calcium bath.

10 Jansen-type metaphyseal chondrodysplasia is a rare genetic disorder with features of short-limbed dwarfism. Circulating levels of PTH and PTHrP are undetectable. The hypercalcemia is severe but asymptomatic.

Bibliography

Bushinsky DA, Monk RD: Calcium, *Lancet* 352:306–311, 1998.
Fouser L: Disorders of calcium, phosphorus, and magnesium. *Pediatr Ann* 24:38–46, 1995.

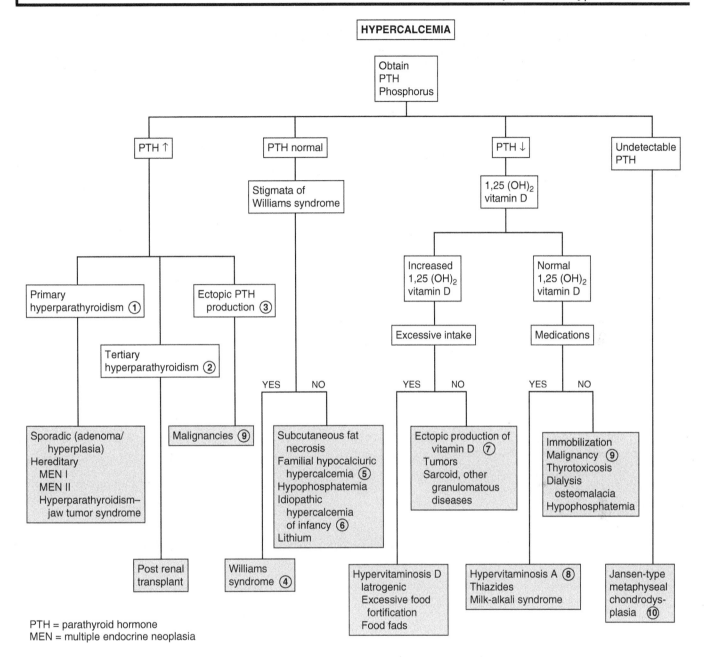

PTH = parathyroid hormone
MEN = multiple endocrine neoplasia

Nelson Textbook of Pediatrics, 19e. Chapter 564

Index